MANUAL OF

Eyes, Ears, Nose, and Throat Emergencies

MANUAL OF
Eyes, Ears, Nose, and Throat Emergencies

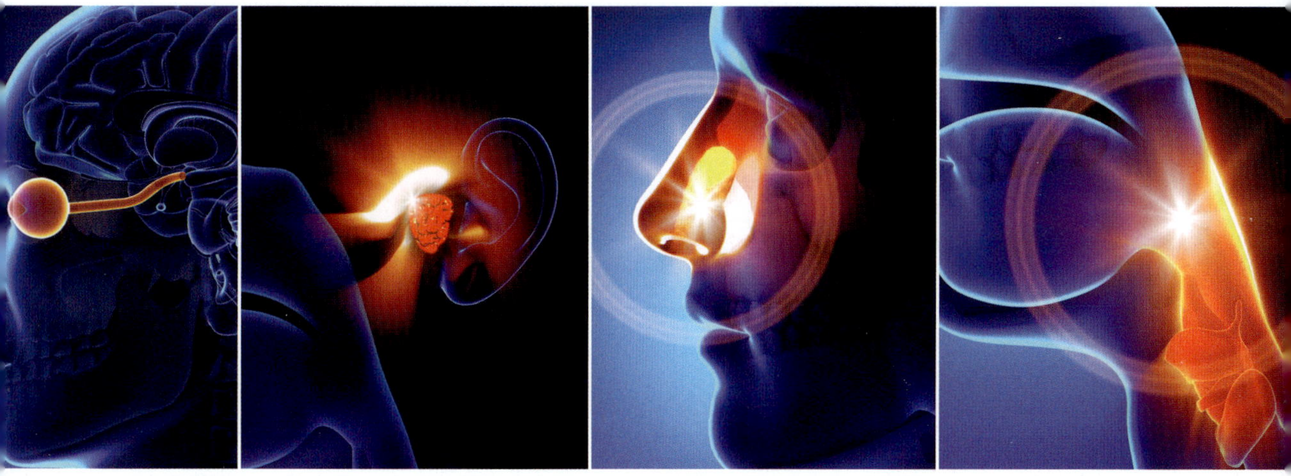

Daniel J. Egan, MD

Associate Professor
Department of Emergency Medicine
Harvard Medical School
Residency Program Director
Harvard Affiliated Emergency Medicine Residency
Mass General Brigham
Boston, Massachusetts

Di Coneybeare, MD, MHPE

Assistant Professor of Emergency Medicine
Columbia University Vagelos College of Physicians and Surgeons
New York, New York

Gareth M. C. Lema, MD, PhD

Associate Professor
Department of Ophthalmology
Icahn School of Medicine at Mount Sinai
Director of Quality, Safety, and Experience
Department of Ophthalmology
Mount Sinai Hospital
New York, New York

Marita S. Teng, MD

Professor
Department of Otorhinolaryngology
Residency Program Director
Icahn School of Medicine at Mount Sinai
New York, New York

Wolters Kluwer

Philadelphia • Baltimore • New York • London
Buenos Aires • Hong Kong • Sydney • Tokyo

Acquisitions Editor: James Sherman
Senior Development Editor: Ashley Fischer
Editorial Coordinator: Christopher Rodgers
Marketing Manager: Kirsten Watrud
Production Project Manager: Justin Wright
Manager, Graphic Arts & Design: Stephen Druding
Manufacturing Coordinator: Beth Welsh
Prepress Vendor: S4Carlisle Publishing Services

9 8 7 6 5 4 3 2 1

Printed in Mexico

Library of Congress Cataloging-in-Publication Data

ISBN-13: 978-1-975183-54-7

ISBN-10: 1-975183-54-1

Library of Congress Control Number: 2022909980

shop.lww.com

QUADM1022

Dedication

This book is dedicated to all the healthcare workers around the country who have been working tirelessly during the COVID-19 pandemic. The authors who contributed to this new text created, wrote, and edited their sections through the pandemic, at a time when many were tirelessly taking care of patients in the new normal of our healthcare system. We want to recognize the sacrifice our colleagues have made and continue to make over the last 2 years as the pandemic continues around the world.

Preface

We are excited and humbled to present the inaugural edition of the *Manual of Eyes, Ears, Nose and Throat Emergencies*. We were delighted to contribute to the new series of educational materials led by Dr. Ron M. Walls, creator of *The Walls Manual of Emergency Airway Management*.

This book is the work of faculty from multiple academic medical centers throughout the United States. The provision of high-quality healthcare requires the collaboration of physicians and providers across multiple specialties. We wanted to capitalize on the expertise of physicians from the three specialties represented in this book of emergency medicine, otorhinolaryngology, and ophthalmology. Bringing these specialties together to focus on the diagnoses relevant to the practice of medicine in emergency or urgent care settings demonstrated the importance of knowledge, collaboration, and unique expertise.

In this new manual, the reader will enjoy a systematic approach to patient complaints and specific diagnoses affecting the eyes and ears, nose, and throat (ENT). Each chapter takes us through the basic understanding of the clinical challenge followed by a discussion of pathophysiology, approach and physical examination, differential diagnosis, and ultimately management. The discussions are rich with relevant information for clinical practice in the emergency department and urgent care settings. We have highlighted critical information through abundant tables and photographic representations of most conditions. Before leaving each chapter, highlights are reinforced with critical tips and pearls followed by a deeper dive into some of the evidence-based topics relevant to the condition.

This manual presents detailed information on topics often distilled into single chapters in other texts. The input of emergency physicians with subspecialty coauthors to each chapter has ensured a peer review mechanism and specialty expertise such that the reader finishes knowing the critical information from emergency medicine and ENT or ophthalmology lenses. We are excited to provide this new resource to our colleagues looking for a consolidated and up-to-date book filled with the latest evidence to provide the highest quality of care for patients in the emergency department or urgent care setting.

Acknowledgments

Successful careers are built on the mentorship of others and the network of colleagues built over time. I am incredibly grateful to Dr. Ron Walls, the series editor of this book and my chair from when I was a resident, for placing his trust in me to execute the first edition of this new manual. His commitment to advancing the specialty of emergency medicine through high-quality educational material is inspiration for those of us who have committed our careers to education. I also want to acknowledge all the trainees in emergency medicine with whom I have worked over my career. As a residency director, it is the privilege of working with the next generation of physicians that motivates me to be a better physician and educator. Finally, I am indebted to my associate editors, Drs. Coneybeare, Lema, and Teng. Watching what began as a concept grow into this collaborative project among our specialties has been a highlight of my career.

—Daniel J. Egan, MD

When Dr. Egan approached me to help him edit this incredible book, I thought he must have been talking to someone else. I am forever grateful for his belief in me, his mentorship, and friendship. I also feel incredibly lucky to have worked with our coeditors Dr. Lema and Dr. Teng; one could not have asked for more wonderful colleagues and collaborators. Thank you to my spouse, Matt, who always maintains a paragon of support for any goal I choose to pursue. And thank you to Eli, our now toddler, born at the very beginnings of this book and mercifully started sleeping through the night when I needed to get through the bulk of editing.

—Di Coneybeare, MD, MHPE

First and foremost, this is for my colleagues in emergency medicine (EM). We started this effort as COVID-19 ravaged New York City and spread across the country. Half of the authors and editors of this text wrote while also juggling the uncertainty and terror of serving on the front line of a global pandemic. Thank you. I have depended on my EM colleagues countless times to help evaluate and treat complicated patients. I hope this manual makes the eye a little less mysterious and much less burdensome. I am grateful to Dr. Dan Egan for the opportunity to work with him on this project. His guidance and leadership were exemplary. Dr. Di Coneybeare's assistance in writing and editing informed my own efforts to guide ophthalmologists in writing to an unfamiliar audience. We could not have done any of this without our many contributors; through this experience I hope I have strengthened relationships with old friends while also forging new friendships among my colleagues. My wife Penny, an emergency physician, has always been an inspiration, role model, and constant source of support. And always with me are my kids, Alessandra and Xavier, who bring me happiness each and every day.

—Gareth M. C. Lema, MD, PhD

This inspiring project has brought to light some of the most important pillars of medical practice: communication, collaboration, and cooperation, all applied in an effort to provide our patients the best possible care. As generations of physicians learn from their teachers and mentors, I would also like to acknowledge the important role of our trainees. Our fellows, residents, and students keep us not only alert and engaged but also humble and honest. Finally, my deepest appreciation and love goes to my family—my partner in life and golf, Greg, and our amazing, talented, and hilarious children, Zoe and Alec. Thank you for the ongoing motivation to be the best version of myself.

—Marita S. Teng, MD

Contributors

Dunia Abdul-Aziz, MD
Instructor
Department of Otolaryngology
Harvard Medical School
Clinician-Scientist
Department of Otolaryngology
Mass Eye and Ear
Boston, Massachusetts

Kirsten Bechtel, MD
Professor of Pediatrics and Emergency Medicine
Department of Pediatrics
Yale School of Medicine
Attending Physician
Children's Emergency Department
Yale New Haven Hospital
New Haven, Connecticut

Laura J. Bontempo, MD, MEd
Associate Professor, Emergency Medicine
Department of Emergency Medicine
University of Maryland School of Medicine
Attending Emergency Physician
Department of Emergency Medicine
University of Maryland Medical Center
Baltimore, Maryland

Samantha F. Bordonaro, MD, FACEP
Assistant Clinical Professor
Department of Emergency Medicine
Jacobs School of Medicine and Biomedical Sciences
Medical Student Clerkship Director
Department of Emergency Medicine
UB/MD Emergency Medicine
Buffalo, New York

Amy B. Caggiula, MD, MAEd
Assistant Professor
Department of Emergency Medicine
George Washington School of Medicine and Health Sciences
Attending Physician
Department of Emergency Medicine
George Washington University Hospital
Washington, District of Columbia

Daniel S. Casper, MD, PhD
Professor of Ophthalmology
Department of Ophthalmology
Columbia University Vagelos College of Physicians and Surgeons
Attending Ophthalmologist
Department of Ophthalmology
New York Presbyterian Hospital
New York, New York

Sirivalli Chamarti, MD
Assistant Professor
Department of Emergency Medicine
Columbia University Vagelos College of Physicians and Surgeons
New York, New York

Khurram Chaudhary, MD
Assistant Professor
Department of Ophthalmology
Renaissance School of Medicine at Stony Brook University
Stony Brook, New York

Christina H. Chien, MD
Assistant Professor
Department of Emergency Medicine
Sidney Kimmel Medical College
Clinical Assistant Professor
Department of Internal Medicine, Division of Pulmonary, Allergy, and Critical Care
Thomas Jefferson University Hospital
Philadelphia, Pennsylvania

Peter W. Clark, MD
Vitreoretinal Surgery Fellow
Department of Ophthalmology
Gavin Herbert Eye Institute
University of California, Irvine Medical Center
Irvine, California

Trudi S. Cloyd, MD, MS
Assistant Professor
Department of Emergency Medicine
Columbia University Vagelos College of Physicians and Surgeons
Attending Physician
Department of Emergency Medicine
New York Presbyterian Hospital
New York, New York

Di Coneybeare, MD, MHPE
Assistant Professor of Emergency Medicine
Columbia University Vagelos College of Physicians and Surgeons
New York, New York

Abbe Craven, MD
Clinical Assistant Professor
Department of Ophthalmology
New York Eye and Ear Infirmary of Mount Sinai
New York, New York

Alison V. Crum, MD
Associate Professor
Department of Ophthalmology
John A. Moran Eye Center
Associate Professor
Department of Ophthalmology
University of Utah School of Medicine
University of Utah Hospital
Salt Lake City, Utah

Avnish Deobhakta, MD
Assistant Professor
Department of Ophthalmology
Icahn School of Medicine at Mount Sinai
Faculty
Department of Ophthalmology
New York Eye and Ear Infirmary of Mount Sinai
New York, New York

Daniel J. Egan, MD
Associate Professor
Department of Emergency Medicine
Harvard Medical School
Residency Program Director
Harvard Affiliated Emergency Medicine Residency
Mass General Brigham
Boston, Massachusetts

Tabitha Ford, MD
Assistant Professor
Department of Emergency Medicine
Larner College of Medicine
Assistant Residency Program Director
Department of Emergency Medicine
University of Vermont Medical Center
Burlington, Vermont

Ashley A. Foster, MD
Instructor
Department of Emergency Medicine and Pediatrics
Harvard Medical School
Assistant Professor
Department of Emergency Medicine
Massachusetts General Hospital
Boston, Massachusetts

Tamiesha A. Frempong, MD, MPH
Assistant Professor, Ophthalmology, Pediatrics and Medical Education
New York Eye and Ear Infirmary of Mount Sinai
New York, New York

Mona Gangar, MD, MS
Assistant Professor
Department of Otorhinolaryngology/Head & Neck Surgery
Albert Einstein College of Medicine
Attending Physician
Department of Otorhinolaryngology/Head & Neck Surgery
Children's Hospital at Montefiore
Bronx, New York

Joshua Gauger, MD, MBA
Assistant Professor
BerbeeWalsh Department of Emergency Medicine
University of Wisconsin School of Medicine and Public Health
Medical Director
Department of Emergency Medicine
UW Health University Hospital
Madison, Wisconsin

Joshua Gentges, DO, MPH
Associate Professor and Research Director
Department of Emergency Medicine
University Of Oklahoma College of Medicine
Emergency Department Attending
Department of Emergency Medicine
Hillcrest Hospital
Tulsa, Oklahoma

Robin N. Ginsburg, MD
Associate Professor of Ophthalmology and Pediatrics
Department of Ophthalmology
Icahn School of Medicine at Mount Sinai
Director of Vitreoretinal Surgery and ROP Service
Department of Ophthalmology
Mount Sinai Hospital
New York, New York

Lora R. Dagi Glass, MD
Assistant Professor
Department of Ophthalmology
Columbia University Vagelos College of Physicians and Surgeons
Columbia University Irving Medical Center
New York, New York

Kyle J. Godfrey, MD
Assistant Professor
Department of Ophthalmology and Neurological Surgery
Joan & Sanford I. Weill Medical College of Cornell University
Assistant Attending
Department of Ophthalmology and Neurological Surgery
New York Presbyterian Hospital
New York, New York

Bradley D. Gordon, MD, MS
Associate Professor
Department of Emergency Medicine
University of Minnesota Medical School
Minneapolis, Minnesota
Staff Physician
Department of Emergency Medicine
Regions Hospital/HealthPartners
St. Paul, Minnesota

Mark Grbic, MD
Assistant Professor
Department of Emergency Medicine
Columbia University Vagelos College of Physicians and Surgeons
Assistant Attending Physician
Department of Emergency Medicine
New York-Presbyterian Hospital
New York, New York

Sanjey Gupta, MD
Professor
Department of Emergency Medicine
Zucker School of Medicine at Hofstra/Northwell
Hempstead, New York
Chairperson
Department of Emergency Medicine
South Shore University Hospital
Bay Shore, New York

Alyssa M. Hackett, MD
Assistant Professor
Department of Otolaryngology
Mount Sinai Hospital
New York, New York

Victoria M. Hammond, MD
Emergency Physician
Crucial Care
St. Petersburg, Florida

David J. Harris, III, MD
Assistant Professor
Department of Ophthalmology
Icahn School of Medicine at Mount Sinai
Staff Surgeon
Department of Ophthalmology
New York Eye and Ear Infirmary of Mount Sinai
New York, New York

Chen He, MD
Assistant Professor
Department of Emergency Medicine
Icahn School of Medicine at Mount Sinai
New York, New York

Samuel N. Helman, MD
Assistant Professor of Clinical Otolaryngology
Department of Otolaryngology - Head and Neck Surgery
Joan & Sanford I. Weill Medical College of Cornell University
New York, New York

Candace E. Hobson, MD
Department of Otolaryngology - Head and Neck Surgery
Emory University School of Medicine
Atlanta, Georgia

Nicholas E. Hoda, MD, PhD
Associate Professor
Department of Emergency Medicine
University of Mississippi School of Medicine
University of Mississippi Medical Center
Jackson, Mississippi

Christopher P. Hogrefe, MD, FACEP, CAQ-SM
Clinical Associate Professor
Department of Emergency Medicine
University of Iowa Carver College of Medicine
Iowa City, Iowa
Adjunct Associate Professor
Department of Orthopaedic Surgery
Northwestern University Feinberg School of Medicine
Chicago, Illinois

Shirley Hu, MD
Facial Plastic and Reconstructive Surgeon
Icahn School of Medicine at Mount Sinai
New York, New York

Rupal S. Jain, MD
Adjunct Assistant Professor
Department of Emergency Medicine
University of Maryland School of Medicine
Baltimore, Maryland
Attending Physician
Department of Emergency Medicine
University of Maryland Capital Region Medical Center
Largo, Maryland

Anne Kane, MD
Assistant Professor
Department of Otolaryngology
University of Mississippi School of Medicine
University of Mississippi Medical Center
Jackson, Maryland

Anne Katz, MD
Assistant Professor of Clinical Emergency Medicine
Emergency Medicine
Joan & Sanford I. Weill Medical College of Cornell University
Assistant Program Director, NYP Emergency Medicine Residency
Emergency Medicine
New York Presbyterian-Weill Cornell Medical Center
New York, New York

Melissa W. Ko, MD, MBA
Professor
Department of Neurology, Ophthalmology, and Clinical Neurosurgery
Indiana University School of Medicine
Neuro-Ophthalmologist
Department of Neurology
Indiana University Health
Indianapolis, Indiana

Paul Y. Ko, MD, MEd
Associate Professor & Associate Dean for Curricular Development & Oversight
Department of Emergency Medicine
Indiana University School of Medicine
Emergency Medicine Physician
Indiana University Health
Indianapolis, Indiana

Anjum F. Koreishi, MD
Assistant Professor
Department of Ophthalmology
Northwestern University
Assistant Professor
Department of Ophthalmology
Northwestern University/Northwestern Medicine
Chicago, Illinois

Zachary Kuschner, MD
Icahn School of Medicine at Mount Sinai
New York, New York

Yan Lee, MD
Assistant Professor
Department of Surgery, Division of Otolaryngology
Yale School of Medicine
Yale New Haven Hospital
New Haven, Connecticut

Ashton Lehmann, MD
Research Instructor in Otolaryngology
Department of Otolaryngology—Head & Neck Surgery
Vanderbilt University Medical Center
Nashville, Tennessee

Gareth M. C. Lema, MD, PhD
Associate Professor
Department of Ophthalmology
Icahn School of Medicine at Mount Sinai
Director of Quality, Safety, and Experience
Department of Ophthalmology
Mount Sinai Hospital
New York, New York

Penelope C. Lema, MD
Associate Professor of Emergency Medicine
Department of Emergency Medicine
Columbia University Vagelos College of Physicians and Surgeons
Vice Chair, Faculty Affairs
Director, Emergency Ultrasound Division
Department of Emergency Medicine
New York–Presbyterian Hospital
New York, New York

Albert Lin, MD
Assistant Professor
Department of Ophthalmology
University of Mississippi School of Medicine
University of Mississippi Medical Center
Jackson, Mississippi

Harrison W. Lin, MD
Associate Professor
Otolaryngology—Head and Neck Surgery
University of California, Irvine, School of Medicine
University of California, Irvine Medical Center
Irvine, California

Yue Ma, MD
Assistant Professor
Department of Otolaryngology Head and Neck Surgery
UCSF School of Medicine
San Francisco, California

Benjamin D. Malkin, MD, FACS
Senior Physician
Department of Head and Neck Surgery
The Permanente Medical Group
Oakland Medical Center
Oakland, California

Douglas P. Marx, MD
Associate Professor
Department of Ophthalmology
Moran Eye Center
Division Chief, Oculofacial Plastic and Reconstructive Surgery
Department of Ophthalmology
University of Utah School of Medicine
Salt Lake City, Utah

Erica Mayland, MD
Baptist Health
Jacksonville, Florida

Brian Milman, MD
Assistant Professor
Department of Emergency Medicine
University of Oklahoma School of Community Medicine
Attending Physician
Department of Emergency Medicine
Hillcrest Medical Center
Tulsa, Oklahoma

Sanjay Mohan, MD
Assistant Professor
Department of Emergency Medicine
Donald and Barbara Zucker School of Medicine at Hofstra/Northwell
Uniondale, New York
Assistant Professor
Department of Emergency Medicine
Northwell Health—Long Island Jewish Medical Center
New York, New York

Kathryn Noonan, MD
Assistant Professor
Clerkship Director
Departments of Otolaryngology and Neurotology
Tufts University School of Medicine
Associate Program Director, Otolaryngology Residency Program
Tufts Medical Center
Boston, Massachusetts

Rodney Omron, MD, MPH
Assistant Professor
Department of Emergency Medicine
Johns Hopkins School of Medicine
Baltimore, Maryland

Alexandra L. Ortego, MD
Assistant Professor
Department of Emergency Medicine
NYU Long Island School of Medicine
Attending Physician
Department of Emergency Medicine
NYU Langone Hospital—Long Island
Mineola, New York

Daniel L. Overbeek, MD
Senior Instructor
Department of Emergency Medicine and Toxicology
University of Rochester School of Medicine and Dentistry
Rochester, New York

David Peak, MD
Assistant Professor
Department of Emergency Medicine
Harvard Medical School
Associate Program Director,
Harvard Affiliated Emergency Medicine Residency Program
Department of Emergency Medicine
Massachusetts General Hospital
Boston, Massachusetts

Enrique Perez, MD, MBA
Director of Otology, Assistant Professor of Otolaryngology
Otolaryngology Head and Neck Surgery
Mount Sinai Hospital
New York Eye and Ear Infirmary of Mount Sinai
New York, New York

Paul Petrakos, DO, MS
Assistant Professor of Ophthalmology
Department of Ophthalmology
Joan & Sanford I. Weill Medical College of Cornell University
Assistant Professor of Ophthalmology
Department of Ophthalmology
New York Presbyterian Hospital
New York, New York

Matthew S. Pihlblad, MD
Assistant Professor
Department of Ophthalmology
University of Pittsburgh School of Medicine
Pediatric Ophthalmologist
Department of Ophthalmology
UPMC Children's Hospital of Pittsburgh
Pittsburgh, Pennsylvania

Brittany Elizabeth Powell, MD
Assistant Professor
Department of Surgery
Uniformed Services University
Bethesda, Maryland
Chief
Department of Ophthalmology
Fort Belvoir Community Hospital
Fort Belvoir, Virginia

Sarah Kate Rapoport, MD
Assistant Professor
Department of Otolaryngology/Head & Neck Surgery
Georgetown University School of Medicine
Georgetown University Hospital
Attending Physician
Department of Surgery, Division of Otolaryngology
Veterans Affairs Medical Center of Washington D.C.
Washington, District of Columbia

Harsha S. Reddy, MD
Associate Professor
Department of Ophthalmology
Icahn School of Medicine at Mount Sinai
Director, Oculoplastic Surgery
Department of Ophthalmology
New York Eye and Ear Infirmary of Mount Sinai
New York, New York

Magdalena Robak, MD
Assistant Professor
Ronald O. Perelman Department of Emergency Medicine
NYU Grossman School of Medicine
New York, New York

Daniel R. Rutz, MD
Assistant Professor
BerbeeWalsh Department of Emergency Medicine
University of Wisconsin-Madison School of Medicine and Public Health
Medical Director
Emergency Department
University of Wisconsin Health—East Madison Hospital
Madison, Wisconsin

Alok T. Saini, MD
Assistant Professor
Department of Otolaryngology—Head and Neck Surgery
University of Kentucky College of Medicine
Assistant Professor
Department of Otolaryngology—Head and Neck Surgery
UK Albert B. Chandler Hospital
Lexington, Kentucky

Sophia Mirza Saleem, MD
Assistant Professor
Department of Ophthalmology
Icahn School of Medicine at Mount Sinai
New York, New York

Soshian Sarrafpour, MD
Clinical Instructor of Glaucoma
Department of Ophthalmology and Visual Science
Yale School of Medicine
New Haven, Connecticut

Jamie Lea Schaefer, MD
Assistant Professor of Surgery, Clinician Educator
Department of Surgery, Division of Ophthalmology
The Warren Alpert Medical School of Brown University
Director of Medical Student Education in Ophthalmology
Oculofacial Plastic Surgeon
Department of Surgery, Division of Ophthalmology
Rhode Island Hospital
Providence, Rhode Island

Neha Shaik, MD
Clinical Assistant Professor
Department of Ophthalmology
Icahn School of Medicine at Mount Sinai
Clinical Assistant Professor
Department of Ophthalmology
New York Ear and Eye Infirmary of Mount Sinai
New York, New York

Sandra Fernando Sieminski, MD
Associate Professor
Department of Ophthalmology
Jacobs School of Medicine and Biomedical Sciences
Chief of Service
Department of Ophthalmology
Erie County Medical Center
Buffalo, New York

Adria Simon, MD
Assistant Professor
Department of Emergency Medicine
Columbia University Vagelos College of Physicians and Surgeons
Assistant Professor
Department of Emergency Medicine
Columbia University Irving Medical Center
New York, New York

Todd Spock, MD
Assistant Professor
Department of Otolaryngology
Icahn School of Medicine at Mount Sinai
New York, New York
Regional Director of Otolaryngology—Head and Neck Surgery
Department of Otolaryngology
NYC HHC Elmhurst Hospital Center
Elmhurst, New York

Katelyn O. Stepan, MD
Assistant Professor
Department of Otolaryngology—Head and Neck Surgery
Northwestern University—Feinberg School of Medicine
Attending Physician
Department of Otolaryngology—Head and Neck Surgery
Northwestern Memorial Hospital
Chicago, Illinois

Mitchell B. Strominger, MD
Professor of Surgery, Ophthalmology and Pediatrics
Department of Surgery, Ophthalmology and Pediatrics
University of Nevada Reno School of Medicine
Chief, Neuro-ophthalmology, Pediatric Ophthalmology
Department of Surgery, Ophthalmology and Pediatrics
Renown Medical Center
Reno, Nevada

Jonathan Strong, MD
Department of Emergency Medicine
Harvard Medical School
Brigham and Women's Hospital
Boston, Massachusetts

Leejee H. Suh, MD
Miranda Wong Tang Associate Professor of Ophthalmology
Department of Ophthalmology
Edward S. Harkness Eye Institute
Director, Cornea and Refractive Surgery Service
Department of Ophthalmology
Columbia University Irving Medical Center
New York, New York

Tjoson Tjoa, MD
Associate Professor
Otolaryngology—Head & Neck Surgery
University of California, Irvine, School of Medicine
Irvine, California

Samuel J. Trosman, MD
Icahn School of Medicine at Mount Sinai
New York, New York

Jimmy Truong, DO, MS
Assistant Professor
Department of Emergency Medicine
Columbia University Vagelos College of Physicians and Surgeons
Columbia University Irving Medical Center
Faculty
Department of Emergency Medicine
NewYork-Presbyterian Hospital
New York, New York

Benjamin C. Tweel, MD
Assistant Professor
Department of Otolaryngology—Head and Neck Surgery
Icahn School of Medicine at Mount Sinai
Assistant Professor
Department of Otolaryngology—Head and Neck Surgery
Mount Sinai Hospital
New York, New York

Vilija J. Vaitaitis, MS, MD
Assistant Professor
Department of Otolaryngology, Head and Neck Surgery
Louisiana State University Health Sciences Center, New Orleans
Otolaryngologist
Department of Otolaryngology, Head and Neck Surgery
University Medical Center, New Orleans
New Orleans, Louisiana

Zoe R. Williams, MD
Associate Professor
Department of Neurosurgery, Ophthalmology and Neurology
University of Rochester School of Medicine
Chief of Neuro-Ophthalmology
Department of Neurosurgery, Ophthalmology and Neurology
Strong Memorial Hospital
Rochester, New York

Juliana Wilson, DO, MPH
Assistant Professor
Department of Emergency Medicine
University of Colorado School of Medicine
Faculty
Emergency Medicine
UCHealth University of Colorado Hospital
Aurora, Colorado

Kei U. Wong, MD
Assistant Professor
Department of Emergency Medicine
Rutgers New Jersey Medical School
Attending Physician
Pediatric Emergency Department, Division of Pediatric Emergency Medicine
University Hospital
Newark, New Jersey

Emmagene Worley, MD
Assistant Professor
Department of Emergency Medicine
Columbia University Vagelos College of Physicians and Surgeons
Attending Physician
Department of Emergency Medicine
NewYork–Presbyterian Hospital
Columbia University Irving Medical Center
New York, New York

Benjamin Wyler, MD, MPH
Assistant Professor
Department of Emergency Medicine
Icahn School of Medicine at Mount Sinai
Attending Physician
Department of Emergency Medicine
Mount Sinai West
New York, New York

Elizabeth J. Yetter, MD
Assistant Professor
Department of Emergency Medicine
Icahn School of Medicine at Mount Sinai
Ultrasound Division Director
Department of Emergency Medicine
Mount Sinai Morningside & Mount Sinai West
New York, New York

Contents

Section 1 Principles of Urgent and Emergent Otorhinolaryngology

CHAPTER 1

ENT Anatomy

Sarah K. Rapoport

THE CLINICAL CHALLENGE

Understanding the structural details of the ear, nose, and throat is imperative for accurate diagnosis of its pathologies. Formulating a conceptual map of these regions can prove invaluable for diagnosing and treating disorders of the ears, nose, and throat, as well as avoiding some of their lurking pitfalls.

The Scalp

The five tissue layers that comprise the scalp (skin, connective tissue composed of superficial fascia, galea aponeurosis, loose areolar tissue, and periosteum or pericranium) form a dense, protective covering for the skull (**Figure 1.1A**). The scalp is thickest in its hair-bearing regions and grows thinner in areas without hair follicles.[1] The frontalis muscle lies beneath the anterior skin and subcutaneous tissue layers of the scalp. This muscle is a continuation of the galea aponeurosis layer anteriorly and helps to protect the pericranium.

Laterally, the galea aponeurosis extends to form the temporoparietal fascia and the superficial musculoaponeurotic system (SMAS). The galea aponeurosis is most dense and adherent to the underlying scalp at the vertex. It gradually becomes looser the more laterally it extends, especially in areas of muscle and fascial attachment. The pliability of this tissue is relevant when you need to repair simple and complex lacerations of the scalp.

The scalp has a luxuriant vasculature system, so even small lacerations can generate copious bleeds. The internal carotid arteries provide tributaries for the arterial vasculature of the forehead and scalp. As demonstrated in **Figure 1.1B**, the supratrochlear artery is a branch of the ophthalmic artery and runs along the anterior forehead. After branching from the ophthalmic artery, the supratrochlear artery emerges from the orbital septum above the trochlear notch, where it travels between the corrugator and frontalis muscles to pass vertically along the forehead to the scalp. Together with its corresponding nerve, a branch of the ophthalmic distribution of the trigeminal nerve (CN V_1), the supratrochlear artery is reliably located 1.7 to 2.2 cm from the midline of the forehead (which usually aligns with the medial border of the eyebrow).[2] The supraorbital artery, also a branch of the ophthalmic artery, runs just lateral and parallel to the supratrochlear artery along the anterior forehead. The supraorbital artery passes through the supraorbital notch, penetrates the corrugator muscle, and then divides into superficial and deep branches that ascend laterally to anastomose with the superficial and deep temporal arteries that supply blood to the remainder of the scalp.

The Paranasal Sinuses

The paranasal sinuses lie deep to the face, scalp, and forehead. Once developed, these paired and aerated cavities occupy the bony spaces around the eyes and nose. The paranasal sinuses serve

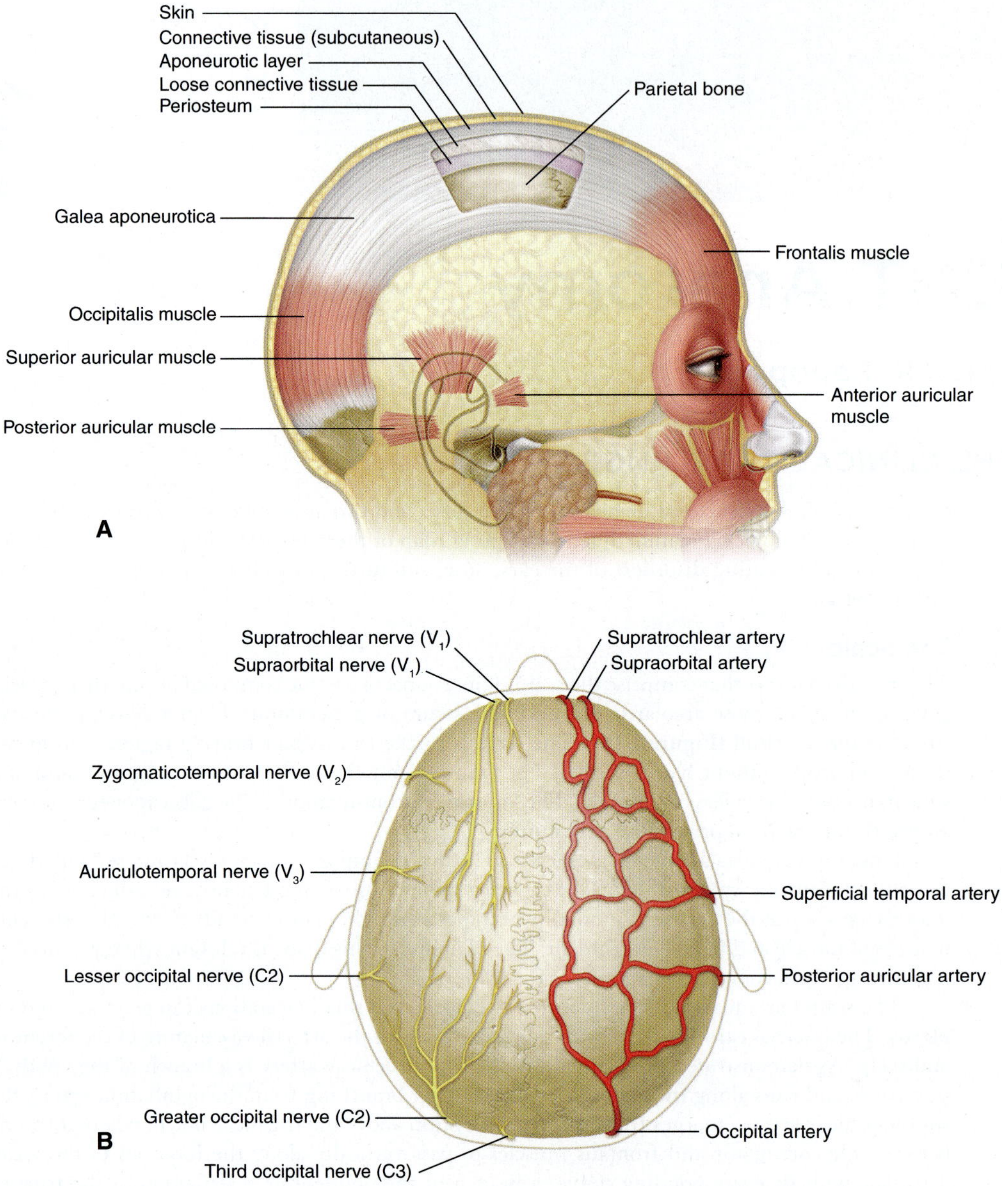

Figure 1.1: A, Lateral view of the layers of the scalp. B, Superior view of the cutaneous innervation and arterial blood supply of the scalp. (From Panksy B, Gest TR. Head. In: Panksy B, Gest TR. *Lippincott Concise Illustrated Anatomy*. Wolters Kluwer; 2014:91-222. Figure 2.9.)

multiple purposes, including decreasing the weight of the skull, acting as pathways to filter inhaled pathogens or allergens, providing drainage outflow tracts for mucus accumulation, and absorbing forceful blunt trauma to the face. These sinuses include the frontal, ethmoid, maxillary, and sphenoid paranasal sinuses, depicted in **Figure 1.2**, and reliably distribute the impact of blunt facial trauma to protect critical structures such as the eyes and brain.[3] These sinuses are lined with respiratory mucosa composed of pseudostratified ciliated columnar epithelium. And firmly adherent to the periosteum or perichondrium of the adjacent bone and cartilage of the sinuses lies a rich capillary network.

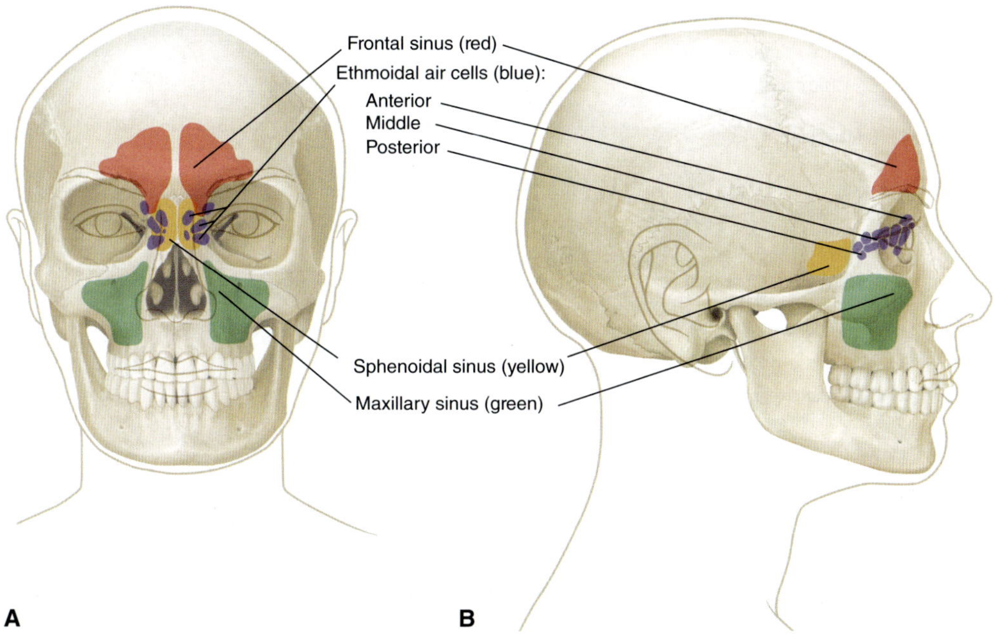

Figure 1.2: Anterior (A) and lateral (B) views of the paranasal sinuses. (From Gest TR. The head and neck. In: Gest TR. *Lippincott Atlas of Anatomy*. 2nd ed. Wolters Kluwer; 2020:324-441. Figure 7.53B and C.)

The Facial Nerve

The facial nerve is a mixed (motor, special sensory, and autonomic) nerve that originates in the brainstem, courses through the temporal bone of the skull, and exits the skull base through the stylomastoid foramen. As a mixed nerve, it has multiple roles: (1) its motor nucleus innervates the muscles of facial expression, digastric, stylohyoid, and stapedius muscles, (2) its superior salivatory nucleus provides preganglionic parasympathetic innervation to the lacrimal and salivary glands, and (3) its solitary tract nucleus receives sensory innervation, sound, and taste (special sensory), respectively, from the posterior superior external auditory ear canal (EAC) and from the anterior two-thirds of the tongue.[4] Violation of the facial nerve along its course can compromise these functions and produce facial paralysis, loss of taste, and hyperacusis. For example, tumors can infiltrate or compress the nerve, infections such as otitis externa or herpes zoster can inflame or compress the nerve, and trauma can directly sever or stretch the nerve.

To reach the mimetic (facial) muscles, the facial nerve travels through the parotid gland, dividing it into its deep and superficial lobes. After exiting the parotid gland, the facial nerve branches into its five principal motor branches: temporal, zygomatic, buccal, marginal mandibular, and cervical (**Figure 1.3**). The facial nerve is located deep to the facial muscles, with three exceptions: the buccinator, mentalis, and levator anguli oris muscles. These three muscles are located underneath the facial nerve and are innervated along their superficial surfaces.

Confirming intact function of the facial nerve in patients presenting with symptoms of the ear, nose, and throat is a mandatory component of a thorough exam. In cases of facial nerve dysfunction or injury, it is critical to determine whether there is adequate eye closure, because it is important to protect the cornea of a patient with facial palsy. The facial nerve innervates the orbicularis oculi muscles, sphincteric muscles that surround the eye. To test orbicularis oculi function, ask the patient to squeeze their eyelids shut tightly, and test the patient's resistance to your elevating the eyelid. If you simply ask a patient to close their eyes, gravity can help lower the eyelid, and the oculomotor nerve will elevate the eyelid via the levator palpebrae superioris, giving the false impression that the patient's eye closure and elevation are adequate when they may actually be impaired.

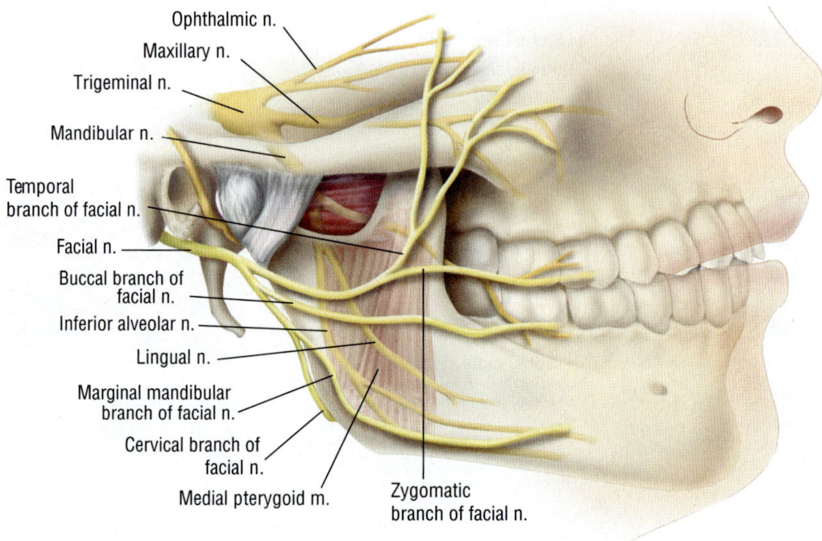

Figure 1.3: The facial nerve exits the stylomastoid foramen—located 1 cm inferior and deep to the external ear's tragal cartilage—at the skull base and then branches into its five motor branches to innervate the muscles of facial expression. (From The Anatomical Chart Company. *Temporomandibular Joint (TMJ) Anatomical Chart*. Wolters Kluwer; 2001.)

The Ear

The external ear, also referred to as the pinna or the auricle, helps funnel sound into the ear canal, where it can be directed to the tympanic membrane (TM) and ossicles to reach the inner ear (cochlea) and auditory nerve. The external components of the ear are illustrated in **Figure 1.4A** and include the helix, antihelix, tragus, antitragus, conchal bowl, and lobule. The superficial temporal and posterior auricular arteries provide the blood supply to the external ear, which is composed of skin, subcutaneous tissue, muscles, and perichondrium that supplies blood to the underlying elastic cartilage. Trauma that damages or elevates the perichondrium off the cartilage risks devascularizing the cartilage, because the cartilage does not contain its own blood vessels and relies on its overlying perichondrium for diffusion of nutrients.[5]

Sensation to the auricle is provided by five nerves, as depicted in **Figure 1.4B**. The auriculotemporal nerve provides sensation to the anterior auricle along its superomedial surface extending along the superior EAC, the lesser occipital nerve provides sensation to the posterior medial surface, the great auricular nerve provides sensation along the lateral auricle extending down to the lobule, the auricular branch of the vagus nerve provides sensation along the conchal bowl and floor of the EAC, and the facial nerve provides scattered points of sensation throughout the conchal bowl.

The EAC provides crucial information and is examined using a handheld otoscope in the emergency setting. For example, in cases of otitis externa, edema of the EAC can prohibit visualization of the distal canal and TM. In the case of a herpes zoster oticus infection, vesicular lesions usually extend along the auricle and EAC.

Although on gross inspection the TM appears to be a thin single membrane, it is actually comprised of three layers that adhere to one another: an outer epidermal layer that is continuous with the skin of the EAC, a middle fibrous layer that gives the TM its stiff tension that contributes to its vibratory capacity, and an inner mucosal layer that is continuous with the mucosal membrane that lines the middle ear. In a healthy patient, one can often see the impression of the ossicles medial to the TM (**Figure 1.5A and B**). Visualizing the membrane as four quadrants (anterior superior, anterior inferior, posterior superior, and posterior inferior) can help when describing anatomic abnormalities of the TM as a result of trauma or infection. For example, when calling an ENT consult in the case of a traumatic TM perforation, one might describe the defect thus: *the perforation extends*

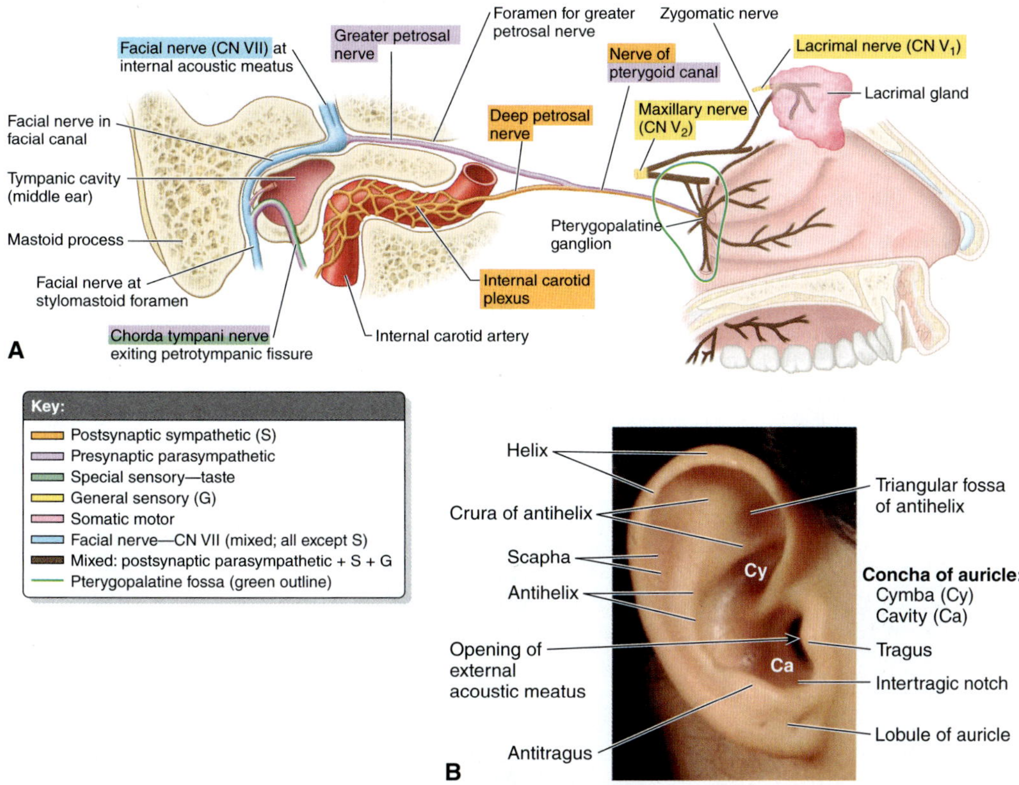

Figure 1.4: A, Anatomy of the external ear. B, Sensory innervation to the external ear. (From Dalley AF II, Agur AMR. Head. In: Dalley AF II, Agur AMR. *Moore's Clinically Oriented Anatomy*. 9th ed. Wolters Kluwer; 2022:839-999. Figure 8.112 and 8.48.)

along the anterior inferior and posterior inferior TM and occupies approximately 50% of the membrane's surface area in this region.[5]

Middle and internal ear structures are not visible on routine examination because these deeper structures are obscured by the TM and skull. However, it is useful to understand the orientation of the ossicles and how they connect to the inner ear. The medial aspect of the TM attaches to the handle of the malleus, and the head of the malleus attaches to the short process of the incus. The lenticular process or long crus of the incus then attaches to the stapes, and the footplate of the stapes adheres to the oval window of the cochlea. This attachment of the stapes footplate to the oval window allows the vibration of the TM produced by sound to travel along the ossicles to reach the cochlea and inner ear (**Figure 1.5C**).

The middle ear cavity and its ossicles also extend into the mastoid bone. This area of the skull's temporal bone contains bony, air-filled sacs that resemble a sponge. When an otitis media (OM) infection accumulates in the middle ear and is unable to drain properly, fluid can track into the mastoid air cells, further extending the infection into the skull.

The Nose

The nose serves an important role in both facial aesthetics and respiratory physiology. The upper one-third of the nose's framework is composed of the nasal bones, and the lower two-thirds is composed of cartilage. The nasal septum also has segments of cartilage and bone and serves as an internal partition between the right and left nasal cavities. Lateral to each side of the nasal septum are three nasal turbinates, known as the superior, middle, and inferior turbinates. The turbinates are oblong structures made of thin bone and covered by respiratory mucosa in the nasal cavities. The turbinates humidify the air as it passes into the upper respiratory system, and their overlying mucosa serve to filter particles such as dust and pollen (**Figure 1.6**).[6]

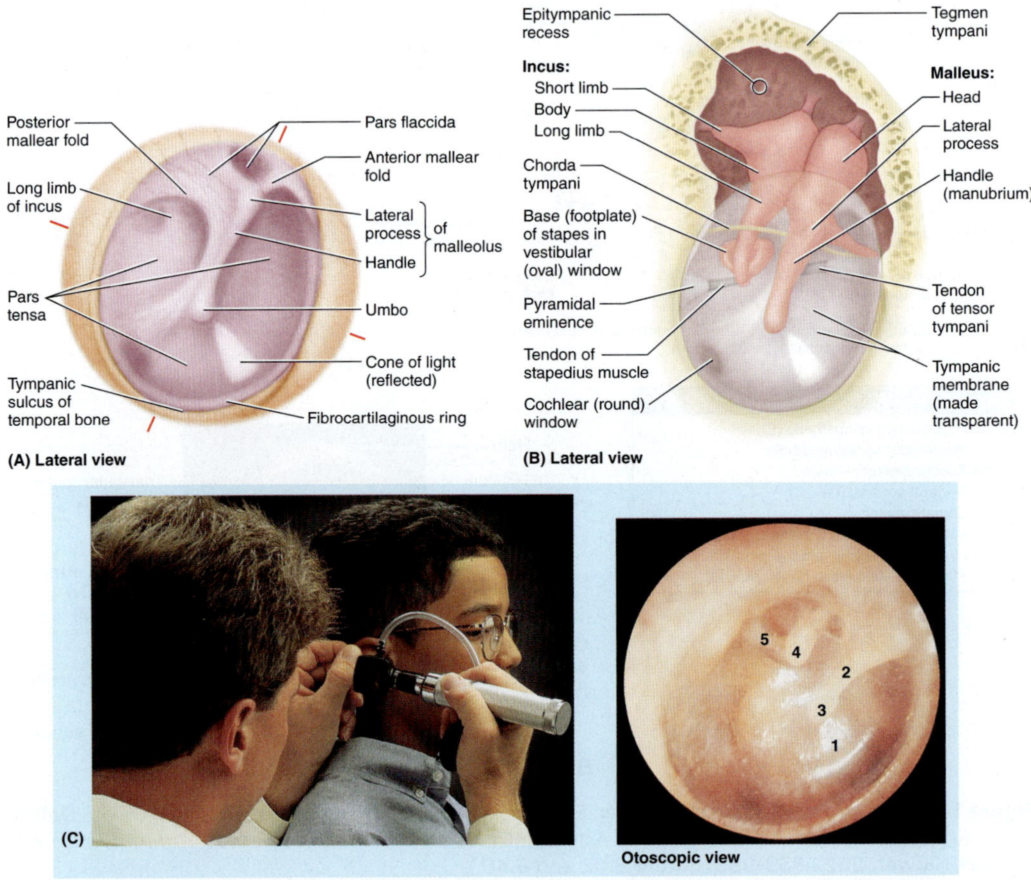

Figure 1.5: A and B, Artistic rendering of an otoscopic view of the tympanic membrane (TM). C, Anatomic view of the TM through an otoscope. Note how the umbo is located at the center of the TM abutting the pars tensa and how the impressions of lateral process and handle of the malleus bone are visible through the TM. Similarly, the outlines of the posterior limb of the stapes and long limb of the incus can often be seen along the TM. 1, cone of light; 2, manubrium; 3, umbo; 4, long limb of incus; 5, posterior limb of stapes. (From Dalley AF II, Agur AMR. Head. In: Dalley AF II, Agur AMR. *Moore's Clinically Oriented Anatomy*. 9th ed. Wolters Kluwer; 2022:839-999. Figure 8.114 and B8.43B.)

Internally, the anterior nasal cavities are continuous with the nose's external skin. Much like the rest of the face, the nose carries a robust blood supply from branches of both the internal and the external carotid arteries. Heat radiating from these vessels humidifies and warms inspired air as it enters the airway. Along the anterior septum, five arterial tributaries of the internal and the external carotid arteries terminate in an arterial plexus called Kiesselbach plexus, the most common source of epistaxis.[6]

The nose carries both special and general nervous innervation. Branches of the first cranial nerve tunnel through the cribriform plate at the roof of the nasal cavity to mediate olfaction through the nose. Patients suffering whiplash or forceful head traumas are at risk for anosmia because of the traumatic shearing of delicate branches of the olfactory nerve as they pass through the cribriform plate. The general sensory innervation of the septum and lateral nasal walls is provided by the nasopalatine nerve, a branch of the maxillary nerve (CN V_2) and the nasociliary nerve, which is a branch of the ophthalmic nerve (CN V_1).

The Mouth and Pharynx

The floor of the anterior nasal cavity is the palatine bone, which serves as the roof of the mouth and oral cavity. The oral cavity is composed of the lips, hard palate, anterior soft palate, the retromolar trigone (area behind the wisdom teeth), the anterior two-thirds of the tongue, the gingiva, and the

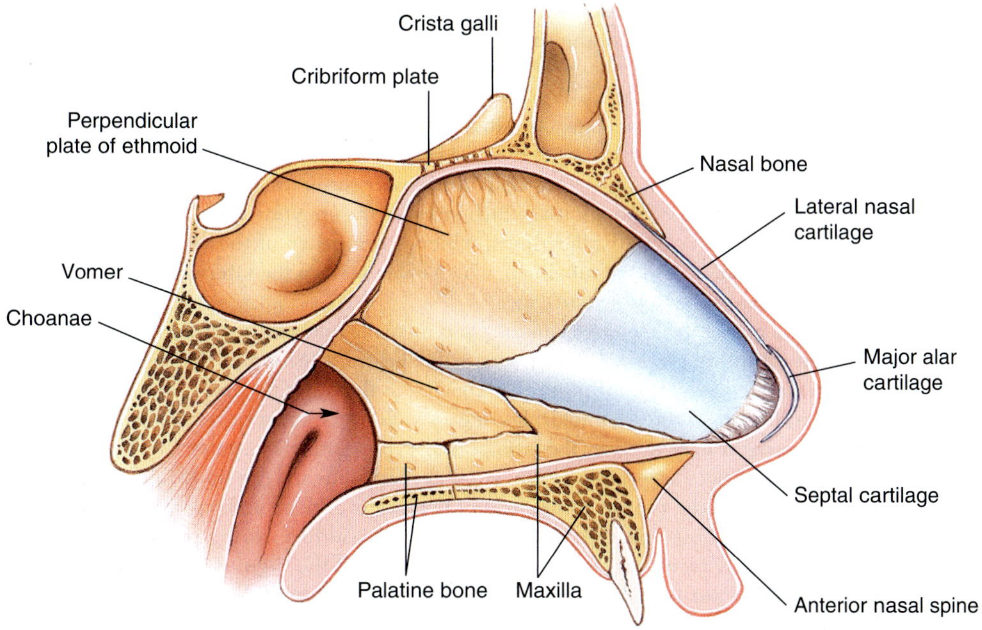

Figure 1.6: The components of the nasal septum. (From The Anatomical Chart Company. *ACC Atlas of Human Anatomy.* Wolters Kluwer; 2001.)

buccal mucosa. Beneath the thin layer of mucosa of the oral cavity lies a muscular diaphragm composed of the mylohyoid muscles that provides structural support to the floor of the mouth and pulls the larynx forward during swallowing. The sublingual and submandibular salivary gland ducts empty into the floor of the mouth beneath the anterior oral tongue.[7]

The oral cavity is contiguous with the oropharynx, which includes the base of the tongue, posterior soft palate and uvula, palatine tonsils, and the pharynx (side and back walls of the throat). The point at which the oral cavity becomes the oropharynx is defined by the hard and soft palate junction, and the line between the anterior two-thirds and posterior one-third of the tongue. During a swallow, the involuntary external pharyngeal muscles—namely, the superior, middle, and inferior constrictor muscles—contract to propel a bolus to the esophagus. These constrictor muscles are unpaired, flat, broad muscles that attach to both the right and the left aspects of the medial pterygoid plate, hyoid bone, and thyroid cartilage, creating the tubular shape of the pharynx.

The posterior and lateral walls of the pharynx extend inferiorly into the pyriform sinuses and posterior cricoid region down to the larynx. The pyriform sinuses serve as gutters for food and saliva to travel from the pharynx into the cervical esophagus.

Sensory innervation of the oral cavity is predominantly supplied by the branches of the trigeminal nerve (CN V). The hard palate is innervated by the greater palatine and nasopalatine nerves, and the soft palate is innervated by the lesser palatine nerve; these are all branches of the maxillary nerve (CN V_2). The floor of the oral cavity and the sensation to the oral tongue are innervated by the lingual nerve, which is a branch of the mandibular division of the trigeminal nerve (CN V_3). The anterior two-thirds of the tongue is also innervated by special sensory fibers from the chorda tympani (CN VII), which mediate taste. And, lastly, the buccal mucosa is innervated by the buccal nerve, a branch of the mandibular division of the trigeminal nerve (CN V_3).[7]

More distally along the pharynx, the pharyngeal branches of the vagus nerve (CN X) provide sensory and motor innervation to all the muscles of the pharynx except the stylopharyngeus, which receives motor innervation from the glossopharyngeal nerve (CN IX). CN IX also mediates the sense of taste for the posterior third of the tongue. The constrictor muscles, which help form the pharynx, facilitate peristalsis during swallow. The pharyngeal branches of the glossopharyngeal nerve provide most of the pharynx with sensory innervation.[8] The laryngeal pharynx is innervated by the vagus nerve. This is the reason why, when you remove earwax along the inferior EAC, innervated by the auricular branch of the vagus nerve, it is common for patients to cough.

The Larynx

As the pharynx extends distally, it connects into the larynx anteriorly and the esophagus posteriorly (**Figure 1.7, left panel**). The larynx bridges the pharynx with the respiratory tract and is responsible for phonation, the cough reflex, and protection of the lower respiratory tract. There are three parts to the larynx (**Figure 1.8**): the supraglottis, which includes the epiglottis and the vestibular mucosal folds that extend to the vocal folds; the glottis, which is comprised of the vocal folds and extends 1 cm below the vocal folds; and the subglottis, which extends from the inferior border of the glottis to the inferior border of the thyroid cartilage.[9]

By acting as a gate at the opening from the pharynx to the trachea, the larynx protects the airway from aspiration during swallowing. This gating is the central function of the epiglottis, a piece of fibroelastic cartilage covered with mucosa that attaches to the inner thyroid cartilage lamina above the anterior commissure of the vocal folds. During a swallow, the superior free edge of the epiglottis flaps over the laryngeal inlet to cover the laryngeal inlet preventing aspiration.[9] In infections of the epiglottis—such as epiglottitis—the epiglottis becomes edematous and can lead to airway obstruction.

The vocal folds are the central component of the larynx and are abducted, adducted, relaxed, and tensed to control phonation. The vocal folds normally adduct during phonation and abduct during respiration. The recurrent laryngeal nerve, a branch of the vagus (CN X) nerve, innervates all muscles responsible for vocal fold movement except the cricothyroid muscle, which is responsible for elevating vocal pitch and is innervated by the superior laryngeal nerve. If the vocal folds do not fully abduct during respiration or if there is abnormal or paradoxical vocal fold motion, there will be turbulent airflow through the glottis. Such patients will present with stridor.

The Neck

Traditionally, anatomic descriptions of the neck have focused on triangles of the neck. These include the submandibular triangle, the carotid triangle, and others. Clinically, the cervical neck is divided into levels based on the patterns of malignant lymphatic spread. The sternocleidomastoid muscle is a paired anterior cervical neck muscle that is often visible and palpable externally. It

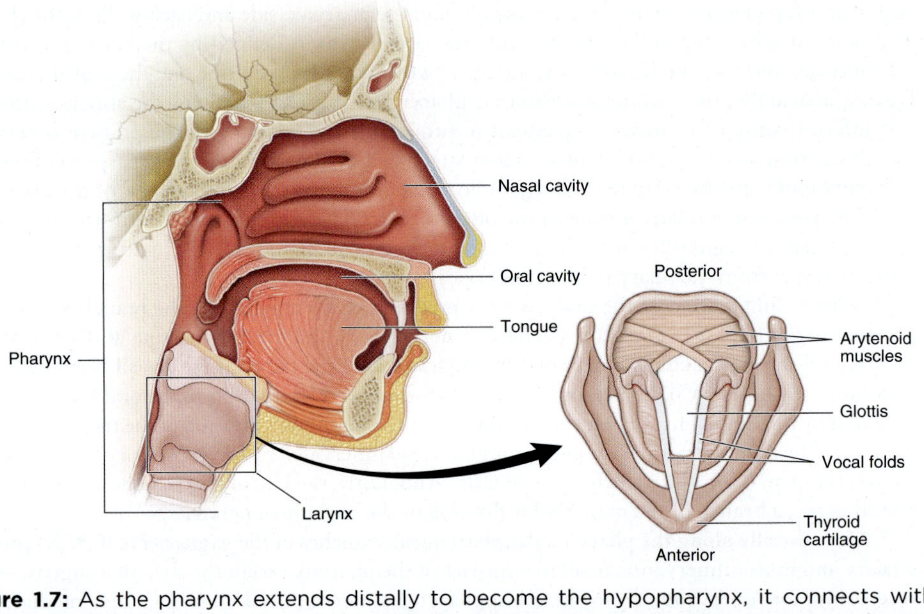

Figure 1.7: As the pharynx extends distally to become the hypopharynx, it connects with the cervical esophagus posteriorly and the larynx anteriorly. The larynx then opens into the trachea and upper airway. (From Bear MF, Connors BW, Paradiso MA. Language. In: Bear MF, Connors BW, Paradiso MA. *Neuroscience: Exploring the Brain*. Wolters Kluwer; 2016: 685-718. Figure 20.1.)

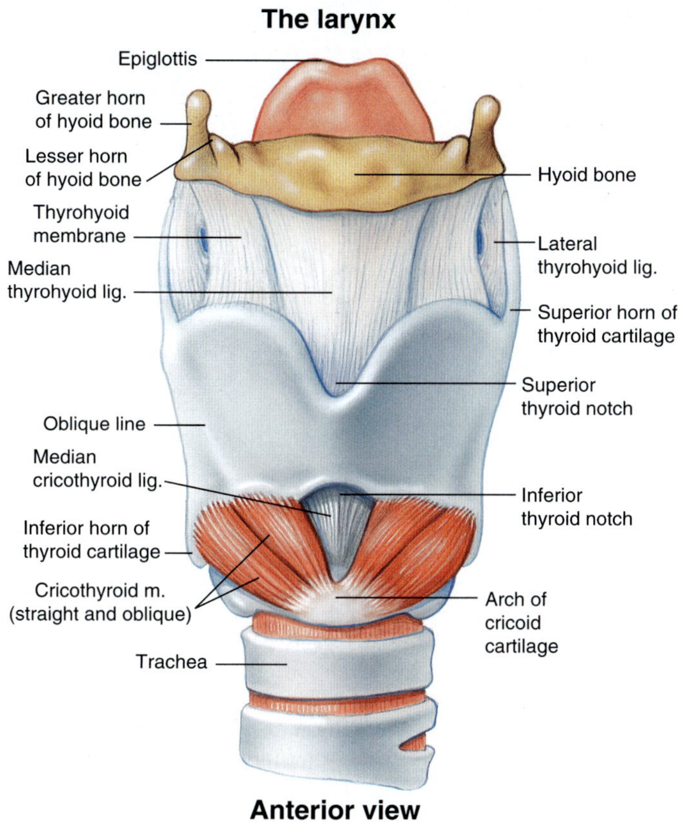

Figure 1.8: Anterior view of the larynx. (From The Anatomical Chart Company. *Pharynx & Larynx Anatomical Chart*. Wolters Kluwer; 2001.)

traverses the cervical neck anteriorly to laterally, originating at the heads of the clavicle and extending superiorly and laterally to attach to the mastoid tip. Medial to these muscles are the hyoid bone, thyroid cartilage, and cricoid bone. These three structures serve as important landmarks of the neck when considering a surgical airway. Ideally a surgical airway, or tracheostomy, is inserted below the level of the cricoid bone, between the first and the second tracheal rings.

References

1. Bradford BD, Lee JW. Reconstruction of the forehead and scalp. *Facial Plast Surg Clin North Am*. 2019;27(1):85-94.
2. Menick FJ. Nasal reconstruction. *Plast Reconstr Surg*. 2010;125(4):138e-150e.
3. Pisano J, Tiwana PS. Management of panfacial, naso-orbital-ethmoid and frontal sinus fractures. *Atlas Oral Maxillofac Surg Clin North Am*. 2019;27(2):83-92.
4. Kochhar A, Larian B, Azizzadeh B. Facial nerve and parotid gland anatomy. *Otolaryngol Clin North Am*. 2016;49(2):273-284.
5. Eagles K, Fralich L, Stevenson JH. Ear trauma. *Clin Sports Med*. 2013;32(2):303-316.
6. Patel RG. Nasal anatomy and function. *Facial Plast Surg*. 2017;33(1):3-8.
7. Madani M, Berardi T, Stoopler ET. Anatomic and examination considerations of the oral cavity. *Med Clin North Am*. 2014;98(6):1225-1238.
8. Sasegbon A, Hamdy S. The anatomy and physiology of normal and abnormal swallowing in oropharyngeal dysphagia. *Neurogastroenterol Motil*. 2017;29(11):e13100. doi:10.1111/nmo.13100
9. Simpson CB, Rosen CA. *Operative Techniques in Laryngology*. Springer; 2008.

CHAPTER 2

Examination of the Ears, Nose, and Throat

Katelyn Stepan
Jimmy Truong

THE CLINICAL CHALLENGE

Examination of the ears, nose, and throat reveals pertinent information regarding their form and function, as well as insight into the condition of the associated alimentary and respiratory tracts. Although many symptoms of the head and neck are manifestations of benign conditions, an attentive history and physical exam are critical to identifying the underlying etiology and potentially more serious underlying disease. A carefully performed physical exam may also allow the provider to avoid unnecessary testing, facilitate appropriate triage and management, and prevent delays in care.

PHYSICAL EXAMINATION

General Appearance

Valuable information can be gathered by simply observing a patient's appearance, behavior, and affect. A patient's vital signs, alertness, orientation, and evidence of toxicity or distress should be noted. Retractions, increased work of breathing, diaphoresis, stridor, or wheezing should alert the physician to evaluate for possible underlying causes.

Head and Facies

The head and facial skeleton should be inspected and palpated for any lesions or asymmetries, as well as evidence of irregularities or step-offs, particularly in the setting of trauma. This includes inspection of the cranial bones, mandible, maxilla, zygomatic arch, orbital rims, and nasal dorsum. The condition of the skin, hair, and scalp should also be noted. The areas overlying the paranasal sinuses may be palpated for tenderness. Conditions involving the temporomandibular joint, which may result in clicking, dislocation, or locking of the jaw, may be assessed by having the patient open and close the jaw while simultaneously palpating both sides of the joint just anterior to the ear canal. Assessment of suboccipital, preauricular, and retroauricular lymph nodes is performed with bilateral palpation. The salivary glands, including bilateral parotid and submandibular glands, are assessed with external palpation and by using bimanual palpation with one hand placed intraorally. With the use of a headlight, the patency of Stensen and Wharton ducts can be inspected intraorally to look for salivary flow during bimanual palpation, when saliva may be "milked" out of the parotid or submandibular glands, respectively.

Ears

The ear exam involves evaluation of the external ear and auricle as well as otoscopic exam of the external auditory canal (EAC) and tympanic membrane (TM). It also entails hearing assessment with the use of tuning forks and evaluation of the vestibular system if clinically indicated.

External Ear

The auricle and postauricular region should be inspected and palpated for any evidence of deformities, lesions, or asymmetries. The preauricular area may be evaluated for evidence of a sinus tract or drainage. Postauricular pain, swelling, fluid collection, ecchymosis, or lymphadenopathy may indicate an underlying infectious or traumatic process.

External Auditory Canal

The EAC should be inspected with an otoscope for discharge, lesions, foreign bodies, and cerumen. Foul odor may also indicate infection.

TM and Middle Ear

Otoscopy should be performed to evaluate the TM and middle ear using the largest speculum to afford the best view. The otoscope can be held like a pen while the little finger rests against the patient's head to ensure stability and to prevent any injury that may occur with sudden patient movement. The speculum is carefully inserted roughly 1 cm into the canal with one hand while the other gently retracts the pinna posterosuperiorly to align the meatus and auditory canal. Landmarks such as the malleus, color, and contour of the TM should be observed. Fluid, air bubbles, and masses involving the middle ear can be appreciated behind the TM. Pneumatic otoscopy can be used to evaluate the mobility of the TM when there is concern for middle ear disorders by gently applying negative or positive pressure from the pneumatic bulb. An immobile TM may be secondary to middle ear fluid or perforation. An otoscope with a working channel can be used to remove any debris or cerumen that may inhibit visualization. In the absence of TM perforation, pressure equalizer (PE) tubes, or otitis externa, warm water irrigation may also be used. Size and location of any perforation and the presence of PE tubes should be noted.

Hearing

Hearing can be grossly evaluated by monitoring the patient's response to questions during the interview. The whispered voice test can also be used to crudely assess hearing by having the patient repeat back numbers, letters or words whispered into the patient's test ear while the patient covers the non-test ear. The examiner stands an arm's length behind the patient and whispers a combination of numbers and letters, asking the patient to repeat them. Each ear is tested separately. Concern for hearing impairment should be raised if the patient is unable to repeat 50% of the numbers or words correctly.

Tuning fork exams can be used to differentiate conductive and sensorineural hearing loss. The Weber and Rinne tuning fork exams are typically performed with a 512 Hz tuning fork. The tuning fork is made to vibrate by gently striking the prongs against a hard surface.

The Weber test is performed by placing the base of the vibrating tuning fork on the middle of the forehead and asking the patient where they hear the sound. With normal hearing, the sound is heard in both ears equally or centrally. This is referred to as a "negative" Weber. A bilateral symmetric loss will also be heard in the midline. A unilateral sensorineural loss will be heard louder in the unaffected ear, while a conductive loss will be heard in the affected ear.

The Rinne test is performed by first placing the vibrating tuning fork against the patient's mastoid bone (bone conduction [BC]) and then positioning the still vibrating base of the tuning fork in the air, 1 to 2 cm away from the external auditory meatus on the same side (air conduction [AC]). The patient is then asked to identify the position in which the sound is louder: "behind" (BC) or "in front of" (AC) the ear. AC is perceived as louder than BC in those with normal hearing in that ear, as well as those with sensorineural hearing loss. BC is perceived to be louder in those with a conductive loss, such as that associated with an effusion or TM perforation. The test is considered "positive" if AC > BC and "negative" if BC > AC. Patients with findings suggestive of hearing loss should be referred to a specialist for a more complete evaluation, including audiometric testing.

Table 2.1 reviews how to interpret findings of the Weber and Rinne tuning fork exams.

TABLE 2.1 Tuning Fork Exam Interpretation

	Sensorineural Hearing Loss	Conductive Hearing Loss
Rinne	AC > BC	BC > AC
Weber	Heard in "good" ear	Heard in "bad" ear

AC, air conduction; BC, bone conduction.

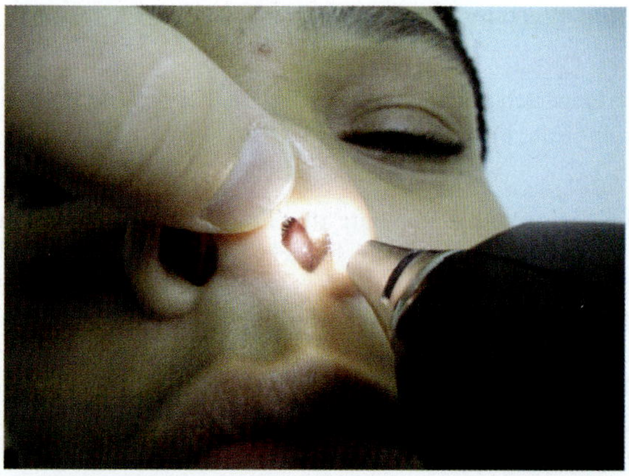

Figure 2.1: Inferior turbinate. Image of pale, boggy inferior turbinate as seen in allergic rhinitis. (Courtesy of Paul S. Matz, MD and from Kelly SF. Nasal swelling, discharge, and crusting. In: Chung EK, Atkinson-McEvoy LR, Lai NL, Terry M, eds. *Visual Diagnosis and Treatment in Pediatrics*. 3rd ed. Wolter Kluwer; 2015:182-188. Figure 23.2.)

Vestibular

Complaints of dizziness, vertigo, or disequilibrium often warrant a detailed and specialized exam. Vestibular testing is performed to determine whether the etiology is central (pathology originating from the cerebellum or brainstem) or peripheral (pathology arising from the inner ear or vestibular nerve). The physical examination evaluates for nystagmus, central oculomotor function, and the vestibulo-ocular reflex. Posture, coordination, and gait are also assessed. More detailed information regarding the workup of vertigo can be found in Chapter 7.

Nose

Examination of the nose begins with gross inspection. Note the shape of its dorsal aspect, the width of the tip, and any deviation from the midline. Examine the tip of the nose with gentle pressure for any tenderness. Examine each nasal vestibule. Anterior rhinoscopy allows for assessment of the nasal septum and inferior turbinates. The patient should be seated and their head tilted backward for better visualization. A nasal speculum is introduced carefully into the nare along the lateral wall, observing the color, vascularity, and any discharge. The nasal septum is evaluated for discoloration, deviation, hematoma, or perforation. The turbinates, attached to the lateral nasal wall, can be evaluated; pathologic findings may range from boggy, edematous, pale, or erythematous **(Figure 2.1)**. Adjacent to the nose are the paranasal sinuses, which can be palpated to elicit any tenderness. Severe tenderness indicates an inflammatory process of the sinuses. Palpation may also reveal step-off deformities in the setting of trauma.

Nasopharynx

The nasopharynx represents the most superior aspect of the pharynx, extending from the skull base superiorly to the soft palate inferiorly. The nasopharynx can be a difficult area to examine and often requires the use of rigid or flexible fiberoptic scope. If available, a flexible scope can be gently introduced through the nose after topical decongestant (neosynephrine) and anesthetic (4% topical lidocaine) are sprayed in bilateral nasal cavities. The Eustachian tube orifice, torus tubarius, fossa of Rosenmuller, and adenoids should be inspected. Any cysts, masses, or asymmetries should be noted.

Oral Cavity

The oral cavity is comprised of the lips anteriorly, cheeks laterally, palate superiorly, floor of the mouth inferiorly, and oropharynx posteriorly. The patient should be asked to remove any oral appliances to allow for better visualization. Observe the lips for color, moisture, ulcers, or irregular skin changes. Look inside the mouth with a good light source and the assistance of a tongue blade. Inspect the oral mucosa, including the gums, for color, ulcerations, or masses. On the hard palate, a midline excessive bone growth is a normal anatomic variant called a torus palatini. Similar excessive bone growth on the anterior lingual surface of the mandible is called torus mandibularis. Examine dentition for decay, discoloration, malalignment, and looseness. Note that there are 32 teeth in an adult. Permanent teeth start appearing by age 6, and the Universal Numbering System is the most common classification method. This numbering system is depicted in **Figure 2.2**.

Each tooth is divided into the crown and the roots, with the outer portion covered by enamel. Directly underneath the enamel is dentin, forming the bulk of the tooth, which can be sensitive with loss of enamel. The pulp of the tooth starts at the tip of the root and spans to the crown. The pulp contains the blood and nerve supply and is encased within the dentin.

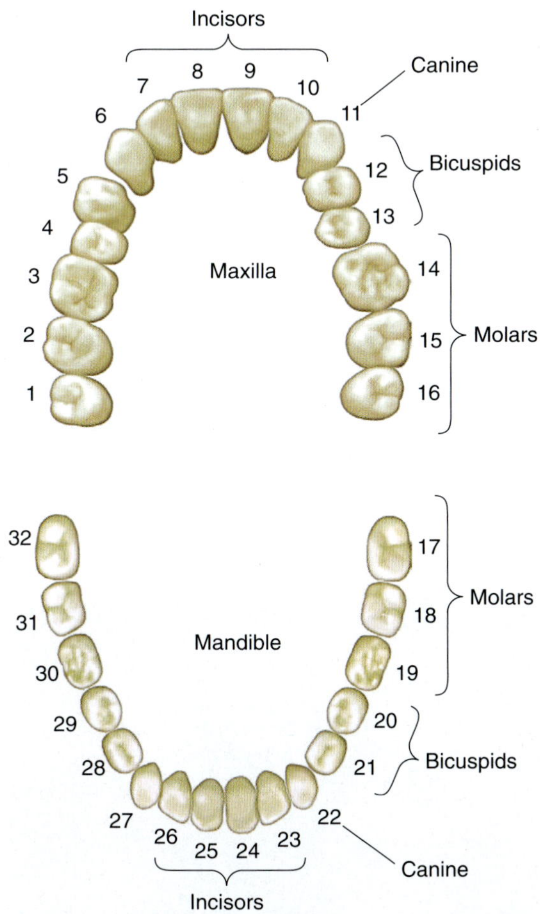

Figure 2.2: The universal tooth numbering system. Numeral 1 starts at the right maxillary third molar; teeth are numbered sequentially up to 32, the right mandibular third molar. (From Hansen SL, Balkin DM. Maxillofacial injuries. In: Britt LD, Peitzman AB, Barie PS, Jurkovich GJ, eds. *Acute Care Surgery*. 2nd ed. Wolters Kluwer; 2019:365-376. Figure 29.2.)

Oropharynx

The oropharynx is posterior to the oral cavity and bound superiorly by the soft and hard palate and inferiorly by the base of the tongue. Observe the soft palate and note the color and consistency. The uvula is assessed for its size, length, color, and position if not midline. The palatine tonsils are directly visualized on both sides of the pharynx. The tonsils may be smooth or have crypts that can collect food, bacteria, and debris. Depressing the tongue with a tongue depressor and asking the patient to say "Ahh" will help to visualize the tonsils. Observe for enlargement, redness, ulcerations, discolorations, and discharge. Inclusion cysts, inflammatory debris, or stones (tonsilliths) will frequently be visible on exam. Normal tonsils vary in size from being barely visible to touching in the midline ("kissing tonsils").

Larynx and Hypopharynx

The larynx, or "voice box," extends from the epiglottis down to the subglottic airway and contains the vocal cords. The hypopharynx is continuous with the oropharynx, extending from the level of the hyoid bone down to the esophageal inlet. The integrity and function of the larynx and hypopharynx play critical roles in maintaining a patient's airway, speech, and swallow. Indirect laryngoscopy with a dental mirror may be performed to evaluate the tongue base, hypopharynx, and larynx. The patient is seated in an upright position while leaning forward slightly at the waist, with the chin in the sniffing position. With one hand, the examiner gently grasps the patient's protruded tongue with a gauze sponge while the other hand is used to position a warmed dental mirror just below the soft palate, allowing visualization of the oropharynx, hypopharynx, and larynx. Flexible fiberoptic laryngoscopy (FFL) may be indicated for a more detailed and dynamic assessment. After decongestant and topical anesthetic are sprayed in the nose, the flexible scope is passed through the nasal cavity to visualize the more distal airway. The patient may be asked to vocalize and swallow during the assessment. Any mucosal irregularities, edema, cysts, or masses should be noted. The mobility and integrity of the vocal cords should also be noted. Normal vocal cords can be seen in **Figure 2.3**.

Neck

The neck and clavicles should be exposed, and the examiner should make note of any asymmetry, masses, skin lesions, or scars. Evaluate lymph nodes in the parotid, preauricular, postauricular, and mastoid regions by palpating the mastoid bone following the trapezius muscle down into the supraclavicular fossa. The neck region can be divided into the anterior and the posterior cervical triangles, with the sternocleidomastoid (SCM) muscle dividing them. Have the patient flex and extend their neck to check for normal range of motion. The thyroid gland is found in the anterior midline of the neck. Asymmetries in the gland are often caused by nodules, and masses superior to the thyroid isthmus along the axis of the larynx may represent remnants of the thyroglossal duct.

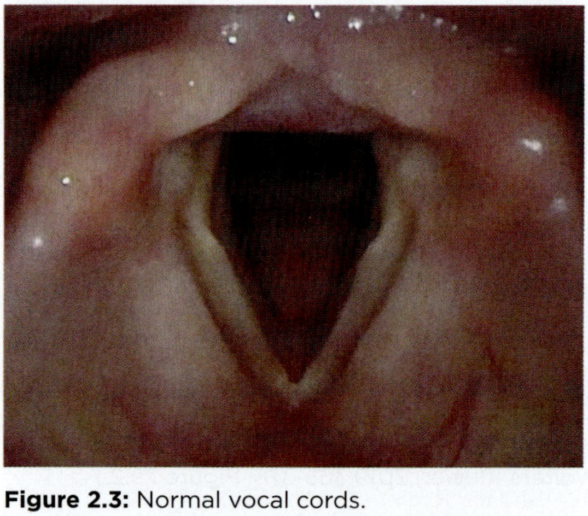

Figure 2.3: Normal vocal cords.

TABLE 2.2 Cranial Nerve Assessment

Cranial Nerve(s)		Function	Assessment
I	Olfactory	Sensory: smell	Smell identification test
II	Optic	Sensory: vision	Visual acuity (Snellen chart), visual field testing, pupillary reaction to light, fundoscopy
III	Oculomotor	Motor: eye movement	Extraocular movements ("H" tracking), pupillary reaction to light and accommodation, ptosis evaluation
IV	Trochlear	Motor: eye movement (superior oblique)	Extraocular movements ("H" tracking)
V	Trigeminal	Sensory: facial, anterior tongue sensation Motor: mastication	Palpate masseter while patient clenches jaw, open mouth against resistance Facial sensation of relevant dermatomes (forehead, cheek, chin)
VI	Abducens	Motor: eye movement (lateral rectus)	Extraocular movements ("H" tracking)
VII	Facial	Sensory: taste Motor: facial expression	Facial expression (raise eyebrows, squeeze eyes shut, scrunch nose, puff out cheeks, smile, pucker lips)
VIII	Vestibulocochlear	Sensory: hearing, balance	Hearing evaluation (whispered voice, tuning fork, audiometry), vestibular testing, gait assessment
IX	Glossopharyngeal	Sensory: pharyngeal sensation Motor: pharynx	Elicit gag reflex
X	Vagus	Sensory: pharynx, larynx, esophagus Motor: palate, pharynx, larynx	Elicit gag reflex Phonation, voice quality, swallow, soft palate elevation
XI	Spinal accessory	Motor: shoulder, neck movement	Shoulder shrug, turn head against resistance
XII	Hypoglossal	Motor: tongue movement	Protrude tongue, move side to side (deviates toward side of weakness)

Neurologic and Cranial Nerve Exam

A complete cranial nerve exam is often indicated in patients presenting with a head and neck complaint. **Table 2.2** provides a brief overview of how a clinical cranial nerve assessment is performed.

PEDIATRIC ISSUES

When examining the pediatric patient, cooperation, patience, and enlisting the help of any available caretaker is key. In some cases, it may be best to examine the patient supine on an examination bed. In newborns and infants, make note of the larger head to body ratio. Examine the head, paying attention to the suture lines and fontanelles. Palpate with care and observe size, asymmetry, shape, and color. In children, also make note of any abnormal facies.

When examining the neck in infants and newborns, palpate the lymph nodes of the neck and assess for masses, noting any congenital cysts. For instance, branchial cleft cysts may present as small dimples or openings anterior to the sternocleidomastoid muscle. Preauricular cysts are pinhole-sized pits anterior to the helix of the ear. Another common cyst is the thyroglossal duct cyst, which moves with swallowing and may present as a small, firm, mobile mass in the midline of the neck above the thyroid cartilage. Check for the position of the thyroid and trachea. Palpate both clavicles for symmetry and tenderness.

Careful examination of the ear begins with determination of the position in relation to the eyes. Note that the canthi of the eye should cross the pinna or auricle. If the pinna or auricle is below this axis, then the patient has low-set ears. Examine the EAC with an otoscope and assess for color, tenderness, and patency. Note that in infancy, the EAC is pointed downward in relation to the more external ear, so it is best examined by pulling downward on the auricle. When examining the ear in children, restraining techniques may need to be employed to best visualize the EAC and TM. With the help of the caregiver and the child in their lap, the child's legs can be secured between their lap. The caregiver then crosses one arm over the child's body, restraining their arms while the other is used to gently steady the child's head in order to facilitate examination of the child's ear. Alternatively, infants and small children may be tightly swaddled in a blanket or sheet (papoosed) to prevent movement during the ear exam.

When evaluating the mouth and pharynx, use a tongue blade and flashlight. Observe the smooth mucosa of the oropharynx. Examine the tongue and oropharynx, which can best be seen while the infant is crying. During nasal exam, ensure the nasal passages are open. Observe that the nose and septum are midline, noting any asymmetry.

TIPS AND PEARLS

- The physical exam should be performed in a standardized approach and tailored based on the clinical scenario.
- Special equipment, such as a flexible endoscope, can aid the examiner in performing a detailed assessment.
- When examining the ear in children, restraining techniques may need to be employed to best visualize the ear canal and TM.

SUMMARY

A detailed history and physical examination is paramount to the evaluation of patients presenting with ears, nose, and throat complaints. The regional anatomy presents a challenge because some structures are not easily accessible by direct visualization without additional equipment or instrumentation. Information obtained from the physical exam provides a framework to develop a differential diagnosis and determine appropriate definitive management.

EVIDENCE

What is the best hearing evaluation in the emergency department or urgent care setting?

The whispered voice test offers a valuable tool for hearing assessment in these settings, because it is the only hearing test that does not require specialized equipment. It has been found to have good specificity and sensitivity for detecting hearing loss in adults 50 to 70 years of age if administered by an experienced practitioner.[1] However, it has reduced sensitivity when administered to children and is therefore not recommended for pediatric screening. This method has a reported 80% sensitivity in detecting hearing impairment greater than or equal to 25 dB hearing loss in children aged 5 to 12 years.[2]

What is the diagnostic accuracy for pediatric acute otitis media?

In a 2019 study, it was found that only 52.1% of pediatric patients diagnosed with acute otitis media (AOM) had symptoms consistent with AOM. The same study found that 31% of those diagnosed with AOM had no supporting physician exam findings, as outlined by the American Academy of Pediatrics. About 90% of patients included in the study were prescribed antibiotics, presenting a concern for overprescribing practices.[3]

References

1. McShefferty D, Whitmer WM, Swan IR, Akeroyd MA. The effect of experience on the sensitivity and specificity of the whispered voice test: a diagnostic accuracy study. *BMJ Open*. 2013;3(4):e002394. doi:10.1136/bmjopen-2012-002394

2. Dempster JH, Mackenzie K. Clinical role of free-field voice tests in children. *Clin Otolaryngol Allied Sci*. 1992;17(1):54-56.

3. Brinker DL Jr, MacGeorge EL, Hackman N. Diagnostic accuracy, prescription behavior, and watchful waiting efficacy for pediatric acute otitis media. *Clin Pediatr (Phila)*. 2019;58(1):60-65. doi: 10.1177/0009922818806312. Erratum in: *Clin Pediatr (Phila)*. 2019;58(4):491.

Suggested Reading

American Academy of Otolaryngology-Head and Neck Surgery. ENT Exam Video Series. Accessed May 8, 2021. https://www.entnet.org/education/ent-exam-video-series/

Bickley, LS. *Bates' Guide to Physical Examination and History Taking*. Lippincott Williams & Wilkins; 2003.

Chan JYK, Tsang RKY, Yeung KW, et al. There is no routine head and neck exam during the COVID-19 pandemic. *Head Neck*. 2020;42(6):1235-1239.

Eggers SDZ, Zee DS. Evaluating the dizzy patient: bedside examination and laboratory assessment of the vestibular system. *Semin Neurol*. 2003;23(1):47-57.

Goebel JA. The ten-minute examination of the dizzy patient. *Semin Neurol*. 2001;21(4):391-398.

James M, Palmer O. Instrumentation and techniques for examination of the ear, nose, throat, and sinus. *Oral Maxillofac Surg Clin North Am*. 2012;24(2):167-174, vii.

Madani M, Berardi T, Stoopler ET. Anatomic and examination considerations of the oral cavity. *Med Clin North Am*. 2014;98(6):1225-1238.

Rosenberg TL, Brown JJ, Jefferson GD. Evaluating the adult patient with a neck mass. *Med Clin North Am*. 2010;94(5):1017-1029.

CHAPTER 3

Communication With ENT Consultants

Yan Lee
Mark Grbic

THE CLINICAL CHALLENGE

For the successful management of a patient in the emergency department (ED) or urgent care setting, clear communication between emergency providers and ENT specialists is paramount. Working within hospital systems, it is also important to be cognizant of a system's limitations and availability of services (eg, in-house consultants, on call physicians, telehealth providers, or no specialty backup). Understanding how to balance all these factors is the keystone of communication with consultants. As with any consultation, the usual goal is to ask for a service outside the scope of practice of the emergency provider or to obtain expert opinion. The objectives of this chapter are to provide a schema for the ENT consultation question and conversation, establish the capabilities and timing of consultation by an otolaryngologist, and clarify when to involve further services to help our patients outside of otolaryngology.

The Consultation Question and Communication

To optimize care of patients with ENT pathologies requires prompt and effective communication. Ideally, there are simple and reliable mechanisms for communication between the ED providers and consultants. Several studies have demonstrated that consults following a specific format help to convey a comprehensive description of the patient as well as a focused reason for consulting a provider (**Figure 3.1**).[1] There are also tools to guide consultants' communication with the requesting provider (**Table 3.1**).[2] These schemas can clarify and anticipate issues that ENT providers will need to know in order to provide appropriate recommendations or prepare for an in-person evaluation. In general, these schemas involve identifying the consultant and consultee, identifying the patient, providing a precise and focused history of present illness, relevant studies or imaging already performed, a clinical question, or a confirmed diagnosis requiring the consultant's expertise.

As with all ED consults, one of the most important considerations is providing the consultant with a specific actionable item for collaboration. These actionable items can be divided into questions regarding diagnosis, specific management options, and patient disposition. Framing the clinical question around what is lacking that the consultant can provide is a key factor in clear communication between services. Asking for clear procedural guidance (eg, help with locating a foreign body in the airway, laryngoscopy for evaluation of angioedema) or for help with disposition and management of a patient (eg, evaluation for admission for mastoiditis, advanced airway management, or surgical intervention for epistaxis) helps to narrow the focus of the consultant to provide optimal care.

Another important aspect of the clinical consultation is anticipating and acknowledging what needs the ENT consultant will have in order to best help you with your patient. Anticipating and performing appropriate imaging, such as computed tomography (CT) evaluation for mastoiditis or

FRONT

C **ontact the consultant courteously**
Caller's name, training level, team, "I am requesting a CONSULT please."

O **rient**
Patient name, medical record number (MRN), floor, and bed

N **arrow question**
Ask a focused question regarding diagnosis (workup, procedures) and/or management (treatments, pre-op)

S **tory**
Patient age, sex, *pertinent* history (HPI), hospital course, relevant labs, radiology, anticipated plan

U **rgency**
When should the patient be evaluated? 30 minutes to 1 hour (emergent), 2 to 3 hours (very urgent), 8 hours (urgent), 24 hours (routine)

L **ater**
Make a follow-up plan with the consultant (how and by when?) and give your pager/cell number

T **hank you!**

BACK

Other tips for calling a consult:

Orient the listener to each component of the call.
Be courteous and polite (even if they are not).
Avoid calling a consult just to be "on board" with no particular question for that service to address.
For diagnostic questions, have a differential in mind.
For diagnostic questions, begin and anticipate the workup.
For therapeutic questions, have an anticipated management plan in mind.
Have pertinent information available (either written) or open on EPIC.
Follow up with the consultant after the initial recommendations to: ask questions and discuss the outcomes of the case (it's your time to learn!).

Figure 3.1: A CONSULT card to facilitate consults from the emergency room. (From Podolsky A, Stern DT, Peccoralo L. The courteous consult: a CONSULT card and training to improve resident consults. *J Grad Med Educ*. 2015;7(1):113-117. Figure 1.)

imaging to localize foreign bodies, can help your consultants make quicker and simpler decisions on cases. ENT consultations usually focus on a wide variety of diagnoses. One study on ENT consultation at a quaternary care hospital revealed that the most common reason for consultation from the ED was facial trauma, followed by airway evaluation, neck infection, then epistaxis, as outlined in **Table 3.2.**[3]

Systems Considerations, Capability of ENT Consultants, and Telemedicine

Because healthcare facilities have variable staffing and care capabilities, it is critical to understand the resources available both for consultation and for definitive care. The scope of practice may vary for consultants available to the ED, so agreements and protocols are important to discuss between services in advance of consultation. For example, if a patient with uncontrolled epistaxis requires ligation, and the on-call ENT does not perform these, the patient may need to be transferred to another facility, or a neurosurgeon/interventional radiologist may need to be called. There are also some diagnoses that may be handled by multiple services (eg, orbital fractures may be evaluated by ENT, ophthalmology, or plastic surgery). Bedside procedures commonly performed by ENT are listed in **Table 3.3.**[3]

TABLE 3.1 Modified Commandments to Facilitate Communication Between Consultant and the Requesting Provider

Commandment	Meaning
1. Determine the question being asked	Ask the person requesting the consult what specific question they are trying to ask; sometimes this is not obvious and you may need to ask probing questions.
2. Establish urgency	Ask if the situation is emergent, urgent, or elective; this may require additional questions during the conversation.
3. See the consult in person	See the patient and perform physical exam whenever possible; "trust but verify."
4. Be brief when appropriate	Consultant may not need to repeat every detail of the history taking and documentation, but should still verify the pertinent details.
5. Be specific	Do not assume that the requesting provider knows details of your recommendations; be as specific as possible about your recommendations.
6. Provide contingency plans	Anticipate issues with your recommendations and provide secondary backup plans.
7. Do not overstep boundaries	Remember that you are the consultant and should not overstep your boundaries (ie, change orders without notifying the requesting/primary provider).
8. Teach as appropriate	Use consultations as an opportunity to discuss patient's case with learning points (only if the requesting provider is amenable).
9. Talk is essential	Having a conversation between requesting provider and the consultant is crucial for optimal patient care and outcomes.
10. Provide follow-up	Even if you feel that the consultation has been completed, provide means for follow-up for any concerns or issues that may arise.

(Derived from Salerno SM, Hurst FP, Halvorson S, Mercado DL. Principles of effective consultation: an update for the 21st-century consultant. *Arch Intern Med.* 2007 Feb 12;167(3):271-275.)

TABLE 3.2 Common Reasons for Consults From the ED to ENT

Requested Consultation Reasons for ENT	
Airway evaluation	107 (20.3%)
Bleeding	5 (0.9%)
Epistaxis	33 (6.3%)
Facial trauma	179 (33.9%)
Facial fracture	97 (18.4%)
Facial laceration	44 (8.3%)
Facial fracture and laceration	38 (7.2%)
Gunshot wound	1 (0.2%)
Infection	103 (19.5%)
Neck mass	7 (1.3%)
Oral lesion	2 (0.4%)
Odynophagia	1 (0.2%)
Other (facial lesion, foreign body in oral cavity)	2 (0.4%)
Otologic	21 (4.0%)
Postoperative	51 (9.7%)
Rhinologic	13 (2.5%)
Tracheotomy	3 (0.6%)

(Derived from Choi KJ, Kahmke RR, Crowson MG, Puscas L, Scher RL, Cohen SM. Trends in otolaryngology consultation patterns at an Academic Quaternary Care Center. *JAMA Otolaryngol Head Neck Surg.* 2017;143(5):472-477.)

TABLE 3.3 Common Procedures Performed by ENT Consultants	
Common Otolaryngology Bedside Procedures	
Flexible laryngoscopy	54.6%
Repair of complex facial laceration	10.8%
Nasal endoscopy	10.7%
Management of epistaxis	9.5%
Incision and drainage of head and neck abscess	6.5%
Needle aspiration	2.0%
Foreign body removal	1.0%
Tracheotomy change	0.8%
Myringotomy and PE tube placement	0.7%
Closed reduction of nasal bone fracture	0.7%
Other (biopsy, cautery of tonsillar fossa, etc.)	3.0%

(Derived from Choi KJ, Kahmke RR, Crowson MG, Puscas L, Scher RL, Cohen SM. Trends in Otolaryngology Consultation Patterns at an Academic Quaternary Care Center. *JAMA Otolaryngol Head Neck Surg*. 2017 May 1;143(5):472-477.)

However, not all ENT diagnoses in the emergency setting require ENT consultants as proceduralists. In some cases, a telehealth consult can be used instead to allow for a more widespread application of ENT needs. According to an evaluation of visits in a general clinic setting, up to 62% of ENT encounters can be eligible for telemedicine applications, particularly those referring to problems within the inner and middle ear, whereas those involving the larynx or external ear were least applicable.[4]

A retrospective review of ENT consultations looked at interventions and the varying services provided by ENT consultants in a metropolitan hospital.[5] These were consultations across all services, not limited to the ED alone. This study found that the chief complaints of epistaxis and angioedema consistently required interventions, 57.5% and 84% respectively. However, they found that other chief complaints such as dysphagia (32.3% intervention rate), dysphonia (16%), otalgia (20.8%), hearing loss (13.3%), and vertigo/dizziness (0%) often did not require intervention, which may be diagnoses amenable for telemedicine evaluation from the ED or follow-up.

TIPS AND PEARLS

- Having a structure to providing consultation is important to clear communication with ENT consultants.
- General system considerations can affect the ability of the ENT consultant to be able to help with given interventions.

EVIDENCE

How has the COVID-19 pandemic changed telemedicine for ENT?

ENT subspecialists have rapidly adopted the telemedicine platform during the COVID-19 pandemic.[6] On average, it takes a program about 23 months to establish a telemedicine program from the beginning.[6] Prior to the pandemic, telemedicine for ENT was utilized primarily by socioeconomically disadvantaged communities or rural communities that otherwise did not have access to subspecialty care.[6] The pandemic has expanded the reach of telemedicine to almost all communities, especially Medicare eligible patients who are particularly vulnerable to COVID-19.[6]

Telemedicine by ENT specialists are often used for two primary purposes relevant to emergency providers: (1) Forward triage: preevaluation of a patient destined for the ED to help with management and disposition; (2) Direct-to-consumer (DTC): screening patients for ED referral versus later outpatient follow-up.[6]

A telemedicine history of present illness should mirror in person visits. The Telemedicine Work Group in the American Academy of Allergy, Asthma & Immunology (AAAAI) provided guidance regarding physical examination of the telemedicine patient, some of which requires patient cooperation, additional help from technology such as smartphone applications that provide digital telemedicine otoscopes, or the aid of another provider such as an emergency physician.[6]

A recent meta-analysis shows improvement in patients' quality of life and noninferiority for patient safety in patients with asthma.[6] As more cases are explored through telemedicine and studied for safety and efficacy, there is doubt that telemedicine will continue to expand. Emergency providers will have to adapt to the changing landscape of subspecialty consultation and establish systems to interface with consultants both in-person as well as on virtual platforms.

References

1. Podolsky A, Stern DT, Peccoralo L. The courteous consult: a CONSULT card and training to improve resident consults. *J Grad Med Educ*. 2015;7(1):113-117. doi:10.4300/JGME-D-14-00207.1. PMID: 26217436; PMCID: PMC4507900.
2. Salerno SM, Hurst FP, Halvorson S, Mercado DL. Principles of effective consultation: an update for the 21st-century consultant. *Arch Intern Med*. 2007;167(3):271-275. doi:10.1001/archinte.167.3.271. PMID: 17296883.
3. Choi KJ, Kahmke RR, Crowson MG, Puscas L, Scher RL, Cohen SM. Trends in otolaryngology consultation patterns at an Academic Quaternary Care Center. *JAMA Otolaryngol Head Neck Surg*. 2017;143(5):472-477.
4. McCool RR, Davies L. Where does telemedicine fit into otolaryngology? An assessment of telemedicine eligibility among otolaryngology diagnoses. *Otolaryngol Head Neck Surg*. 2018;158(4):641-644.
5. Mors M, Bohr C, Fozo M, Shermetaro C. Consultation intervention rates for the otolaryngology service: a large metropolitan hospital experience. *Spartan Med Res J*. 2020;4(2):11596.
6. Hare N, Bansal P, Bajowala SS, et al. Work group report: COVID-19: unmasking telemedicine. *J Allergy Clin Immunol Pract*. 2020;8(8):2461-2473.e3.

CHAPTER 4

Infections of the Ear: Otitis Media and Externa, Mastoiditis

Rupal S. Jain
Candace E. Hobson

INTRODUCTION

Infections of the external and middle ear (otitis externa and otitis media) are common reasons for presentation to urgent care facilities or emergency departments (EDs). A foundational understanding of the anatomy of the ear and the pathophysiology of these infections is key to their successful management.

Anatomically, the ear is divided into the external, middle, and internal ear. The external ear consists of the auricle (pinna) and the external auditory canal (EAC). The auricle is the portion of the ear that protrudes from the head and is composed of cartilage covered by skin. The EAC, also known as the ear canal, is approximately 25 mm in length. The outer third of the EAC consists of an outer layer of skin with underlying skin follicles, cerumen and sebaceous glands, and cartilage. A thin layer of skin directly overlying bone comprises the medial two-thirds of the EAC. The tympanic membrane (TM) separates the external from the middle ear. The middle ear is an air-filled space containing the hearing ossicles (malleus, incus and stapes), the facial nerve, and the chorda tympani nerve. The middle ear communicates with the mastoid via the aditus ad antrum and with the nasopharynx via the eustachian tube. The inner ear consists of the cochlea and the vestibular labyrinth, the neural structures of hearing and balance.

THE CLINICAL CHALLENGE

Otitis Media

Acute otitis media (AOM) is a painful infectious process of the air-filled space of the middle ear, marked by the presence of both infected fluid and inflamed mucosa. It is a clinical diagnosis that is especially challenging owing to reliance on symptoms that are neither sensitive nor specific. Adding to the challenge, the physical examination is often limited owing to inadequate visualization of the TM secondary to obstructing cerumen, operator inexperience with otoscope, and/or lack of patient/child cooperation with examination. AOM is grossly overdiagnosed and unnecessarily treated, largely because of the aforementioned limitations, and this problem is compounded by the significant overlap of symptoms with the common cold, and patient preference for antibiotic treatment.[1] Furthermore, the gold standard test for the diagnosis of otitis media is pneumatic otoscopy—a diagnostic maneuver not routinely taught to many providers.

MASTOIDITIS

Mastoiditis is a nonspecific term describing an inflammatory process of the mastoid. Because the middle ear and mastoid air spaces are confluent, AOM and serous otitis media typically result in some degree of mastoid inflammation. Technically, however, mastoiditis is a complication of otitis media caused by osteitis of the mastoid air cells resulting in breakdown of bony septations and coalescence of air cells. The full term for this condition, "acute coalescent mastoiditis," is often simply referred to as "mastoiditis."

Untreated, mastoiditis can lead to abscess formation, bone resorption, and invasive spread of the infection. Part of the diagnostic challenge is that initial findings may be subtle and variable based on the involved pathogen and patient age group. The classic postauricular symptom, tender and erythematous postauricular swelling as well as anteroinferior displacement of auricle, were present in only 10% of patients in a 2012 retrospective study.[2] Accurate diagnosis relies on a combination of clinical symptoms, physical exam and otoscopic findings, and supportive evidence on computed tomography (CT) or magnetic resonance imaging (MRI).[3]

Otitis Externa

Acute otitis externa (AOE) affects patients of all ages with a lifetime prevalence of 10%.[4,5] Otitis externa is inflammation or infection of the EAC, which may extend to involve the auricle or TM. AOE, also known as "swimmer's ear," is a cellulitis of the skin of the EAC. When otitis externa persists for over 3 months, it is considered chronic. Chronic otitis externa may be the result of inadequately treated AOE but is often associated with chronic dermatologic conditions. Distinguishing the nature and etiology of otitis externa is key to effective management.

PATHOPHYSIOLOGY

Otitis Media

AOM occurs most commonly in patients 6 to 24 months old, with most cases occurring in patients under the age of 5.[6] In developed countries, the incidence of AOM in adults is less than 1%.[7] Children are more susceptible to AOM owing to their shorter and more vertical eustachian tubes. Acute infection usually occurs in the setting of a recent viral upper respiratory infection, as inflammation and edema impede normal flow through the eustachian tube and allow pooling in the middle ear, creating conditions favorable for infection. In pediatric studies, AOM is most often associated with viral pathogens isolated from middle ear aspirates.[8] The most commonly responsible bacterial pathogens are *Streptococcus pneumoniae*, nontypeable strains of *Haemophilus influenzae*, and *Moraxella catarrhalis*. In the less commonly infected adult population, further organisms include Group A *Streptococcus*, *Pseudomonas aeruginosa*, and *Staphylococcus aureus*.

Mastoiditis

The mastoid is an air-filled space of the temporal bone that lies posterior to the ear canal and middle ear. Acute coalescent mastoiditis is the most common intratemporal complication of AOM, which most typically occurs in young children following an episode of AOM. As purulent fluid from the middle ear collects in the mastoid air cells, osteitis, bony erosion, and coalescence of the mastoid air cells occurs. The most common offending organisms are *S pneumoniae, Streptococcus pyogenes, S aureus,* and *P aeruginosa.*[9]

By contrast, chronic mastoiditis is chronic inflammation of the mastoid air cells occurring in the setting of chronic otitis media; this sometimes requires elective surgical intervention. These patients present with chronic otorrhea, otalgia, and hearing loss and are not typically acutely ill.

Otitis Externa

AOE is an infection of the skin of the EAC that often occurs owing to a break in the EAC skin and cerumen barrier. Cerumen provides a protective lipid film overlying the skin of EAC that is slightly acidic and thus inhibits bacterial or fungi proliferation. Often, instrumentation of the ear, whether by a physician or by the patient with a Q-tip, fingernail, or bobby pen, disrupts this protective layer and, additionally, causes microtrauma to the underlying skin and allows for the entrance of pathogenic organisms. The introduction of moisture (irrigation, swimming, sweat) further contributes by creating a moist, warm, dark space that is ideal for bacterial or fungal proliferation. *P aeruginosa* and *S aureus* are the most common AOE pathogens.[2,5]

APPROACH/THE FOCUSED EXAM

Acute Otitis Media

AOM is a clinical diagnosis; therefore, laboratory and imaging tests are not routinely necessary. Symptoms of AOM may include current or recently resolved upper respiratory infection (URI) symptoms (rhinorrhea, cough), unilateral or bilateral otalgia, decreased or muffled hearing, and otorrhea. On examination, the patient may have fever, retracted or bulging TM (**Figure 4.1A**), erythematous (from inflammation) or a yellow/white (from effusion) hue to the TM (**Figure 4.1B**), reduced TM motion on pneumatic otoscopy, and TM perforation (especially if the patient presents with otorrhea). Facial paralysis, meningismus, mastoid tenderness, or toxic appearance may be late signs suggestive of spread of the infection beyond the ear. In severe cases, intracranial complications may include meningitis, intracranial abscess, lateral sinus thrombosis, and otitis hydrocephalus.

Mastoiditis

Presenting signs and symptoms of acute coalescent mastoiditis include fever, otalgia, and mastoid tenderness, erythema, pain, and edema. There may be protrusion of the auricle with loss of the postauricular sulcus. Otoscopy may demonstrate purulent otorrhea or an intact TM with evidence of AOM.

CT or MRI of the temporal bones with contrast demonstrating partial-to-complete opacification of the mastoid air cells and erosion of mastoid air cell bony septa confirms the diagnosis (**Figure 4.2**). If infection spreads through the outer mastoid cortex, a subperiosteal (postauricular) abscess or Bezold (sternocleidomastoid) abscess may develop.

Otitis Externa

Often, patient history alone can suggest a diagnosis of AOE. Patients may describe symptoms that begin with itching and fullness and progress to pain (otalgia), decreased hearing, drainage (otorrhea), and swelling of the auricle. In most cases, there are clear predisposing factors for AOE, including EAC trauma (Q-tips, scratching, recent ear cleaning, or hearing aid), water exposure (swimming, humid environments), dermatologic conditions (eczema, psoriasis), and medical comorbidities (diabetes, immunosuppression).

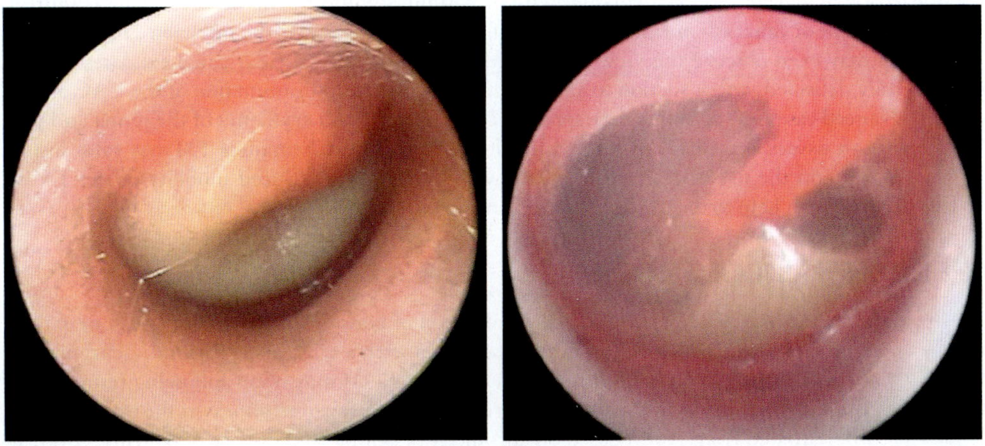

A **B**

Figure 4.1: A, Acute otitis media with bulging TM. B, Acute otitis media with fluid level. (Courtesy of Alejandro Hoberman, MD, Children's Hospital of Pittsburgh of UPMC. In: Johnson J. *Bailey's Head and Neck Surgery.* 5th ed. Wolters Kluwer; 2014. Figure 99.1AB.)

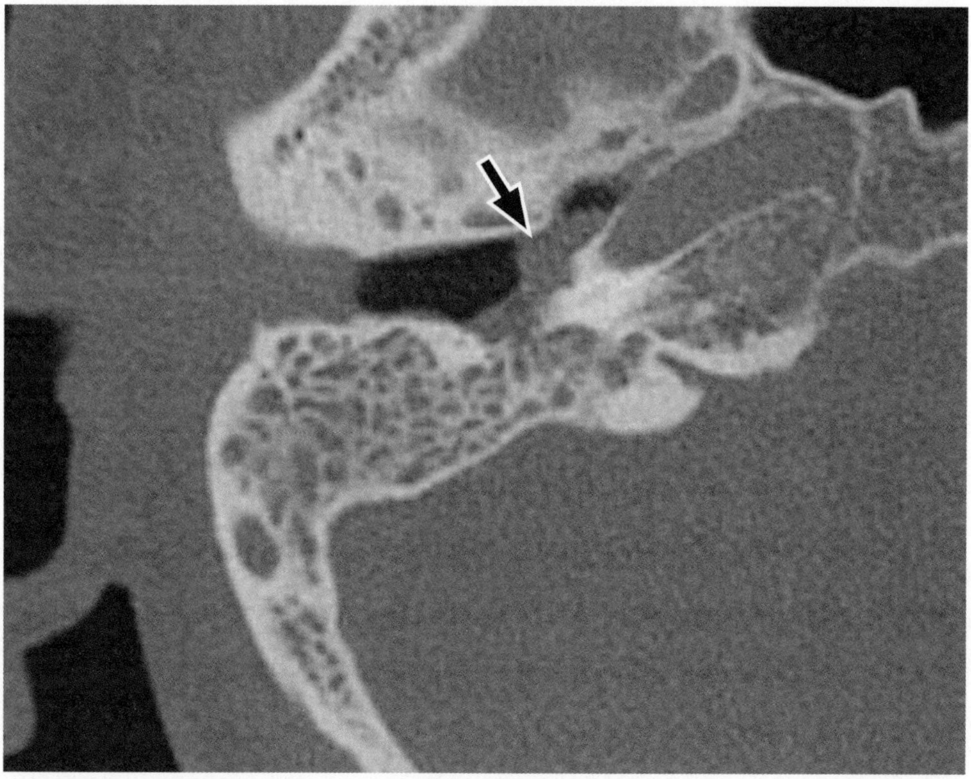

Figure 4.2: Acute mastoiditis. Axial bone window computed tomography image demonstrates opacification of the mastoid air cells. The mastoid bony septations and cortex remain intact without erosion. The patient also has otitis media, with opacity in the middle ear (arrow). (From Juliano AF, Vargas SO, Robson CD. Head and Neck. In: Lee E. *Pediatric Radiology: Practical Imaging Evaluation of Infants and Children*. 1st ed. Wolters Kluwer; 2018:163-260. Figure 3.98.)

Examination should begin by inspecting the auricle for edema, erythema, or chronic skin changes. Tugging traction of the auricle or pushing on the tragus may cause pain. On otoscopy, the ear canal may appear erythematous with or without significant edema or exudates (**Figure 4.3**). The amount of canal edema and formation of exudates increases as the infection progresses; canal edema may even obscure the view of the TM entirely. Ideally, the ear canal exudates should be carefully debrided with a suction to allow for a more thorough examination of the EAC and TM. In advanced cases, the cellulitis may spread to cause edema and erythema of the pinna and preauricular soft tissues as well as cervical lymphadenopathy. An erythematous TM may raise suspicion for AOM, and the use of pneumatic otoscopy, demonstrating reduced mobility of the TM with insufflation, can help to distinguish AOM from AOE.

DIFFERENTIAL DIAGNOSIS

- Serous otitis media (SOM): SOM is a collection of nonpurulent fluid (an effusion) in the middle ear space. This may occur in association with a URI, allergic rhinitis, chronic eustachian tube dysfunction, or air travel. In children, SOM may occur following resolution of AOM. Symptoms of SOM include hearing loss and pressure/fullness of the ear. This can be differentiated from AOM based on chronicity of symptoms, absence of pain and fever, and the exam finding of a straw-colored middle ear effusion (vs purulent in AOM).
- Cholesteatoma: A collection of squamous epithelium (skin) in the middle ear and/or mastoid that occurs secondary to eustachian tube dysfunction or a TM perforation. Patients may be asymptomatic or may present with chronic/recurrent otorrhea, pain, and hearing

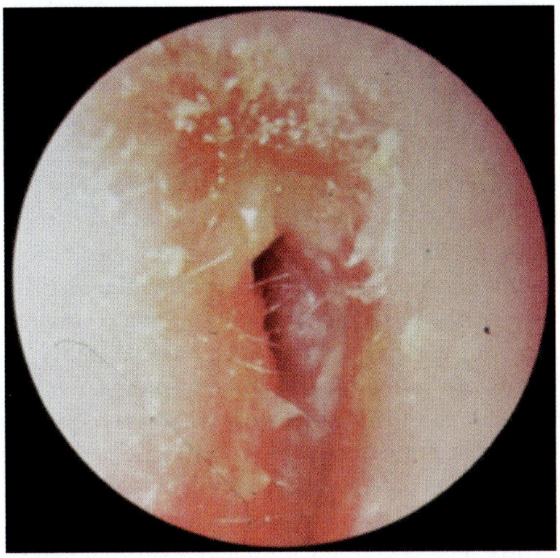

Figure 4.3: Otitis externa. Note the swollen, erythematous canal, filled with exudate. (From *Stedman's Medical Dictionary for the Health Professions and Nursing*. Illustrated (standard edition). 6th ed. Lippincott Williams & Wilkins; 2007.)

loss. Examination may reveal a polyp in the ear canal or retraction of the TM containing pearly white skin debris. Referral to an ENT specialist is required, as surgery is often indicated.

- Bullous myringitis: Mimics AOM but is distinguished by the presence of vesicles or bullae on the TM. Pathogens are most commonly viral but may also be bacterial.
- Acute otitis media: an infection in the middle ear can cause otorrhea if the TM is not intact (perforation or tympanostomy tube in place). It is important to visualize the TM to determine whether the drainage is coming from the EAC or the middle ear. If there is a known perforation/tube, or if the status of the TM is unknown, topical aminoglycosides, polymyxin, and acetic acid should not be utilized because of the theoretical risk of ototoxicity.[5]
- Fungal otitis externa: Fungal OE tends to occur following treatment (or overtreatment) of bacterial AOE. Fungal spores (black dots) or hyphae may be observed on exam. Fungal debris may appear white, black, or as a gray plug (**Figure 4.4**). *Aspergillus* and

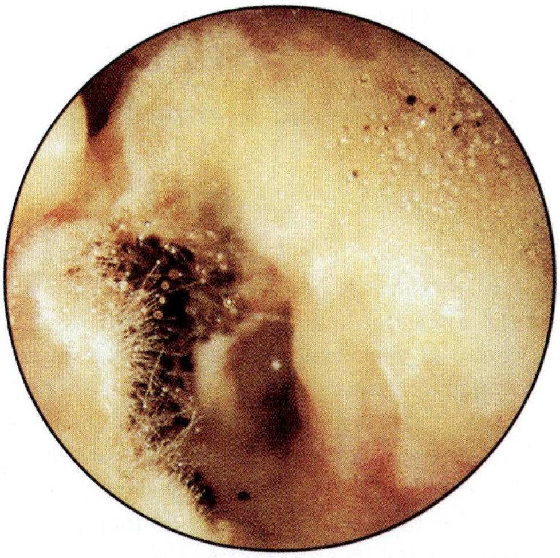

Figure 4.4: Fungal otitis externa. (Used with permission from Handler SD, Myer CM. *Atlas of Ear, Nose and Throat Disorders in Children*. BC Decker; 1998:24.)

Candida are the most frequent offenders.[2] The principles of treatment are similar to those of AOE—aural toilet (debridement), dry ear precautions, and an antifungal ototopical. If the TM is intact, clotrimazole or other antifungal drops may be prescribed. Alternatively or additionally, an oral antifungal can be prescribed. ENT consultation should be considered.

- Malignant (necrotizing) otitis externa (MOE): MOE is osteomyelitis of the temporal bone that can progress to involve the surrounding skin and soft tissue, cranial nerves, and the skull base. MOE typically affects elderly, diabetic, or immunocompromised patients. Patients may present with pain out of proportion to exam, granulation tissue in the EAC, or, in advanced cases, a cranial neuropathy (facial paresis/paralysis most commonly). Left untreated, MOE can be a life-threatening condition. Patients with persistent OE symptoms despite appropriate treatment with ototopical antibiotics should be suspected of having MOE. An otolaryngologist should be consulted if MOE is suspected, because it requires long-term systemic antibiotic treatment, often with the input of an infectious disease specialist.
- Dermatoses: These patients often have a history of allergy, atopy, or chronic dermatitis of the ear and/or other parts of the body and often present with complaints of ear itching.
  - Atopic dermatitis: The skin of the auricle or ear canal may appear dry, flaky, scaly, erythematous, hyperpigmented, or lichenified. Treatment includes use of moisturizers (mineral oil), topical steroid creams/ointments, and steroid-containing oil ear drops (fluocinolone acetonide oil).
  - Seborrheic dermatitis: Greasy scales overlying plaques may be observed. Dandruff or scaly plaques of the scalp are common. Secondary infection with *Malassezia* yeast may occur.[3] Treatment includes use of topical antifungal and anti-inflammatory creams or ointments.
- Herpes Zoster: Like AOE, patients present with otalgia, but otoscopy reveals vesicles of the EAC. Herpes Zoster infection occurs secondary to reactivation of the varicella-zoster virus. If facial paralysis develops, the condition is called herpes zoster oticus (HZO) or Ramsay Hunt syndrome. Management includes prompt treatment with an oral antiviral (acyclovir, valacyclovir, or famciclovir) in combination with oral steroids.
- Cutaneous Malignancy: Squamous cell carcinoma or basal cell carcinoma of the auricle or EAC may present with otalgia, aural fullness, and decreased hearing similar to otitis externa. It is important to examine the skin of the auricle and EAC for raised or ulcerated skin lesions.
- Temporomandibular joint (TMJ) arthralgia: TMJ pain is a common cause of referred otalgia because the anterior wall of the EAC is adjacent to the TMJ. Patients may point directly to the TMJ (just anterior to the tragus) as the site of discomfort, with pain often radiating to the angle of the jaw, temple, or neck. Patients may report a history of bruxism/clenching, popping/clicking of TMJ, pain with chewing or recent dental procedure. Conservative treatment includes warm compresses, nonsteroidal anti-inflammatory drugs (NSAIDs), and a dental guard. Referral to a dentist or oral surgeon should be considered.

MANAGEMENT

Acute Otitis Media

In general, outpatient antibiotics are the mainstay of therapy for adults with AOM (**Table 4.1**). It is important to treat the associated fever and pain with an analgesic such as a nonsteroidal anti-inflammatory medication or acetaminophen. In children, because at least 25% of cases are viral, and because a percentage of cases are self-limiting, patients can be safely discharged home with only observation of symptoms.[10] Immediate antibiotics are recommended in patients aged under 6 months, 6 to 23 months with bilateral otitis media, over 6 months with severe symptoms (moderate/severe ear pain, pain greater than 48 hours, fever greater than 39 °C). The first-line treatment is amoxicillin 80 to 90 mg/kg/day. Duration of therapy varies from 5 to 7 days for children greater than 2 years old with nonsevere symptoms to 10 days for children younger than 2 years of age or those with severe symptoms. Refer to Table 4.1 for further antibiotic guidance. In patients who do not meet criteria for immediate treatment, providers can consider observation followed by

TABLE 4.1 Antibiotic Guidance for Treatment of Acute Otitis Media

First-line therapy *Adults* *Pediatrics*	• Amoxicillin/clavulanate 875/125 mg PO BID • Amoxicillin 40–45 mg/kg PO q12h
Second-line therapy *(If the patient is immunocompromised, had a recent hospitalization, used antibiotics in the past 30 d, has concurrent purulent conjunctivitis or has worsening symptoms after 2–3 d of first-line treatment)*	• Amoxicillin-clavulanate 40 mg/kg amoxicillin/6.4 mg/kg clavulanate PO q12h
Recurrence of infection in children *If recurrence occurs >15 d after completion of prior antibiotics* *If recurrence occurs <15 d of completion of antibiotics, the infection is likely due to persistence of the original pathogen*	• Amoxicillin-clavulanate 40 mg/kg amoxicillin/ 6.4 mg/kg clavulanate PO q12h • Ceftriaxone 50 mg/kg IM or IV daily for 3 d ***Or*** • Levofloxacin 10 mg/kg PO q12h3 for 10 d for children 6 mo to 5 y ***Or*** 10 mg/kg PO daily for 10 d for children ≥5 y (maximum 750 mg/d)
In penicillin-allergic patient with a mild-delayed reaction, alternatives include cephalosporins	• Cefdinir 7 mg/kg PO q12h ***Or*** • Cefpodoxime 5 mg/kg PO q12h
In penicillin-allergic patient with a significant delayed reaction or immediate reaction, alternatives include	• Azithromycin 5-10 mg/kg daily × 5 d • Clindamycin 30–40 mg/kd/d divided into 4 doses
For adults, antibiotics are the mainstay of therapy	• Amoxicillin 875 mg with clavulanate 125 mg PO q12h for 5–7 d

prescribed antibiotics if symptoms persist or worsen in 48 to 72 hours. The observation option is often termed wait-and-see prescription (WASP).

Mastoiditis

Treatment of acute coalescent mastoiditis involves ENT consultation, hospital admission, and administration of parenteral antibiotics. In adults, first-line treatment is typically ceftriaxone with or without vancomycin. Children who have had antibiotic treatment within the past 6 months should additionally receive either intravenous ceftazidime, cefepime, or piperacillin-tazobactam. Duration of parenteral IV antibiotic treatment is 7 to 10 days before transitioning to oral antibiotics. Treatment may also include a myringotomy, placement of a tympanostomy tube, and, in some cases, mastoidectomy. In cases of a subperiosteal or Bezold abscess, mastoidectomy will include incision and drainage of the abscesses. Patients suspected of having chronic mastoiditis who are not acutely ill may be referred instead for outpatient ENT evaluation.

Acute Otitis Externa

The principles of management of AOE are aural toilet (careful removal of canal debris under direct visualization by an experienced provider), ototopical antimicrobials, and adherence to dry ear precautions. Mild or early infections may be effectively treated with an antiseptic solution—acetic acid or vinegar-alcohol solutions that do have antimicrobial properties. For moderate to severe bacterial infections, topical antibiotic preparations include ciprofloxacin, ofloxacin, neomycin, polymyxin, gentamicin, and tobramycin. Many of these ototopical antibiotics are also available in steroid-containing preparations (eg, ciprofloxacin-dexamethasone or ciprofloxacin-hydrocortisone); however, cost may limit the practicality of these medications. In cases where obstructive canal edema is present, placement of a wick will facilitate the effective instillation of drops into the EAC. If the infection has spread to involve the pinna or face, an oral antibiotic should also be prescribed. Until the infection has resolved, it is prudent that the patient keep the ear dry. This can be accomplished by avoidance of water exposure with the use of an ear plug or placement of a Vaseline-coated cotton ball at the external meatus with water exposure (showering, swimming).

TIPS AND PEARLS

- TM rupture, mastoiditis, facial paralysis, meningitis, brain abscess, and venous sinus thrombosis (see **Chapter 8**) may occur as a consequence of AOM.
- Suspect acute coalescent mastoiditis in patients with otalgia, otorrhea, fevers, a protruding auricle, and CT demonstrating mastoid opacification with loss of mastoid bony septations. ENT should be consulted in these cases.
- Suspect AOE in a patient with otalgia and otorrhea, especially in the setting of recent microtrauma (Q-tips, ear cleaning) or water exposure.
- Follow AOE treatment principles: (1) aural toilet (debride EAC of exudates), (2) application of ototopical antimicrobial drops, and (3) adherence to dry ear precautions.
- In treatment of AOE with a nonintact TM, ototoxic agents should be avoided.
- Consider fungal infection in cases of recurrence or worsening of symptoms after treatment with ototopical antibiotics.
- Consider MOE, a potentially life-threatening osteomyelitis, in cases of AOE unresponsive to therapy, especially in elderly, diabetic, or immunocompromised patients presenting with severe pain.
- Persistent granulation tissue following treatment of AOE may represent cutaneous malignancy and needs referral for biopsy.

EVIDENCE

Are antibiotics required for treatment of AOM?

In meta-analyses and systematic reviews of pediatric patients, the benefit of providing immediate antibiotics over initial observation and analgesics alone are modest.[11] For healthy children older than 6 months with mild symptoms and unilateral AOM, consider WASP for antibiotics and repeat evaluation in 48 to 72 hours. Adults should be managed with immediate antibiotic treatment.

Are oral antibiotics necessary in AOE?

Unlike other skin and soft tissue infections, oral should *not* be prescribed as primary treatment of AOE, unless there is extension of infection beyond the ear canal. Ototopical administration of an antimicrobial achieves a 100 to 1000 times higher local concentration of antimicrobial than that of systemic antimicrobials. Additionally, this localized high concentration reduces the risk of creating resistant organisms. Finally, use of a topical antimicrobial reduces the risk of adverse effects of a systemic antimicrobial.[5]

References

1. Legros JM, Hitoto H, Garnier F, Dagorne C, Parot-Schinkel E, Fanello S. Clinical qualitative evaluation of the diagnosis of acute otitis media in general practice. *Int J Pediatr Otorhinolaryngol.* 2008;72(1):23-30.
2. Chien JH, Chen YS, Hung IF, et al. Mastoiditis diagnosed by clinical symptoms and imaging studies in children: disease spectrum and evolving diagnostic challenges. *J Microbiol Immunol Infect.* 2012;45(5):377-381.
3. Kornilenko L, Rocka S, Balseris S, Arechvo I. Clinical challenges in the diagnosis and treatment of temporal bone osteomyelitis. *Case Rep Otolaryngol.* 2017;2017:4097973.
4. Raza SA, Denholm SW, Wong JC. An audit of the management of acute otitis externa in an ENT casualty clinic. *J Laryngol Otol.* 1995;109(2):130-133.
5. Rosenfeld RM, Schwartz SR, Cannon CR, et al. Clinical practice guideline: acute otitis externa. *Otolaryngol Head Neck Surg.* 2014;150(1 Suppl):S1-S24.
6. Pichichero ME. Otitis media. *Pediatr Clin North Am.* 2013;60(2):391-407.
7. Monasta L, Ronfani L, Marchetti F, et al. Burden of disease caused by otitis media: systematic review and global estimates. *PLoS One.* 2012;7(4):e36226.

8. Ruohola A, Meurman O, Nikkari S, et al. Microbiology of acute otitis media in children with tympanostomy tubes: prevalences of bacteria and viruses. *Clin Infect Dis*. 2006;43(11):1417-1422.
9. Saunders JE, Raju RP, Boone JL, Hales NW, Berryhill WE. Antibiotic resistance and otomycosis in the draining ear: culture results by diagnosis. *Am J Otolaryngol*. 2011;32(6):470-476.
10. American Academy of Pediatrics Subcommittee on Management of Acute Otitis Media. Diagnosis and management of acute otitis media. *Pediatrics*. 2004;113(5):1451-1465.
11. Venekamp RP, Sanders S, Glasziou PP, Del Mar CB, Rovers MM. Antibiotics for acute otitis media in children. *Cochrane Database Syst Rev*. 2013;(1):CD000219.

CHAPTER 5

External Ear: Perichondritis, Lacerations, Auricular Hematoma

Rupal S. Jain
Samuel N. Helman

INTRODUCTION

The external ear is a defining anatomical feature susceptible to several pathologies. It consists of a uniquely shaped and bent elastic cartilage covered by thin skin and connects inferiorly with a lobule that is absent of cartilage but contains fibro-fatty tissue and a robust vascular supply. The ear cartilage is elastic and 1.0 to 3.0 mm thick depending on its location.[1] The ear protrudes at an angle of 25° to 30° from the skull base.[1] The cartilaginous regions of the external ear receive their blood supply through the tightly adherent overlying perichondrium, which is important to remember in treating trauma patients. The ear is robustly vascular and supplied by a helical arcade that is anteriorly and posteriorly supplied from the superficial temporal artery (STA) and posterior auricular artery (PAA), respectively. Although venous drainage can vary, blood is generally felt to egress via the postauricular vein into the external jugular, superficial temporal, and retromandibular venous systems.[1,2] The external ear is innervated from branches of the trigeminal, vagus, facial, and great auricular nerves.

CLINICAL CHALLENGES

Perichondritis

The cartilage of the external ear is easily damaged owing to the lack of overlying subcutaneous tissue and relative avascularity. Onset of infection can be insidious, and misdiagnosis and mistreatment are common. This pitfall can be avoided by examining specifically for redness and painful swelling of pinna sparing the lobule, suggesting the diagnosis of perichondritis (**Figure 5.1**).[3]

Ear Laceration and Auricular Hematoma

Traumatic ear laceration and auricular hematoma can disrupt key cosmetic features of the external ear. Because of the external ear's extensive arterial supply, healing can occur even in highly disruptive injury. However, cartilage injury can lead to structural deformation during healing, resulting in tissue loss and a potentially challenging reconstructive dilemma. Therefore, in both laceration and hematoma, early intervention is critical.

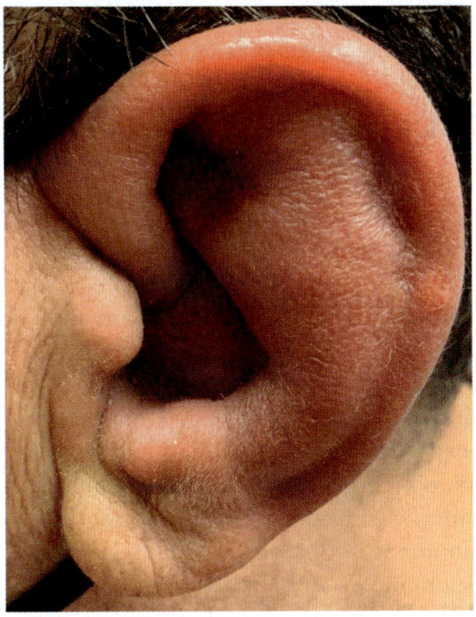

Figure 5.1: Classic presentation of perichondritis with inflammatory change to the auricle and sparing of the lobule. (Courtesy of Kirkland Lozada MD, Philadelphia, PA.)

PATHOPHYSIOLOGY

Perichondritis

Perichondritis is an infection of the connective tissue overlying the cartilage of the pinna, called the perichondrium, manifested by pain, erythema, warmth, and swelling. Perichondritis is a bit of a misnomer, because concomitant chondritis (infection of the cartilage) is common.[4] There is often an inciting injury or trauma with hematoma formation, ear piercing, surgery, burns, insect/human bite, frostbite, or even a minor scratch 3 to 4 weeks preceding the development of perichondritis. The pinna receives less humoral circulation, resulting in delayed healing and resorption of edema/exudates, which can lead to abscess formation and eventual necrosis.[5] *Pseudomonas aeruginosa* is the most common causative pathogen. Other pathogens include *Escherichia coli, Staphylococcus aureus*, and *Proteus* species.[6] Without proper treatment, accumulation of pus between the perichondrium and underlying cartilage diminishes blood supply to the cartilage and can lead to deformity of the ear (see "Auricular Hematoma" section).

It is important to distinguish infectious from inflammatory perichondritis. Inflammatory perichondritis does not respond to antibiotic therapy and is characterized by relapsing symptoms. Relapsing polychondritis (RPC) is immune-mediated and associated with inflammation in various cartilaginous structures (ie, unilateral or bilateral perichondritis, episcleritis, scleritis, nasal cartilage inflammation, and inflammation of large airways and other organs).[7]

Auricular Hematoma and Laceration

The exposed nature of the ear places it at high risk of deformity during head injury. Trauma can occur in the form of shearing forces and laceration and can lead to hematoma. The hematoma disrupts the attachment of the perichondrium to the underlying cartilage and therefore its vascular supply.[2,8] Laceration, in turn, often causes exposed cartilage and can lead to necrosis, erosive chondritis, and infection.

Formation of a hematoma disrupts blood supply to underlying cartilage, leading to necrosis, fibrosis, and disfigurement. Mixed martial artists are especially prone to auricular hematoma because they do not utilize any form of ear protection or head gear. Neurodegenerative diseases can precipitate falls and resultant laceration or hematoma. Auricular hematoma, particularly recurrent auricular hematoma, in patients not involved in sports, should raise concern for home violence and child abuse.[9] Without treatment, the steady influx of fibroblast infiltration leads to fibrous tissue and neocartilage formation, creating the so-called "cauliflower ear," a visible long-term sequela of the injury seen in wrestlers, boxers, mixed martial artists, and participants in contact sports.[10]

APPROACH/THE FOCUSED EXAM

The history of a trauma patient should include the context of the injury and the likelihood for future episodes. Tetanus vaccination history should be elicited. Head and neck bony and soft tissue anatomy should be carefully examined for associated injuries, and the patient should be assessed for Battle sign, which may indicate the presence of a skull base fracture.[8] An otoscopic examination evaluates for hemotympanum, and a tuning fork examination should be considered in patients who endorse hearing loss.

In patients presenting with preceding trauma or other penetration of skin, development of redness and painful swelling of the pinna should prompt the emergency provider to consider perichondritis. Patients often experience an initial dull indolent ache with redness and swelling involving the helix and antihelix, which later may progress to involve the entire cartilage, producing a "loss of contours" appearance.[4] On examination, it is important to carefully assess for fluctuance, which indicates the development of abscess and necessitates ENT consultation for incision and drainage. In later stages, spontaneous fluid may drain from the wound and an eventual deformity of the ear known as "cauliflower ear" can form. This deformity may occur even after proper hematoma incision and drainage but is far more likely in cases where continued chondritis and necrosis are allowed to occur unabated.

Generally, perichondritis is unlikely to cause critical illness, and evaluation for an alternative cause with systemic illness is important. However, in an immunocompromised host, pseudomonal infection can progress rapidly and spread to involve the parotid gland, facial nerve, external auditory canal, middle ear, temporal bone, and central nervous system (CNS).

DIFFERENTIAL DIAGNOSIS

Perichondritis

Perichondritis is distinguished by its localized infection to the pinna sparing lobule involvement. This differentiates it from otitis externa, which similarly can present with cellulitic changes and tenderness of the tragus and pinna. Both mastoiditis and perichondritis can lead to an increase of the auriculocephalic angle. Redness and painful swelling over the mastoid process would be specific to mastoiditis. Malignancy, although uncommon, should always be considered in patients presenting with ear pain coupled with unhealing cutaneous lesions, or a deep persistent pain without a history of trauma or infection.

Auricular Hematoma and Laceration

Auricular hematoma is distinguished by loss of normal anatomical landmarks owing to the presence of a ballotable hematoma or edema. Patients presenting several weeks after the index injury may start to demonstrate signs of fibrous tissue and neocartilage formation leading to the clinically distinct cauliflower ear deformity. Auricular laceration is more straightforward to recognize. Attention should be paid to whether the laceration is simple or complex, the layers of tissue involved, whether the injury is "through and through" the underlying perichondrium or cartilage, and the presence of a missing anatomic segment. Cartilaginous injury is especially important to identify and is frequently better distinguished once the wound has been irrigated and debrided. Nerve injury, such as facial anesthesia or paralysis, can occur with penetrating injuries.

MANAGEMENT

Analgesia

The patient should be positioned supine in a comfortable position, and the external ear and skin in a 2.0-cm radius to the ear prepared with chlorhexidine 2% or povidone-iodine solution. The anesthetic agent, either 1% to 2% lidocaine with or without 1:100 000 epinephrine or 0.5%

bupivacaine, is then prepared. The use of adrenaline- or epinephrine-containing anesthetic is controversial and should be done with caution in laceration injuries in which blood supply is compromised. The auricular block is achieved using a 25- or 27-gauge 1.5-inch needle on a 10-mL syringe. The needle is inserted and aspirated to prevent vascular injection of anesthetic. In the authors' practice, a partial ring block may be employed to densely anesthetize the ear. The injection sites are located 0.5 cm anterior to the tragus; 0.5 cm inferior to the ear, just posterior to the lobule; and 0.5 cm posterior to the helical root. Here, approximately 2 to 3 mL of anesthetic is injected in each site (**Figure 5.2**).

Auricular Laceration

An external ear laceration should be carefully examined for the extent of injury, subsite involvement, and the presence of foreign body. Soft tissue and cartilaginous defects should be noted. For more deformed auricular injuries, the contralateral ear should be examined as a framework for repair. In cases where the ear is simply abraded, management should include debridement and irrigation, and application of topical petroleum-based jelly. Neomycin-based antimicrobials should not be used owing to ototoxicity.[11]

Auricular lacerations refer to soft tissue transection with or without loss of a full-thickness segment.[11] After appropriate anesthesia, wounds should be copiously irrigated and debrided. Basic linear lacerations can be closed primarily using 5-0 sutures to approximate the perichondral layer and the cartilage edge.[11] In cases of cartilaginous malunion, a 6-0 nonabsorbable suture is adequate to close cartilaginous lacerations. Superficial wounds involving the pinna or helix can be approximated and closed using 5-0 or 6-0 nonabsorbable sutures in a running or interrupted fashion.[11] Loose approximation of the wound edges is essential given the expected edema following repair. In select patients in whom follow-up for suture removal is ensured, nonabsorbable monofilament suture, used in an interrupted horizontal or vertical mattress fashion, can be used and removed after 5 to 7 days. Although many auricular lacerations can be closed primarily, larger lacerations may require wedge excision or relaxing incisions to allow for tension-free approximation (**Figure 5.3**). In conditions of exposed perichondrium or cartilage, wounds require coverage to offset the risk of chondritis and infection. Skin grafts or soft tissue flaps may be used in these cases, requiring specialty consultation (**Figure 5.4**). The patient is provided a tetanus vaccine if necessary. Owing to controversy regarding postclosure antibiotic prophylaxis, the authors recommend the use of antibiotics against *Pseudomonas* in clearly contaminated wounds, in patients with deficient immune

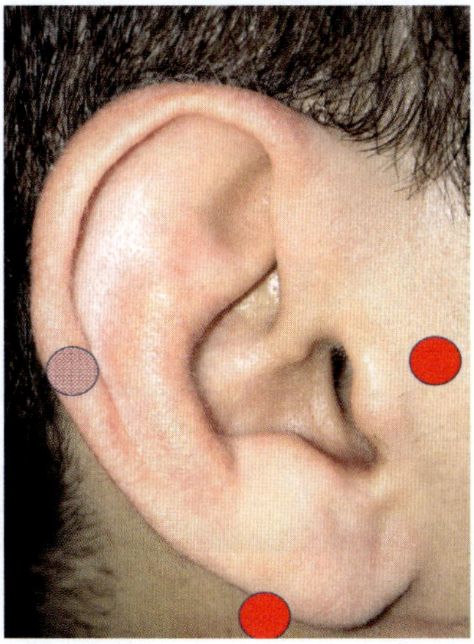

Figure 5.2: Auricular block injection sites. Red filled circles indicate injection sites. The shaded circle is an injection site over the mastoid and behind the pinna. Each site should receive 2 mL of 1% lidocaine with 1:100 000 epinephrine to achieve full auricular block.

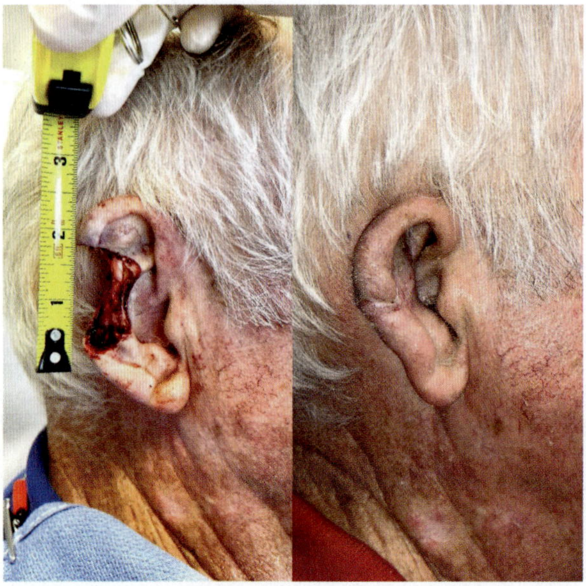

Figure 5.3: Large, full-thickness defect in the middle third of helix and antihelix. An M-plasty reduction of the conchal bowl was employed to reduce overall defect closure size and prevent lateral deflection of the reconstructed ear. Excess cartilage was removed and the ear was closed in a layered fashion. A small cartilage batten was placed over the incision line posteriorly and a Mustarde suture to further prevent lateral deflection of the ear. Postoperative photo was taken 1 month afterward. (Courtesy of Lucas Bryant MD, Nashville, TN.)

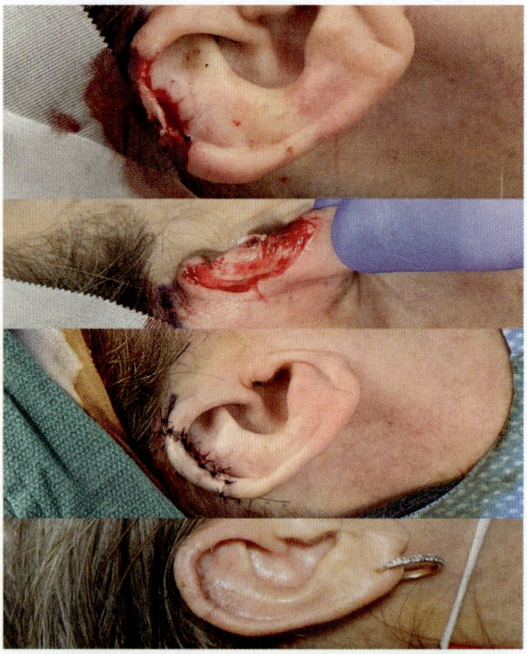

Figure 5.4: Top to bottom: Superior helix defect with some cartilage loss. The helical skin was undermined and the cartilage sculpted. The exposed cartilage was then buried in a subcutaneous pocket over the mastoid. After 3 weeks, the ear was elevated and the wound closed. The skin defect over the mastoid was closed with wide undermining and tissue advancement similar to a second-stage microtia reconstruction. The sulcus of the helix was maintained through thinning of the skin during stage 1, and through the placement of through-and-through 5-0 chromic sutures at stage 2. Final image was taken 1 week postoperatively. (Courtesy of Lucas Bryant MD, Nashville, TN.)

systems and human bite wounds, and in lacerations with significant cartilaginous disruption.[1,4] Follow-up is recommended in a week or sooner in cases of high infection risk.

Auricular Avulsions (Near Total and Total)

Avulsion is defined by the loss of a portion or the entirety of the auricle with no skin bridge or soft tissue attachment to its native original structure. The robust vascular arcade allows for ear survival with only a small remnant skin bridge. There are several methods to repair partial or total avulsion, typically requiring operative intervention by a specialist. With total avulsion, the amputated segment should be meticulously cleaned and rinsed with saline or diluted povidone-iodine solution in preparation for repair.

Auricular Hematoma

Prompt hematoma evacuation is essential. Small acute hematomas can be managed with needle aspiration alone and bolster dressing. Large hematomas require open management with incision and drainage and placement of a drain or bolster. Hematomas that are discovered several days post injury have likely coagulated and require an incision to remove clot. One week post injury, the clot begins to break down and again becomes amenable to aspiration.

For hematoma drainage, an 18-gauge needle may be used to evacuate the hematoma contents into a 10-mL syringe. The needle is placed into the largest area of the hematoma while two fingers milk the hematoma. If unsuccessful owing to clot formation or recollection, a small stab incision can be made at the needle puncture site, and a hemostat utilized to break up the clot. A pressure dressing is placed, and the wound is reevaluated for reaccumulation in 24 hours (**Figures 5.5** and **5.6**).[8] Alternatively, drainage can be performed using an 18-gauge angiocatheter, and the catheter can be left in the hematoma cavity.[10] The drained ear is further compressed manually to express additional blood. In general, incisions should be performed along the helical rim or in an anatomic crease for maximal cosmesis. Once the blood products are removed, the sub-perichondrial space is copiously irrigated with saline. The wound is then compressed and bolstered to eliminate dead space and the incision is closed. Compression dressings can take several forms, including bolstered and compressive antibiotic impregnated gauze, sutured bolster, and through-and-through absorbable sutures tied to the anterior pinna.[10,12] If bolsters, buttons, casts, or sutures are used, these should

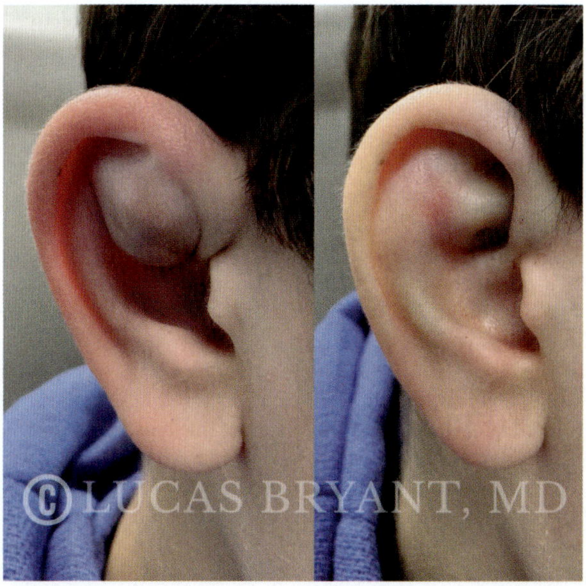

Figure 5.5: Auricular hematoma from trauma. This was drained under local anesthetic with incision. Aquaplast was used to mold a customized bolster into the scapha and was kept in place for 1 week using through-and-through 4-0 nylon mattress sutures. (Courtesy of Lucas Bryant MD, Nashville, TN.)

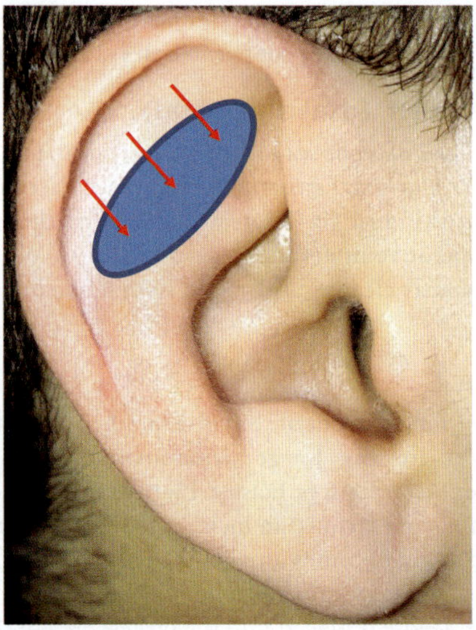

Figure 5.6: Ear bolster placement. Blue oval delineates ideal location for bolster placement after drainage of an auricular hematoma. The red arrows identify sites for placement of the horizontal mattress sutures.

be contoured to the underlying cartilaginous landmarks. The application of an auricular bolster significantly reduces the risk of reaccumulation.[12]

In cases where a compressive bolster is not used, antibiotic ointment may be placed over the suture sites and the ear dressed and bandaged. In general, bolsters, drains, or catheters should be removed in 3 to 5 days. Some thermoplastic splints can be left to bolster the ear for 3 to 7 days for acute auricular hematoma or 7 to 10 days for recurrent or large hematomas present for more than 6 hours.[9] Following either aspiration or incision and drainage, patients should be sent home with antistaphylococcal antibiotics. Patients should abstain from blood thinners if possible and avoid nonsteroidal anti-inflammatory medications.[10] Posttreatment, patients should abstain from contact sports for at least 5 days; if that is not possible, they should wear protective head and ear gear.[9] Hematoma patients should follow-up within 24 to 48 hours to assess for reaccumulation.[8]

Perichondritis

Treatment of perichondritis begins with prevention because this is a difficult infection to manage and carries significant potential for disfigurement. Preventative measures after a traumatic injury or open wound include the following: gently washing twice daily with soap and water followed by complete drying and application of topical antibacterial ointment; keeping hair away from the ear; and minimizing active debridement of eschars and crust.

The mainstay of perichondritis treatment is antibiotic treatment. In general, perichondritis can be treated with outpatient oral antibiotics such as ciprofloxacin (or other fluoroquinolone), for its antipseudomonal as well as antistaphylococcal activity with good tissue penetration.[13] For an adult, a typical regimen would be ciprofloxacin 750 mg PO q12h for 14 days. In addition to antibiotics, any foreign body such as chondral piercings should be removed. Consideration of ENT consultation for incision and drainage should be made if there is associated fluctuance/evidence of abscess formation in order to prevent necrosis of underlying cartilage. Admission for parenteral antibiotics should be considered if there is high community *Pseudomonas* resistance to fluoroquinolones, relative/absolute contraindication to fluoroquinolone use, or concern for ability to comply with outpatient treatment. Parenteral antibiotic regimens for admitted patients include piperacillin/tazobactam 4.5 g IV q6h or cefepime 2 g IV q8h + clindamycin 600 mg IV q8h. For severe cases, ENT consultants may determine the need for necrotic tissue debridement and adjunct therapies. In cases of severe pain, analgesia may be obtained by performing a nerve blockade or local field block as mentioned earlier, especially if incision and drainage of abscess are required.

TIPS AND PEARLS

- In auricular laceration and hematoma, early management and follow-up are essential for best outcomes. Following primary intervention, patients should receive follow-up anywhere from 1 day to 5 days for auricular hematoma—depending on the extent of injury and need for follow-up—and for 1 week in the case of lacerations.
- Perichondritis is a clinical diagnosis and requires prompt diagnosis, distinction from otitis externa based on sparing of the lobule, and treatment to prevent focal cartilage necrosis and disfigurement. Standard therapy is an oral antipseudomonal antibiotic like ciprofloxacin.

EVIDENCE

Is antipseudomonal coverage always required for treatment of perichondritis?

There are two retrospective studies that describe two different approaches. In one study, all patients with perichondritis were treated empirically for *P. aeruginosa*.[4] In a more recent retrospective study of 112 patients, for nonabscessed perichondritis, empiric treatment with antibiotics covering *S. aureus* alone (without antipseudomonal coverage) was found to be sufficient.[6] A randomized control trial is needed for definitive guidance; however, currently the recommendation is to cover empirically for *P. aeruginosa*; this is supported by the majority of recent case series and retrospective studies.

Is fluoroquinolone use safe in pediatric patients and warranted in treatment of perichondritis?

Although fluoroquinolone use in pediatrics has been traditionally restricted owing to risk of arthropathy and risk to growing cartilage, this risk is likely overestimated by small case series or single case reports and anecdotal evidence.[14] In line with the most recent update from the American Academy of Pediatrics (AAP), there is not enough compelling evidence to withhold fluoroquinolones in pediatric patients.[14]

References

1. Lavasani L, Leventhal D, Constantinides M, Krein H. Management of acute soft tissue injury to the auricle. *Facial Plast Surg*. 2010;26(6):445-450.
2. Bai H, Tollefson TT. Treatment strategies for auricular avulsions: best practice. *JAMA Facial Plast Surg*. 2014;16(1):7-8. doi:10.1001/jamafacial.2013.1622
3. Kullar P, Yates PD. Infections and foreign bodies in ENT. *Surgery*. 2012;30(11):590-596. doi:10.1016/j.mpsur.2012.09.005
4. Prasad HK, Sreedharan S, Prasad HS, Meyyappan MH, Harsha KS. Perichondritis of the auricle and its management. *J Laryngol Otol*. 2007;121:530-534.
5. Pattanaik S. Effective, simple treatment for perichondritis and pinna haematoma. *J Laryngol Otol*. 2009;123(11):1246-1249. doi:10.1017/S0022215109005635
6. Klug TE, Holm N, Greve T, Ovesen T. Perichondritis of the auricle: bacterial findings and clinical evaluation of different antibiotic regimens. *Eur Arch Otorhinolaryngol.* 2019;276:2199-2203. doi:10.1007/s00405-019-05463-z
7. Kent PD, Michet CJ Jr, Luthra HS. Relapsing polychondritis. *Curr Opin Rheumatol*. 2004;16(1):56-61. doi:10.1097/00002281-200401000-00011
8. Eagles K, Fralich L, Stevenson JH. Ear trauma. *Clin Sports Med*. 2013;32(2):303-316. doi:10.1016/j.csm.2012.12.011
9. Greywoode JD, Pribitkin EA, Krein H. Management of auricular hematoma and the cauliflower ear. *Facial Plast Surg*. 2010;26(6):451-455. doi:10.1055/s-0030-1267719
10. Brickman K, Adams DZ, Akpunonu P, Adams SS, Zohn SF, Guinness M. Acute management of auricular hematoma: a novel approach and retrospective review. *Clin J Sport Med*. 2013;23(4):321-323.

11. Osetinsky LM, Hamilton GS 3rd, Carlson ML. Sport injuries of the ear and temporal bone. *Clin Sports Med*. 2017;36(2):315-335. doi:10.1016/j.csm.2016.11.005
12. Dalal PJ, Purkey MR, Price CPE, Sidle DM. Risk factors for auricular hematoma and recurrence after drainage. *Laryngoscope*. 2020;130(3):628-631.
13. Liu ZW, Chokkalingam P. Piercing associated perichondritis of the pinna: are we treating it correctly? *J Laryngol Otol*. 2013;127(5):505-508. doi:10.1017/S0022215113000248
14. Rivera-Morales MD, Rodríguez-Belén JL, Vera A, Ganti L. Perichondritis: not all ear pain is otitis. *Cureus*. 2020;12(10):e11141. doi:10.7759/cureus.11141

CHAPTER 6

Sudden Hearing Loss

Enrique Perez
Laura J Bontempo

THE CLINICAL CHALLENGE

The rapid onset of unilateral or bilateral hearing loss can be a devastating event. Beyond the immediate sensory disorientation, which can lead to difficulty with sound localization and the ability to understand speech, particularly in noisy environments, persistence of hearing loss can significantly impact quality of life. This impact is even more pronounced in patients who experience hearing loss along with other common coexisting symptoms such as vertigo and tinnitus.[1]

Sudden hearing loss is a subjective complaint of rapid-onset unilateral or bilateral hearing impairment. It is characterized as sensorineural, conductive, or mixed types, depending on the underlying mechanism. Acute-onset sensorineural hearing loss (SNHL) can be further classified as sudden sensorineural hearing loss if the onset is rapid and the magnitude is severe. Sudden SNHL is defined as hearing loss of 30 decibels or greater across at least three consecutive frequencies within 72 hours.[2]

Approximately 15 000 to 60 000 annual visits for sudden hearing loss present to the emergency department (ED), urgent care, or primary care facilities annually.[2] Alexander et al. found the annual incidence of sudden SNHL in the United States to be 5 to 27 per 100 000 people, increasing with advancing age.[3] This figure may underrepresent the incidence of sudden hearing loss because patients may not seek care if they experience spontaneous hearing recovery.

PATHOPHYSIOLOGY

Whether sudden or not, SNHL is generally considered a byproduct of cochlear and/or auditory neural pathway dysfunction and hence is termed "nerve-type hearing loss." Damage to cochlear hair cells or ischemic injury to the auditory nerve are two common pathophysiologic processes shared by various conditions leading to SNHL. Whereas sudden SNHL may be idiopathic, non-idiopathic forms of sudden SNHL include Meniere disease, noise-induced hearing loss, labyrinthine fistulas, congenital hearing loss, cerebrovascular accidents, and vestibular schwannomas.[3] Furthermore, although most cases of sudden SNHL occur unilaterally, various conditions may be associated with bilateral sudden SNHL. Bilateral loss is very rarely idiopathic, so its presence should prompt further investigation into possible underlying etiologies. **Table 6.1** lists a multitude of diseases associated with bilateral sudden SNHL and their various associated features.[2]

When possible, SNHL must be differentiated from conductive hearing loss (CHL). Natural conduction of sound through the ear canal occurs via pressure changes in a column of air that leads to displacement of the tympanic membrane (TM) and subsequent movement of the coupled middle ear ossicular chain. Through a highly synchronized mechanism, this movement leads to a mechanical fluid wave in the intracochlear fluid compartments via the piston-like function of the stapes,

TABLE 6.1 Selected Conditions That May Be Associated With Bilateral Sudden Sensorineural Hearing Loss

Cause	Other Features
Infection (viral, including herpes simplex virus, varicella zoster virus, human immunodeficiency virus, and others; bacterial; mycoplasma; Lyme; tuberculosis; syphilis; fungal)	Headache, fever, other cranial nerve palsies, abnormal cerebrospinal fluid commonly seen in meningitis; pinna or ear canal vesicles and facial weakness are often seen in varicella zoster virus (Ramsay Hunt syndrome/herpes zoster oticus)
Autoimmune inner ear disease	Hearing fluctuation, vertigo
Ototoxic medication	Vestibular loss, oscillopsia
Trauma	Temporal bone fracture with possible Battle sign; cochlear concussion without visible fracture; barotrauma
Lead poisoning	Learning disabilities, other stigmata of lead poisoning
Genetic disorders	May be syndromic or nonsyndromic and may present later in life
Mitochondrial disorders, including MELAS (metabolic encephalopathy, lactic acidosis, and stroke-like episodes) and others	Confusion, stroke-like spells, elevated lactate, MRI white matter changes; others with variable phenotypes
Stroke	Vertigo, dysarthria, facial weakness, ataxia, nystagmus, unilateral numbness, abnormal CT or MRI or MR angiogram of the vertebrobasilar vasculature
Cogan syndrome	Non-syphilitic interstitial keratitis of the cornea, hearing loss, vertigo
Neoplastic (neurofibromatosis II, bilateral vestibular schwannomas, carcinomatous meningitis, intravascular lymphomatosis, others)	Abnormal brain MRI, cerebrovascular imaging study, or cerebrospinal fluid
Sarcoidosis	Pulmonary symptoms, bilateral vestibular loss, elevated angiotensin-converting enzyme level, abnormal Gallium scan
Hyperviscosity syndrome	Mucous membrane bleeding, neurologic and pulmonary symptoms, associated retinopathy

CT, computed tomography; MR, magnetic resonance; MRI, magnetic resonance imaging.

From Chandrasekhar SS, Tsai Do BS, Schwartz SR, et al. Clinical practice guideline: sudden hearing loss (update). *Otolaryngol Head Neck Surg*. 2019;161(1_suppl):S1-S45. Table 7.

the most medial ossicle in the ossicular chain. Disruption in any of these coupled mechanisms for sound conduction will diminish the sound energy delivered to the cochlea and lead to a CHL. Common example of conditions leading to sudden CHL include cerumen impactions, ear canal foreign bodies, ossicular chain disruption secondary to trauma, eardrum perforations, and acute otitis media (AOM). Chronic otitis media with or without cholesteatoma and otosclerosis are other fairly common otologic conditions leading to CHL, but their onset is generally gradual. Sudden hearing loss may also present as a combination of SNHL and CHL. This is termed mixed hearing loss, as may be the case with some AOM infections. Ultimately, a hearing test or audiogram must be carried out to confirm a specific diagnosis.

While a patient with complaints of sudden hearing loss may have any one of the three forms of hearing loss, it is most important to recognize sudden SNHL in a timely fashion. Unlike most forms of sudden CHL, sudden SNHL is considered an "otolaryngologic emergency" because it may become an irreversible condition unless urgently intervened upon.[4]

Noise-induced hearing loss is perhaps one of the most common causes of non-idiopathic sudden SNHL. Although often unilateral, it can also be bilateral depending on the circumstances of the noise exposure. Luckily, most forms of noise-induced sudden hearing loss reverse spontaneously within 24 to 48 hours. Nonetheless, recurring exposure to hazardous noise can often lead to progressive SNHL over time.

APPROACH/THE FOCUSED EXAM

History

Historical features that will help a clinician narrow the differential diagnosis of a patient with sudden hearing loss include unilaterality or bilaterality, symptom recurrence, associated trauma, and the presence or absence of associated symptoms.

Clinicians can make a fairly accurate determination on whether a patient is likely experiencing SNHL or CHL based on history alone. Whether sudden or not, CHL is more often associated with a history of penetrating or nonpenetrating trauma, or infectious symptoms such as ear drainage and otalgia. The patient may also report a history of recurring infections or prior otologic procedures. On the contrary, SNHL is more often associated with other inner ear-like symptoms such as vertigo, tinnitus, or aural fullness.

Vertigo complaints are present in 30% to 60% of cases of sudden SNHL.[5-7] This may also indicate a poor hearing prognosis and is often associated with worse degrees of hearing loss.[6] New-onset tinnitus is present in almost every case of sudden SNHL, and while having little bearing on the prognosis, it can lead to functional and psychological distress.[8] Importantly, when evaluating patients with acute hearing loss, it is critical to remember that erroneously labeling a case of sudden SNHL as sudden CHL can lead to delays in treatment and potentially worse hearing outcomes.

A basic examination of the ear must be carried out in all cases of sudden hearing loss, including otoscopic evaluation of the ear canals and TMs. If the ear exam demonstrates a cerumen impaction, it must be removed for the proper assessment of sudden hearing loss. If there are no concerns for an underlying TM perforation, such as a history of ear drainage, trauma, or recent ear surgery, gentle irrigation can be performed to flush out the cerumen. When possible, pneumatic otoscopy can aid in making a diagnosis by providing information on the compliance of the TM and, indirectly, the middle ear. The absence of TM movement during pneumatic otoscopy supports the presence of an effusion and, therefore, the diagnosis of CHL.

Confirmation of hearing loss will require formal audiometric testing. In the ED and urgent care settings with limited resources, clinical guidelines recommend the use of a tuning fork during the initial evaluation of a patient with sudden hearing loss.[2] The traditional tuning fork tests to differentiate SNHL from CHL are the Weber and Rinne tests. A detailed explanation of these tests is provided in Chapter 2. Please review the "Evidence" section at the end of the chapter for information on tuning fork test accuracy.

DIFFERENTIAL DIAGNOSIS

In cases of CHL, the clinician may find evidence of cerumen impaction, a perforated TM, middle ear effusion, middle ear or external auditory canal infection, debris in the ear indicating cholesteatomatous disease, bony exostosis, or even a foreign body such as a cotton swab tip. In trauma patients, CHL can be associated with temporal bone fractures and subsequent ossicular injury. In these patients, an acute hemotympanum will be apparent and injury to the ear canal and TM is commonly seen with longitudinal fractures. By contrast, cases of SNHL will often demonstrate an intact ear canal and TM.

A system-based examination including a neurologic and cranial nerve exam should be carried out in every patient presenting with sudden hearing loss. A focal neurologic finding in a patient with sudden hearing loss likely indicates a central nervous system (CNS) etiology, such as a cerebral vascular accident (CVA). Examples of such findings include ipsilateral facial numbness/paralysis, nystagmus, dysarthria, ipsilateral Horner syndrome (miosis, ptosis, and anhidrosis), diplopia, contralateral body numbness, dysmetria, and ataxia.[8,9] Although the presence of vertigo or imbalance is common in sudden SNHL related to peripheral causes, corresponding exam findings such as nystagmus that is up-beating, direction-changing, or worsened with fixation suggest CNS involvement.[10,11] On the contrary, CVAs rarely present with isolated hearing loss. Most CVA-related sudden SNHL is caused by disruption in the blood supply from the vertebrobasilar and anterior inferior cerebellar arteries (AICA).[12] Other inflammatory and autoimmune conditions such as multiple sclerosis and sarcoidosis can present with sudden SNHL along with other focal neurologic findings.[13]

Recurrent episodes of unilateral sudden SNHL may be associated with Meniere disease. Although Meniere disease is more commonly associated with acute vertigo attacks, it may present as isolated hearing loss in atypical or earlier forms of the disease. Rare conditions such as autoimmune inner ear disease and Cogan syndrome can lead to recurrent episodes of bilateral sudden SNHL and require management separate from that of idiopathic sudden SNHL.

MANAGEMENT

In cases of CHL associated with evidence of an active, complicated ear infection or significant temporal bone trauma, further testing such as computed tomography (CT), magnetic resonance imaging (MRI), or laboratory tests should be carried out as necessary. CT and MRIs with vessel imaging should also be considered in any patient demonstrating focal neurologic signs or symptoms beyond hearing loss. Based on appropriateness criteria established by the American College of Radiology (ACR) and other high-level evidence in the sudden hearing loss literature, the American Academy of Otolaryngolog-Head and Neck Surgeons (AAO-HNS) guideline provides a strong recommendation against routinely ordering a CT head in the initial evaluation of patients with presumptive idiopathic sudden SNHL.[2]

In the absence of any concerning neurologic findings, patients should be referred for a dedicated internal auditory canal contrast MRI following audiometric confirmation of sudden SNHL. MRI of the internal auditory canals is the preferred study for ruling out retrocochlear pathology such as vestibular schwannomas, which may present with isolated sudden hearing loss.[14] These MRIs can be completed as nonurgent outpatient studies.

If a reversible cause of sudden hearing loss is identified through history, exam, or diagnostic studies, it should be corrected in the primary, urgent, or emergency care settings. Examples include the removal of cerumen or a nonpenetrating ear canal foreign body or the treatment of uncomplicated otitis media with or without effusion. Follow-up with the patient's primary care physician is usually sufficient; evaluation by a specialist is generally not necessary. Patients with sudden hearing loss not resolved by interventions or not anticipated to resolve following treatment of an infection should be referred to an otolaryngologist for further management.

All forms of unresolved sudden hearing loss merit prompt follow-up and the AAO-HNS guidelines give a clear recommendation to obtain, or refer to a clinician who can obtain, audiometry within 14 days of symptom onset in all cases of sudden hearing loss.[2] The time requirement for this recommendation is based on the evidence for treatment of sudden SNHL and its efficacy.

Based on thorough review of the literature, the AAO-HNS guideline states that clinicians may offer corticosteroids as initial therapy to patients with sudden SNHL.[2] Both systemic oral and localized intratympanic (IT) steroid therapy are potentially effective in restoring hearing in this patient population. In either case, the majority of the trials demonstrating a therapeutic benefit use a 1- to 2-week window from symptom onset as enrollment criteria to initiate treatment. Evidence of an early intracochlear inflammatory process in sudden SNHL further supports the early use of steroids to diminish irreversible damage. Nevertheless, there is evidence of benefit up to 6 weeks postonset of hearing loss.[2] Because a definitive diagnosis of sudden SNHL may not be confirmed in the ED or urgent care setting, clinical judgment must be used to determine the risks and benefits of initiating systemic steroids in cases with high suspicion for this diagnosis. Effective dosages include Prednisone 1 mg/kg/d (maximum dose of 60 mg/d), Methylprednisolone 48 mg/d, or Dexamethasone 10 mg/d. These should be taken as full dose for 7 to 14 days followed by a taper over a similar period of time.[2] IT steroid injections should be done by an otolaryngologist, so prompt outpatient follow-up is a necessity.

Aside from antibiotics for acute ear infections and cases of penetrating trauma leading to CHL, other forms of CHL previously listed do not require immediate intervention and can be further evaluated and managed by an otolaryngologist in follow-up.

Most conditions leading to sudden CHL will eventually undergo surgical management or nonsurgical management with hearing aid amplification. With the exception of a suspected labyrinthine fistula, which may require a fairly urgent, but not emergent, surgical repair after further evaluation, most conditions leading to sudden SNHL will be treated nonsurgically.

TIPS AND PEARLS

- While sudden hearing loss can be very frightening to a patient, prompting an ED, urgent care, or primary care visit, there is often a 14-day time window for optimal intervention, even in cases of sudden SNHL. One exception is sudden hearing loss associated with penetrating ear trauma that would require a same-day evaluation.
- All patients with sudden hearing loss require a full neurologic examination. Focal neurologic findings may indicate a CNS etiology such as a CVA. Tinnitus and vertigo often accompany sudden hearing loss and, without other associated findings, do not suggest a CNS etiology.
- A history and directed physical exam will reveal most causes of reversible CHL such as cerumen impaction, infection, and nonpenetrating foreign bodies.
- The mainstay of therapy for patients with sudden SNHL is corticosteroid treatment for 1 to 2 weeks followed by a taper, although the evidence is inconclusive as to any long-term benefit. Earlier initiation of this treatment is thought to lead to better outcomes. Therefore, if steroids are used, treatment should be started early if follow-up can be assured within 1 week of symptoms onset.

EVIDENCE

Does the proper use of tuning fork testing help providers differentiate the type or severity of hearing loss?

In a study of sudden SNHL patients, Shuman et al. showed that despite unreliable results 20% of the time, the sensitivity of the Weber test was 99% for patients whose Weber test lateralized away from the suspected side of hearing loss.[15] Based on metanalysis data, the Rinne has a sensitivity of 16% to 87% and specificity of 55% to 100% to detect CHL when a 512-Hz tuning fork is used.[16] When the two tests are consistent with each other, the sensitivity can be as high as 95%.[17]

The Weber and Rinne tests have a similarly poor predictive value in the diagnosis of CHL in children.[18]

Does early treatment with steroids affect long-term hearing outcomes in patients with sudden SNHL?

The evidence supporting the benefit of corticosteroid treatment to improve outcomes in patients with sudden SNHL is limited and outcome results are mixed. A Cochrane review of systemic steroid (oral, intravenous, or intramuscular) use in sudden SNHL did not show conclusive benefits to hearing outcomes.[19] Data supports that IT steroids offer early benefits to hearing recovery but long-term outcomes have not been shown to conclusively differ between patients receiving IT steroids plus systemic steroids versus those receiving systemic steroids alone.[20] In children, a delay in initiation of steroid therapy greater than 6 days after symptom onset was associated with lower odds of hearing improvement.[21] Although currently there is no conclusive evidence that systemic or IT steroids affect hearing loss outcome, if the clinician decides to treat with steroids, this treatment should be initiated as soon as possible and ideally within 2 weeks of the onset of symptoms.

References

1. Carlsson PI, Hall M, Lind KJ, et al. Quality of life, psychosocial consequences, and audiological rehabilitation after sudden sensorineural hearing loss. *Int J Audiol*. 2011;50:139-144.
2. Chandrasekhar SS, Tsai Do BS, Schwartz SR, et al. Clinical practice guideline: sudden hearing loss (update). *Otolaryngol Head Neck Surg*. 2019;161(1_suppl):S1-S45.

3. Alexander TH, Harris JP. Incidence of sudden sensorineural hearing loss. *Otol Neurotol*. 2013;34: 1586-1589.

4. Byl FM Jr. Sudden hearing loss: eight years' experience and suggested prognostic table. *Laryngoscope*. 1984;94:647-661.

5. Rauch SD. Clinical practice: idiopathic sudden sensorineural hearing loss. *N Engl J Med*. 2008;359:833-840.

6. Fetterman BL, Saunders JE, Luxford WM. Prognosis and treatment of sudden sensorineural hearing loss. *Am J Otol*. 1996;17:529-536.

7. Niu X, Zhang Y, Zhang Q, et al. The relationship between hearing loss and vestibular dysfunction in patients with sudden sensorineural hearing loss. *Acta Otolaryngol*. 2016;136:225-231.

8. Amarenco P, Rosengart A, DeWitt LD, Pessin MS, Caplan LR. Anterior inferior cerebellar artery territory infarcts: mechanisms and clinical features. *Arch Neurol*. 1993;50:154-161.

9. Lee H, Cho YW. Auditory disturbance as a prodrome of anterior inferior cerebellar artery infarction. *J Neurol Neurosurg Psychiatry*. 2003;74:1644-1648.

10. Oas JG, Baloh RW. Vertigo and the anterior inferior cerebellar artery syndrome. *Neurology*. 1992;42:2274-2279.

11. Lee H, Kim JS, Chung EJ, et al. Infarction in the territory of anterior inferior cerebellar artery: spectrum of audiovestibular loss. *Stroke*. 2009;40:3745-3751.

12. Hausler R, Levine RA. Auditory dysfunction in stroke. *Acta Otolaryngol*. 2000;120:689-703.

13. Atula S, Sinkkonen ST, Saat R, et al. Association of multiple sclerosis and sudden sensorineural hearing loss. *Mult Scler J Exp Transl Clin*. 2016;2:2055217316652155.

14. St Martin MB, Hirsch BE. Imaging of hearing loss. *Otolaryngol Clin North Am*. 2008;41:157-178.

15. Shuman AG, Li X, Halpin CF, Rauch SD, Telian SA. Tuning fork testing in sudden sensorineural hearing loss. *JAMA Intern Med*. 2013;173:706-707.

16. Kelly EA, Li B, Adams ME. Diagnostic accuracy of tuning fork tests for hearing loss: a systematic review. *Otolaryngol Head Neck Surg*. 2018;159(2):220-230. doi:10.1177/0194599818770405

17. Boatman DF, Miglioretti DL, Eberwein C, Alidoost M, Reich SG. How accurate are bedside hearing tests? *Neurology*. 2007;68(16):1311-1314. doi:10.1212/01.wnl.0000259524.08148.16

18. Behn A, Westerberg BD, Zhang H, Riding KH, Ludemann JP, Kozak FK. Accuracy of the Weber and Rinne tuning fork tests in evaluation of children with otitis media with effusion. *J Otolaryngol*. 2007;36(4):197-202. doi:10.2310/7070.2007.0025

19. Wei BP, Stathopoulos D, O'Leary S. Steroids for idiopathic sudden sensorineural hearing loss. *Cochrane Database Syst Rev*. 2013;(7):CD003998.

20. Crane RA, Camilon M, Nguyen S, Meyer TA. Steroids for treatment of sudden sensorineural hearing loss: a meta-analysis of randomized controlled trials. *Laryngoscope*. 2015;125:209-217.

21. Wood JW, Shaffer AD, Kitsko D, Chi DH. Sudden sensorineural hearing loss in children-management and outcomes: a meta-analysis. *Laryngoscope*. 2021;131(2):425-434. doi:10.1002/lary.28829

CHAPTER 7

Acute Vertigo

Harrison Lin
Rodney Omron

Dizziness is a common chief complaint in the emergency department (ED) that poses unique diagnostic challenges.[1] The feeling of "dizziness" can be described in many ways, many of which fall into the subcategory of a vestibular syndrome (VS). The patient's description of dizziness as lightheadedness versus spinning offers minimal benefit in diagnosing the underlying disease.[1]

The differential diagnosis of dizziness in the ED is broad, with no single cause accounting for the majority of cases, so some rarely encountered diseases need to be considered in every dizzy patient. A systematic approach or direct feedback about every dizzy patient is critical to avoid misdiagnosis.[2]

Many of the most reliable diagnostic tools for dizziness, such as the Dix-Hallpike test for benign positional vertigo, are simple to perform bedside. By contrast, overreliance on advanced imaging without a systematic problem-based history and physical has been shown to increase length of stay, increase the cost of care, and falsely reassure providers that a life-threatening cause has been ruled out.

PATHOPHYSIOLOGY

See **Figure 7.1**[3] and the section that follows.

Type	Prevalence	Pathophysiology
Benign paroxysmal positional vertigo (BPPV)	High	Caused by calcium carbonate debris that erodes or becomes dislodged from the macula epithelium within the utricle; 90% of BPPV is related to the posterior canal because it is closest to the utricle.[4]
Vestibular migraine (VM)	High	A key mechanism is the activation of the trigeminovascular system. The labyrinthine vessels are innervated by the trigeminal nerve terminals.[5]
Vestibular neuritis (VN)	Moderate	The most popular theory is that of a viral cause, but the evidence for it remains circumstantial. VN interferes with the vestibulo-ocular reflex, thus allowing the head impulse test to cause a catch-up saccade when present.[1]
Ménière disease (MD)	Low	The prevalence of MD is 5-500 per 100 000 habitants, and familial MD is around 9% of cases. It is suspected from human temporal bone studies that MD is due to excessive accumulation of endolymph within the cochlear duct and the sacculus.[5]

(continued)

Type	Prevalence	Pathophysiology
Perilymphatic fistula	Low	Communication between the perilymph of the cochlea/ vestibule and outside the inner ear is usually from the round or oval window. The etiology is trauma or congenital.
Labyrinthitis	Low	The etiology is viral, bacterial, or autoimmune causing dizziness and hearing loss.
Vestibular schwannoma	Low	It is the most common neoplasm of the cerebellopontine angle in adults. These tumors derive from myelinating Schwann cells of the vestibular division of the vestibulocochlear (eighth cranial) nerve.
Stroke	Low	A stroke occurs in 3.2% of all dizziness presentations to the ED. It is common from the anterior inferior cerebellar artery.[1]

Approach/The Focused Exam

Triage-Titrate-Tests

The Triage-Titrate-Test (3-TTT) algorithm is a systematic way to approach the dizzy patient.

- **Triage:** comprehensive review of systems to rule out stroke and to discover non-neurologic etiologies of dizziness.
- **TiTrATE**: (**Ti**ming, **Tr**iggers, **A**nd **T**argeted History/**E**xamination): Timing classifies symptoms into brief versus continuous. Triggers are aggravating factors (eg, vertigo with laying down). Targeted history/examination uses history elements (eg, trauma) to differentiate between the underlying causes of vertigo and lead to very specific physical examination maneuvers to better characterize the dizziness into peripheral versus central (see **Table 7.1**).
- **Tests:** Ancillary tests such as labs and imaging are then ordered based on the history and examination.[1]

Triage

Seeking associated factors and symptoms in addition to the chief complaint of dizziness is known as the **Triage** step in determining the underlying etiology. See Table 7.1 for other signs. Any one of the "deadly D" findings (**dysarthria, dysphagia, dysphonia, dysmetria,** and **diplopia**) should provoke a high suspicion of stroke. Also, any acute hearing loss, neck or head trauma, severe ataxia, or unilateral lean suggests a central cause.

Timing and Triggers

Symptoms should be classified as intermittent or persistent, each of which can further be divided into triggered or not triggered.

Intermittent = **episodic vestibular syndrome (EVS)**—seconds, minutes, or hours of vertigo. It usually has a duration of fewer than 30 seconds. Relapsing symptoms that last for weeks are not considered new onset and therefore fall in the chronic category.[1]

- **Triggered = triggered episodic vestibular syndrome (t-EVS)**
- **Not Triggered = spontaneous episodic vestibular**

Persistent = **acute vestibular syndrome (AVS)**—continuous and persistent at rest. AVS can be further grouped into diseases triggered by a trauma or toxin (t-AVS) or spontaneously (s-AVS).[1]

- **Triggered = triggered acute vestibular syndrome (t-AVS)**
- **Not Triggered = spontaneous acute vestibular syndrome (s-AVS)**

Intermittent and Triggered (t-EVS)

Intermittent and triggered (t-EVS) is vertigo that is brief, lasting seconds to minutes, and is triggered by something. The patient will say *no* to the question, "Are you dizzy right now without moving?" The trigger is often a change in head position but may also be a loud sound or valsalva.[1]

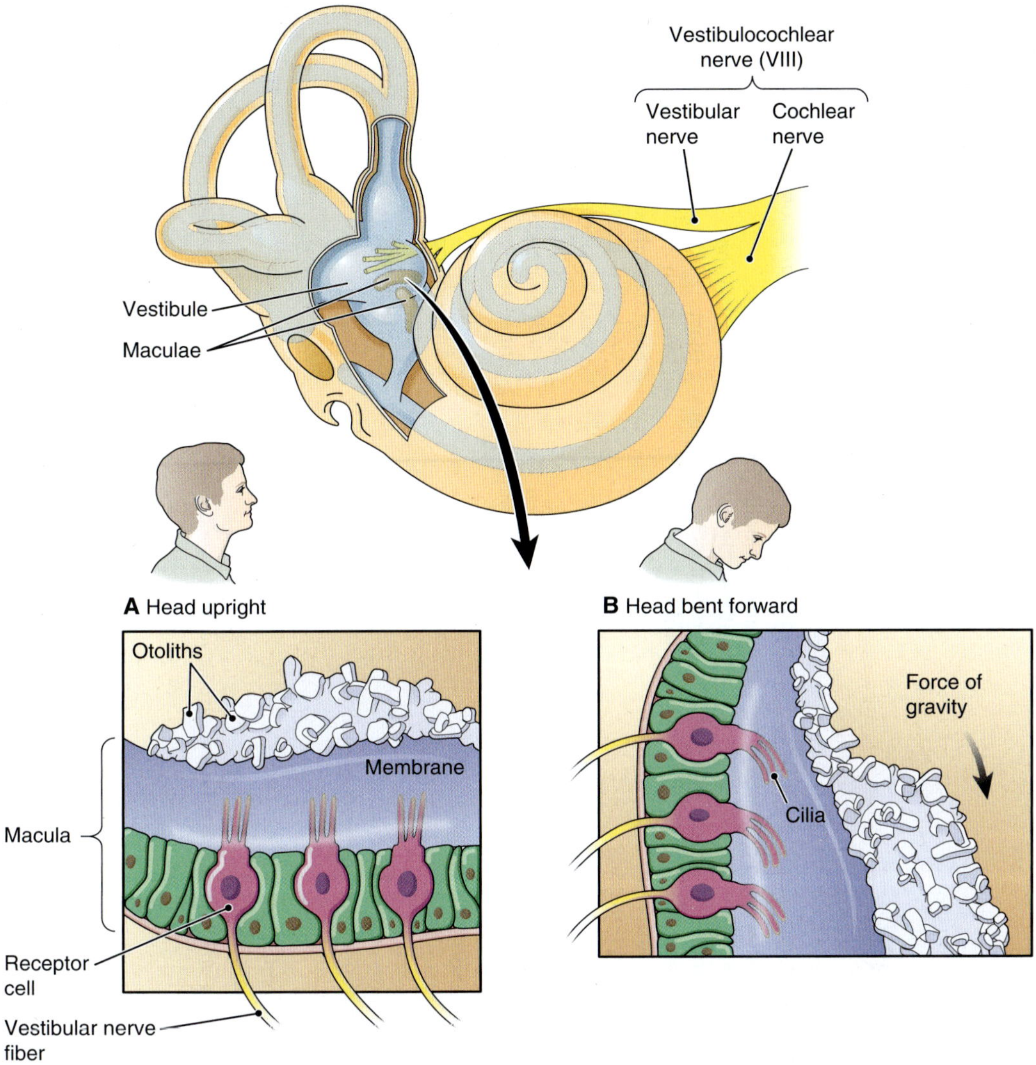

Figure 7.1: The vestibular system comprises peripheral vestibular system, the ocular system, the brainstem, cerebellum, and cortex as well as postural muscles. A disruption of any part of this complex system causes dizziness. The peripheral vestibular system is composed of the **utricle, the saccule,** and **the lateral, anterior,** and **posterior semicircular canals**. The entire apparatus is encased by **temporal bone**. The **macula** and **crista ampullaris** are sensory neuroepithelia. Each contains rod-shaped sensory mechanoreceptors called **hair cells**. The **utricle** and **saccule** are structures that sense the position of the head, each contain macula. The exterior of the macula is coated with a gel-like membrane embedded with calcium carbonate particles called **otoliths**. Semicircular canals are oriented at right angles to each other. **Endolymph** flows through these canals, and at the end of each is a dilation called the **ampulla**, at the base of which is the crista ampullaris. The crista ampullaris is coated with the **cupula**, which is thicker than the gelatinous material on the macula and does not contain otoliths. (From Cohen BJ, Hull KL. *Memmler's Structure and Function of the Human Body*. 12th ed. Wolters Kluwer; 2020. Figure 10.12.)

The most common causes of t-EVS are orthostatic hypotension and benign paroxysmal positional vertigo (BPPV) (**Table 7.2**). In cases where BPPV is suspected, the clinician should be looking for orthostatic hypotension in patients with positional triggers. Orthostatic hypotension (*must* have a change in blood pressure) should be distinguished from orthostatic dizziness (*no* change in blood pressure but a subjective feeling of light-headedness with standing), which may suggest decreased flow to the brain caused by a transient ischemic attack (TIA), cranial vascular stenosis, or intracranial hypotension.[1]

TABLE 7.1 The Targeted History That Suggests a Cause for Acute Vertigo (Based on 3-TTT)

Dizzy + Other Symptoms (TRIAGE)	Intermittent and Spontaneous (s-EVS)	Intermittent and Triggered (t-EVS)	Persistent and Spontaneous (s-AVS)	Persistent and Triggered by Trauma or Toxin (t-AVS)
Altered mental status Loss of consciousness Neck pain Abdominal pain Dyspnea Palpitations New medications Fever Abnormal glucose	Vestibular migraine Ménière disease Panic attacks Vasovagal syncope Transient ischemic attack Subarachnoid hemorrhage Arrhythmia	Horizontal canal—benign paroxysmal positional vertigo Posterior canal—benign paroxysmal positional vertigo Posterior fossa tumor Orthostatic hypotension Transient ischemic attack/stroke Cranial vascular stenosis Intracranial hypotension Alcohol intoxication Myocardial infarct Unstable angina Pulmonary embolism Hypoglycemia Carbon monoxide poisoning Gastrointestinal/retroperitoneal bleed Dehydration Sepsis Adrenal insufficiency Diabetic ketoacidosis	Acute vestibular neuritis Multiple sclerosis Transient ischemic attack Stroke	**Trauma** Barotrauma Blast Whiplash Skull fracture concussion Vertebral artery dissection Direct vestibular nerve/labyrinthine concussion Mechanical disruption of the inner ear **Toxin** Aminoglycoside (gait unsteadiness, oscillopsia) Carbon monoxide poisoning

3-TTT, Triage-Titrate-Test; s-AVS, spontaneous acute vestibular syndrome; s-EVS, spontaneous episodic vestibular syndrome; t-AVS, triggered acute vestibular syndrome; t-EVS, triggered episodic vestibular syndrome.

TABLE 7.2 Discharge Features for Common Vestibular Causes of Vertigo

Type of Vertigo	Targeted Examination	Benign	Danger	Discharge Criteria
Intermittent and triggered (t-EVS)	Orthostatic vitals; positional Tests for nystagmus	BPPV	Posterior fossa mass	• No headache, auditory, neurologic, syncope • Symptoms occur when tipping the head forward/back/rolling, not limited to rising • Asymptomatic with head stationary, symptoms reproduced by positional test • Characteristic, canal-specific peripheral type nystagmus only triggered by positional tests • Therapeutic response to canal-specific repositioning maneuvers
Intermittent and spontaneous (s-EVS)	Head, neck, and cranial nerve history, hearing history	Vestibular migraine Ménière disease	Transient ischemic attack	• No cardiorespiratory symptoms or loss of consciousness • No dangerous D symptoms (dysarthria, dysphagia, dysphonia, dysmetria, diplopia) • No papilledema, Horner syndrome, cranial nerve abnormalities • No pain especially in the posterior neck • Strong/long history of prior dizziness episodes (at least five over last 2 yr) • Clear precipitant with the episode or $ABCD^2$ risk ≤ 3 • Migraine: history of migraine, classic visual aura, or photophobia with most attacks • Ménière disease: history of unilateral fluctuating hearing loss or tinnitus with most attacks
Persistent and spontaneous (s-AVS)	HINTS; ear; hearing examination	Vestibular neuritis	Stroke	• Maximum one prodromal spell <48 hr before the onset • No excessive vomiting or gait disorder • No pain, hearing loss, or neurologic symptoms • No papilledema, Horner syndrome, cranial nerve abnormalities • No headache • Stands and walked unassisted • HINTS plus hearing/ear examination • SEND HIM ON HOME • SEND—Straight eyes, no deafness • HIM—Head impulses miss (unilateral abnormal impulse opposite nystagmus direction) • ON—One-way nystagmus (unidirectional nystagmus worse in a gaze toward fast phase) • HOME—healthy otic and mastoid examination

BPPV, benign paroxysmal positional vertigo; HINTS, HI = head impulse, N = unidirectional nystagmus, s-AVS, spontaneous acute vestibular syndrome; s-EVS, spontaneous episodic vestibular syndrome; TS = test of skew; t-AVS, triggered acute vestibular syndrome.

Adapted from NOVEL. The David Newman-Toker neuro-ophthalmology collection. Accessed May 10, 2021. https://novel.utah.edu/Newman-Toker/

BPPV must be differentiated from central paroxysmal positional vertigo (CPPV), which often stems from posterior fossa mass lesions, strokes, and alcohol intoxication. CPPV has a specific type of nystagmus on examination that distinguishes it from BPPV (see video at https://collections.lib.utah.edu/details?id=1213448).[6] Other etiologies include intravascular volume loss such as gastrointestinal, retroperitoneal bleed, dehydration, myocardial infarct, sepsis, adrenal insufficiency, and diabetic ketoacidosis (**Figure 7.2** and Table 7.1).

Intermittent and Not Triggered (s-EVS)

Intermittent and not triggered (s-EVS) is brief (lasting minutes to hours) and comes and goes without a trigger. The patient will say *no* to the question, "Are you dizzy right now without moving?" A thorough history is required to differentiate causes of s-EVS because most patients are asymptomatic at the time of presentation—no trigger will cause symptoms. Included in this group are benign disorders such as vestibular migraine (VM), panic attacks, vasovagal syncope, and MD. Dangerous causes include TIA, subarachnoid hemorrhage, arrhythmia, myocardial infarct, unstable angina, pulmonary embolism, hypoglycemia, and carbon monoxide poisoning.[1]

- MD typically does not exhibit the entire classic triad of unilateral tinnitus, reversible sensorineural hearing loss, and aural fullness. In patients presenting with low-frequency sensorineural hearing loss with aural symptoms and vertigo attacks, MD is probable.
- New-onset vertigo, hearing loss, and tinnitus may herald anterior inferior cerebellar artery (AICA) territory ischemia.[1]
- VM is the second most common cause of dizziness next only to BPPV and the most often missed cause of s-EVS. These patients present similarly to posterior stroke, and have an increased risk of stroke, it is often necessary to perform a central workup before assigning the diagnosis of VM. VM diagnosis requires five attacks of vestibular symptoms, migraine headache history, and migraine-like symptoms (eg, photophobia, phonophobia, visual aura) associated with at least half of the episodes. Symptoms typically last for at least 5 minutes but can persist for days. Ironically, this condition is rarely associated with headaches.
- Neurally mediated syncope is usually associated with light-headedness and often includes dizziness or vertigo. The diagnosis is confirmed as an outpatient with a tilt table test.[1] Central causes of this include TIA. Also, cardiac arrhythmias may explain light-headedness/dizziness without a trigger, so providers should have a low threshold for recommending echocardiogram and cardiology follow-up (see Figure 7.2 and Table 7.1).

Persistent and Triggered (t-AVS)

Persistent and triggered (t-AVS) vertigo is often a sequela of blunt head trauma or because of a toxin. The patient will say *yes* to the question, "Are you dizzy right now without moving?" Physical examination findings vary based on the type of trauma or toxin (see Table 7.1). Blunt head trauma, blast injury, whiplash, and barotrauma all cause direct injury to the vestibular nerve, labyrinth, or inner ear. Whiplash can also cause vertebral artery dissection. Patients with traumatic brain injuries experience post-concussive syndrome, which is a type of t-AVS. Types of toxins that cause t-AVS include alcohol, anticonvulsant drugs such as phenytoin, and aminoglycosides such as gentamicin. Gentamicin is usually associated with gait unsteadiness and bouncing vision while walking (oscillopsia) (see Figure 7.2 and Table 7.1).

Persistent and Not Triggered (s-AVS)

Persistent and not triggered (s-AVS) vertigo is persistent and has no underlying trauma or toxin. The patient will say *yes* to the question, "Are you dizzy right now without moving?" s-AVS lasts for days to weeks, accompanied by gait instability, nystagmus, and symptoms worsened with head motion. The most common cause of s-AVS is acute vestibular neuritis (VN).

Targeted Examination + Tests

Nystagmus

One important element of the physical examination in the dizzy patient is the observation of nystagmus (**Figure 7.3**). Nystagmus suggests a central cause if it is in any direction other than unidirectional lateral or upgoing rotary. Upbeating, downbeating, and direction changing are particularly

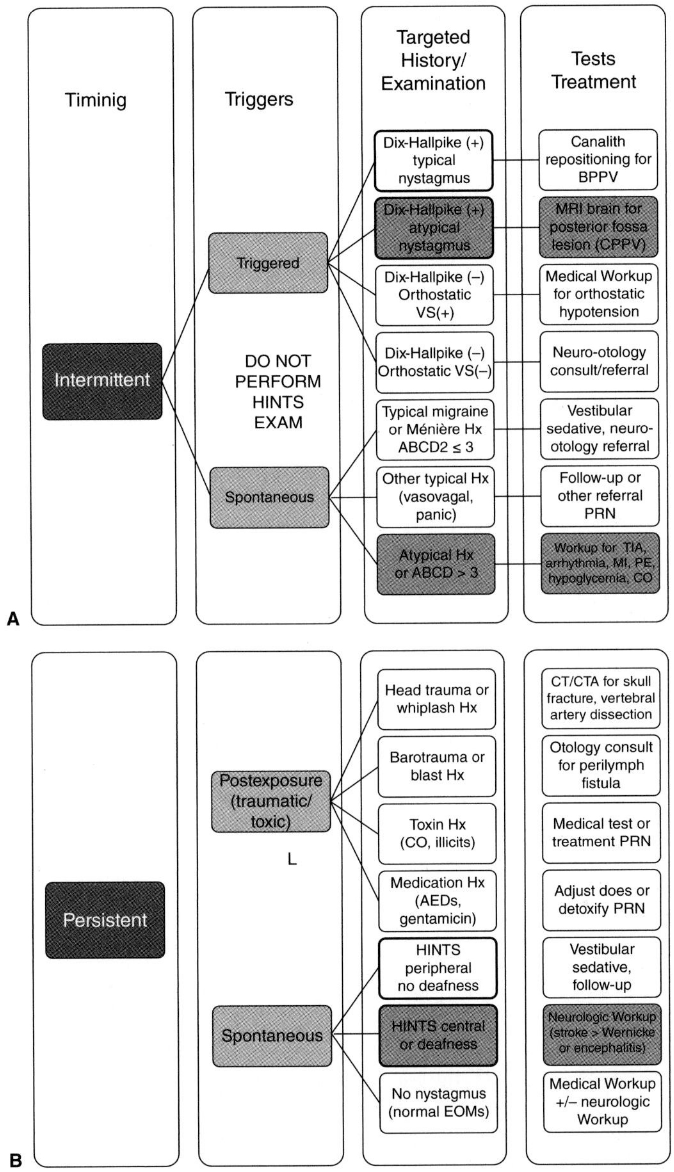

Figure 7.2: TiTrATE algorithm for differential diagnosis and workup of dizziness and vertigo. The TiTrATE algorithm divides acute dizziness and vertigo into four key categories: A, t-EVS and s-EVS forms of EVS and B, t-AVS and s-AVS forms of AVS. Each syndrome determines a targeted bedside examination, differential diagnosis, and tests, regardless of symptom type (vertigo, presyncope, unsteadiness, or nonspecific dizziness). Some steps may occur after the ED visit, as part of follow-up, or during inpatient hospital admission. Bolded color in the Targeted and Tests columns denotes risk of a dangerous disorder. Bold outlines denote evidence-based, targeted eye examinations that discriminate between benign and dangerous causes. AED, antiepileptic drug; BPPV, benign paroxysmal positional vertigo; CO, carbon monoxide; CPPV, central paroxysmal positional vertigo; CT, computerized tomography; CTA, computed tomography angiography; ED, emergency department; EOM, extraocular movement; Hx, history; HINTS, HI = head impulse, N = unidirectional nystagmus, TS = test of skew; MI, myocardial infarction; MRI, magnetic resonance imaging; PE, pulmonary embolus; PRN, pro re nata (as needed); s-AVS, spontaneous acute vestibular syndrome; s-EVS, spontaneous episodic vestibular syndrome; t-AVS, triggered acute vestibular syndrome; t-EVS, triggered episodic vestibular syndrome; TIA, transient ischemic attack; VS, vital signs. (Adapted from Newman-Toker DE, Edlow JA. TiTrATE: A Novel, Evidence-Based Approach to Diagnosing Acute Dizziness and Vertigo. *Neurol Clin*. 2015;33(3):577-579, viii.)

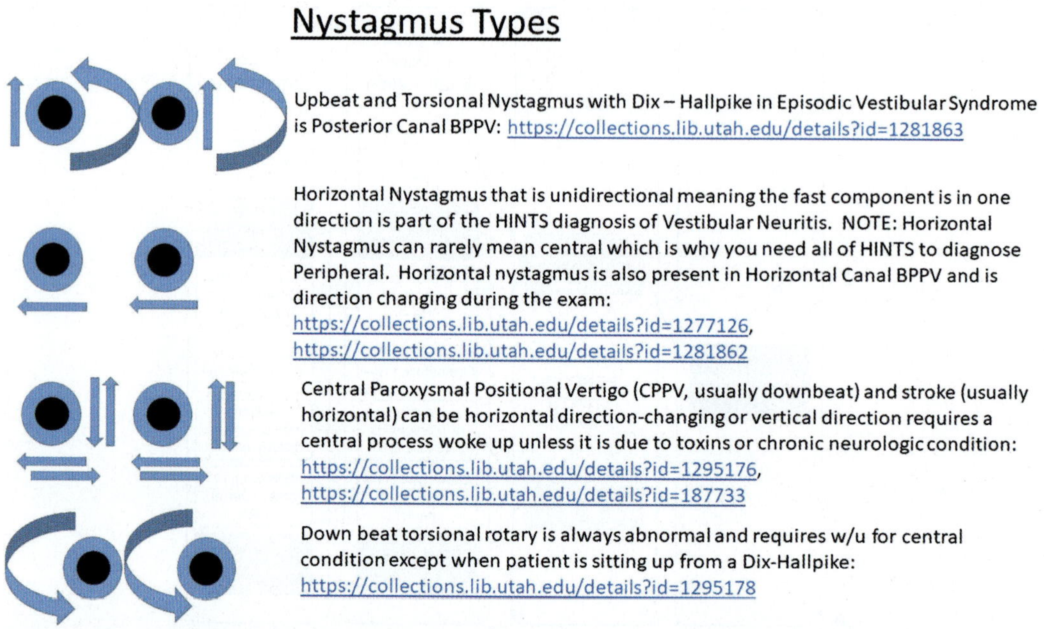

Figure 7.3: Primer on different nystagmus types. BPPV, benign paroxysmal positional vertigo; CPPV, central paroxysmal positional vertigo; HINTS, HI = head impulse, N = unidirectional nystagmus, TS = test of skew. (Video links from the Dan Gold Collection. NOVEL. The Dan Gold neuro-ophthalmology collection. Accessed May 10, 2021. https://novel.utah.edu/Gold/)

concerning for a central cause. Visual fixation minimizes peripheral nystagmus; therefore, to appreciate a peripheral process, visual fixation must be removed. To do this, ask the patient to look left or right instead of having them follow your finger. Alternatively, consider using a penlight test (intermittently shining a light into the patient's eye while watching for nystagmus), Frenzel goggles (one-way lens), or simply placing a sheet of blank paper in front of the patient's field of view during examination.[7]

Dix-Hallpike Maneuver

BPPV, the most common form of t-EVS, is always of brief duration and only triggered by position changes. In 90% of cases of BPPV, the condition occurs because of otolith particles entering the semicircular canals, with the posterior canal being the most common.[4,7] Treatment involves performing the Epley maneuver to move the otolith back to its canal of origin (see "Management" section).

In the Dix-Hallpike maneuver, the patient is laid down and the affected ear is placed down in the plane of the posterior semicircular canal, resulting in upbeat torsional nystagmus (**Figure 7.4**). Sometimes the Dix-Hallpike is not positive though they have a classic story for BPPV. In such cases, consultation with a neurologist is reasonable.

Supine Roll

The much less common horizontal canal BPPV can be evoked using the supine roll test. Lie the patient supine with their head 30° from horizontal. If the right ear is affected, rotating to the right provokes horizontal nystagmus beating to the right, and rotating to the left then beats to the left with less intense effect as the particle rolls from side to side in the Horizontal plane (**Figure 7.5**). Anterior canal BPPV is exceedingly rare; it causes downbeat torsional nystagmus and, if recognized, requires ruling out a central cause. (See the following stroke mimicking an anterior canal BPPV: https://collections.lib.utah.edu/details?id=1213448.)[6]

The test for diagnosing acute VN is summarized as HINTS Plus *no* hearing loss (HI = head impulse, N = unidirectional nystagmus, TS = test of skew).

- A delayed saccade is expected with VN on the head impulse test (described subsequently), which indicates a disrupted vestibulo-ocular reflex.

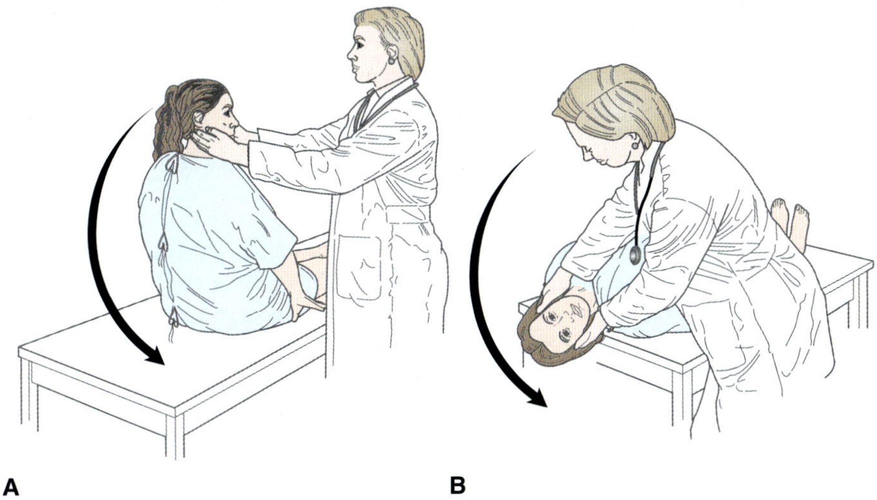

Figure 7.4: Dix-Hallpike to the right going from the sitting (A) to the head-hanging right position (B) Dix-Hallpike to the left. (From Seffinger M. *Foundations of Osteopathic Medicine*. 4th ed. Wolters Kluwer; 2019. Figure 48.5.)

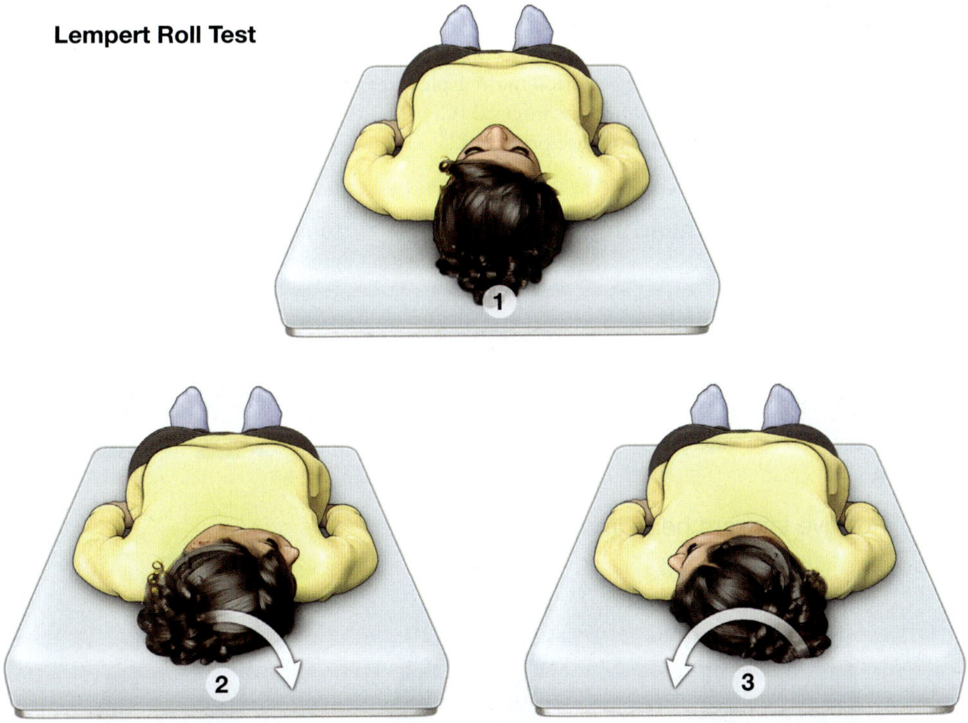

Figure 7.5: Supine roll test. The patient's head is moved rapidly from the straight supine position (1) to the right side (2). Observe for horizontal nystagmus and note the direction and intensity. Then move the patient's head back to the straight position (1) for 15 seconds. Then move the head from straight to the head left position (3) and note any nystagmus and its direction and intensity. If the nystagmus is of the geotropic type, the side resulting in the strongest nystagmus is taken to be the affected side.

- Unidirectional, gaze-evoked nystagmus is also because of a disrupted vestibulo-ocular reflex.
- If no nystagmus is present, it is bidirectional nystagmus; or if there is vertical or pure torsional component, consider a central etiology.[1]
- No skew deviation on eye examination is suggestive of a central cause.
- Plus there is no hearing loss, which if present is suggestive of a central cause.

The Head Impulse Test

The vestibulo-ocular reflex allows the retina to stay focused on an object while the head is in motion. The left and right vestibular nuclei normally have an equal discharge rate. However, if one of the nuclei is affected, unidirectional horizontal nystagmus develops toward the affected side, and a lateral catch-up saccade is seen on movement of the head away from the affected side (see **Figure 7.6**). The head impulse test assesses disruption of the vestibulo-ocular reflex.[3] A cerebellar/posterior stroke (usually from the AICA) preserves the vestibulo-ocular reflex because it affects both the left and right vestibular nuclei and the labyrinth.[8] When the vestibular nerve is inflamed and the head is moved, there is a delay in refixation called a "saccade." Central etiologies, such as a stroke, may cause a saccade as well, so the rest of HINTS + no hearing loss must be performed. If horizontal nystagmus is not present, one cannot reliably diagnose acute VN, and a central cause should be pursued. See the following videos to demonstrate the HINTS examination in total. (Demonstration of the steps of HINTS in someone without vertigo: https://collections.lib.utah.edu/details?id=1209722.[6] HINTS in VN: https://collections.lib.utah.edu/details?id=1277126.[6])

Management

Posterior Canal BPPV: Epley Maneuver

The treatment involves using an Epley maneuver as a means of displacing the otolith from the canal back to the utricle (**Figure 7.7**). The 2014 updated Cochrane review based on 11 trials reported complete resolution of vertigo more often in the Epley treatment group when compared with sham (odds ratio [OR] 4.42; 95% confidence interval [CI], 2.62 to 7.44).[9] Table 7.2 summarizes the discharge criteria for the different disease processes.[10]

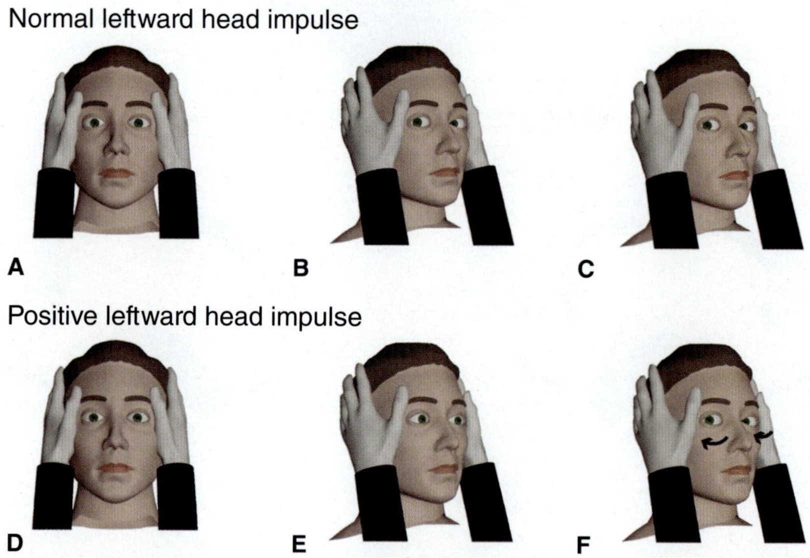

Figure 7.6: The head impulse test. The top panel illustrates a normal (negative) head impulse test. The subject fixes on a near target (the examiner's nose). A, When the head is turned left, the intact left horizontal VOR produces an equal and opposite eye movement that returns the eye to the target (B, C). The bottom panel shows a VOR deficit (D). E, When the head is turned leftward, the eyes initially move with the head. F, A refixation saccade, or catch-up saccade, returns the eye to the target. VOR, vestibulo-ocular reflex.

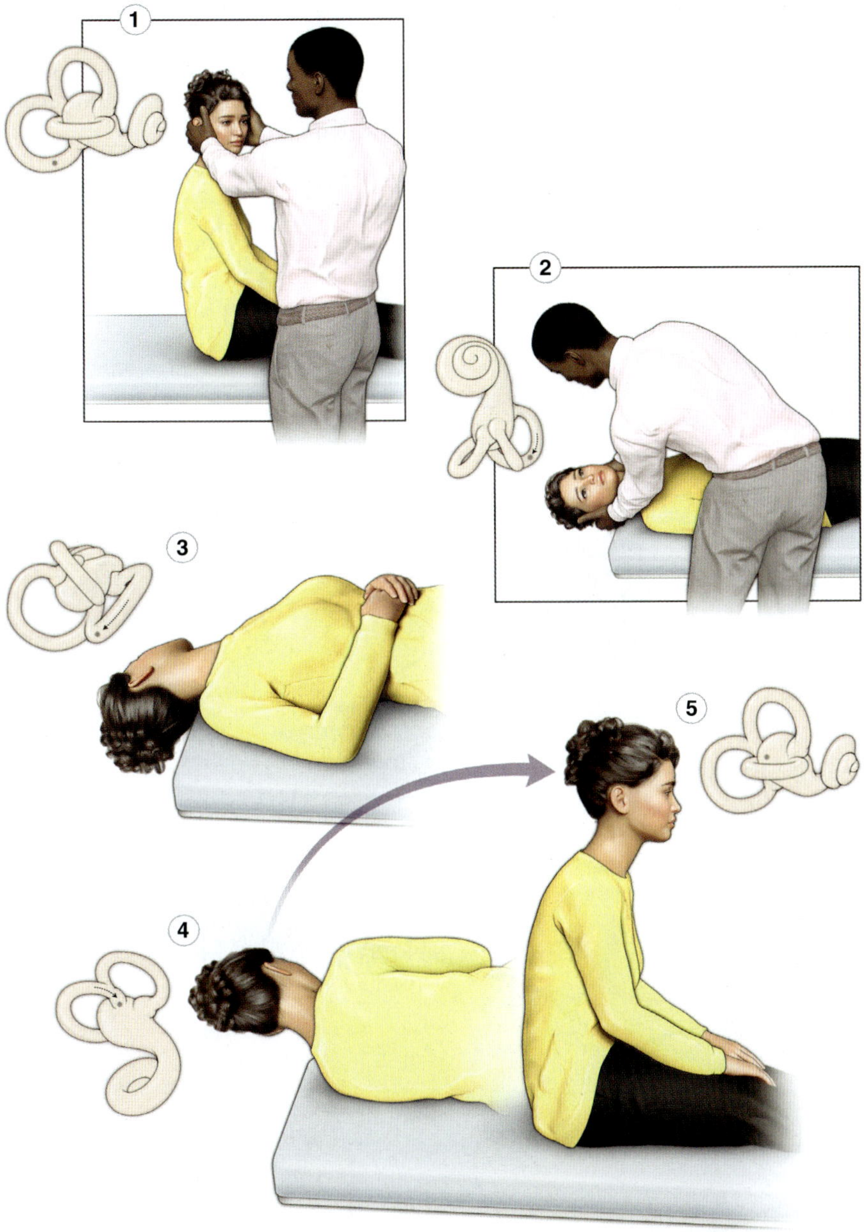

Figure 7.7: Canalith (Canalolith) repositioning maneuver for right side. Steps: (1) Have the patient sit on a table positioned so that they may be laid back to the head-hanging position with the neck in slight extension. Stabilize the head and move it 45° toward the side to be tested. (2) Move the head, neck, and shoulders all together to avoid neck strain. Observe the eyes for nystagmus; hold them open, if necessary. If nystagmus is seen, wait for all nystagmus to abate and hold the position for another 15 seconds. (3) While the head is slightly hyperextended, turn the head 90° toward the opposite side, and wait 30 seconds. (4) Roll the body to the lateral body position, turn the patient's head toward the ground so that the patient is facing straight down, and hold for 15 seconds. (5) While maintaining the head position unchanged relative to the shoulders, have the patient sit up and hold on to the patient for 5 seconds or so to guard against momentary dizziness upon sitting up. This maneuver may be repeated several times or until symptoms and nystagmus cannot be reproduced. As an alternative, a clinician can use the Semont maneuver, where the patient is laid from side to side.

Horizontal Canal BPPV: Lempert 360° Roll

The treatment for horizontal canal BPPV is called the Lempert 360° roll maneuver/BBQ roll test (**Figure 7.8**). Horizontal canal BPPV is a self-limited disease process. Another technique, forced prolonged positioning, involves instructing patients to sleep on the unaffected ear for many hours. About 90% of cases resolve in 1 week, and all resolve within 4 weeks.[7]

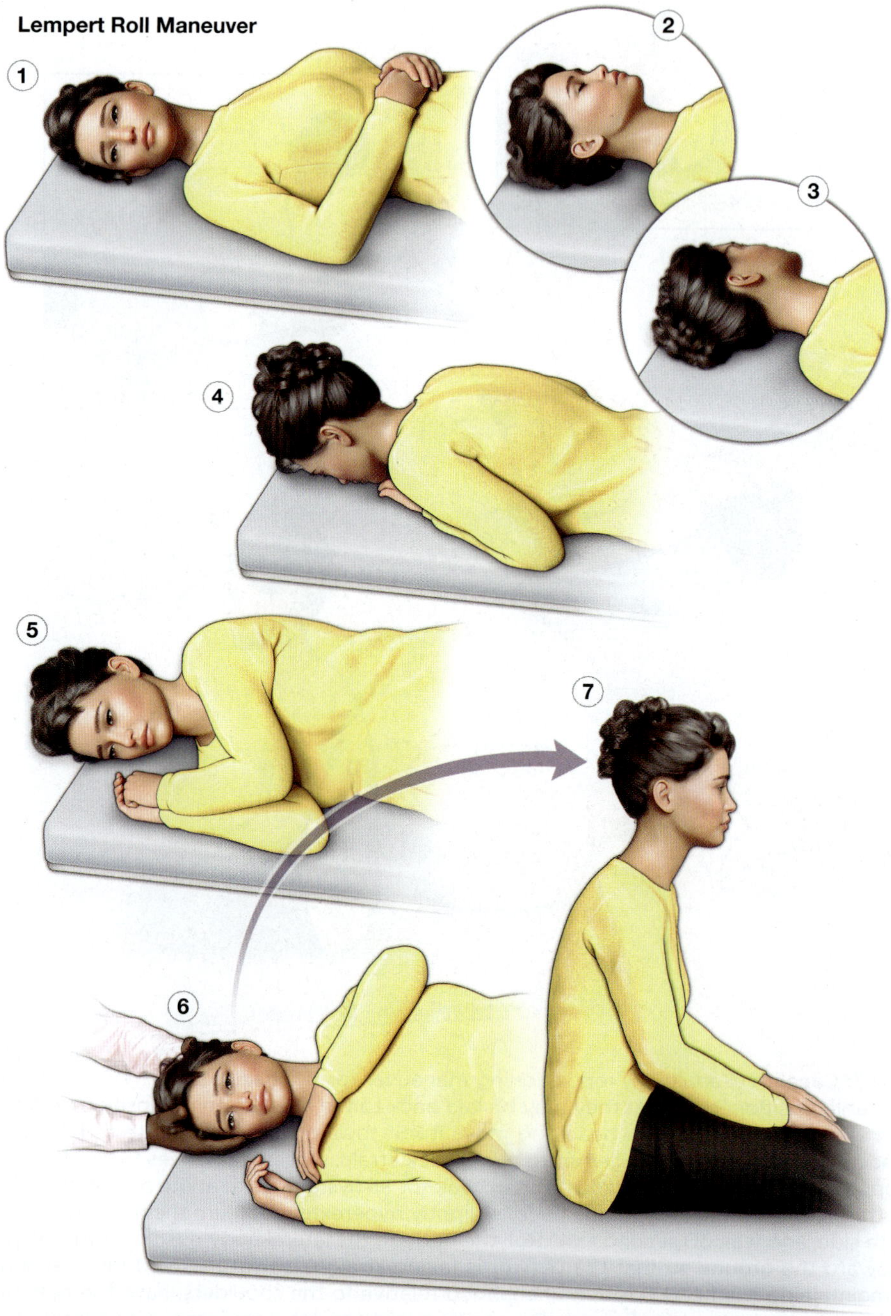

Figure 7.8: The Lempert 360° roll maneuver for the treatment of right horizontal canal benign paroxysmal positional vertigo with geotropic-type nystagmus. Numbers 1 to 7 depict the sequential steps in the maneuver.

Vestibular Neuritis

The traditional treatment is intravenous or oral steroids, though evidence of efficacy is limited.[7]

Computed tomography of the head without contrast is not indicated for dizziness unless there is a concern for hemorrhage. Magnetic resonance imaging (MRI) also has poor sensitivity in the first 24 hours, given the small vessels that are typically affected in dizziness owing to stroke.

TIPS AND PEARLS

1. Learn the Epley maneuver: OR of 4.24.
2. Use a systematic approach: 3-TTT.
3. When in doubt, walk the patient.
4. On the HINTS examination, the presence of any one of the exclusion criteria warrants workup for a central cause. You do not need to perform all of HINTS → If they have any one of the exclusion criteria, they need a neurology consult/MRI/admission.
5. Although migraine is a common cause of vertigo, it is important to rule out central causes in these patients. Therefore, the diagnosis often requires full workup including an MRI unless presentation is classic for VM.
6. Ideally, observe nystagmus in a dark room without visual fixation on a finger. Peripheral causes of nystagmus can be suppressed by fixation.
7. If there is horizontal nystagmus with episodic vertigo, it is horizontal canal BPPV rather than the more common posterior canal BPPV, and therefore needs a simple but effective BBQ roll test to fix.
8. For a Dix-Hallpike or a supine roll, it is important to wait 10 seconds after moving the head to allow the otolith to roll, causing the appropriate nystagmus.
9. Hearing loss and ataxia should raise suspicion for a serious cause.
10. Remember the deadly D's (dysarthria, dysphagia, dysphonia, dysmetria, diplopia), which may signify stroke.

EVIDENCE

TiTrATE has been shown to work at the hands of a neurologist, but does it have benefit in the hands of physicians? A recent paper demonstrated that after a 9-hour course, internal medicine interns using the 3-TTT method performed better than graduating residents at more accurately diagnosing dizziness with fewer unnecessary tests.[11]

Is the HINTS examination better than MRI? HINTS is more effective at ruling out stroke than MRI and has the reliability to rule in acute VN, thus saving on unnecessary tests. Recently, it was shown that the addition of hearing loss to HINTS called "HINTS PLUS" even further increased its sensitivity to 99% from 96% (LR+ 32, LR− 0.01) without decreasing its specificity.[12] A recent meta-analysis showed that HINTS in the hands of emergency providers was not reliable to rule out stroke when compared to official neurology consultation.[13]

If I cannot figure out how to perform the HINTS+ examination, can I test for truncal ataxia and rule out stroke that way? The lack of ataxia has a 90% sensitivity at ruling out stroke though it will not rule in acute VN, and there is a chance you may miss a stroke mimicking a benign cause if you do not perform HINTS+.[14] Therefore, if you use truncal ataxia as your test of choice, have a low threshold for advanced imaging/admission/neurology follow-up.

References

1. Newman-Toker DE, Edlow JA. TiTrATE: a novel, evidence-based approach to diagnosing acute dizziness and vertigo. *Neurol Clin*. 2015;33(3):577-599. doi:10.1016/j.ncl.2015.04.011

2. Omron R, Kotwal S, Garibaldi BT, Newman-Toker DE. The diagnostic performance feedback "calibration gap": why clinical experience alone is not enough to prevent serious diagnostic errors. *AEM Educ Train*. 2018;2(4):339-342. doi:10.1002/aet2.10119

3. Khan S, Chang R. Anatomy of the vestibular system: a review. *NeuroRehabilitation*. 2013;32(3): 437-443. doi:10.3233/NRE-130866
4. Fife TD, von Brevern M. Benign paroxysmal positional vertigo in the acute care setting. *Neurol Clin*. 2015;33(3):601-617. doi:10.1016/j.ncl.2015.04.003
5. Seemungal B, Kaski D, Lopez-Escamez JA. Early diagnosis and management of acute vertigo from vestibular migraine and Ménière's disease. *Neurol Clin*. 2015;33(3):619-628. doi:10.1016/j.ncl.2015.04.008
6. NOVEL. The Dan Gold neuro-ophthalmology collection. Accessed May 10, 2021. https://novel.utah.edu/Gold/
7. Welgampola MS, Bradshaw AP, Lechner C, Halmagyi GM. Bedside assessment of acute dizziness and vertigo. *Neurol Clin*. 2015;33(3):551-564. doi:10.1016/j.ncl.2015.04.001
8. Kerber KA, Newman-Toker DE. Misdiagnosing dizzy patients: common pitfalls in clinical practice. *Neurol Clin*. 2015;33(3):565-575. doi:10.1016/j.ncl.2015.04.009
9. Bhattacharyya N, Gubbels SP, Schwartz SR, et al. Clinical practice guideline: benign paroxysmal positional vertigo (update). *Otolaryngol Head Neck Surg*. 2017;156(3_suppl):S1-S47. doi:10.1177/0194599816689667
10. NOVEL. The David Newman-Toker neuro-ophthalmology collection. Accessed May 10, 2021. https://novel.utah.edu/Newman-Toker/
11. Kotwal S, Fanai M, Fu W, et al. Real-world virtual patient simulation to improve diagnostic performance through deliberate practice: a prospective quasi-experimental study. *Diagnosis*. 2021;8(4): 489-496. doi:10.1515/dx-2020-0127
12. Kattah JC, Talkad AV, Wang DZ, Hsieh Y-H, Newman-Toker DE. HINTS to diagnose stroke in the acute vestibular syndrome: three-step bedside oculomotor examination more sensitive than early MRI diffusion-weighted imaging. *Stroke*. 2009;40(11):3504-3510. doi:10.1161/STROKEAHA.109.551234
13. Ohle R, Montpellier RA, Marchadier V, et al. Can emergency physicians accurately rule out a central cause of vertigo using the HINTS examination? A systematic review and meta-analysis. *Acad Emerg Med*. 2020;27(9):887-896. doi:10.1111/acem.13960
14. Carmona S, Martínez C, Zalazar G, et al. The diagnostic accuracy of truncal ataxia and HINTS as cardinal signs for acute vestibular syndrome. *Front Neurol*. 2016;7:125. doi:10.3389/fneur.2016.00125

CHAPTER 8

Tympanic Membrane Perforation: Traumatic, Infectious

Rupal S. Jain
Dunia Abdul-Aziz

THE CLINICAL CHALLENGE

The tympanic membrane (TM) is a thin, three-layered tissue that divides the external auditory canal from the middle ear. The TM functions to amplify and transmit sound vibration to the ossicles, which in turn transmit that acoustic stimulation to the inner ear (cochlea). Perforations of the TM therefore lead to varying degrees of predominantly conductive, or mechanical, hearing loss, depending on their sizes and locations. Although most perforations heal spontaneously within 4 weeks, morbidity associated with TM perforations is reduced with early identification, treatment of underlying infection or disease, recognition of more complicated/severe cases, and appropriate referral.

TM perforation occurs most commonly as a complication of a middle ear infection, but it can also occur owing to rapid changes in pressure (barotrauma), blunt and penetrating trauma, acoustic trauma, and middle ear disease (eg, cholesteatoma). The diagnosis of TM perforation is mainly clinical, relying on history and physical examination findings. Clinicians must have a high index of suspicion in children with acute otitis media (AOM) with drainage and in adult patients with trauma. Complete visualization of the TM may not always be possible with a limited otoscopic examination. Certain features of the history may suggest perforation, such as symptoms of AOM, followed by aural purulence or blood, which relieves the pain. Direct visualization of the TM is important to distinguish otorrhea caused by otitis externa (OE) from otorrhea caused by otitis media (OM) with perforation, because management differs. Certain topical antibiotics containing gentamicin, neomycin, or tobramycin are ototoxic and cause sensorineural hearing loss; these should be avoided in the setting of perforation. Although most cases of TM perforation have a favorable prognosis, ENT follow-up is required to ensure healing, recovery of hearing, and intervention for progressive and destructive cases that may necessitate surgical intervention.

PATHOPHYSIOLOGY

Traumatic Perforation

Traumatic TM perforation or rupture often presents with acute pain in response to an exposure. Examples include barotrauma (eg, scuba diving or rapid changes in pressure during air travel), acoustic trauma (eg, loud blast), blunt trauma (eg, open-handed slap across the ear), penetrating trauma (eg, cotton swabs), chemical and thermal burns (eg, slag injuries), and iatrogenic injury (eg, during cerumen/foreign body removal).[1] Any of these forces transmitted to the less-than-one-millimeter-thick TM can cause either a partial tear or a complete rupture, impeding conduction of sound vibrations. Studies have suggested that larger-sized perforations, perforations in the posterior or anterior quadrants, and perforations that contact the manubrium of the malleus portend more severe hearing loss.[2]

Infectious Perforation

Infectious TM perforations most commonly result from an acute middle ear infection, or AOM. They can also result from OE, which may be bacterial and/or fungal (otomycosis), as well as superinfection of chronic middle ear disease (chronic OM, cholesteatoma). In AOM, which is defined by a suppurative process of short-term or sudden onset with infected fluid in the middle ear and associated inflammation of the middle ear mucosa, the increased pressure from middle ear infection results in spontaneous rupture through the TM. The most common infectious pathogen associated with AOM with TM perforation is nontypeable *Haemophilus influenzae* (approximately 50% of cases) followed by *Streptococcus pneumoniae* and *Moraxella catarrhalis*.[3] Viral infection can cause TM perforation, either as the primary infectious agent or as a coinfection with a bacterium. Severe outer ear infections, usually fungal, can also result in TM perforation, with *Aspergillus niger* and then *Candida* being the most common culprits in these cases.[4]

Risk factors for developing TM perforation in the setting of infection include severity of infection, duration of infection, recurrent infections, underlying otologic disease (eg, cholesteatoma) and prior surgery or trauma to the TM and middle ear (eg, tympanostomy tube placement). These factors can be gathered in the history and increase the suspicion for perforation.

APPROACH/THE FOCUSED EXAM

TM perforation is a clinical diagnosis defined by the presence of a hole in the TM (**Figure 8.1A** and **B**). The exam should note the size and location of the perforation. Size should be described as a percentage relative to the entire TM. Location should be described relative to the manubrium of the malleus. On pneumatic otoscopy, the perforated TM is immobile, because a pressure seal cannot be formed. A 512 Hz tuning fork can help distinguish the conductive versus sensorineural nature of the hearing loss; with a TM perforation, a conductive hearing loss pattern (Weber lateralizes to the affected ear, Rinne negative [bone conduction louder than air conduction] in severe cases) is expected. Details of the tuning fork exam are more completely described in Chapter 2.

AOM with TM perforation is characterized by an erythematous and bulging TM, with drainage emanating from the middle ear. In these cases, the ear canal is typically filled with pus but is not itself markedly inflamed. In contrast, perforations that arise from AOE typically manifest with a tender, edematous, and erythematous ear canal. In cases of otomycosis, fungal elements are characteristically seen in the ear canal along with perforation. The ear canal may be occluded with purulent or bloody discharge, obscuring a view of the TM. It is important to be cautious when clearing cerumen, debris, and drainage from the canal. Irrigation should be avoided owing to potential contamination of water in the middle ear space. If there is blood or pus present, ENT should be consulted before evacuation. Similarly, penetrating foreign bodies should not be removed without ENT consultation in order to determine the need for operative removal of foreign bodies to minimize risk of further damage and injury.

Patients may complain of vertigo and have evidence of nystagmus or gait disturbance on physical examination. The examination should also exclude other potential diagnoses like cholesteatoma (**Figure 8.1C**), TM retraction (**Figure 8.1D**), and granulation tissue.

Imaging is not routinely necessary, because TM perforation is a clinical diagnosis. Computed tomography (CT) imaging of the temporal bone may be indicated in the setting of perforation with complicating factors such as facial nerve palsy, severe/profound hearing loss, vestibular symptoms (nausea, vertigo, ataxia, nystagmus), cholesteatoma, concern for a retained foreign body, or in cases of severe head trauma with skull fracture. In the latter setting, opacification of the mastoid air cells and fracture line(s) may be apparent on head CT.

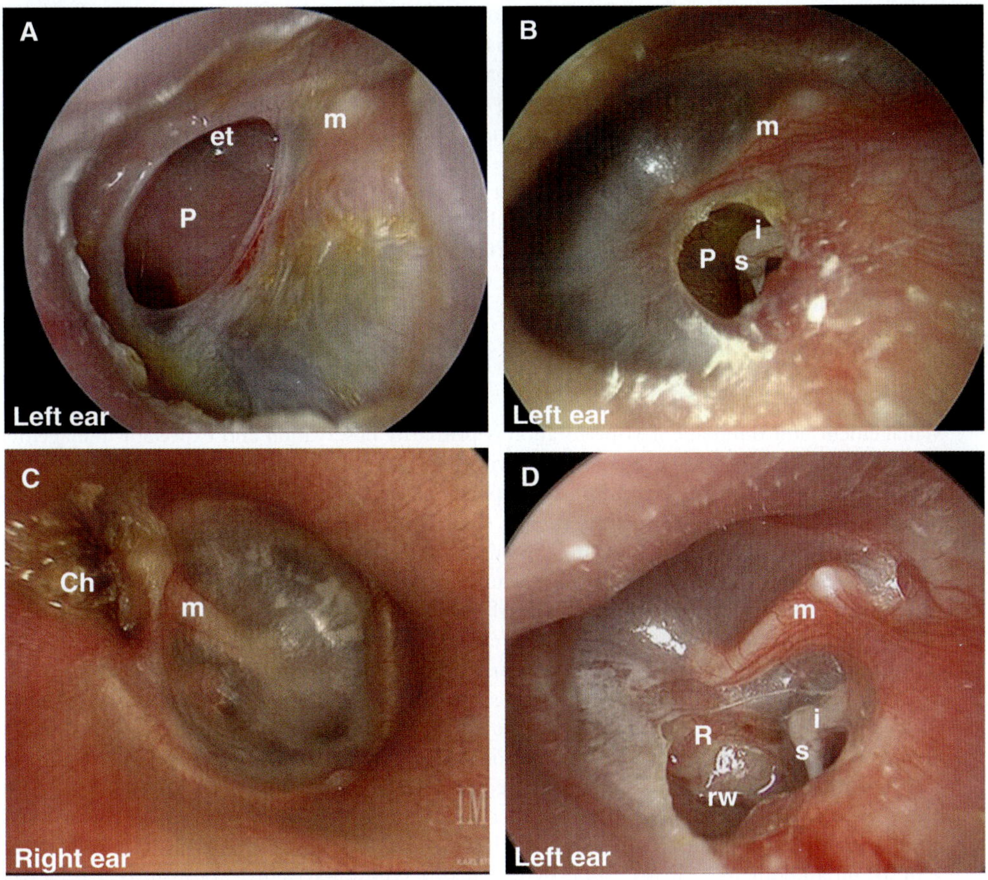

Figure 8.1: Tympanic membrane (TM) pathologies. Endoscopic views of TM highlighting perforations and other diseases of the TM. A: Anterior TM perforation (P) relative to the malleus (m) extending to the anterior margin toward the eustachian tube (et). B: Posterior TM perforation (P) with visualization of the incus (i) and stapes (s). C: Retracted TM with superior defect and impacted debris consistent with attic cholesteatoma (Ch). D: TM retraction (R) without true perforation. The retracted TM is thin and translucent, giving the illusion of a perforation. Retraction extends to the incus (i), stapes (s), and cochlear promontory, with round window (rw) niche in view.

DIFFERENTIAL DIAGNOSIS

In the case of a traumatic TM perforation, it is also important to evaluate for other associated injuries with similar symptomatology, including:

- *Basilar skull fracture*: Patients with raccoon eyes, Battle sign (mastoid ecchymosis), and CSF rhinorrhea should be evaluated with CT scan for this complication of blunt or penetrating trauma.
- *Dislocation of the ossicular chain/fracture of the stapedial footplate*: Usually presents with more severe hearing loss. Noncontrast CT images of the temporal bones identify joint separation of the ossicles.
- *Perilymph fistula*: The presence of an abnormal connection between the middle and the inner ear is detected by vestibular signs such as vertigo, nystagmus, vomiting, and ataxia. On physical examination, patients may have the fistula (Hennebert) sign. With this sign, nystagmus is elicited by applying intermittent pressure on the tragus or with sealed pneumatic otoscopy to simulate pressure changes in the ear canal, suggesting that the labyrinth (inner ear) is connected or stimulated.

TM perforation should be distinguished from a retraction pocket, which is an area of the TM that has been pulled into the middle ear owing to dysventilation (Figure 8.1A-D). Retraction pockets typically occur in the posterior superior aspect of the TM (pars flaccida) but can also occur at other sites of the TM. Underlying eustachian tube dysfunction with resultant chronic negative pressure in the middle ear can give rise to retraction. Posterior TM retractions can extend to, abut, or erode through the incus and stapes, giving the illusion of perforation. It is important to recognize TM retractions, as they can result in hearing loss and cholesteatoma formation if epithelium is trapped in the pockets. These patients deserve full outpatient ENT evaluation.

After a TM perforation has healed or at the site of prior tympanostomy tube, the TM may heal thinly, in only two layers (epithelial and mucosal layer); this "dimeric" TM is thin, nearly translucent, and may give the illusion of a perforation. Pneumatic otoscopy can help elucidate this scenario, as a mobile TM would be observed.

MANAGEMENT

Traumatic Perforation

Management of a traumatic TM perforation is primarily observation and expectant management. Most perforations heal without intervention within 4 weeks, and associated conductive hearing loss resolves. Two main factors predict failure to spontaneously heal: the size of perforation and the occurrence of secondary infection. Therefore, in the ED or urgent care setting, patients must receive instructions for the prevention of water exposure to the affected ear to prevent secondary suppurative OM. Measures include avoidance of swimming and occlusion of the ear canal with petroleum-impregnated cotton when showering. Prophylactic antibiotics are not indicated in the case of dry trauma (eg, a blow to the side of the face). However, antipseudomonal ototopical antibiotics should be prescribed in cases of trauma with suspected entry of water into the middle ear (eg, barotrauma while scuba diving) as prophylaxis against OE. It is reasonable to administer tetanus prophylaxis as well.

Other standard precautions include avoidance of forceful nose blowing or valsalva. Pain should be managed with acetaminophen or nonsteroidal anti-inflammatory drugs.

In simple cases, follow-up can be arranged with ENT for otoscopic evaluation of TM healing and to perform audiometry for improved hearing acuity after 4 weeks. Prompter evaluation by ENT is required for patients with significant hearing loss (decreased perception of normal speech, >40 dB on audiometry), suspected perilymph fistula (vestibular signs), concern for basilar skull fracture, or facial nerve injury. Finally, certain patterns of trauma (eg, bilateral auricular hematoma) or other presentations where the injury does not match the history of reported mechanism should raise concern for physical abuse, particularly in the pediatric population.

Infectious Perforation

Central to management of infectious TM perforation is treatment of the underlying etiology. In cases of AOM with TM rupture, treatment should be with oral and ototopical antibiotics. In a case of AOE complicated by TM rupture, treatment should focus on removal of the infectious debris in the ear canal and ototopical antimicrobial therapy. In the unique setting of otomycosis with TM rupture, clotrimazole is the most common solution used but can be irritating to the middle ear mucosa, resulting in burning sensation.[4] Water precautions should be maintained until the infection has resolved and TM perforation healed. In recalcitrant cases, culture-directed therapy should be considered, guided by sampling of the fluid in the ear canal. Patients should follow up with an ENT specialist to ensure resolution of infection and to monitor the perforation. In patients with recurrent infection or other complicating factors (cholesteatoma, large perforation, significant hearing loss, facial nerve weakness, mastoiditis, or abscess), ENT referral is recommended.

TIPS AND PEARLS

- In cases of TM perforation with complicating pathology such as facial nerve weakness, vertigo, profound hearing loss, concern for acute mastoiditis, trauma with presence of blood in the canal, or penetrating foreign body, ENT consultation is urgently warranted.
- Most cases of TM perforation heal without intervention within 4 weeks. Nonemergent follow-up is required to ensure healing, recovery of hearing, or intervention for cases of nonhealing perforations.

- The size of the perforation predicts the potential to heal as well as the degree of long-term hearing loss.
- In the pediatric patient with traumatic TM perforation, the potential for child abuse should be considered if supported by additional history or physical exam findings.

EVIDENCE

Does size or location of perforation affect degree of hearing loss?

Conductive hearing loss from TM perforation occurs more significantly in the lower frequencies of sound. The degree of hearing loss is greater with increasing size of perforation, but location of perforation matters less in terms of hearing effect.[5]

Are antibiotics required for prophylaxis in traumatic perforation?

Unlike perforations caused by a suppurative complication of AOM, traumatic TM perforations are often dry and do not require systemic antibiotics. One prospective study demonstrated that ototopical antibiotics shortened the duration of perforation and increased the rate of spontaneous healing but did not prevent the development of AOM or improve hearing.[6] Antibiotics are therefore not routinely indicated. Topical fluoroquinolones such as ciprofloxacin or ofloxacin should, however, be prescribed in cases of a contaminated perforation, especially with water exposure.

References

1. Carniol ET, Bresler A, Shaigany K, et al. Traumatic tympanic membrane perforations diagnosed in emergency departments. *JAMA Otolaryngol Head Neck Surg*. 2018;144(2):136-139. doi:10.1001/jamaoto.2017.2550
2. Aslıer M, Özay H, Gürkan S, Kırkım G, Güneri EA. The effect of tympanic membrane perforation site, size and middle ear volume on hearing loss. *Turk Arch Otorhinolaryngol*. 2019;57(2):86-90. doi:10.5152/tao.2019.4015
3. Marchisio P, Esposito S, Picca M, et al. Prospective evaluation of the aetiology of acute otitis media with spontaneous tympanic membrane perforation. *Clin Microbiol Infect*. 2017;23(7):486.e1-486.e6. doi:10.1016/j.cmi.2017.01.010. Epub 2017 Jan 19. PMID: 28110050.
4. Koltsidopoulos P, Skoulakis C. Otomycosis with tympanic membrane perforation: a review of the literature. *Ear Nose Throat J*. 2020;99(8):518-521. doi:10.1177/0145561319851499. Epub 2019 May 29. PMID: 31142158.
5. Mehta RP, Rosowski JJ, Voss SE, O'Neil E, Merchant SN. Determinants of hearing loss in perforations of the tympanic membrane. *Otol Neurotol*. 2006;27(2):136-143. doi:10.1097/01.mao.0000176177.17636.53. PMID: 16436981; PMCID: PMC2918411.
6. Lou Z, Lou Z, Tang Y, Xiao J. The effect of ofloxacin otic drops on the regeneration of human traumatic tympanic membrane perforations. *Clin Otolaryngol*. 2016;41(5):564-570. doi:10.1111/coa.12564

CHAPTER 9

Facial Paralysis

Kathryn Noonan
Anne Katz

THE CLINICAL CHALLENGE

Facial paralysis, whether partial or complete, causes significant morbidity, impairing the ability to smile, blink, eat, and even taste. Moreover, the alteration of one's physical appearance can have significant psychosocial implications, leading to social isolation and depression.[1]

The facial nerve is primarily responsible for motor innervation of the muscles of facial expression but also carries special sensory fibers supplying taste and parasympathetic fibers controlling salivary function and lacrimation. It can be injured anywhere along its complex course from the brainstem, through the temporal bone and into the face.

FACIAL NERVE ANATOMY

The central portion of the facial nerve includes the supranuclear tracts, facial nucleus (lower pons) and brainstem components. Importantly, the superior portion of the motor nucleus, which innervates the upper face, receives bilateral central innervation from the corticobulbar tracts. This anatomy explains why a patient with a stroke or acute central pathology will have forehead-sparing paralysis.[2]

The intracranial segment of the facial nerve enters the skull base at the internal acoustic meatus, transverses the internal auditory canal, then exits the meatal foramen to form the labyrinthine segment on its way to the geniculate ganglion. The nerve is commonly injured in this perigeniculate location owing to localized inflammation and swelling within a narrow bony channel (**Figure 9.1**). At the geniculate ganglion, it joins the greater superficial petrosal nerve to supply parasympathetic innervation for the lacrimal, salivary, nasal, palatine, and pharyngeal mucous glands. The tympanic and mastoid segments of the nerve then travel through the middle ear and mastoid to exit at the stylomastoid foramen. The extratemporal segment courses through the parotid gland and ultimately give rise to the five nerves that are responsible for facial motor function—the temporal, zygomatic, buccal, mandibular, and cervical branches.[3]

PATHOPHYSIOLOGY

A facial nerve injury can present as weakness, spastic or flaccid paralysis, depending on the extent of damage. Severity of weakness can be described using the House-Brackmann scale. Incomplete paralysis, or a lower House-Brackmann score, indicates an excellent prognosis, whereas complete paralysis is associated with poorer outcomes and requires an urgent referral to a specialist (**Table 9.1**).

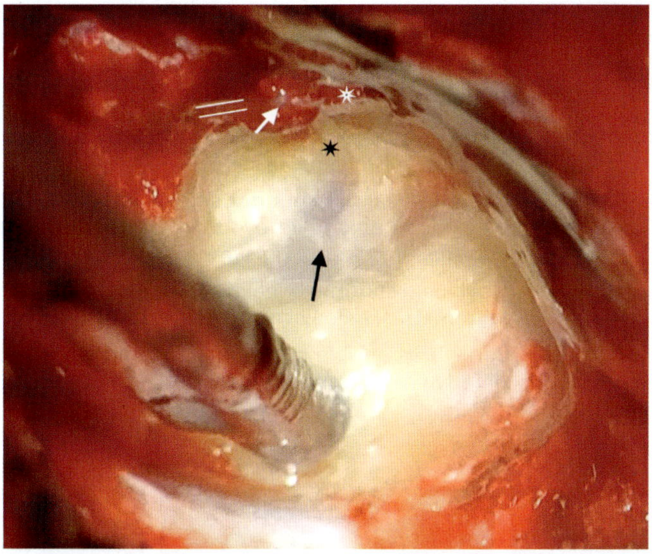

Figure 9.1: Surgical representation of the facial nerve and its course as seen during a facial nerve decompression for a patient with complete right paralysis from Bell palsy. The geniculate ganglion (white arrow) is noted to be inflamed and edematous. Black arrow: internal auditory canal, black star: labyrinthine segment of facial nerve, white arrow: geniculate ganglion, parallel lines: greater superficial petrosal nerve, white star: tympanic segment of facial nerve.

The degree of injury predicts recovery and dictates management. Neuropraxia is the mildest form of injury, where the nerve remains intact but a conduction block exists. It is usually a result of compression or interrupted blood flow to the nerve, and although it may take days to months, a complete recovery is expected. Axonotmesis, a more severe form of injury, involves disruption of the nerve axon with preservation of the epineurium or support structures. Neurotmesis is the most severe form of nerve injury and results from complete disruption of nerve fibers.

Over the first 72 hours, axons distal to the injury suffer Wallerian degeneration, which often results in worsening of paralysis over the first few days. After 72 hours, electroneuronography (ENoG) can be used to quantify the extent of weakness, and electromyography (EMG) can look for voluntary movement.

APPROACH/THE FOCUSED EXAM

Common complaints of facial neuropathy include facial droop, eye irritation, taste changes, and lacrimal dysfunction. Patients should be questioned about constitutional symptoms, ear pain, otorrhea, hearing loss, tinnitus, dizziness, hyperacusis, and rashes. In addition, a history of recent trauma, surgery, travel, tick bites, and cutaneous or parotid malignancies should be obtained. It is also critical to ask about recurrent episodes.[4]

On physical exam, facial motor function is assessed by asking the patient to close the eyes, elevate the brows, smile, and puff cheeks (**Figure 9.2**). The degree of paralysis should be noted with a detailed description or using the House-Brackmann Scale (see Table 9.1). Additionally, any evidence of synkinesis should be noted. The presence of vesicles or crusted lesions in the external auditory canal, palate, and face may indicate Ramsey-Hunt syndrome. The parotid gland should be palpated carefully to evaluate for masses. The ear should be examined for evidence of otitis media and externa.

A complete neurologic exam should be performed to distinguish an upper motor neuron facial nerve palsy from a lower motor neuron palsy. Central lesions are more likely to spare the forehead, present as a spastic paralysis, and have focal extremity weakness or numbness. Paralysis caused by

TABLE 9.1 House-Brackmann Grading System for Facial Paralysis

Grade	Description	Characteristics
I	Normal	Symmetric function
II	Mild dysfunction	Slight weakness noticeable on close inspection, complete eyelid closure with minimal effort
III	Moderate dysfunction	Obvious weakness but not significantly disfiguring, may or may not be able to lift eyebrow, complete eyelid closure with maximal effort, strong asymmetric smile
IV	Moderately severe dysfunction	Obvious disfiguring weakness, incomplete eyelid closure, asymmetric smile with maximal effort
V	Severe dysfunction	Barely perceptible movement, incomplete eyelid closure, can slightly move corner of mouth
VI	Complete paralysis	No movement

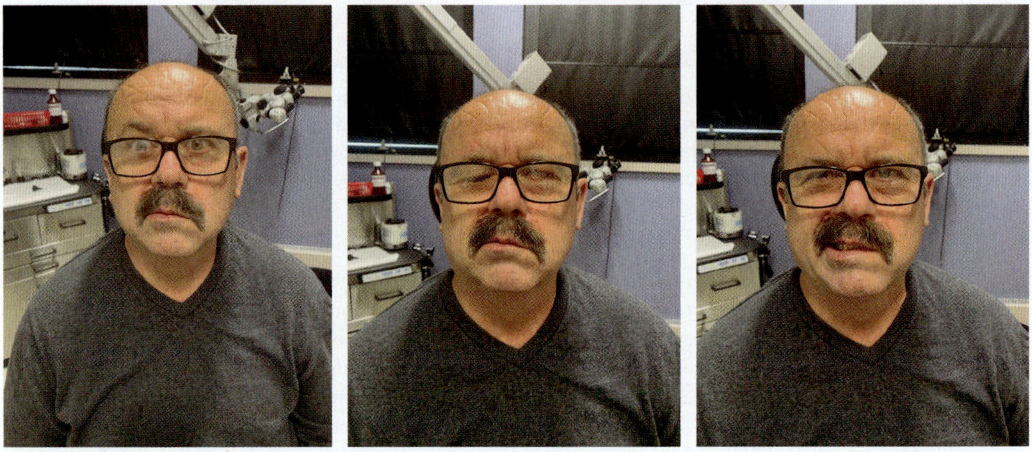

A B C

Figure 9.2: Patient with left facial paralysis from Bell palsy. (A) asymmetric at rest, (B) incomplete eye closure, (C) asymmetric smile.

peripheral lesions will typically include the forehead and present with flaccid paralysis. Central causes of facial palsies are commonly vascular in etiology but may also be neoplastic, infectious, or autoimmune.

Particular attention should be paid to vestibular and auditory function. Any additional cranial nerve palsies, dysphagia, or diplopia should be noted. Any localizing findings warrant additional workup that often involves magnetic resonance imaging (MRI) with and without contrast of the head and internal auditory canal. Interestingly, patients with Bell palsy (BP) may complain of accompanying numbness, which is thought to be caused by the connections between the maxillary branch of the trigeminal nerve and the sphenopalatine ganglion. Additionally, decreased sensation over the ipsilateral conchal bowl may be reported if the facial nerve is affected proximal to the stylomastoid foramen.[5]

DIFFERENTIAL DIAGNOSIS

The differential diagnosis for acute facial paralysis is broad and can be divided into categories: idiopathic, infectious, traumatic, neoplastic, systemic/autoimmune, metabolic, otologic, iatrogenic, and central (**Table 9.2**).

TABLE 9.2 Differential Diagnosis for Acute Facial Paralysis

Idiopathic Bell palsy	**Central Causes** Stroke Brainstem tumor
Infectious Ramsay Hunt syndrome Lyme disease Other viruses: HIV, HSV-6, EBV, CMV, Syphilis, TB Acute otitis media Skull base osteomyelitis (malignant otitis externa) Petrous apicitis	**Systemic/Autoimmune** Sarcoidosis, SLE, Bachet, Wegner Melkersson-Rosenthal syndrome Guillain Barre syndrome Multiple sclerosis Amyloidosis
Traumatic Temporal bone fractures Soft tissue injury to cheek	**Surgical** Neurosurgical procedure Ear surgery Parotid surgery
Neoplastic Vestibular and facial schwannoma Hemangioma Parotid neoplasms Temporal bone neoplasms Cholesteatoma	**Metabolic** Pregnancy Hypothyroidism

BP, also known as idiopathic facial paralysis, is the most common cause of facial paralysis. It is characterized by its acute onset (less than 72 hours) with no associated neurologic or other physical exam findings. BP does not require laboratory studies or additional imaging, but, importantly, is clinically a diagnosis of exclusion. The annual incidence of BP ranges from 11.5 to 40.2 per 100 000 and frequently occurs between the ages of 15 and 45. Hypertensive, diabetic, immunocompromised, obese, and pregnant patients are at increased risk for developing BP.[6]

Ramsay Hunt syndrome (RHS) results from reactivation of latent herpes zoster within the geniculate ganglion of the facial nerve. It accounts for 12% of cases of facial paralysis and typically has a poorer prognosis than BP.[7] RHS is characterized by ipsilateral facial paralysis, vesicles along the dermatome of CN7 (auditory canal and pinna), and otalgia. It can also affect the vestibulocochlear nerve (CN8), resulting in tinnitus, hearing loss, and vertigo.

Early disseminated Lyme disease can cause either unilateral or bilateral facial nerve palsies. Other cranial nerves, such as the abducens nerve (CN6), can be impaired as well. Lyme titers should be considered in endemic areas to assist with the diagnosis, although empiric treatment in the emergency department (ED) may be necessary, because serologic testing cannot always definitively diagnose or exclude Lyme disease.

Recurrent paralysis or other neurologic defects accompanying facial paralysis may signify neoplastic and central etiologies, which can be further differentiated with imaging.

MANAGEMENT OF BP

Management of acute facial paralysis depends on the diagnosis. Most patients with acute facial paralysis will have no identifiable cause and can be diagnosed and managed as BP.

Steroids

In randomized controlled trials, high-dose oral corticosteroids prescribed within 72 hours of symptom onset resulted in improved recovery and shorter duration of weakness.[8] Potent corticosteroids relieve the inflammation and edema that causes compression of the facial nerve as it travels through the narrow fallopian canal. The BP Clinical Practice Guideline recommends 10 days of oral steroid therapy with Prednisolone 50 mg × 10 days or Prednisone 60 mg × 5 days with 5-day taper by 10 mg/d in all patients over 16 years of age.[8] Initiation of steroids after 72 hours is less clearly beneficial, and, given the potential adverse effects, risks, and benefits of corticosteroid use, should be considered on a case-by-case basis.

Antivirals

An antiviral may be offered within 72 hours of symptom onset in combination with a corticosteroid, although no strong evidence exists for this practice. Antivirals are frequently used owing to the possible benefit of improved long-term sequelae with minimal adverse reactions. Patients can be prescribed valacyclovir 1000 mg 3 times daily for 1 week or acyclovir 400 mg 5 times daily.

Eye Care

In cases of incomplete eyelid closure, eye protection is critical to prevent corneal abrasions, ulcerations, and exposure keratitis, which result from both incomplete eyelid closure and decreased tear production from the lacrimal gland. Typically, patients with a House-Brackmann score of 4 or above require eye care. Preservative-free artificial tears should be applied at least 4 times a day and as needed for symptomatic dry, scratchy eyes. A moisture chamber can be worn to prevent injury to the eye, or the eye can be taped shut, approximating the lower lid to the lateral aspect of the lateral canthus. Lubricating ointment should be used in the eye while sleeping to keep it maximally protected.

Surgical Decompression

Early surgical decompression of the facial nerve can be considered in patients with complete paralysis, but it is not recommended in cases of partial or incomplete paralysis.

Labs and Imaging in the ED

Routine imaging with computed tomography or MRI is not recommended for idiopathic facial paralysis. However, any red flags suggestive of a stroke, such as dysphagia, extremity weakness, numbness other than ipsilateral CN5, ataxia, or diplopia, warrant advanced imaging and neurologic consultation. Furthermore, any obvious facial masses or recent head trauma should prompt additional imaging. Lyme titers should be considered in endemic areas.

Referral From the ED

All patients with a diagnosis of suspected lower motor neuron facial paralysis should be referred to neurology for close monitoring within 1 to 2 weeks. Severe cases with House-Brackmann scores of 5 to 6 should be referred for urgent ENT consultation within the week. Patients presenting with House-Brackmann scores of 4 to 6 or otherwise complaining of eye discomfort should be referred to ophthalmology. Any patients with associated tinnitus, vertigo, or subjective hearing loss should have a formal hearing evaluation with an audiogram.

TIPS AND PEARLS

- BP is a diagnosis of exclusion.
- Steroids and eye care improve long-term outcomes.
  - **In patients with concomitant cranial nerve VI and VII palsies,** consider early disseminated Lyme disease, multiple sclerosis, petrous apicitis, or pontine stroke.[9]
  - **Bilateral cranial nerve VII palsies.** The presence of a bilateral facial palsy may be attributable to Lyme, sarcoidosis, syphilis, Parkinson disease, Melkersson-Rosenthal syndrome, metastatic disease, HIV, or multiple sclerosis.
  - **Cranial nerve VII and VIII palsies.** The presence of facial palsy with tinnitus, hearing loss, or vertigo may be attributable to RHS or cerebellopontine angle tumor and should be referred for a hearing evaluation.

EVIDENCE

What is the efficacy of steroids in the treatment of BP?

A recent Cochrane review found moderate to high-quality evidence from randomized controlled trials showing significant benefit from treating BP with corticosteroids. Seven trials including 895 participants found that 17% of the steroid group had incomplete recovery compared to 28% of the control group. There was also a reduction in synkinesis in the steroid group. Additionally, in the three trials that reported adverse events from steroids, none were considered serious. Combined analysis found no difference in adverse events between the corticosteroid and placebo groups.[10]

Do antivirals, in addition to steroids, improve clinical outcomes for the treatment of BP?

Multiple meta-analyses of randomized trials have shown that antivirals alone do not improve clinical outcomes. When antivirals are added to steroids, the outcomes are less clear. The most recent meta-analysis from Cochrane, including 14 trials with over 2488 participants with mild, moderate, or severe unilateral BP, concluded that the combination of antivirals and corticosteroids may have little to no effect on rates of recovery compared to corticosteroids alone.[11] However, it did conclude that the combination of antivirals and corticosteroids probably reduces the late sequelae of BP such as synkinesis and crocodile tears (tearing while eating/salivating).

Should imaging be obtained in patients with facial paralysis?

In a retrospective review of 147 patients with facial palsy who underwent MRI, compared to 300 non-palsy controls, peri-geniculate enhancement was found to be specific for BP; however, this did not change management.[12] Additionally, this MRI enhancement can be confused with small tumors, leading to additional unnecessary workup. Therefore, imaging is indicated only if symptoms suggest a possible alternative diagnosis to BP, such as multiple cranial nerve involvements, 3 to 6 months without signs of improvement, bilateral involvement, or slow progressive onset. In these patients, MRI with and without contrast with thin cuts of the internal auditory canal and inclusion of the parotid is recommended.[13]

References

1. Owusu JA, Stewart CM, Boahene K. Facial nerve paralysis. *Med Clin North Am*. 2018;102(6):1135-1143.
2. George E, Richie MB, Glastonbury CM. Facial nerve palsy: clinical practice and cognitive errors. *Am J Med*. 2020;133(9):1039-1044.
3. Reich SG. Bell's palsy. *Continuum (Minneap Minn)*. 2017;23(2, Selected Topics in Outpatient Neurology):447-466.
4. Chweya CM, Anzalone CL, Driscoll CLW, Lane JI, Carlson ML. For whom the Bell's toll: recurrent facial nerve paralysis, a retrospective study and systematic review of the literature. *Otol Neurotol*. 2019;40(4):517-528.
5. Gilchrist JM. Seventh cranial neuropathy. *Semin Neurol*. 2009;29(1):5-13.
6. Vakharia K, Vakharia K. Bell's palsy. *Facial Plast Surg Clin North Am*. 2016;24(1):1-10.
7. Monsanto RD, Bittencourt AG, Bobato Neto NJ, Beilke SC, Lorenzetti FT, Salomone R. Treatment and prognosis of facial palsy on Ramsay Hunt syndrome: results based on a review of the literature. *Int Arch Otorhinolaryngol*. 2016;20(4):394-400.
8. Baugh RF, Basura GJ, Ishii LE, et al. Clinical practice guideline: Bell's palsy executive summary. *Otolaryngol Head Neck Surg*. 2013;149(5):656-663.
9. Tsukita K, Sakamaki-Tsukita H, Suenaga T. Combined abducens and peripheral facial nerve palsy. *Intern Med*. 2018;57(21):3223-3224.
10. Madhok VB, Gagyor I, Daly F, et al. Corticosteroids for Bell's palsy (idiopathic facial paralysis). *Cochrane Database Syst Rev*. 2016;7(7):CD001942.
11. Gagyor I, Madhok VB, Daly F, Sullivan F. Antiviral treatment for Bell's palsy (idiopathic facial paralysis). *Cochrane Database Syst Rev*. 2019;9(9):CD001869.
12. Kinoshita T, Ishii K, Okitsu T, Okudera T, Ogawa T. Facial nerve palsy: evaluation by contrast-enhanced MR imaging. *Clin Radiol*. 2001;56:926-932.
13. Su BM, Kuan EC, St John MA. What is the role of imaging in the evaluation of the patient presenting with unilateral facial paralysis? *Laryngoscope*. 2018;128:297-298.

CHAPTER 10

Epistaxis

Trudi Cloyd
Alok Saini

THE CLINICAL CHALLENGE

Approximately 60% of the US population will experience epistaxis during their lifetime, with one-tenth of these patients seeking medical attention. Epistaxis occurs in a bimodal distribution, with peaks at age 2 to 10 and 50 to 80 years, and peak incidence occurring among those older than 70. Although rarely a direct cause of mortality, epistaxis can represent management challenges to the emergency provider, especially in elderly patients and in those with underlying medical conditions.

PATHOPHYSIOLOGY

The mucosal lining of the nose is richly vascularized, with blood vessels arising from branches of both internal and external carotid arteries. Kiesselbach plexus, at the anteroinferior portion of the septum, is an anastomosis of branches of the sphenopalatine, greater palatine, anterior ethmoid, and superior labial arteries, and it is the most common site of bleeding in epistaxis. Anterior bleeds are generally less challenging to manage given the ease of accessibility for cauterization, topical treatment, or application of pressure. By contrast, Woodruff plexus, a conglomeration of thin-walled veins on the lateral nasal wall just under the posterior aspect of the inferior turbinate, is much harder to reach. These posterior venous bleeds, accounting for less than 10% of epistaxis cases, are significantly more difficult to identify and manage.

The etiologies of epistaxis are numerous, but in most cases (80%) there is no identifiable cause. Nasal dryness may be a contributing factor in any case of epistaxis. In children, digital trauma is a common cause. Other causes of epistaxis include recent or distant surgery involving the nose or sinuses, vascular lesions, benign or malignant neoplasms, inherited or acquired coagulopathies, anticoagulant use, chronic uncontrolled hypertension, and trauma.

APPROACH/THE FOCUSED EXAM

Initial evaluation of the epistaxis patient focuses on assessing the patient's airway, breathing, and circulation and determining whether emergent airway management is necessary. In patients with hemodynamic instability or significant ongoing epistaxis, large bore intravenous access should be obtained for fluid resuscitation and a complete blood count drawn to assess for degree of hemorrhage. Type and screen with ABO cross-match should be considered, because transfusions may be necessary, particularly in patients with existing comorbidities and concomitant cardiovascular disease.

A targeted history should be obtained to determine severity, frequency, duration, and laterality of the nosebleed. Underlying etiologic factors such as coagulopathy (eg, hereditary, hepatic impairment, renal insufficiency), malignancy, preceding trauma or surgery, or anatomic abnormalities should be identified to help direct further workup and management. Additionally, a focused review of medications, specifically anticoagulants, antiplatelet agents, and nonsteroidal anti-inflammatory medications, should be performed, because these may require escalation of therapy to achieve hemostasis. Social history including drug (eg, intranasal cocaine) and alcohol use, as well as smoking, are also important to address with the patient.

Particular attention should be paid to a history of endonasal surgical intervention. True posterior arterial bleeds are quite uncommon and usually associated with recent endoscopic surgery, which can expose arteries in the posterior aspect of the sinonasal cavity. Nasal packing may be necessary in this situation as a temporizing or definitive treatment measure, but a recent history of surgical intervention likely warrants ENT consultation, because packing may have negative consequences for surgical outcomes. In the absence of prior endoscopic surgery, a suspected posterior arterial bleed often instead represents a brisk bleed from a more posterior location of the anterior nose.

Anterior epistaxis will often be clinically obvious. In cases of posterior epistaxis, blood may be traveling from the nasopharynx to the oropharynx, resulting in blood being expelled from the mouth. The source might initially be unclear, as upper gastrointestinal (GI) and pulmonary causes of bleeding could present similarly. Posterior bleeding may also involve larger vessels, resulting in large-volume epistaxis that can present from both nares.

Proper preparation and setup are critical for the effective examination of the patient with epistaxis. A headlamp is essential for visualization, because it allows use of both hands during the assessment and intervention. The provider should have a face mask with eye protection, gloves, a nasal speculum (**Figure 10.1**), and a Frazier suction tip at bedside. Additional materials for epistaxis treatment such as nasal decongestants, cottonoids, absorbable and nonabsorbable packing materials, procoagulants, and silver nitrate should be readily available. An organized approach to epistaxis treatment will include an orderly progression from less invasive to more invasive therapies.

Encourage the patient to sit up and lean forward to avoid swallowing or aspirating blood. Firm pressure should be applied over Kiesselbach plexus by compressing the soft alar regions of the external nose against the anterior septum for a minimum of 10 minutes. A nasal decongestant can be applied to the nose prior to the initiation of pressure. In most cases, bleeding is minor and will stop with pressure alone.

If pressure fails to resolve the epistaxis, the nares should be cleared of clot using a Frazier tip suction before applying a topical vasoconstrictor such as 0.5% phenylephrine hydrochloride or 0.05% oxymetazoline. The solution can be administered as a spray or applied on a cottonoid. Nasal decongestants can help with vasoconstriction to slow bleeding but will also decongest the nose, allowing for a more thorough nasal evaluation, which may facilitate identification of the site of bleeding. Using a headlamp, anterior rhinoscopy may be performed with a nasal speculum to visualize an anterior bleeding point. If identified, the area can be anesthetized with local anesthesia (such as lidocaine or tetracaine applied via cottonoid) prior to being cauterized directly with either chemical cautery (silver nitrate) or electrocautery.

If no source of bleeding can be identified, or if cauterization is unsuccessful, progression to nasal packs may be required. Ideally, unilateral packing is preferred for patient comfort, although there are instances where bilateral nasal packing is required in order to maximize applied pressure. A variety of absorbable and nonabsorbable packing materials are available,[1] but absorbable packing materials have been shown to be effective.[2] Some materials may require lubrication to make insertion easier. Generally, all nasal packing will be inserted by sliding the pack posteriorly along the floor of the nose, preferably with bayonet forceps (**Figure 10.2**). Some packing materials may require administration of saline after insertion for expansion. Inflatable packs require introduction of air via syringe to provide gentle, low-pressure tamponade to the bleeding site. It is beyond the scope of this chapter to debate the merits of all individual packing materials available. Absorbable packing material provides the benefit of avoiding the rebleeding often seen with removal of nonabsorbable packing. Nonabsorbable nasal packing, if employed, should be left in place for 24 to 72 hours before removal. Local complications of nasal packing include sinusitis, septal perforation, and alar necrosis. On removal of packing, the nasal septum should be reexamined and bleeding points cauterized.

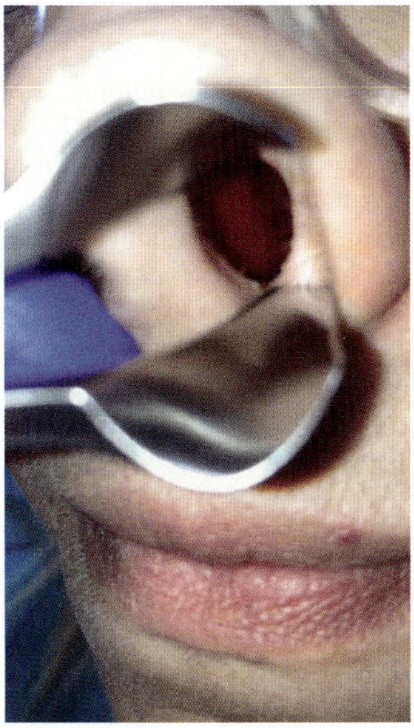

Figure 10.1: Nasal speculum exposing left anterior septum.

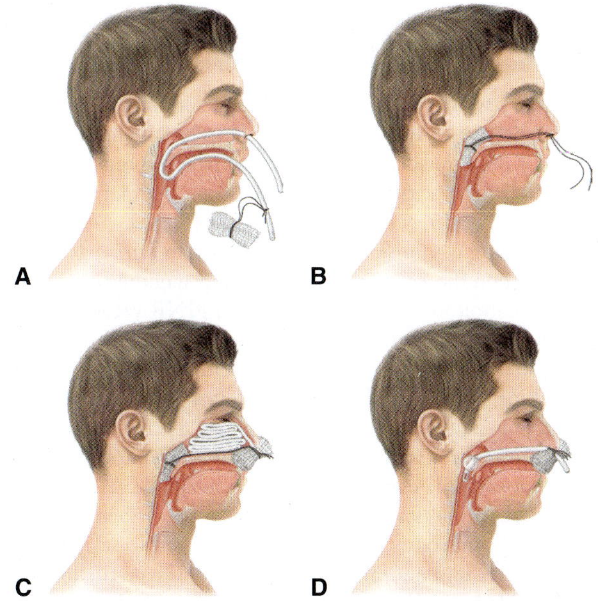

Figure 10.2: Nasal packing: packing to control bleeding from the posterior nose. A: Catheter inserted and packing attached. B: Packing drawn into position as catheter is removed. C: Strip tied over bolster to hold packing in place with anterior pack installed "accordion pleat" style. D: Alternative method, using balloon catheter instead of gauze packing. (From Britt LD, Peitzman AB, Barie PS, Jurkovich GJ. *Acute Care Surgery*. 2nd ed. Wolters Kluwer; 2019. Figure 29.1.)

Topical hemostatic agents such as tranexamic acid (TXA), Surgicell, and Floseal can be used alone or as adjuncts to standard treatment of epistaxis. TXA is an antifibrinolytic agent that works by competitive inhibition, preventing the binding of plasminogen to fibrin and the subsequent fibrinolysis that ensues. Evidence on topical use of TXA is mixed, with most recent evidence demonstrating that it is no more effective than placebo in the largest randomized controlled trial to date.[3] Alternatively, oxidized regenerated cellulose (eg, Surgicell) and Floseal are hemostatic agents that can be topically applied and are effective for both anterior[4] and posterior[5] epistaxis. The latter has been shown to be as effective for anterior epistaxis as nasal packing in randomized controlled trials, although it is often less readily available in the emergency department owing to cost.[6] Oxidized regenerated cellulose products (eg, Surgicell) might represent a more accessible option in the emergency department.

If bleeding continues despite appropriate anterior nasal packing, consultation with ENT should be obtained. Traditional teaching would suggest placement of a posterior pack. This can be done with specific inflatable packs that have both anterior and posterior balloon components, a gauze, and a red rubber catheter, or even with a foley catheter. In one well-described technique, a foley catheter is passed from the nose to the oropharynx before being insufflated. Gentle traction is then applied to the catheter proximally at the nares to provide tamponade of the posterior bleeding source. This is typically combined with traditional anterior nasal packing. Care must be taken when securing the red rubber catheter or foley to the anterior tip of the nose in order to prevent pressure necrosis of the ala or columella. Generally, the use of a posterior packing is rare, and the decision to use one should be on a case-by-case basis with the help of an ENT consultant. Advancements in endonasal surgery likely obviate the need for posterior packs in most cases. For example, an endoscopic approach with electrocauterization or an endoscopic sphenopalatine artery ligation can be performed at many institutions. Alternatively, in other situations, embolization via angiography may be considered.

TIPS AND PEARLS

- Epistaxis secondary to coagulopathies or antiplatelet/anticoagulant medication rarely responds to local treatment. Although direct therapy with chemical or electrocautery may be attempted, it is often unsuccessful, and nasal packing may be preferred. If significant hemorrhage occurs in the setting of antiplatelet use, platelet transfusion may be necessary. Patients on warfarin or direct oral anticoagulants (DOACs) can pose a significant challenge given their underlying comorbidities. The decision to pursue warfarin anticoagulant reversal should be based on the severity of epistaxis and whether it is controlled with packing, as well as the indication for anticoagulant use and INR value if on warfarin. Continued severe epistaxis despite local therapy should trigger further discussion with the hematologist and consideration of factor replacement or systemic TXA.
- Absorbable packing may be preferable to nonabsorbable packing in many circumstances. Utilizing absorbable packing obviates the need for a return trip to the emergency room (ER) or ENT specialist for packing removal and is often more comfortable for the patient. A variety of nonabsorbable packing options are available.
- Antistaphylococcal antibiotics typically have been prescribed with any nasal packing to prevent toxic shock syndrome. However, the data used to support antibiotic use are based on small retrospective and nonrandomized trials.[1,7] Given the low incidence of sinusitis and a lack of attributable toxic shock syndrome on case review, prophylactic antibiotics after packing may not be necessary, but further research is needed to confirm this.
- When attempting to cauterize the nose anteriorly, patience is key. It is often useful to have a number of 0.5 by 3 inch cottonoids soaked in nasal decongestant available. Careful application of a soaked cottonoid to the bleeding site with the addition of gentle pressure can easily slow, if not stop, even brisk anterior bleeding. Taking the time to slow the bleeding can aid in the effectiveness of cautery application. Additionally, multiple applications of cautery may be required, with topicalized cottonoids used in between applications.

EVIDENCE

When should coagulation studies be obtained in the patient with epistaxis?

Coagulation studies (prothrombin time [PT]; activated partial thromboplastin time [aPTT], and international normalized ratio [INR]) should not be routinely performed in patients with epistaxis.[8] The interpretation of results is highly dependent on antithrombotic therapy, and DOACs such as dabigatran, apixaban, and rivaroxaban can produce variable effects on the usual coagulation screen. Patients on warfarin should be assessed for supratherapeutic INR levels, and in cases with moderate to severe bleeding, reversal may be required. In addition, patients with suspected or known underlying coagulopathy should have coagulation tests performed.

What evidence-based management strategies exist for patients on antithrombotic agents during an episode of epistaxis?

Given the lack of universally accepted grading system for severity of epistaxis, research on acute management of epistaxis is often insufficient, particularly with respect to patients on antithrombotic therapies. In these patients, the initial assessment should ascertain the indication of the antithrombotic agent. A comprehensive risk assessment must be performed prior to withdrawal or alteration of any current treatment. Special attention should be paid to antithrombotic therapy for recent cardiac stents, new venous thromboembolism, and metallic heart valves, because these represent high-risk scenarios for medication adjustment.

In 2016, a systematic literature review examined 29 articles to determine evidence-based management strategies for antithrombotic agents during an episode of epistaxis.[8] Overall, they found a lack of evidence on this topic and highlighted the need for further research. However, they provided early guidance informed by international guidelines on anticoagulants and bleeding in other conditions. Although individuals taking antiplatelet medications are at an increased risk for developing epistaxis, the withdrawal of antiplatelet agents is unlikely to help in the acute setting.[8] Platelet transfusion might be beneficial in cases of severe, life-threatening epistaxis, but there are currently no completed trials addressing this question. Patients on vitamin K antagonists, the most common being warfarin, should have an INR level obtained during epistaxis. There is increasing evidence that these medications can be continued in mild and moderate epistaxis, provided that the INR is not supratherapeutic. Many guidelines suggest that vitamin K be administered if the INR level is greater than 6 and bleeding is moderate or uncontrolled.[8] In the case of life-threatening nasal hemorrhage for patients on DOACs, prothrombin complex concentrate (PCC) should be given for rapid reversal. Fresh frozen plasma may be considered if PCC is unavailable.

The use of DOACs, including both direct thrombin inhibitors and factor Xa inhibitors, has increased over the last decade, complicating the management of the anticoagulated epistaxis patient. Unlike other antithrombotic agents, these medications have a relatively short half-life (8-12 hours), and withholding them can be very effective.[8] However, close consideration for indication should determine whether these medications can and should be stopped.

Does uncontrolled hypertension worsen outcomes or complicate treatment in epistaxis?

The effect of hypertension on epistaxis is a question often posed in clinical practice. It is a common observation that patients presenting to the emergency department with epistaxis are also noted to have elevated blood pressure, and it is often debated whether this is the cause or a secondary effect of the epistaxis. Many patients will have elevated blood pressure at presentation because of anxiety caused by bleeding or even "white coat syndrome."

Chronic hypertension is known to disrupt normal endothelial function owing to increased tension on vessel walls, increasing the risk of rupture. However, the correlation between hypertension and the severity or frequency of epistaxis remains unclear. Although multiple studies have attempted to answer this question, consensus has not been achieved because of multiple confounders such as age and anticoagulant medications.[9]

Providers are often asked whether it is necessary to treat elevated blood pressure during an episode of epistaxis. Given the limited quality of evidence directly linking hypertension to an acute causal role in epistaxis, we do not suggest acutely lowering the blood pressure as treatment for epistaxis given the risk to end-organ perfusion. There is currently no evidence to support or refute treatment of hypertension during epistaxis. However, the relative risks and benefits must be considered in treating the refractory or severe epistaxis on an individualized basis.[10]

Are prophylactic antibiotics necessary after nasal packing?

Prophylactic antibiotics are often recommended after nasal packing to reduce the risk of sinusitis, otitis media, and/or toxic shock syndrome. However, the data used to support antibiotic use are based on small retrospective and nonrandomized trials.[1,7] The incidence of the complications is low, with sinusitis only rarely seen. There have also been no cases of toxic shock syndrome reported in the medical literature from anterior nasal packing. The overall risks are minimal in comparison to the known risks of systemic antibiotics, which include anaphylaxis, Stevens-Johnson syndrome, *Clostridium difficile* infection, or other gastrointestinal intolerance.

Is there a role for topical TXA in the management of acute epistaxis?

Although TXA has proven efficacy across multiple other applications for reducing acute blood loss, its role in the management of epistaxis remains unclear. In 2018, Cochrane published a review of six randomized controlled trials (692 participants) using TXA for control of epistaxis and found moderate-quality evidence that either oral or topical TXA, in addition to usual standard care, reduces the risk of rebleeding when compared to placebo with usual care.[11] The review found moderate quality evidence suggesting that topical TXA is better than other topical agents at stopping bleeding in the first 10 minutes. However, the authors concluded that further research was needed given the advancement in other management techniques, specifically cautery and packing. A subsequent large multicenter, double-blind, placebo-controlled trial (496 participants) published in 2021 found no increased efficacy with topical TXA when compared to placebo.[3] The study examined the topical application of TXA after first aid with routine compression and topical vasoconstrictor on soaked cottonoid held in place by a disposable nasal clip for 10 minutes. No statistical difference was observed in subsequent rates of packing, admission to hospital, transfusion, or recurrent episodes of epistaxis.

References

1. Iqbal IZ, Jones GH, Dawe N, et al. Intranasal packs and haemostatic agents for the management of adult epistaxis: systematic review. *J Laryngol Otol.* 2017;131:1065-1092.
2. Milinis K, Swords C, Hardman JC, et al. Dissolvable intranasal haemostatic agents for acute epistaxis: a systematic review and meta-analysis. *Clin Otolaryngol.* 2021;46:485-493.
3. Reuben A, Appelboam A, Stevens KN, et al. The use of tranexamic acid to reduce the need for nasal packing in epistaxis (NoPAC): randomized controlled trial. *Ann Emerg Med.* 2021;77(6):631-640.
4. Mathiasen RA, Cruz RM. Prospective, randomized, controlled clinical trial of a novel matrix hemostatic sealant in patients with acute anterior epistaxis. *Laryngoscope.* 2005;115:899-902.
5. Kilty SJ, Al-Hajry M, Al-Mutairi D, et al. Prospective clinical trial of gelatin-thrombin matrix as first line treatment of posterior epistaxis. *Laryngoscope.* 2014;124:38-42.
6. Murray S, Mendez A, Hopkins A, et al. Management of persistent epistaxis using Floseal hemostatic matrix vs. traditional nasal packing: a prospective randomized control trial. *J Otolaryngol Head Neck Surg.* 2018;47:3.
7. Cohn B. Are prophylactic antibiotics necessary for anterior nasal packing in epistaxis? *Ann Emerg Med.* 2015;65:109-111.
8. Musgrave KM, Powell J. A systematic review of anti-thrombotic therapy in epistaxis. *Rhinology.* 2016;54:292-301.
9. Kikidis D, Tsioufis K, Papanikolaou V, et al. Is epistaxis associated with arterial hypertension? A systematic review of the literature. *Eur Arch Otorhinolaryngol.* 2014;271:237-243.
10. Payne C, Feldstein D, Anne S, et al. Hypertension and epistaxis: why is there limited guidance in the nosebleed clinical practice guidelines? *Otolaryngol Head Neck Surg.* 2020;162:33-34.
11. Joseph J, Martinez-Devesa P, Bellorini J, et al. Tranexamic acid for patients with nasal hemorrhage (epistaxis). *Cochrane Database Syst Rev.* 2018;(12):CD004328.

CHAPTER 11

Rhinitis, Sinusitis, Including Orbital and Cranial Complications, Invasive Fungal Rhinosinusitis

Ashton Lehman
Di Coneybeare

INTRODUCTION

Rhinitis, rhinosinusitis, and their suppurative complications present commonly in the emergency department (ED). Rhinitis alone afflicts 10% to 40% of the general population globally and more than 60 million Americans annually, whereas rhinosinusitis afflicts about one in six Americans annually.[1-3]

The sinonasal region—including the nasal cavity and bilateral paranasal sinuses—serves as a conduit for air movement while heating and humidifying inspired air; a filter for airborne particulate matter; a detection system for odorants, irritants, and temperature changes; and a defense system capable of triggering innate and adaptive immune system responses.[4] This region is susceptible to a heterogeneous group of infectious and inflammatory conditions, many of which result in overlapping symptomatology in children and adults.[5]

When rhinosinusitis inflammation or infection extends beyond the paranasal sinuses and nasal cavity to involve neurologic, ophthalmologic, osseous, or soft tissue regions, it is considered complicated. Although rare, such complications (eg, orbital cellulitis, orbital abscesses, meningitis, and brain abscesses) can lead to significant morbidity and mortality.[6] Given this potential risk, accurate and expeditious diagnosis and prompt management of sinonasal conditions are critical in ED and urgent care settings.

THE CLINICAL CHALLENGE

Because the sinus and nasal structures abut each other sharing continuous mucosa, many consider diseases of the sinonasal region along a pathologic spectrum.[1,2] However, treatment options may differ dramatically depending on the underlying pathophysiology, location, and the severity of disease. Allergic and nonallergic rhinitis often share similar symptoms.[3] Likewise, viral rhinitis and rhinosinusitis have significant symptomatologic overlap with acute bacterial rhinosinusitis.[2] Differentiating between viral and bacterial rhinosinusitis is challenging to emergency providers. Physical exam findings are often subtle, and many serious suppurative complications of bacterial rhinosinusitis may present without the overt neurologic deficits that traditionally signify their presence.[6] Imaging from computed tomography (CT) will result in similar findings in patients with a common cold as well as in patients with bacterial rhinosinusitis.[5] Furthermore, nasal microbiologic results may be misleading; even patients with viral illness may be colonized by common nasopharyngeal flora. For example, *Staphylococcus aureus* can be present in up to 30% of healthy adults, and fungi are almost ubiquitous.[5,6]

Uncertainty in diagnosis may lead to inappropriate antibiotics, therapeutics, and costly imaging.[6] When to start antibiotics vexes providers the most. Viral infections most commonly afflict patients presenting with rhinosinusitis, and even in the case of bacterial rhinosinusitis, about two-thirds of patients will improve without any pharmaceutical intervention.[5] However, if left untreated, serious bacterial rhinosinusitis may progress to life-threatening intracranial and extracranial suppurative complications.

PATHOPHYSIOLOGY

Rhinitis is defined by allergic or nonallergic inflammation of the nasal mucosa. The epithelial layer of the nasal mucosa overlies submucosal layers and filters the external world for the body's immune system.[2] Submucosal layers secrete mucous that protects the nasal airway as a physical barrier and through production of various glycoproteins with antimicrobial and antioxidant properties.[2] Epithelial cilia brush mucous posteriorly that has trapped environmental foreign particles.[2] In allergic rhinitis, an IgE-mediated process, patients respond to allergens by activating epithelial cells, instigating downstream inflammatory reactions. Excessive mucous production and increased vascular permeability result in congestion and nasal drainage. By contrast, inflammation from nonallergic rhinitis is, by definition, not IgE-mediated. Common causes of nonallergic rhinitis that can directly activate inflammatory reactions include infection (viral or bacterial), food- or drug-triggered, and idiopathic (formally known as vasomotor rhinitis).[2,5]

The mucosa that lines the nasal cavity extends throughout the four paranasal sinuses on each side (**Figure 11.1**): frontal, maxillary, sphenoid, and ethmoid.[1] Sinus secretions drain via a complex and connected system of ostia that is contiguous through all the paranasal sinuses.[6] Pathology of the sinuses is thus caused by inflammation of its mucosa, obstruction of its ostia, structural abnormalities, direct extension of pathology from adjacent structures, and/or ciliary dysfunction.[6] Because the nasal and sinus mucosa are contiguous, pathology in either region almost always affects the other, and hence inflammation is often referred to as "rhinosinusitis."[3]

Bacterial infections of the sinuses are often caused by stasis of sinonasal mucous, which fosters a breeding ground for bacteria. Infections are mostly polymicrobial, often representative of nasal and oropharyngeal flora. Common pathogens include *Streptococcus pneumoniae, Haemophilus influenzae B, Moraxella catarrhalis, S aureus,* anaerobes, and fungi.

Intracranial complications of sinusitis can be caused by seeding via septic emboli from diploic veins originating at the base of the skull penetrating the dura or via direct extension through ostia of the skull or from rhinosinusitis-related osteomyelitis.[6] Orbital and other extracranial complications of rhinosinusitis occur primarily via direct extension associated with infections of the ethmoid and maxillary sinuses.[6]

Fungi thrive in the setting of hyperglycemia and acidosis, and this explains why acute invasive fungal infections of the sinonasal region occur almost exclusively in patients with poorly controlled diabetes or those otherwise immunocompromised.[1,7] *Aspergillus, Mucor,* and *Rhizopus* are implicated in most patients with acute invasive fungal rhinosinusitis.

APPROACH/THE FOCUSED EXAM

During history-taking, noteworthy elements include the presence, character, and time course of symptoms as well as history of neurosurgery or sinonasal surgery. Specific relevant historical features and important comorbid conditions can be found in **Table 11.1**.

Examination of the sinonasal region includes an external evaluation of the nose, internal evaluation with anterior rhinoscopy and rigid nasal endoscopy, evaluation of facial soft tissues, orbits, oral cavity, and relevant neurologic function. Note edema, erythema, warmth, fluctuance, drainage, or changes in sensation of the facial soft tissues overlying the nasal, maxillary, and frontal regions. Orbital findings such as epiphora (ie, excessive tearing), lid abnormalities, proptosis, extraocular movements, visual acuity, light perception/sensitivity, pupil reactivity, and red desaturation should be assessed. The status of dentition and the presence of fistulae or palatal changes should be noted.

The workup of sinonasal pathology may include imaging in cases with a suspected complication or alternative diagnosis (eg, nonsinonasal causes of facial pain, potential malignant processes

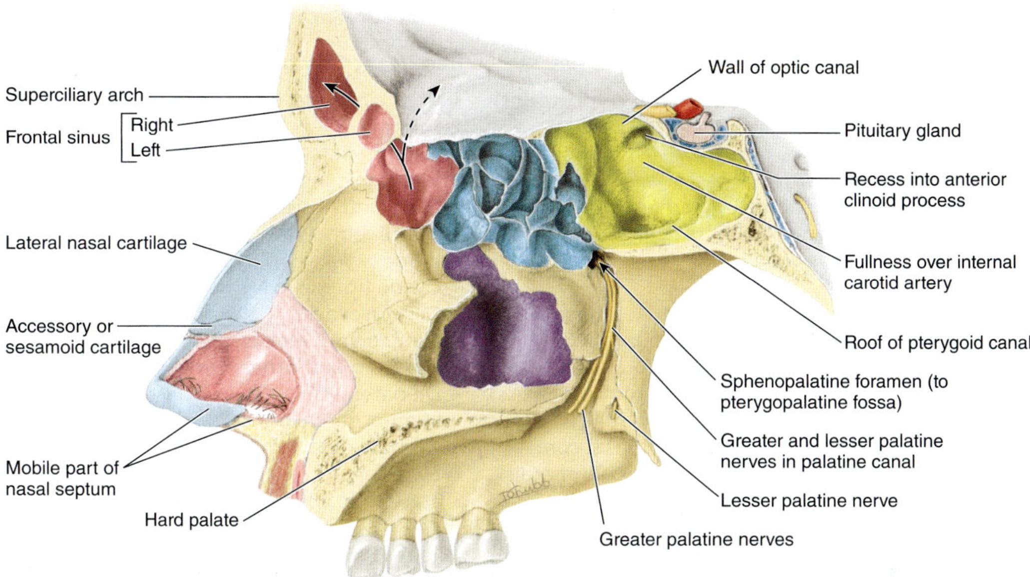

(A) Sagittal depiction of paranasal sinuses

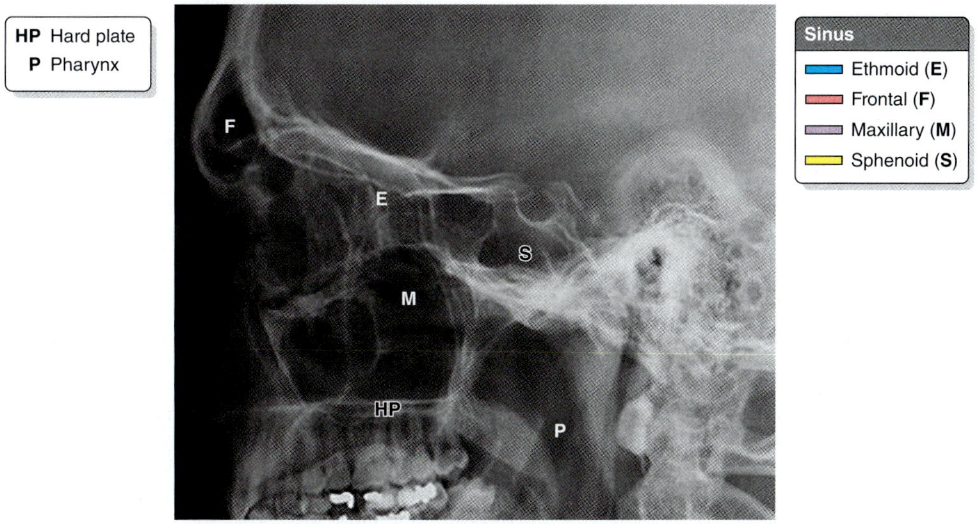

(B) Lateral radiograph

Figure 11.1: A. Sagittal depiction of paranasal sinuses. The paranasal sinuses of the right side have been opened from a nasal approach and color coded. An anterior ethmoidal cell (pink) is invading the diploë of the frontal bone to become a frontal sinus. An offshoot (broken arrow) invades the orbital plate of the frontal bone. The sphenoidal sinus in this specimen is extensive, extending (1) posteriorly, inferior to the pituitary gland, to the clivus; (2) laterally, inferior to the optic nerve (CN II), into the anterior clinoid process; and (3) inferiorly to the pterygoid process but avoiding the pterygoid canal (which is seen rising as a ridge on the floor of the sinus). The maxillary sinus is pyramidal. B. Radiograph of cranium. Air densities (dark areas) associated with paranasal sinuses, nasal cavity, oral cavity, and pharynx are demonstrated. (From Head. In: Moore KL, Dalley AF II, Agur AMR. *Moore's Clinically Oriented Anatomy*. 9th ed. Wolters Kluwer; 2023:839-999. Figure 8.109.)

signified by concomitant neurologic deficits).[2] If an orbital or intracranial complication is suspected, suggested by severe headache, facial swelling, cranial nerve palsies, proptosis, impaired extraocular movements, or impaired visual acuity, contrast-enhanced CT is the initial imaging modality of choice.[5,6] Depending on the presentation and the findings on initial CT imaging, magnetic resonance imaging (MRI) may be pursued. MRI often offers superior resolution of soft tissues, intracranial complications, and orbital complications/pathology.[4,6]

TABLE 11.1 History and Comorbid Conditions

Important Features in History of Present Illness	Important Comorbid Conditions
• Location of nasal drainage (anterior or posterior) • Characteristic of drainage (clear or purulent) • Facial pain/pressure • Change in/loss of smell or taste • Atopic-related reactions (eg, itchy/watery eyes, watery rhinorrhea, sneezing, urticaria) • Fever • Headache • Neck stiffness • Change in vision (including diplopia) • Light sensitivity • Neurologic symptoms (sensory or motor deficits) • Current and recent medications including sinonasal-targeted treatments, eg, nasal sprays • Environmental exposures (eg, chemicals, metals, irritants)	• Prior sinonasal infections • Asthma • Aspirin-exacerbated respiratory disease • Idiopathic intracranial hypertension • Obstructive sleep apnea • Hydrocephalus • Intracranial neoplasm • Cystic fibrosis • Cilia disorders • Human immunodeficiency virus infection and other immune deficiencies • Diabetes • Lymphoreticular malignancy • Chronic renal failure • Liver failure • Traumatic injuries

TABLE 11.2 Chandler Classification for Orbital Complications of Rhinosinusitis

Chandler Class	Orbital Complication	Common Findings
I	Preseptal cellulitis	Eyelid edema/erythema, tenderness, normal extraocular movements, normal visual acuity
II	Orbital cellulitis	Eyelid edema/erythema, proptosis, chemosis, may have some impairment of extraocular movements, often normal visual acuity
III	Subperiosteal abscess (ie, pus collection between medial periorbita and adjacent bone)	Marked proptosis, chemosis, impaired extraocular movements, may have visual impairment
IV	Orbital abscess (ie, pus collection in orbital tissue)	Severe proptosis, often ophthalmoplegia, severe visual impairment
V	Cavernous sinus thrombosis *(technically, an intracranial complication)*	Often bilateral presentation with orbital pain, severe proptosis, ophthalmoplegia, severe visual impairment, multiple cranial nerve palsies (III, IV, V1-2, VI), papilledema, retroocular headache, fevers

The presence of clear rhinorrhea, especially if unilateral, should raise the possibility of a cerebrospinal fluid (CSF) leak (see Chapter 21). In the presence of fluctuant forehead swelling, consider a Pott puffy tumor. This is a form of frontal bone osteomyelitis in which frontal sinusitis erodes the anterior bony table of the sinus, resulting in a subperiosteal abscess, which can also be associated with intracranial complications.

Orbital complications of rhinosinusitis are organized by the Chandler classification system (**Table 11.2**).[4] A high index of suspicion must be maintained in patients with chronic or acute rhinosinusitis presenting with the findings in Table 11.2. A low threshold should exist for ophthalmology consultation when orbital findings are encountered.

Intracranial complications of rhinosinusitis include meningitis, venous thromboses, and abscesses in the epidural, subdural, or parenchymal spaces (**Table 11.3**). Their clinical presentations can be silent, nonspecific with high fever and severe headache, or more specific with neck stiffness, nausea and vomiting, and altered mental status.[4] CT, MRI, or lumbar puncture may be pursued. When the presentation raises suspicion for an intracranial complication, the cavernous and dural venous sinuses also ought to be evaluated for thrombosis with CT or MRI.[6]

TABLE 11.3 Intracranial Complications of Rhinosinusitis

Intracranial Complication	Common Findings
Meningitis	Headache, high fevers, neck stiffness, seizures, mental status changes; MRI: meningeal enhancement
Epidural abscess	Headache (often sole initial symptom), fever, altered mental status, local tenderness; CT: crescent-shaped collection in the epidural space; MRI: hyperintense on T2, variable intensity on T1
Subdural abscess	Headache, fever, seizures, focal neurologic deficits, lethargy, rapid deterioration; CT: collection along a hemisphere or the falx; MRI: low signal on T1, high signal on T2, peripheral enhancement
Brain abscess	Headache, fever, vomiting, lethargy, seizures, focal neurologic deficits, frontal deficits (eg, changes in mood/behavior); MRI: cystic lesion with distinct hypointense, strongly enhancing capsule on T2
Venous thrombosis	Headache, fever, focal neurologic deficits; CT angiography or MRI: angiography/venography: filling defects within venous sinuses

Invasive fungal rhinosinusitis should be considered in patients who are immunocompromised (eg, diabetes, chemotherapy, posttransplant, human immunodeficiency virus [HIV] infection), although this can also rarely occur in immunocompetent patients. Invasive fungal rhinosinusitis may present with nasal congestion, painless nasal ulceration, bloodless insensate sinonasal tissue, periorbital or facial swelling, impaired extraocular movements, focal numbness, palatal fistulization, fever, and altered mental status.[4] CT imaging may appear similar to viral or bacterial rhinosinusitis in the paranasal sinuses, but bony erosion on CT imaging is often seen after fungal invasion has progressed. MR imaging may help localize necrotic nonenhancing areas within thickened mucosa and extension beyond the paranasal sinuses.[6] Definitive diagnosis requires biopsy.[6] To speciate fungi, culture with sporulation is often required, so fungal cultures are best obtained prior to any antifungal treatment.[4]

DIFFERENTIAL DIAGNOSIS

The differential diagnosis for sinonasal pathology presents along a spectrum of diseases that is wide ranging in severity and often characterized by overlapping symptoms. Considerations for differential diagnoses for rhinitis and rhinosinusitis presentations can be divided into common, life-threatening, and special populations (**Tables 11.4** and **11.5**).

MANAGEMENT

Rhinitis

In cases of allergic rhinitis, management often entails some combination of the following: allergen avoidance, saline nasal irrigations, oral and nasal antihistamines, nasal steroid sprays, oral decongestants, oral antileukotrienes, nasal mast cell stabilizers, and consideration of immunotherapy. In infectious rhinitis, management consists of supportive treatment for viral rhinitis versus antibiotic treatment for bacterial rhinitis. As in many infectious sinonasal pathologies, the duration and selection of antibiotics depend on the underlying cause. In atrophic rhinitis, a rare form of rhinitis caused by atrophy of the nasal mucosa paradoxically producing excess mucous, management involves saline nasal irrigations, topical antibiotics, and nasal ointments. In rhinitis medicamentosa (rebound nasal congestion caused by overuse of decongestant medications), management involves discontinuation of the culprit topical decongestant, which may be better tolerated with a short-term course of oral steroids while weaning off the decongestant. In vasomotor rhinitis, management often consists of anticholinergic nasal sprays, and referral for consideration of surgical intervention may be pursued if the symptoms are recalcitrant to medical management.

TABLE 11.4 Differential Diagnosis for Patients with Rhinitis Symptoms

Common	Life-Threatening	Special Populations
Allergic rhinitis Viral infectious rhinitis Idiopathic rhinitis Atrophic rhinitis Rhinitis Medicamentosa Nasal polyps or other structural abnormalities	CSF rhinorrhea	Foreign bodies (P)

CSF, cerebrospinal fluid; P, pediatrics.

TABLE 11.5 Differential Diagnosis for Patients with Rhinosinusitis Symptoms

Common	Life-Threatening	Special Populations
Viral rhinosinusitis Bacterial rhinosinusitis Migraine/headaches Dental pain/abscess Mucoceles	Orbital cellulitis/subperiosteal abscess/abscess Meningitis Osteomyelitis Cavernous sinus thrombosis Intracranial abscess Mucopyocele Malignancy	Invasive fungal rhinosinusitis (I) Pott puffy tumor (P)

I, immunocompromised; P, pediatrics.

Rhinosinusitis

Uncomplicated chronic rhinosinusitis treatment has been extensively studied, the review of which is beyond the scope of this chapter. Acute viral rhinosinusitis is frequent, self-limited, and rarely complicated by secondary bacterial infection.[5] Thus, management is generally geared toward symptomatic relief, often including some combination of analgesics, antipyretics, saline nasal irrigations, oral decongestants, topical decongestants (limited to 3-5 days of use), antihistamines, mucolytics, expectorants/antitussives, and steroids (topical and possibly oral).[5] The management of acute bacterial rhinosinusitis initially involves saline nasal irrigations, analgesics, antibiotics, and intranasal topical steroids.[4] Systemic steroids and decongestants are not supported by evidence.[4] In multiple recent systematic reviews, upfront antibiotics for uncomplicated acute bacterial rhinosinusitis appears to offer a small clinical benefit, with no apparent differences in rates of complications between antibiotic and placebo groups.[4,5] If antibiotics are initiated, the recommended initial selection is amoxicillin with or without clavulanate.[5] In patients with penicillin allergy, alternative antibiotic options are trimethoprim-sulfamethoxazole, doxycycline, or a macrolide. When safe follow-up is assured, a trial of watchful waiting can be explored, and antibiotics may be initiated for nonimprovement by 7 days if is the condition worsens or a complication is detected at any point.[5]

Orbital and Intracranial Complications

Complications in rhinosinusitis can be divided between minor (mucocele, osteitis, bony erosion/expansion, and osseous metaplasia) and major (Pott puffy tumor, orbital and intracranial complications).[4]

In Pott puffy tumor, treatment includes broad-spectrum systemic antibiotics, surgical drainage of the abscess and of the frontal sinus, and debridement of sequestered bone.[4]

Orbital complications of rhinosinusitis are managed stepwise, beginning with preseptal cellulitis (technically, an eyelid rather than orbital condition) to orbital (postseptal) cellulitis. Details of the management of these conditions are discussed in Chapter 30.

Sinogenic cavernous sinus thrombosis (technically, an intracranial complication) is managed with parenteral antibiosis, surgical intervention of the involved sinus(es), saline nasal irrigations, topical decongestants, and possible systemic steroids.[6] The addition of anticoagulants in the treatment of these complications is controversial, and specialty consultation ought to be pursued for consideration of this.[6]

For intracranial abscesses, surgical drainage of diseased sinuses is recommended as soon as possible. A craniotomy, burr hole, or image-guided aspiration is often pursued at the same time for neurosurgical drainage of the abscess.[4,6]

Invasive Fungal Rhinosinusitis

Acute invasive fungal rhinosinusitis management involves prompt surgical debridement, often serially, to remove grossly infected/necrotic tissue and reduce fungal load. Also, culture-directed systemic antifungal treatment is initiated and, if possible, underlying immunosuppression reversed.[4]

TIPS AND PEARLS

- Most patients presenting with symptoms of rhinitis or rhinosinusitis will have causes of benign origin. Treatment should focus primarily on education, reassurance, and symptom management.
- In patients who have symptoms concerning for an intracranial complication, MRI is more sensitive compared with CT and should be pursued if available.
- Patients with poorly controlled diabetes or other immunocompromising conditions have increased propensity for complications.

EVIDENCE

How is viral rhinosinusitis differentiated from acute bacterial rhinosinusitis?

Although guidelines for presumed bacterial rhinosinusitis are based largely on duration of symptoms (varying from 5 to 10 days), there is little clinical evidence to suggest that duration is a good indicator. In a systematic review that evaluated the diagnostic reliability of symptoms to differentiate viral versus bacterial rhinosinusitis, only one study in over 4000 unique publications presented with high directness of evidence.[8] This review found that the value of duration could not be concluded owing to bias and that purulent nasal discharge also poorly differentiates between viral and bacterial infections.[8] Duration guidelines are thus derived from the natural course of viral illness, specifically that of rhinovirus.[3] Some criteria suggest that "high fever" also suggests a diagnosis of bacterial rhinosinusitis, but "high fever" is not universally defined.[1,3] Overall, guidelines are extrapolations of pathophysiology, benefit and harm analysis in the setting of poor evidentiary support, and expert consensus.[1,3] Generally speaking, acute bacterial rhinosinusitis can be diagnosed if the patient experiences symptoms such as purulent nasal discharge, nasal obstruction, and facial pain/fullness that worsen/fail to improve within 10 days of symptom onset.[1]

When should antibiotics be initiated for acute bacterial rhinosinusitis?

The initiation of antibiotics for acute bacterial rhinosinusitis has been intensely studied, and guidelines are based on systematic reviews of many double-blind randomized controlled trials.[1] In the absence of a complicated infection, clinicians have the option of watchful waiting for up to 7 days.[1] In randomized controlled trials, most patients that met clinical criteria improved in the placebo arm, and those in the antibiotic arm only received modest benefit while demonstrating increased rates of adverse events.[1] However, these studies excluded those with "severe" disease, and "severe" was often not clearly defined.[1] These studies also did not decipher what clinical characteristics or other indicators may reveal which patients would benefit most from early antibiotics.[1] Therefore, antibiotic initiation may be dependent on the patient's disease severity at the discretion of the clinician, the ability to monitor the patient's disease progression, and shared decision-making incorporating the patient's preferences.[1]

When should imaging be obtained in patients presenting with symptoms of rhinosinusitis?

Imaging for uncomplicated acute bacterial rhinosinusitis via plain film, CT, or MRI is universally not recommended, because viral syndromes can produce the same imaging results as bacterial infections.[5] Furthermore, meta-analyses have confirmed that imaging offers poor sensitivity and specificity in its diagnostic ability.[5] The risk of radiation exposure, increased length of stay in the ED, and the additional costs render imaging even less appealing. Imaging should not be obtained unless there is clinical suspicion for a complication or an alternative diagnosis requiring exclusion.[5]

When is anticoagulation indicated (and contraindicated) in intracranial venous sinus thrombotic complications of rhinosinusitis?

The use of anticoagulants in the management of rhinosinusitis-related intracranial venous sinus thromboses remains controversial.[4,9] The proposed theoretical benefits of anticoagulation use in these cases include preventing thrombus propagation, inhibiting platelet function, and promoting antibiotic penetration of the thrombus. However, given the rarity of these complications, no randomized controlled trials or prospective studies exist to guide the use of anticoagulation. Furthermore, most existing case series have focused on septic cavernous sinus thromboses specifically, as sigmoid or superior sagittal sinus thromboses are even more rare.[9] Prior case series comparing septic cavernous sinus thrombosis management with antibiotics alone versus antibiotics plus anticoagulation have not convincingly demonstrated decreased mortality, but anticoagulation has proven some reduction in morbidity (eg, reduced rates of blindness, stroke, and cranial nerve deficits), whereas the occurrence of hemorrhagic complications remains rare.[9,10] Noteworthy contraindications to anticoagulation therapy include radiographic evidence of hemorrhagic sequelae, comorbid meningitis (increased risk of intracerebral bleeding), lack of perceived likelihood of thrombus propagation, and suspected elevated risk of septic embolic event(s). The decision to include anticoagulation is thus nuanced and should be made in collaboration with specialty consultants (eg, neurology or hematology).[10]

References

1. Wyler B, Mallon WK. Sinusitis update. *Emerg Med Clin North Am.* 2019;37:41-54.
2. Morjaria JB, Caruso M, Emma R, Russo C, Polosa R. Treatment of allergic rhinitis as a strategy for preventing asthma. *Curr Allergy Asthma Rep*. 2018;18:23.
3. Dykewicz MS, Wallace DV, Amrol DJ, et al. Rhinitis 2020: a practice parameter update. *J Allergy Clin Immunol*. 2020;146:721-767.
4. Orlandi RR, Kingdom TT, Hwang PH, et al. International consensus statement on allergy and rhinology: rhinosinusitis. *Int Forum Allergy Rhinol*. 2016;6(Suppl 1):S22-S209.
5. Rosenfeld RM, Piccirillo JF, Chandrasekhar SS, et al. Clinical practice guideline (update): adult sinusitis. *Otolaryngol Head Neck Surg*. 2015;152:S1-S39.
6. Hoxworth JM, Glastonbury CM. Orbital and intracranial complications of acute sinusitis. *Neuroimaging Clin N Am*. 2010;20:511-526.
7. Eifan AO, Durham SR. Pathogenesis of rhinitis. *Clin Exp Allergy*. 2016;46:1139-1151.
8. van den Broek MF, Gudden C, Kluijfhout WP, et al. No evidence for distinguishing bacterial from viral acute rhinosinusitis using symptom duration and purulent rhinorrhea: a systematic review of the evidence base. *Otolaryngol Head Neck Surg*. 2014;150:533-537.
9. Ziegler A, Patadia M, Stankiewicz J. Neurological complications of acute and chronic sinusitis. *Curr Neurol Neurosci Rep*. 2018;18:5.
10. van der Poel NA, Mourits MP, de Win MML, Coutinho JM, Dikkers FG. Prognosis of septic cavernous sinus thrombosis remarkably improved: a case series of 12 patients and literature review. *Eur Arch Otorhinolaryngol*. 2018;275:2387-2395.

CHAPTER 12

Sialolithiasis/Sialadenitis

Vilija Vaitaitis
Sanjey Gupta

THE CLINICAL CHALLENGE

Patients with salivary gland disease often present to the emergency department (ED) or urgent care setting with acute onset of pain or swelling of the affected salivary gland. In addition to pain and glandular swelling, patients with sialolithiasis or sialadenitis can also present with fever, trismus, difficulty swallowing, local erythema, change in salivary flow/consistency, or leukocytosis.

PATHOPHYSIOLOGY

The salivary gland system is comprised of paired parotid, submandibular, and sublingual glands and numerous minor salivary glands. The parotid glands are located between the ramus of the mandible and the external auditory canal, with the tail of the parotid inferior to the ear lobule, dipping below the jawline. The parotid gland is drained by Stensen duct, which passes over the masseter muscle and pierces the buccinator muscle, then drains into the mouth through an opening in the buccal mucosa near the second maxillary molar on each side. The submandibular glands are located in the submandibular triangle just under the mandible and drain into the midline floor of the mouth, just behind the incisors, via Wharton duct (**Figure 12.1**).

Sialolithiasis is the condition in which stones (calculi) form within a salivary duct, leading to obstruction. It is the most common cause of salivary gland swelling, with an incidence of 1 in 10 000 to 30 000. The primary age range for diagnosis is 30 to 60 years, with a higher incidence in males. Approximately 80% to 85% of stones occur in the submandibular gland, 15% in the parotid gland, and greater than 5% in the sublingual and other glands (**Figure 12.2**).[1] Sialolithiasis is characterized by recurrent pain and swelling of the gland, often exacerbated at mealtime, when salivary flow is greatest.[2]

Sialolithiasis is a leading cause of sialadenitis, or inflammation of the salivary gland(s). However, sialadenitis can be caused, or exacerbated, by several other preexisting conditions, including ductal strictures, diabetes mellitus, hypothyroidism, Sjögren syndrome, gout, and renal failure. Medications that reduce salivary flow, especially those with anticholinergic properties, can also contribute to the development of sialadenitis.[3]

Sialadenitis of one or multiple salivary glands results in pain, swelling, erythema overlying the gland, trismus, purulent drainage from the duct, and, potentially, abscess formation. Parotitis, which is sialadenitis limited to the parotid gland, often results from dehydration, obstruction, or retrograde migration of bacteria through the duct. The parotid is the gland most commonly affected by inflammation.[4]

Similarly to sialithiasis, several medical conditions are also known to predispose patients to acute infectious sialadenitis, including hepatic or renal failure, diabetes, hypothyroidism,

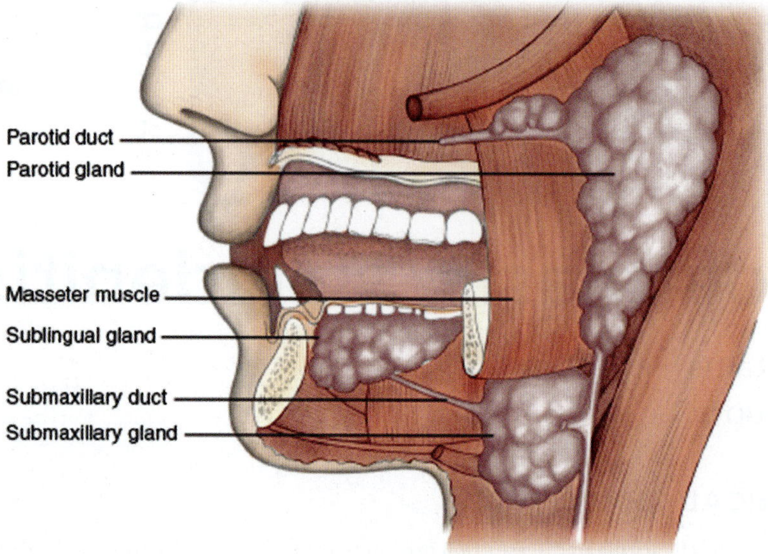

Figure 12.1: This figure demonstrates the location of the parotid gland and its corresponding Stensen duct. The submandibular gland is inferior to the mandible and is drained by Wharton duct, which empties into the floor of the mouth. (From Lippincott Nursing Solutions/Lippincott Nursing Advisor. Wolters Kluwer; 2015.)

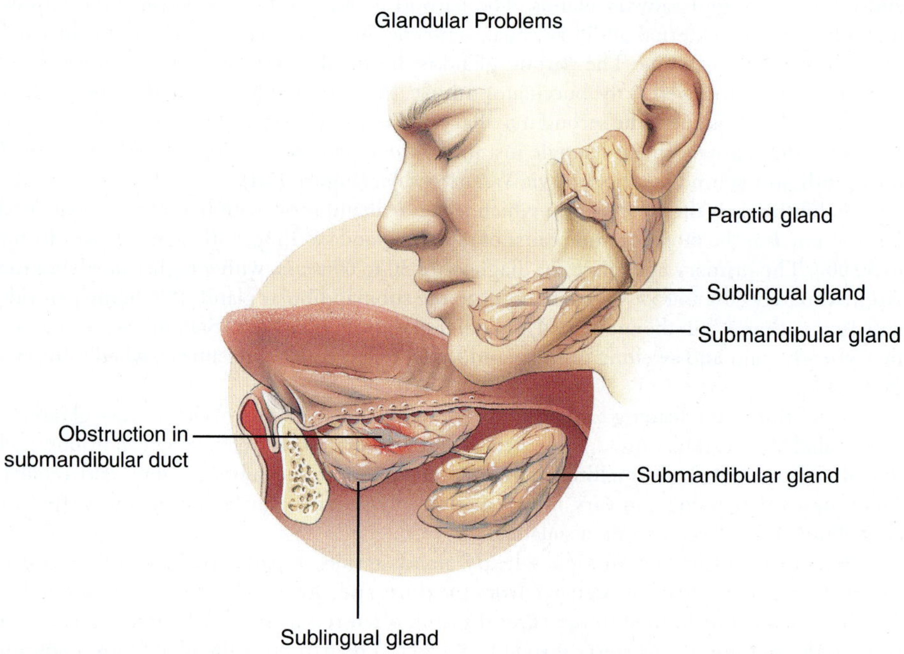

Figure 12.2: Salivary calculus or stone obstructing the outflow through a salivary gland duct, leading to pain and swelling. (From The Anatomical Chart Company. *Disorders of the Teeth and Jaw Anatomical Chart.* Wolters Kluwer; 2005.)

malnutrition, human immunodeficiency virus (HIV), Sjögren syndrome, anorexia or bulimia, hyperlipoproteinemia, hyperuricemia, cystic fibrosis, lead poisoning, and Cushing syndrome.[5] Medications such as diuretics, beta-blockers, tricyclic antidepressants, and phenothiazines can also lead to dehydration and subsequent sialadenitis.[4,5]

APPROACH/THE FOCUSED EXAM

The clinical diagnosis of sialolithiasis can be difficult, because a stone may not be evident unless obstruction of a salivary duct and subsequent gland swelling/sialadenitis occurs. An obstructing stone often presents with unilateral salivary gland swelling and worsening pain or swelling that occurs with eating.[6] The physical exam should include a bimanual palpation of the floor of the mouth, pushing up on the submandibular gland with one hand while intraorally palpating the floor of mouth with the other. An affected gland is firm or tender, and in the case of submandibular gland swelling, the floor of the mouth may be elevated, tender, or inflamed. In sialadenitis, palpation of the gland often leads to expression of pus from the intraoral gland orifice.[7] For the parotid gland, the path of Stensen duct should be palpated (**Figure 12.3**). This palpation can sometimes reveal an obvious calcification, although in acute inflammation stones are frequently nonpalpable owing to the overlying soft tissue edema and induration (**Figure 12.4**). Furthermore, inflamed, firm, irregular glandular tissue can often mimic calcifications.

When the parotid gland is involved, it is important to perform a thorough ipsilateral facial nerve exam. A facial nerve palsy is rarely associated with sialolithiasis or sialadenitis and more often suggests a malignancy, warranting further workup.[8]

Diagnostics

If the clinical exam is not conclusive, multiple imaging modalities can be utilized to assist in the diagnosis of sialolithiasis or sialadenitis (**Figure 12.5**). Ultrasound is a noninvasive and fairly easy modality that can identify calcifications, masses, or fluid collections within the glands. Ultrasound utilized by radiology or clinicians have sensitivities ranging between 71% and 94% for the detection of salivary calculi.[9]

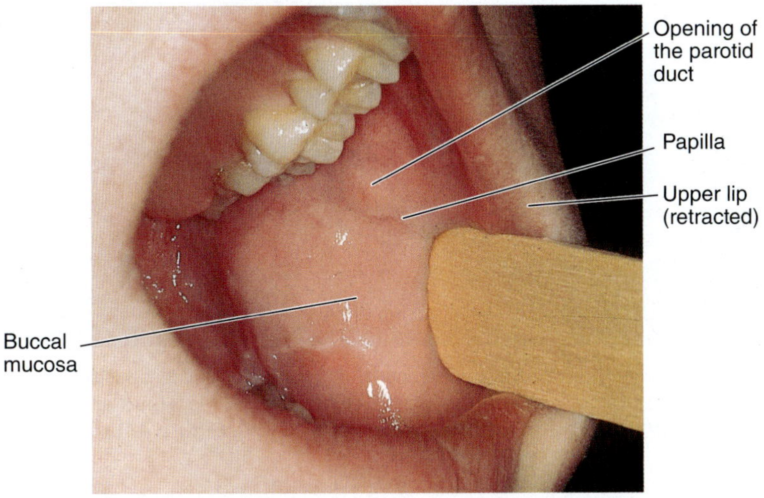

Figure 12.3: Examination of the parotid (Stensen) duct. (From Bickley LS, Szilagyi PG, Hoffman RM, Soriano RP. *Bates' Guide To Physical Examination and History Taking*. 13th ed. Wolters Kluwer; 2021. Figure 14.8.)

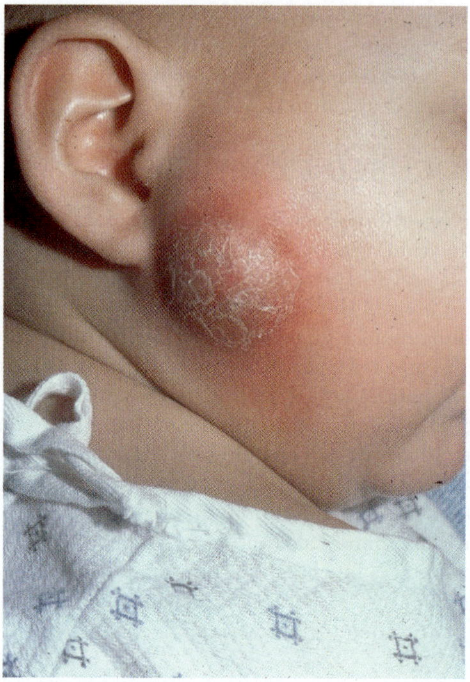

Figure 12.4: Appearance of a parotid gland abscess in a child. (Courtesy of late Peter Sol, MD, and from Leite KR. Lumps on the face. In: Chung EK, Atkinson-McEvoy LR, Lai NL, Terry M, eds. *Visual Diagnosis and Treatment in Pediatrics.* 3rd ed. Wolters Kluwer; 2015:81-88. Figure 11.5.)

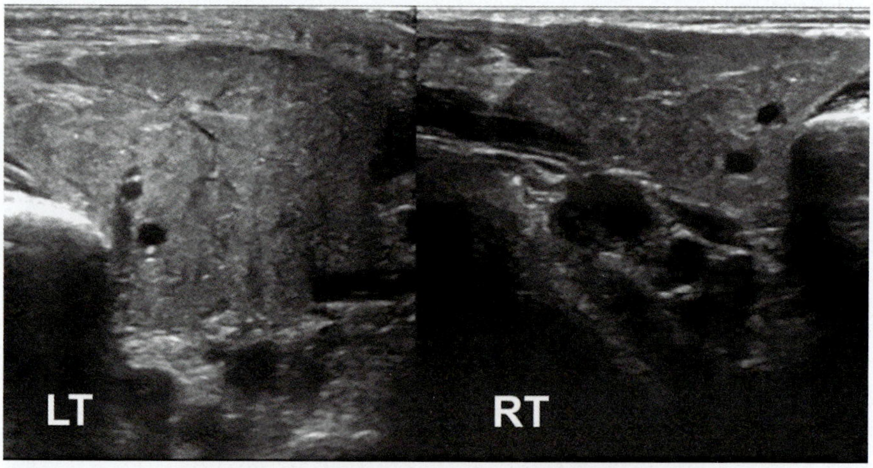

Figure 12.5: Ultrasound demonstrates an enlarged left parotid gland caused by inflammation in comparison to a benign right-sided parotid gland. (From Siegel MJ. Head and neck. In: Siegel MJ, ed. *Pediatric Sonography.* 5th ed. Wolters Kluwer; 2019:112-155. Figure 4.11.)

Computed tomography (CT) is also useful to identify the above lesions and is better than ultrasound for assessing the ducts and surrounding tissues for cellulitis.[10] CT of the head and neck is the diagnostic modality of choice to investigate undifferentiated jaw swelling, with high sensitivity for identifying both sialolithiasis and sialadenitis, as well as numerous other diseases in the differential diagnosis.[11] Noncontrast CT detects stones with high accuracy, but contrast-enhanced CT allows for more detailed exploration of the soft tissue surrounding the gland and is more likely

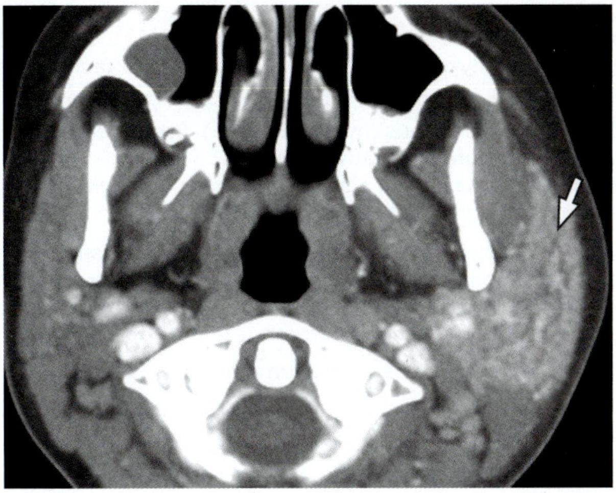

Figure 12.6: Contrast-enhanced CT revealing left parotid inflammation. (From Juliano AF, Vargas SO, Robson CD. Head and neck. In: Lee E, ed. *Pediatric Radiology: Practical Imaging Evaluation of Infants and Children.* 1st ed. Wolters Kluwer; 2018:163-260. Figure 3.151A.)

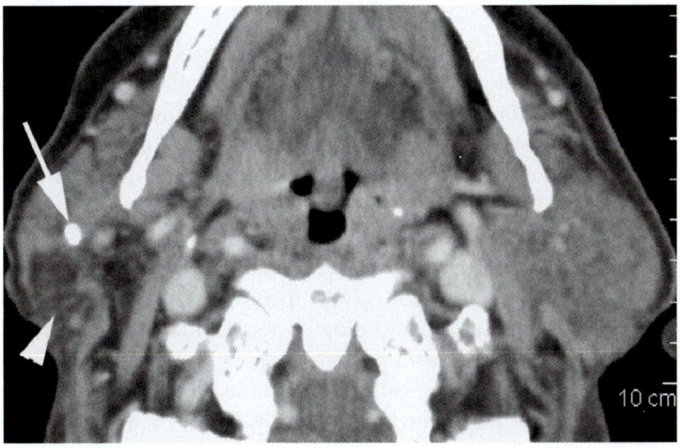

Figure 12.7: CT imaging revealing parotid calculus (long white arrow) and inflammation (white arrowhead). (From Mancuso AA, Vaysberg M. Parotid infections. In: Mancuso AA, ed. *Head and Neck Radiology.* 2nd ed. Wolters Kluwer; 2011:1530-1543. Figure 177.1J.)

to reveal a neoplasm or abscess if present (**Figures 12.6** and **12.7**).[12] Magnetic resonance imaging (MRI) can be used to assess the glands but is often unnecessary in the acute setting of sialadenitis or sialolithiasis.

DIFFERENTIAL DIAGNOSIS

Patients of all ages can be affected by salivary gland swelling, and the disease process has a broad differential diagnosis (**Table 12.1**).

Management

Uncomplicated sialolithiasis can be managed conservatively with intense hydration, warm compresses/heating pads, gland massage after each meal, and use of sialogogues like lemon or vitamin C drops.[13] If a stone is visible or palpable near the duct opening, direct intraoral removal may be

TABLE 12.1 Causes for Salivary Gland Swelling

Viral etiologies	Mumps (paramyxovirus), Epstein-Barr virus, coxsackievirus, influenza A, and parainfluenza
Bacterial etiologies	*Staphylococcus aureus* (most common), *Streptococcus species, Haemophilus influenza*, and gram negative bacteria. **Anaerobic bacteria can also be causative, including** *peptostreptococcus, bacteroides, porphyromonas*, and *prevotella*.
Noninfectious	Cystic fibrosis, collagen vascular disease, alcoholism, diabetes, uremia, gout, sarcoidosis, hepatic or renal failure, hypothyroidism, malnutrition, HIV, Sjögren syndrome, anorexia, bulimia, hyperlipoproteinemia, hyperuricemia, lead poisoning, Cushing syndrome
Oncologic	Benign and malignant salivary tumors
Medications	Diuretics, beta-blockers, tricyclic antidepressants, phenothiazines, anticholinergics, chemotherapy
Iatrogenic	Postoperative hematoma, seroma, or sialocele. Radiation

Derived from Brook I. Diagnosis and management of parotitis. *Arch Otolaryngol Head Neck Surg.* 1992;118(5):469-471.

attempted with a local anesthetic.[1] More complicated cases will warrant an ENT evaluation and invasive treatments, including sialendoscopy, or surgery involving endoscopic or open approaches to the calculi or gland.[7]

Suppurative sialadenitis without abscess formation can be treated with warm compresses/heating pads, hydration, sialogogues, oral hygiene with chlorhexidine 0.12% mouth rinses 3 times a day to reduce intraoral bacterial counts, and antibiotic therapy directed at gram-positive and anaerobic organisms.[1] Most cases without abscess formation resolve with outpatient management.[14] Patients with concern for sepsis or at risk for dehydration or those who have failed a course of oral antibiotics should be admitted for further management with intravenous antibiotics and hydration.

Surgical intervention should be considered when abscess formation occurs, conservative treatment failure occurs, the facial nerve is involved, infection spreads to deep neck spaces, or a high risk of worsening infection exists.[15] Depending on location and severity, abscess drainage can be achieved via bedside needle drainage or operative incision and drainage. Often, when a stone is involved, if it is relatively accessible, surgical drainage is the preferred method because stone removal and abscess evacuation can be performed concurrently. However, with deeper stones, it is preferable to temper the infection with antibiotics and favor an interval less invasive drainage procedure to allow for definitive stone removal in the future.

For patients experiencing chronic sialadenitis, defined as recurrent or persistent salivary gland inflammation, referral to ENT for possible sialendoscopy or open surgery should be considered.[1] In more extreme cases, the entire gland may be removed for disease resolution.[7] Further, any patient found with a mass in the parotid or submandibular gland should be referred to ENT for further workup.

TIPS AND PEARLS

- Sialolithiasis and sialadenitis can successfully be treated in the outpatient setting with the use of heat/warm compresses, sialogogues, glandular massage, and antibiotics in cases of infection.
- Noncontrast and contrast-enhanced CT have high and equivalent sensitivity in the detection of salivary gland calculi in the face of jaw swelling, but contrast CT will better define abscesses or neoplasms.
- Parotid masses or facial nerve palsy should be immediately referred to ENT for further workup given the concern for malignancy.

EVIDENCE

What is the best diagnostic modality to detect salivary duct stones in the presence of jaw or facial swelling?

Contrast-enhanced CT of the neck has a sensitivity of 96%, specificity of 100%, positive predictive value of 100%, negative predictive value of 96.8%, and accuracy of 98% in the detection of salivary gland stones and provides an added benefit for the evaluation of the surrounding soft tissue.[12] Non-contrast CT also has an equivalent sensitivity in the detection of salivary duct calculi.[12] Ultrasound has the benefit of no ionizing radiation but is highly operator dependent and has a sensitivity of 77%, specificity of 95%, positive predictive value of 94%, negative predictive value of 78%, and accuracy of 85% for stone detection in a recent study.[9]

What is the role of sialendoscopy?

Sialendoscopy is a minimally invasive technique that can be performed in both a clinic and an operative room setting to manage obstructive and inflammatory salivary ductal disease. Sialendoscopy utilizes small endoscopes to evaluate the salivary duct. Through working channels on the endoscope, the duct can be irrigated with saline and/or steroids. Although not currently US Food and Drug Administration (FDA) approved, some otolaryngologists also use lithotripsy to break up obstructive stones within the duct to allow them to pass.[16-18] Of note, sialendoscopy cannot be performed during acute infection, owing to risk of duct injury.

What autoimmune or systemic conditions affect the salivary glands, and what is the best management?

Autoimmune and systemic diseases, including Sjögren syndrome and immunoglobulin G4-related disease both affect the salivary glands through an immune-mediate response to the gland parenchyma and/or ductal tissues. The role of interventional sialendoscopy in the treatment of autoimmune mediated inflammation of the glands is currently understudied but is showing promise that it can be a beneficial adjunct in those refractory to other standard rheumatologic therapies.[19]

References

1. Wilson K, Meier J, Ward D. Salivary gland disorders. *Am Fam Physician*. 2014;89(11):882-888.
2. Pasha R, Golub J. *Otolaryngology Head & Neck Surgery: Clinical Reference Guide*. 4th ed. Plural Publishing; 2014.
3. Huoh K, Eisele D. Etiologic factors in sialolithiasis. *Otolaryngol Head Neck Surg*. 2011;145(6):935-939.
4. Brook I. Diagnosis and management of parotitis. *Arch Otolaryngol Head Neck Surg*. 1992;118(5):469-471.
5. Jafek B, Murrow B. *ENT Secrets*. 3rd ed. Elsevier Mosby; 2005.
6. Diebold S, Overbeck M. Soft tissue disorders of the mouth. *Emerg Med Clin North Am*. 2019;37(1):55-68.
7. Kraaij S, Karagozoglu K, Forouzanfar T et al. Salivary stones: symptoms, aetiology, biochemical composition and treatment. *Br Dent J*. 2014; 217(11):E23.
8. Hajiioannou J, Florou V, Kousoulis P, Kretzas D, Moshovakis E. Reversible facial nerve palsy due to parotid abscess. *Int J Surg Case Rep*. 2013;4(1):1021-1024.
9. Terraz S, Poletti P, Dulguerov P, et al. How reliable is sonography in the assessment of sialolithiasis? *Am J Roentgenol*. 2013;201(1):W104-W109.
10. Razek A, Mukherji S. Imaging of sialadenitis. *Neuroradiol J*. 2017;30(3):205-215.
11. Huang F, Caton R, Colla J. Point-of-care ultrasound diagnosis of acute sialolithiasis with sialadenitis. *Clin Pract Cases Emerg Med*. 2017;1(4):437-438.
12. Purcell Y, Kavanagh G, Cahalane A, Carroll A, Khoo S, Killeen R. The diagnostic accuracy of contrast-enhanced CT of the neck for the investigation of sialolithiasis. *Am J Neuroradiol*. 2017;38(11):2161-2166.
13. Duong L, Kakiche T, Ferré F, Nawrocki L, Bouattour A. Management of anterior submandibular sialolithiasis. *J Oral Med Oral Surg*. 2019;25(2):16.
14. Lucerna A, Espinosa J. Acute submandibular sialadenitis. *Emerg Med*. 2017;49(3):131-134.
15. Kim Y, Lee D, Yoon T, Lee J, Lim S. Parotid abscess at a single institute in Korea. *Medicine*. 2018;97(30):e11700.

16. Kim JE, Lee SS, Lee C, et al. Therapeutic effect of intraductal saline irrigation in chronic obstructive sialadenitis. *BMC Oral Health.* 2020;20(1):86.
17. Lele SJ, Hamiter M, Fourrier TL, Nathan C-A. Sialendoscopy with intraductal steroid irrigation in patients with sialadenitis without sialoliths. *Ear Nose Throat J*. 2019;98(5):291-294.
18. Capaccio P, Torretta S, Pignataro L, Koch M. Salivary lithotripsy in the era of sialendoscopy [La litotrissia salivare nell'era della scialoendoscopia]. *Acta Otorhinolaryngol Ital*. 2017;37(2):113-121.
19. Gallo A, Martellucci S, Fusconi M, et al. Sialendoscopic management of autoimmune sialadenitis: a review of literature [Trattamento scialendoscopico delle scialoadeniti autoimmuni: revisione della letteratura]. *Acta Otorhinolaryngol Ital*. 2017;37(2):148-154.

CHAPTER 13

Pharyngitis/Tonsillitis/ Peritonsillar Abscess

Daniel R. Rutz
Samuel J. Trosman

INTRODUCTION

In the outpatient setting, evaluation of sore throat is one of the most common reasons adults and children seek medical care. Approximately 2 million annual emergency department (ED) visits are caused by acute pharyngitis and tonsillitis.[1] Although most of these cases are relatively mild, ED and urgent care providers must be attentive to historical and physical clues signaling dangerous, life-threatening conditions such as deep space neck infections. Peritonsillar abscess (PTA) is a well-known deep space neck infection and a serious complication of bacterial pharyngitis or tonsillitis. Occurring in approximately 30 per 100 000 individuals aged 5 to 59 years, peritonsillar infection can obstruct the upper airway or spread contiguously to surrounding structures in the neck. An understanding of age-specific disease prevalence, throat and neck anatomy, carefully chosen diagnostics, and procedural competency are all required to effectively manage pharyngitis, tonsillitis, and PTA.

PATHOPHYSIOLOGY

The pharynx is the portion of the throat behind the oral cavity, extending from the posterior of the nose to the area behind the larynx and above the esophagus. The palatine tonsils are collections of lymphoid tissue located on the lateral walls of the oropharynx, between the palatoglossal and palatopharyngeal folds. Inflammatory conditions of the pharynx that spare the tonsillar tissues are termed pharyngitis, whereas tonsillitis refers to inflammation of the palatine tonsils. If both structures are involved, the term tonsillopharyngitis is appropriate.

Viruses and β-hemolytic Group A Streptococcus (GAS) account for most cases of acute pharyngitis and tonsillitis. Up to 25% to 50% of acute pharyngitis cases are attributable to respiratory viruses. GAS is responsible for 30% of cases of pharyngitis in children and approximately 15% to 25% of cases in adults. Viruses and GAS circulate widely in the general population and are transmitted through inhalation of droplets. These organisms bind to respiratory epithelium and have direct cytotoxic effects, causing local and systemic inflammatory responses. In addition to sore throat, viral pharyngitis causes fever, coryza, conjunctivitis, nasal congestion, rhinorrhea, fatigue, malaise, and cough. Bacterial pharyngitis causes sore throat, painful swallowing, chills, and fever. Headache, nausea, and vomiting are common as well.

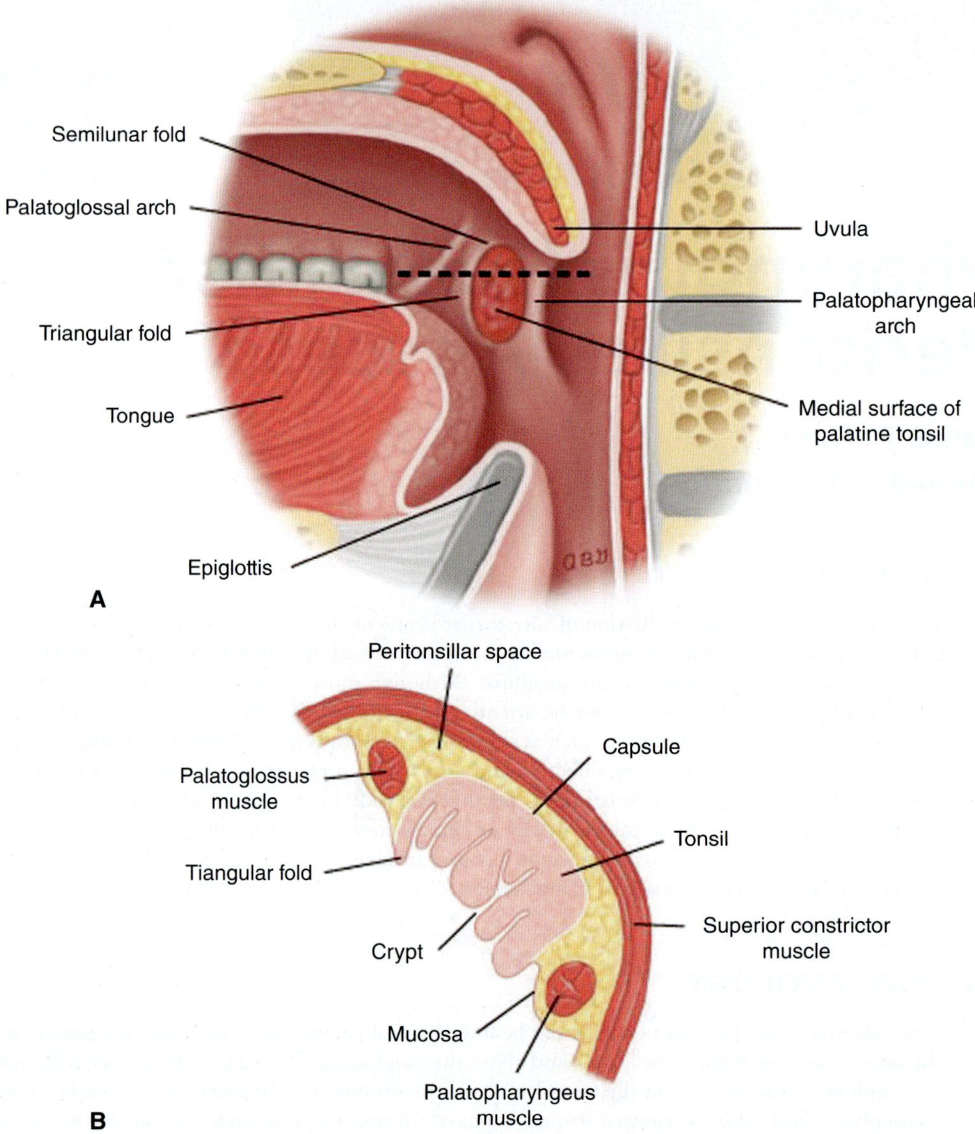

Figure 13.1: Tonsillar anatomy. Panel A shows a sagittal view of the palatine tonsil within the oropharynx. A cross section through the tonsil (dashed line) is shown in Panel B. (*Anatomy of the palatine tonsil*; Graphic 72358 Version 6.0 © 2022 UpToDate, Inc. and/or its affiliates. All Rights Reserved.)

PTA is a purulent infection in the peritonsillar space, which is a potential space adjacent to the superior pharyngeal constrictor muscle and the tonsillar pillars (**Figure 13.1**). The pathophysiology involves progression of bacterial pharyngitis or tonsillitis spilling into the peritonsillar space, causing phlegmonous changes and subsequent abscess formation. PTA usually manifests in the superior portion of the tonsil but can manifest as loculations of purulence inferiorly or laterally as well.

APPROACH/THE FOCUSED EXAM

A careful clinical examination can help differentiate pharyngitis, tonsillitis, and PTA. Using a tongue blade and having the patient yawn or say "ahh" will elevate the palate and uvula, providing

TABLE 13.1 Concerning Exam Findings for Presence of Upper Airway Obstruction or Deep Space Neck Infection

Signs of Upper Airway Obstruction
• Stridor • Muffled or "hot potato" voice • Assuming a tripod position • Tachypnea • Pooling of oropharyngeal secretions
Signs of Deep Space Neck Infection
• Trismus • Inability to flex or extend neck • Torticollis • Crepitus • Dysphagia • Ill appearance (high fever, rigors)

Adapted from Yoon PJ, Scholes MA, Herrmann BW. Ear, nose, & throat. In: Hay WW Jr, Levin MJ, Abzug MJ, Bunik M, eds. *Current Diagnosis & Treatment: Pediatrics.* 25th ed. McGraw-Hill; 2021.

a better view of the oropharynx, palatine tonsils, and peritonsillar tissue. Pharyngitis clinically appears as erythematous and inflamed pharyngeal mucosa. Acute tonsillitis manifests as redness and swelling of the tonsils and tonsillar pillars. Tonsillar exudate may be present, and clinicians may palpate tender cervical lymph nodes. A PTA causes marked unilateral swelling of the peritonsillar soft tissue, deviation of the uvula away from the affected side, and palpable fluctuance. Patients may also present with trismus owing to spasm of the interior pterygoid muscle and with a muffled or "hot potato" voice owing to throat swelling. Unilateral otalgia caused by referred pain also suggests peritonsillar infection, phlegmon, or abscess. In severe cases, symptoms of upper airway obstruction such as respiratory distress, drooling, stridor, and tripod positioning may occur (**Table 13.1**). Bedside laryngoscopy, often performed by clinicians familiar with this technique, or in consultation with otolaryngology, can confirm anatomic findings of airway obstruction. These patients may rapidly decompensate and may need emergent intubation or tracheostomy in the operating room.

DIFFERENTIAL DIAGNOSIS

Although pharyngitis and tonsillitis are most often attributable to viral infection or β-hemolytic GAS, providers should consider a broad differential diagnosis for patients presenting with sore throat.

Commonly transmitted seasonal respiratory viruses, notably rhinovirus, adenovirus, coronaviruses and influenza virus, are the most common causes of viral pharyngitis. These do not require special testing and have a self-limited course. SARS-CoV-2, the virus that causes COVID-19, can also manifest as pharyngitis. Other viral agents include Epstein-Barr virus (EBV), human immunodeficiency virus (HIV), and herpes simplex virus (HSV). EBV causes infectious mononucleosis and is transmitted through oral contact, often in adolescence and young adulthood. Clinically, it appears as tonsillopharyngitis with tonsillar exudate and posterior cervical lymphadenopathy and is associated with high fever, malaise, and fatigue. Patients placed on penicillin-based antibiotics for treatment of presumed streptococcal infection may develop a rash when infected with EBV. Clinicians should examine for splenomegaly and take note of atypical lymphocytes on blood work to aid in the diagnosis of EBV. The acute phase of HIV infection occurs approximately 2 to 4 weeks post exposure and may present with fever, a nonexudative pharyngitis, and cervical adenopathy as part of a flulike syndrome. Physicians should consider this diagnosis in patients with high-risk behaviors or patients with coexisting sexually transmitted infections. The presence of oropharyngeal or tongue ulcers should prompt an evaluation for HSV pharyngitis.

β-Hemolytic GAS accounts for almost 25% of adult cases of tonsillopharyngitis. Other important but less common bacteria include Group C or Group G *Streptococcus*, *Fusobacterium*, *Mycoplasma pneumonia, Neisseria gonorrhoeae,* and *Chlamydia pneumoniae*. *Fusobacterium* is the causative agent of a rare disease process, Lemierre syndrome, also known as septic thrombophlebitis of the internal jugular vein. *Fusobacterium* is an oropharyngeal anaerobe that colonizes young patients. Lemierre Syndrome presents as pharyngitis with tonsillar exudates, jaw pain, and possible swelling of the neck or angle of the jaw. Unvaccinated patients or those from developing countries are at risk for pharyngitis owing to *Corynebacterium diphtheriae*, which causes pharyngitis with a gray membrane that bleeds when prodded.

The differential diagnosis for PTA includes other causes of deep space neck infections and upper airway obstruction. Retropharyngeal abscess, common in early childhood, also causes high fever, throat pain, and trismus. It may also produce neck stiffness caused by torticollis, especially with attempted neck extension, and less prominent peritonsillar soft tissue swelling on examination of the throat. A parapharyngeal abscess can cause a toxic appearance and neck stiffness, as well as displacement of the pharyngeal wall or bulging of the posterior tonsillar pillar. Although less common in individuals vaccinated against *Haemophilus influenzae B*, upper airway obstruction resulting from acute epiglottitis is a diagnostic consideration in this patient population. Young children with epiglottitis attributable to *Haemophilus influenzae B* may present with symptoms of impending airway obstruction with tripod positioning, drooling, stridor, and tachypnea. Older children, adolescents, and adults with epiglottitis may exhibit severe sore throat, dysphagia, and drooling without signs of airway obstruction.

Finally noninfectious considerations of throat pain and swelling include acute angioedema, anaphylaxis, head and neck trauma, or head and neck tumors.

MANAGEMENT

Viral tonsillopharyngitis can be diagnosed clinically based on history and physical examination. RT-PCR testing of SARS-CoV-2 can be obtained to evaluate for COVID-19 if suspected. Other cases where viral testing may be appropriate include evaluation of possible influenza, EBV, and acute HIV. Routine cases of viral pharyngitis are treated symptomatically with oral hydration, antipyretics, analgesics, and rest. In the ED, dehydrated patients or those who cannot take oral fluids should be given IV fluids.

The decision to test for GAS via rapid antigen diagnostic testing (RADT) can be guided by the presence of modified Centor criteria for GAS. These include: (1) tonsillar exudates, (2) tender anterior cervical adenopathy, (3) absence of cough, (4) history of fever, and (5) age 3 to 14 years. When only one criterion is present, GAS is unlikely. When two to three of the five criteria are present, there is an intermediate (11%-35%) likelihood of GAS, and testing should be considered. A score of 4 or 5 points is associated with a 51% to 53% likelihood of GAS infection. RADT have an overall sensitivity of 86% and a specificity of 94% to 96% but are slightly less sensitive in the adult population (77%-92%), so high-risk patients should undergo throat culture testing to avoid false-negative rapid results. High-risk patients include those with immune compromise, with history of acute rheumatic fever (RF), living in congregate facilities, or with high Centor scores (≥3).

Testing for atypical bacterium such as *Chlamydia pneumoniae*, *Neisseria gonorrhoeae*, *Mycoplasma pneumoniae*, *Fusobacterium* species, or rarer causes of pharyngitis, such as *Clostridium diphtheriae* are indicated for patients with risk factors, high provider suspicion, or those in whom treatment for GAS is not curative.

Current infectious disease guidelines recommend antimicrobial treatment of GAS infections.[2] Penicillin is the recommended first-line drug for GAS, with IM Benzathine Penicillin, Penicillin VK, or amoxicillin being appropriate candidates. For nonanaphylactic penicillin-allergic patients, a cephalosporin or clindamycin may be used, although resistance to these agents has been reported. In immunocompetent patients, administration of corticosteroids increases the likelihood of complete pain resolution at 24 hours (absolute reduction 20.8%; number needed to treat [NNT] 5; relative risk [RR] 2.4, 95% confidence interval [CI] 1.3-4.5) and at 48 hours (absolute reduction 24.4%; NNT 5; RR 1.5, 95% CI 1.3-1.8).[3] Antibiotics modestly reduce the risk of local complications such as acute otitis media and PTA. In large meta-analysis of randomized trials comparing antibiotics to placebo in adults and children with streptococcal pharyngitis, antibiotics reduced the rate of acute otitis media within 14 days (0.47% vs 2.0%; risk ratio [RR] 0.30, 95% CI 0.15-0.58) and PTA at two months (0.24% versus 2.3%; RR 0.15, 95% CI 0.05-0.47).[4]

The two major nonsuppurative complications of GAS pharyngitis are RF and poststreptococcal glomerulonephritis (PSGN). Antibiotics have never been shown to prevent PSGN, and the evidence for prevention of rheumatic fever in developed countries is not compelling. Early data on effectiveness of antibiotics for prevention of RF was skewed based on studies of young men in military barracks where there was a high incidence of RF compared with the general population.[5] Newer estimates place the incidence of RF much lower at approximately 300 cases per 2.2 million individuals without antibiotics compared with 75 per 2.2 million with antibiotics, indicating an NNT of 10 000 to prevent one case of RF, and an NNT of 20 000 to prevent one case of rheumatic heart disease.[6] The decline in RF in developed countries is likely a combination of improved sanitation and living conditions, along with changes in the protein structure of circulating GAS that makes it less likely to cause RF.

The diagnosis of PTA can be made clinically by physical exam (**Figure 13.2**) or radiographically via point-of-care ultrasound (POCUS) or contrast-enhanced computed tomography (CT) scan of the neck. Where there is diagnostic uncertainty, as is the case with peritonsillar cellulitis or another deep space infection, bedside endoscopic POCUS performed after the administration of local anesthesia is a useful modality to identify a peritonsillar fluid collection consistent with PTA (**Figure 13.3**). CT scan of the neck with IV contrast can readily distinguish PTA from other mimics such as peritonsillar cellulitis, phlegmon, retropharyngeal or parapharyngeal abscess, Lemierre disease, or other deep space neck infections. A PTA will appear as a hypodense area with rim enhancement, often with mass effect on the surrounding soft tissue.

Treatment of PTA requires needle aspiration or incision and drainage (I&D) followed by antibiotics. Local anesthesia is achieved with topical or nebulized lidocaine, and procedural sedation should be considered in the pediatric population. The area of maximum fluctuance can be aspirated with a needle, evacuating pus until swelling is improved. Alternatively, a mucosal incision is made and the abscess pocket bluntly entered and drained. These two approaches have similar efficacy rates when successfully evacuating the purulent fluid collection, although I&D is typically performed by an ENT consultant. Complications of either procedure include bleeding, aspiration of blood or abscess contents into the airway, and intractable pain. A feared complication, albeit exceedingly rare, is carotid artery injury. Patients should be observed after aspiration or I&D for ability to tolerate liquids and antibiotics. Improvement is rapid, with most patients experiencing subjective decrease in pain and throat swelling in the first 24 hours after successful drainage. Antibiotics should cover GAS and *Staph aureus*, with consideration for methicillin-resistant *Staph aureus* if local disease prevalence is high. Amoxicillin-clavulanic

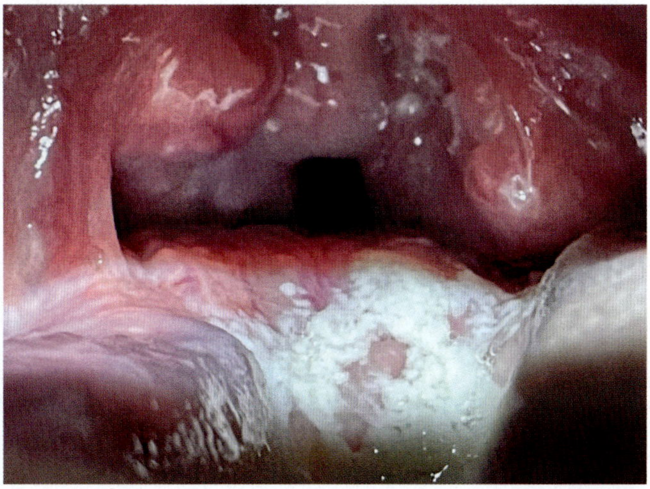

Figure 13.2: Left-sided peritonsillar abscess. Abscess is in the left superior peritonsillar space, evident as increased mucosal swelling in that region and effacement of the left tonsillar pillar. (Courtesy of Dr. Samuel J. Trosman, The Mount Sinai Hospital.)

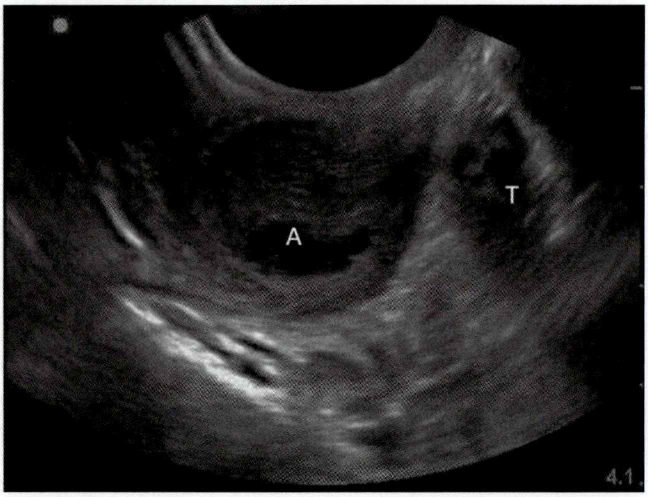

Figure 13.3: Point-of-care endoscopic ultrasound demonstrating peritonsillar abscess (A) adjacent to palatine tonsil (T). Abscess appears as nodular structure with hyperechoic border and mixed hypoechoic and anechoic center consistent with purulent fluid collection. (Courtesy of Dr. David R. Rutz, University of Wisconsin Department of Emergency Medicine, Emergency Ultrasound.)

acid or clindamycin should be prescribed for 14 days.[7] Treatment failure or multiple recurrent PTAs are indications for tonsillectomy. Patients with concern for airway compromise caused by swelling or inability to tolerate liquids and antibiotics caused by pain should be admitted to the hospital for parenteral fluids and IV antibiotic therapy. Data on administration of steroids is incomplete with respect to PTA, but small studies suggest efficacy in symptomatic improvement.[8,9] The decision to give steroids should be considered in the context of the patient's immune status, age, and comorbid illnesses.

PEDIATRIC ISSUES

Respiratory viruses account for most cases of pharyngitis in the pediatric population. Testing for GAS is not recommended for patients under 3 years old owing to the much higher incidence of viral pharyngitis in this age group unless they have a risk factor for infection such as close contact with a sibling that has tested positive.

EVIDENCE

How should the Centor score be used in the evaluation and treatment of GAS tonsillopharyngitis?

First published in 1981, modified in 1998, and validated in the early 2000s, the Centor is an easy-to-use and prospectively validated decision tool when applied to patients with sore throat of 3 days' duration or less. In early studies on small patient populations, a higher Centor score was associated with increased chance of testing positive for GAS. A retrospective study evaluated over 140 000 patients aged 15 years or older presenting to an urgent care setting and found that the modified score performed well compared with the smaller validation studies. In this study, 95% confidence intervals overlapped between the retail health chain derived scores and probabilities of testing positive. For patients scoring 0-1, the Infectious Diseases Society of America (IDSA) recommends against testing or treatment of GAS (1%-10% likelihood of GAS). For a score of 2-3, RADT testing is recommended with antibiotic treatment if positive (11%-53% likelihood of GAS). Empiric treatment with antibiotics is warranted if patients fulfill all of the Centor criteria.[10]

How should rapid antigen diagnostic tests (RADTs) be interpreted, and when should throat cultures be obtained?

RADTs are the mainstay for diagnosis of GAS in the pediatric and adult population owing to their high specificity, ease of performance, and rapid turnaround. However, the sensitivity for most RADT is 70% to 90% compared with gold standard throat culture (90%-95% sensitive when performed correctly). A tradeoff for higher sensitivity with throat culture is delay in diagnosis. Specificity is quite high for most RADT, approaching 95%, meaning that false positive tests from RADT are rare. Therefore, clinicians can be confident in prescribing antibiotics for GAS based on positive RADT. In the pediatric population, owing to lower sensitivity and higher disease prevalence, a negative RADT should have confirmatory throat culture. Accuracy in diagnosis is also important because of the increased risk of rheumatic heart disease. In the adult population, however, a negative RADT should generally be considered a true negative.

Is endoscopic POCUS safe and reliable for diagnosis and guidance for PTA aspiration?

Diagnosis of PTA can be challenging based on exam alone, as unilateral peritonsillar swelling and uvular deviation can be seen with peritonsillar cellulitis and phlegmon, without a discrete purulent fluid collection. Endoscopic POCUS, when utilized correctly, can assist in fluid collection identification and mitigate unnecessary needle aspiration or I&D. In a retrospective review of 43 suspected PTA patients presenting to an ED, endoscopic POCUS performed by ED sonologists correctly identified 34 PTA with only one false-positive. There were no reported aspiration complications in this study.[11] A randomized trial comparing endoscopic POCUS with traditional landmark-based guidance for PTA aspiration yielded greater success in the POCUS group.[12]

Which technique is better, needle aspiration or incision and drainage, for treatment of PTA?

Both needle aspiration and I&D are acceptable treatment options for management of PTA, but neither has been shown in high-quality studies to be superior to the other. A Cochrane review evaluated 11 studies involving 674 patients with PTA undergoing either I&D or needle aspiration.[13] This review rated the quality of evidence as *very low* owing to flawed study design and risk of bias but demonstrated a trend toward a lower recurrence rate of PTA in patients having undergone I&D.

How effective are corticosteroids in the management of peritonsillar abscesses?

Evidence for steroid effectiveness for PTA is mixed. In one study, 41 patients were randomized to a single dose of IV dexamethasone compared with placebo.[8] Both groups underwent needle aspiration for intervention of PTA. The patients in the dexamethasone treatment group reported decreased pain at 24-hour follow-up compared with placebo.[8] However, there was no significant difference in pain at 48 hours or 7-day follow-up periods. No significant side effects were encountered in either group. An older study on hospitalized patients with PTA demonstrated a clinical benefit with IV steroids for symptoms of throat pain, trismus, and dysphagia.[9] Large double-blind placebo-controlled studies are needed to more thoroughly address this question.

References

1. Niska R, Bhuiya F, Xu J. National Hospital Ambulatory Medical Care Survey: 2007 emergency department summary. *Natl Health Stat Report*. 2010;(26):1-31.
2. Shulman ST, Bisno AL, Clegg HW, et al. Clinical practice guideline for the diagnosis and management of group a streptococcal pharyngitis: 2012 update by the Infectious Diseases Society of America. *Clin Infect Dis*. 2012;55(10):e86-e102. doi:10.1093/cid/cis629
3. de Cassan S, Thompson MJ, Perera R, et al. Corticosteroids as standalone or add-on treatment for sore throat. *Cochrane Database Syst Rev*. 2020;2020(5). doi:10.1002/14651858.CD008268.pub3
4. Spinks A, Glasziou PP, del Mar CB. Antibiotics for sore throat. *Cochrane Database Syst Rev*. 2013;2013(11). doi:10.1002/14651858.CD000023.pub4

5. Denny FW, Wannamaker LW, Brink WR, Rammelkamp CH Jr, Custer EA. Prevention of rheumatic fever: treatment of the preceding streptococcic infection. *J Am Med Assoc*. 1950;143(2): 151-153. doi:10.1001/jama.1950.02910370001001
6. McMurray K, Garber M. Taking chances with strep throat. *Hosp Pediatr*. 2015;5(10):552. doi:10.1542/hpeds.2015-0101
7. Apostolopoulos NJ, Nikolopoulos TP, Bairamis TN. Peritonsillar abscess in children. Is incision and drainage an effective management? *Int J Pediatr Otorhinolaryngol*. 1995;31(2):129-135. doi:10.1016/0165-5876(94)01077-B
8. Chau JKM, Seikaly HR, Harris JR, Villa-Roel C, Brick C, Rowe BH. Corticosteroids in peritonsillar abscess treatment: a blinded placebo-controlled clinical trial. In: *Laryngoscope*. Vol 124. John Wiley and Sons; 2014:97-103. doi:10.1002/lary.24283
9. Ozbek C, Aygenc E, Tuna EU, Selcuk A, Ozdem C. Use of steroids in the treatment of peritonsillar abscess. *J Laryngol Otol*. 2004;118(6):439-442. doi:10.1258/002221504323219563
10. Snow V, Mottur-Pilson C, Cooper RJ, Hoffman JR. Principles of appropriate antibiotic use for acute pharyngitis in adults. 2001. www.annals.org
11. Lyon M, Blaivas M. Intraoral ultrasound in the diagnosis and treatment of suspected peritonsillar abscess in the emergency department. *Acad Emerg Med*. 2005;12(1):85-88. doi:10.1197/j.aem.2004.08.045
12. Costantino TG, Satz WA, Dehnkamp W, Goett H. Randomized trial comparing intraoral ultrasound to landmark-based needle aspiration in patients with suspected peritonsillar abscess. *Acad Emerg Med*. 2012;19(6):626-631. doi:10.1111/j.1553-2712.2012.01380.x
13. Chang BA, Thamboo A, Burton MJ, Diamond C, Nunez DA. Needle aspiration versus incision and drainage for the treatment of peritonsillar abscess. *Cochrane Database of Syst Rev*. 2016;2016(12). doi:10.1002/14651858.CD006287.pub4

CHAPTER 14

Deep Space Neck Infections: Retropharyngeal Abscess, Ludwig Angina, Lemierre Syndrome

Amy Caggiula
Tjoson Tjoa

INTRODUCTION

The anatomy of the deep space of the neck allows for the rapid spread of infections along fascial planes. Owing to their proximity to several vital airway and circulatory structures, these infections were usually fatal prior to the modern antibiotic age (**Figure 14.1**). The region posterior to the alar fascia extends from the oropharyngeal region into the posterior mediastinum to the level of the diaphragm. Because of this potential highway of rapid spread, this compartment is referred to as the "danger space." Even now, deep space neck infections pose unique diagnostic and management obstacles, because it is often difficult to visualize affected structures on physical exam. Edema and obscuration of anatomic landmarks add to the challenge. Without prompt diagnosis and initiation of treatment, morbidity and mortality remain high.

THE CLINICAL CHALLENGE

Retropharyngeal Abscess

Retropharyngeal abscess (RPA) is generally considered a disease of children, affecting approximately 4.6/100 000 in the United States annually. Most RPAs present in children under age 6,[1] because retropharyngeal lymph nodes involute around years four to five of life. A true RPA in an adult patient is most often caused by a penetrating injury into the retropharyngeal space. Otherwise, similar infections in adults, usually stemming from pharyngeal or dental origin, generally result in parapharyngeal rather than RPAs.

Owing to its anatomic location, physical exam diagnosis of RPA can be challenging but important to consider. A missed diagnosis of a deep space neck infection, particularly those involving the retropharyngeal space, can have devastating consequences for the surrounding vasculature, mediastinum, airway, and esophagus. If left untreated, infections in the retropharyngeal space lead to mediastinitis, thrombophlebitis of the internal jugular vein (Lemierre syndrome), erosion into the carotid arteries, sepsis, and death.

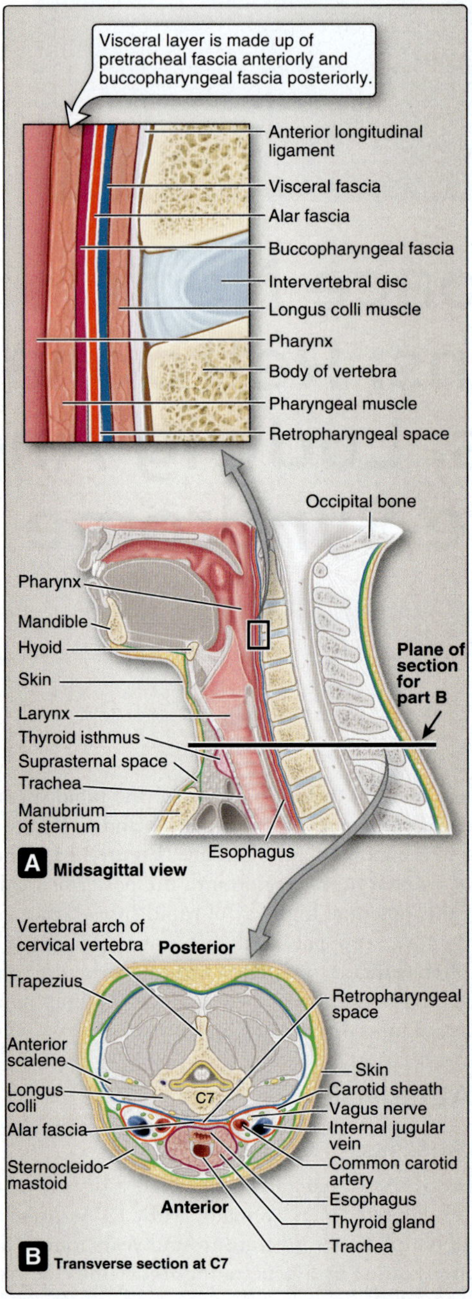

Figure 14.1: Fascial layers and spaces in the neck. A, Note structures forming retropharyngeal space. B, Compartments and fascial arrangement. Superficial cervical fascia: yellow, subcutaneous tissue of neck. Layers of deep cervical fascia: green, investing layer; violet, visceral layer; blue, prevertebral layer; red, alar fascia and carotid sheath. (From Moore KL, Dalley AF II, Agur AMR. *Clinically Oriented Anatomy*. 8th ed. Wolters Kluwer; 2018. Figure 9.4. Based on Gest TR. *Lippincott Atlas of Anatomy*. 2nd ed. Wolters Kluwer; 2020. Plate 7.14.)

Ludwig Angina

Ludwig angina is a rapidly progressive cellulitis involving the floor of the mouth and soft tissues of the neck. Before the widespread use of antibiotics, this gangrenous infection was frequently fatal. Mortality remains high, even in more modern times, and can range from 8% to 50% depending on the promptness of diagnosis and aggressive early management.[2] Most fatalities are caused by airway compromise rather than overwhelming sepsis. The degree of edema and tongue displacement can pose a significant airway challenge, so swift identification and advanced airway planning is crucial to preventing morbidity and mortality.

Lemierre Syndrome

Lemierre syndrome describes a condition of thrombophlebitis of the internal jugular vein and bacteremia secondary to an anaerobic infection, typically originating in the oropharynx. It can ultimately lead to the development of life-threatening septic emboli. It was first described by Andre Lemierre in 1936 through a series of 20 patients with throat infection that exhibited a 90% mortality rate.

Lemierre syndrome predominantly affects healthy young adults and in most cases is caused by *Fusobacterium necrophorum*, a gram-negative, non-spore-forming obligate anaerobe. In the antibiotic era, the prevalence of this disease has decreased dramatically, although there has been a recent uptick in the number of case reports.[3] Delays in treatment are common, likely because of the high frequency of routine throat infections that are appropriately not treated with antibiotics. Lemierre syndrome can be life-threatening, with mortality rates between 5% and 22%, highlighting the importance of prompt recognition of the condition.[3]

PATHOPHYSIOLOGY

Retropharyngeal Abscess

The retropharyngeal space is bounded posterolaterally by the deep layer of the deep cervical fascia and anteriorly by the buccopharyngeal fascia (also referred to as the middle layer of the deep cervical fascia). This compartment contains lymph nodes that drain surrounding structures, specifically the nasopharynx, tonsils, adenoids, sinuses, and middle ear. Early infections are often contained by this series of fascial planes, but with progression of infection, these compartments can become overwhelmed by increasing pressure from abscess and pus formation, allowing the infection to spread across planes into nearby structures.

RPAs in children usually develop due contiguous or hematogenous spread from bacterial infections of the nasopharynx, middle ear, or (rarely) dentition. These infections are most often polymicrobial, with *Staphylococcus aureus* and Group A Streptococcus the most commonly isolated bacteria.[4,5] Anaerobic species are less frequently encountered but have also been cultured, particularly in cases arising from an odontogenic source.

Ludwig Angina

Most Ludwig angina cases arise from an odontogenic source, particularly the first or second molar teeth (teeth numbers 19 and 30 are the most frequently reported source). Poor dentition, history of recent dental extraction, other infections of the pharynx, alcoholism, malnutrition, history of immunocompromise, poorly controlled diabetes mellitus (DM), and recent oral or maxillofacial trauma are risk factors for the development of this infection.

Ludwig angina spreads rapidly and contiguously to surrounding compartments via fascial planes. Infection most often originates in the submylohyoid space, which is divided from the sublingual space by the mylohyoid muscle. Together, these compartments form the submandibular space. When bacteria inoculates the submylohyoid region, it can spread superiorly and posteriorly into the sublingual space, causing elevation of the tongue and potential airway compromise.

Cultures from fluid aspirates usually demonstrate mixed oral flora but can vary depending on underlying risk factors, disease processes, and concomitant infections (**Table 14.1**). *Klebsiella* species are frequently present in patients with a history of alcoholism, and dental anaerobes are often cultured when the patient has a concurrent dental abscess or history of recent extraction.

Lemierre Syndrome

Lemierre syndrome is most commonly associated with a recent history of acute pharyngitis or tonsillitis, although case reports have demonstrated other sources of infection, including otitis media, mastoiditis, sinusitis, or dental infection.[3] The most common initial clinical presentation is that of a throat infection, followed by unilateral neck tenderness and swelling 4 to 12 days afterward.

TABLE 14.1 Common Disease-Causing Pathogens of Ludwig Angina

• Staphylococcus epidermidis • Streptococcus viridans • Klebsiella pneumoniae • Bacteroides • Actinomyces	• Peptostreptococcus • Enterococcus species • Fusobacterium • Streptococcus anginosus • Staphylococcus aureus

F. necrophorum is the most common offending organism, with other *Fusobacterium* species, anaerobic *Streptococci*, *Bacteroides* species, and *Klebsiella pneumoniae* all being reported as causative agents. Although *F. necrophorum* occurs naturally in the human oropharynx, the current consensus is that *Fusobacterium* should always be treated as a pathogen. It is thought that infection of the oropharynx renders the mucosa more vulnerable to penetration by the bacteria, which can then exert its effects through endotoxins. There is an association between Lemierre syndrome and recent Epstein-Barr viral infection, which may represent an alteration of T cell-mediated immunity.

Regardless of how *Fusobacterium* and other anaerobes become invasive, once they penetrate the mucosal lining, the bacteria can migrate through lymphatics or hematogenously. *F. necrophorum* produces hemagglutinin, which has been shown to aggregate human platelets in vitro, resulting in intravascular coagulation and thrombocytopenia.[3] Venous thrombosis first occurs in the peritonsillar veins, then extends proximally into the larger veins, and ultimately into the internal jugular vein. The release of septic emboli from the internal jugular vein can result in widespread dissemination of bacteria through septic metastases, most commonly into the pulmonary capillaries, which can present as cavitary nodules or empyema. Septic emboli can affect the joints, resulting in septic arthritis; muscles, liver and spleen, resulting in abscesses; and even the central nervous system in the form of abscesses or meningitis.

APPROACH/THE FOCUSED EXAM

Retropharyngeal Abscess

Early diagnosis of RPA can be difficult because several disease entities present similarly, and inflamed overlying structures can obscure direct visualization of the posterior pharynx. As such, the medical provider must have a high index of suspicion for deep space infection with specific signs and symptoms (**Table 14.2**).

Physical exam for RPA includes a thorough head, eyes, ears, nose, and throat (HEENT) exam, including early and frequent airway assessment. Because infections in the retropharyngeal space can compress vital airway structures, immediate airway management is sometimes indicated. Further, rapid clinical deterioration of an initially well-appearing child is possible, so repeated evaluation of the patient's neurologic and respiratory status is critical. Physical exam should also include inspection, palpation, and mobility of the neck, and assessment of the cervical, submandibular, and submental lymph nodes. If edema or significant trismus limits the physical exam, fiberoptic laryngoscopy may be indicated to visualize the throat and surrounding structures.

TABLE 14.2 Signs and Symptoms of Retropharyngeal Abscess (RPA)

Symptoms	Physical Exam Findings
• Sore throat • Fever • Odynophagia • Dysphagia • Lethargy	• Limited neck mobility/torticollis • Unilateral swelling of the posterior pharynx • Anterior or lateral neck tenderness to palpation • Cervical lymphadenopathy • Inability to swallow secretions/drooling • Hoarseness • Stridor

Computed tomography (CT) imaging with IV contrast of the neck is often useful, providing vital information regarding location, size, and extent of the abscess. Further, it can demonstrate the presence and/or degree of airway compromise by surrounding inflammation.

Ludwig Angina

Initial examination should include a detailed HEENT exam focusing on the oral cavity, pharynx, teeth, salivary glands, neck, and lymph nodes. Physical examination may be challenging, particularly in the presence of significant trismus and/or edema. Because the first and second mandibular molars are a frequent source of the infection, direct palpation of the tooth surfaces and the gums around those teeth should be performed with a tongue depressor whenever possible. Signs and symptoms suggesting airway compromise (**Table 14.3**) should prompt early consultation with ENT and anesthesia for rapid surgical intervention and airway management.

Lemierre Syndrome

Because Lemierre syndrome is often a sequela of a prior throat infection, the diagnosis can elude clinicians owing to the high incidence of relatively self-limiting oropharyngeal infections and nonspecificity of symptoms. Affected patients are often young (age 16-30 years) and otherwise healthy, with a 2:1 male-to-female ratio. The presence of a fever and worsening status more than a week after the onset of symptoms is often what raises the clinical suspicion for Lemierre syndrome (**Table 14.4**).

Laboratory investigation typically reveals a leukocytosis with primary neutrophilia and a high c-reactive protein. Signs of organ failure, such as elevated liver enzymes, could be a sign of septic emboli. Ultimately, definitive diagnosis of Lemierre syndrome should be made based on the following[6]:

1. A recent pharyngeal illness
2. Thrombosis of the internal jugular vein or findings of *F. necrophorum* in blood cultures
3. Septic emboli

Contrast-enhanced CT scan of the neck is the most appropriate initial imaging modality. It typically reveals a distended internal jugular vein with filling defects and enhancement of the vessel wall.[7] Ultrasonography can be performed at bedside and is more cost-effective and avoids radiation but is less sensitive than CT for recently formed thrombus.

Many microbiology laboratories have a difficult time growing anaerobic bacteria, and *F. necrophorum* can require a longer incubation period than other organisms.[6] Additionally, there are high rates of false negative cultures owing to the liberal use of antibiotics in the outpatient treatment of pharyngitis and tonsillitis. In fact, it has been suggested that *F. necrophorum* is present in all patients with Lemierre syndrome but that it goes undetected for these reasons.

TABLE 14.3 Signs and Symptoms of Ludwig Angina

Symptoms	Physical Exam Findings
• Neck pain • Fever • Dentalgia • Dysphagia • Trismus • Drooling	• Anterior neck swelling/induration • Elevation or protrusion of the tongue • Tense induration of the submandibular area • Edema of the floor of the mouth • Stridor • Lymphadenopathy

TABLE 14.4 Signs and Symptoms of Lemierre Syndrome

Symptoms	Physical Exam Findings
• Recent sore throat • Fever • Pleuritic pain • Dyspnea • Lethargy	• Unilateral neck pain and swelling • Induration at angle of mandible • Trismus • Oxygen desaturation • Tachycardia or tachypnea • Septic shock

TABLE 14.5 Differential Diagnosis (DDx) for Retropharyngeal Abscess (RPA)

• Tonsillitis • Peritonsillar cellulitis or abscess • Pharyngitis (bacterial or viral) • Suppurative lymphadenitis • Parapharyngeal abscess • Epiglottitis	• Bacterial tracheitis • Croup • Uvulitis • Lymphoma • Airway obstruction • Foreign body ingestion

DIFFERENTIAL DIAGNOSIS

Retropharyngeal Abscess

The differential diagnosis (DDx) for RPA is broad and includes any disease entity that could lead to swelling and compression in the retropharyngeal space and surrounding structures (**Table 14.5**). Because patients presenting with RPA are usually febrile and ill-appearing, the DDx can be limited to infectious and inflammatory processes.

Ludwig Angina

Ludwig angina is a clinical diagnosis, but it can be difficult to differentiate on physical exam from other disease entities causing swelling of the oral cavity, pharynx, and neck. **Table 14.6** details inflammatory processes that should also be considered in the right clinical setting.

Lemierre Syndrome

Lemierre syndrome is a diagnosis specifically determined by the presence of internal jugular vein thrombosis and septic emboli, so there are few other diseases that fit these criteria. However, the clinical presentation is nonspecific and can often be mistaken for other throat and neck infections, as well as other causes of sepsis (see **Table 14.7**).

MANAGEMENT

Retropharyngeal Abscess

Once diagnosed, management of RPA involves both medical and surgical interventions. If the patient's airway is at risk at presentation, awake fiberoptic nasotracheal intubation is the modality of choice. In well-appearing children without evidence of complications, hospital admission to the hospital with IV antibiotics and close observation can be considered. Indications for immediate operative management include sepsis, descending infection, airway compromise, or no improvement after 48 hours of high-dose intravenous antibiotics.

Initial antibiotic choice should cover both aerobic and anaerobic species. A regimen consisting of a broad-spectrum penicillin (eg, ampicillin-sulbactam 50 mg/kg/dose IV q6h) **plus** vancomycin 17.5 mg/kg/dose IV q6h should be used for patients in whom methicillin-resistant staphylococcus aureus (MRSA) is suspected. Clindamycin 10 mg/kg/dose IV q8h can be used in penicillin-allergic patients as a monotherapy, but recent studies have demonstrated a rise in clindamycin-resistant *S aureus* isolated from deep space neck infections.[1,8]

TABLE 14.6 Differential Diagnosis (DDx) for Ludwig Angina

• Angioedema • Oral cavity malignancy • Other head and neck cancer • Lymphoma • Parotitis • Dental abscess	• Epiglottitis • Peritonsillar abscess • Submandibular abscess • Diphtheria • Lemierre syndrome • Sublingual hematoma

TABLE 14.7 Differential Diagnosis (DDx) for Lemierre Syndrome

• Pharyngitis (bacterial or viral) • Cervical lymphadenitis • Parapharyngeal abscess	• Sepsis • Lymphoma • Disseminated intravascular coagulation

Ludwig Angina

Initial management of Ludwig angina focuses on protection of the patient's airway because airway obstruction is the most common cause of mortality in this patient population. In patients without acute signs of obstruction, serial assessments of the airway and hemodynamic status are appropriate. These patients should be managed with IV antibiotics and close observation in an intensive care setting, with otolaryngology and anesthesia consultations. With any sign of worsening airway symptoms, such as stertor, stridor, increased work of breathing, or cyanosis, airway intervention is required. If safe transport is possible, airway management should occur in the operating room setting. Mask ventilation can be difficult owing to neck swelling, so preoxygenation is often performed with high-flow nasal cannula and/or nonrebreather. If possible, intubation should be performed with the patient awake and breathing, ideally using a flexible laryngoscope for guidance. Traditional supine direct laryngoscopy is often challenging in these patients owing to trismus and tongue elevation. Preparations should be made for an awake tracheostomy or cricothyrotomy as well, because extensive infections may result in edema that alters the normal anatomy of the supraglottis and renders fiberoptic intubation difficult.

Medical management includes obtaining cultures and rapid initiation of antibiotic therapy. Antibiotics should cover gram-positive, gram-negative, and anaerobic bacteria. Ampicillin-sulbactam is the most commonly prescribed antibiotic in immunocompetent individuals, but coverage should be broadened to include pseudomonas and MRSA in populations deemed high risk for these pathogens.

The use of steroids in the initial management of Ludwig angina is controversial. Although steroids exert a strong anti-inflammatory effect on the airway and improve antibiotic penetration, they may also mask some manifestations of infection. Several case reports have shown a decrease in the need for airway management with the use of steroids, and a recent review of the literature by McKinnon et al. revealed that most authors choose to utilize steroids along with antibiotics for these patients.[9]

Surgical drainage should be performed in patients who fail to improve with antibiotics or with visible abscesses on imaging. Surgery is aimed at decompressing the fascial compartments of the neck, debriding any necrotic tissue, and draining purulent fluid collections.[2] Additionally, dental extraction of the causative teeth is critical for the prevention of recurrence. Tracheostomy is often performed at the time of surgical washout.

Lemierre Syndrome

Once the diagnosis of Lemierre syndrome is confirmed or highly suspected, the mainstay of treatment is medical. Accessible abscesses can and should be treated with surgical drainage, but intravenous antibiotics with anaerobic coverage are first line. Although multiple different antibiotic regimens have been reported, *Fusobacterium* resistance to penicillin has rarely been reported, so a beta-lactamase resistant penicillin such as piperacillin/tazobactam is commonly used either as monotherapy or in combination with metronidazole. Carbapenem has also been reported to be effective, either as monotherapy or with metronidazole. Antibiotic duration is advised to be at least 6 weeks, given the high rate of relapse during treatment, with transition to oral antibiotics when clinically appropriate.

The role of anticoagulation in Lemierre syndrome is controversial. The risks and benefits of anticoagulation therapy for internal jugular vein thrombophlebitis have not been properly assessed in controlled studies, and the low incidence of Lemierre syndrome has made prospective trials impossible.[6] Case reports have demonstrated that uncomplicated Lemierre syndrome without extensive clot burden resolves with appropriate antibiotic and supportive therapy and does not require anticoagulation. Some authors argue for anticoagulation in cases of clot progression while on antibiotics or when the clot burden is significant, such as with retrograde cavernous sinus thrombosis or septic pulmonary emboli.

TIPS AND PEARLS

- RPA is a disease of childhood, because the retropharyngeal lymph nodes usually involute before age 6. After childhood, similar infections present in the parapharyngeal space.
- Initial antibiotic regimen for RPA should be broad and cover both aerobic and anaerobic species. Attention should be paid to hospital or regional antibiotic resistance patterns, particularly regarding methicillin- and clindamycin-resistant *S aureus*.
- Ludwig angina is a rapidly progressive infection of the floor of mouth, often from an odontogenic source, that can compromise the patient's airway.
- Airway assessment and serial observation is critical for these patients, and they should be monitored in an intensive care setting with otolaryngology and anesthesiology consulted.
- IV antibiotics are first-line treatment, and steroids, surgical drainage, and tooth extraction are often included in the definitive treatment of Ludwig angina.
- Lemierre syndrome is internal jugular vein thrombosis and septic emboli, often following an infection in the oropharynx of young, healthy individuals.
- *F. necrophorum* is the most common causative agent, an obligate anaerobe. The mainstay of therapy is IV antibiotics with anaerobic coverage, often a beta-lactamase-resistant penicillin, with or without metronidazole.

EVIDENCE

When do children need surgical management for an RPA?

Multiple studies have demonstrated the efficacy of medical management alone in the treatment of RPA. Treatment failure and need for surgical intervention is more frequent in younger children, those with airway compromise at presentation, abscesses greater than 2.5 cm, and in patients admitted to the intensive care unit.[1]

Are steroids indicated in the management of RPA?

A recent multicenter retrospective study of a large cohort (n = 2258) of patients with RPA demonstrated that corticosteroids are an important adjuvant to antibiotic therapy.[10] Patients who received corticosteroids were less likely to require surgical drainage than those who did not (22.2% vs 51.5%; $P < .001$). Although this study had several limitations, administration of steroids should be considered in patients presenting to the emergency department (ED) with RPA.

Why is the incidence of Lemierre syndrome increasing?

There has been an increase in the reporting of Lemierre syndrome over the past decade, with 102 studies published between 1950 and 2007 and 121 studies the following decade.[3] Whether this is attributable to an increased incidence of the syndrome or an increase in reporting is unknown, but theories around this phenomenon have included a trend of primary care physicians not prescribing antibiotics for uncomplicated pharyngitis, greater clinical awareness of the condition, improved laboratory methods of isolating anaerobic bacteria, and a possible population shift.[11]

References

1. Adil E, Tarshish Y, Roberson D, Jang J, Licameli G, Kenna M. The public health impact of pediatric deep neck space infections. *Otolaryngol Head Neck Surg*. 2015;153(6):1036-1041.

2. Bridwell R, Gottlieb M, Koyfman A, Long B. Diagnosis and management of Ludwig's angina: an evidence-based review. *Am J Emerg Med*. 2021;41:1-5.

3. Karkos PD, Asrani S, Karkos CD, et al. Lemierre's syndrome: a systematic review. *Laryngoscope*. 2009;119(8):1552-1559.
4. Brown NK, Hulten KG, Mason EO, Kaplan SL. *Staphylococcus aureus* retropharyngeal abscess in children. *Pediatr Infect Dis J*. 2015;34(4);454-456.
5. Abdel-Haq N, Quezada M, Asmar B. Retropharyngeal abscess in children: the rising incidence of methicillin-resistant staphylococcus aureus. *Pediatr Infect Dis J*. 2012;31(7):696-699.
6. Johannesen KM, Bodtger U. Lemierre's syndrome: current perspectives on diagnosis and management. *Infect Drug Resist*. 2016;14;9:221-227.
7. Gama R, Sousa M, Castro F, Condé A. Lemierre's syndrome: a forgotten life-threatening entity. *BMJ Case Rep*. 2020;13(10):e236201.
8. Lawrence R, Bateman N. Controversies in the management of deep neck space infection in children: an evidence-based review. *Clin Otolaryngol*. 2017;42(1):156-163.
9. Tami A, Othman S, Sudhakar A, McKinnon BJ. Ludwig's angina and steroid use: a narrative review. *Am J Otolaryngol*. 2020;41(3):102411.
10. Goenka PK, Hall M, Shah SS, et al. Corticosteroids in the treatment of pediatric retropharyngeal and parapharyngeal abscesses. *Pediatrics (Evanston)*. 2021;148(5). doi:10.1542/peds.2020-037010
11. Chapman SC, Andraska E, Kulkarni RN, et al. Lemierre's Syndrome: an atypical presentation. *Ann Vasc Surg*. 2019;60:479.e1-479.e4.

CHAPTER 15

Angioedema

Zachary Kuschner
Yue Ma

THE CLINICAL CHALLENGE

Angioedema is nonpitting edema that often involves orofacial, glossopharyngeal, and laryngeal structures and that can lead to airway obstruction and death. Angioedema accounted for approximately 100 000 emergency department (ED) during the period 2001 to 2009 with an age-adjusted death rate of approximately 0.6 per million per year in 2010.[1,2] The clinical challenge presented with angioedema is 2-fold: airway and medical management. Localized extravasation of fluid from the vascular compartment into surrounding subcutaneous and submucosal tissue caused by histamine or bradykinin release deranges airway anatomy, making intubation difficult. Furthermore, there are multiple underlying pathophysiologic causes of angioedema, each with unique therapies. Differentiation of various angioedema syndromes is critical to allow for pathology reversal and ease airway management.

PATHOPHYSIOLOGY

Angioedema is categorized by the underlying pathophysiologic mechanism that provoking the capillary leak state: either mast cell degranulation producing histamine, or the kallikrein-kinin system producing bradykinin. Increased capillary permeability in the mucosal, submucosal, and subcutaneous tissues allows extravasation of fluid into the extracellular space, causing the physical presentation of angioedema.

Histamine Mediated Angioedema (HMA)

Histamine-mediated angioedema (HMA) is a component of anaphylaxis, an allergic response at the severe end of a broad clinical spectrum of histamine-mediated allergic reactions. In HMA, as with less severe allergic reactions, intracellular storage vesicles within basophils and mast cells release histamine in response to cross-linking of immunoglobulin E (IgE) antibodies provoked by antigen binding. The effects of histamine may be either local or diffuse and can produce edema, bronchial smooth muscle constriction, increased airway sputum production, pulmonary edema, and vasodilatory shock. In the gastrointestinal tract, histamine increases smooth muscle contraction and acid secretion. Histamine stimulation of subcutaneous nerve endings produces urticaria and pruritis. A variety of non-IgE-mediated triggers, including, but not limited to, opiates, salicylates, cyclooxidase inhibitors, iodinated contrast, exercise, and cold temperature, may directly stimulate histamine release.

Bradykinin-Mediated Angioedema (BMA)

Bradykinin, an end-product of the kallikrein-kinin system, is an important component of the physiologic response to tissue injury. It induces smooth muscle relaxation, activates the complement system, and stimulates coagulation. Bradykinin is metabolized by angiotensin converting enzyme (ACE) and carboxypeptidase N, and its production is regulated at multiple steps by C_1-inhibitor (C_1-INH)—also known as C_1 esterase.

Hereditary angioedema (HAE) is an autosomal dominant deficiency of C_1-INH resulting in increased levels of C_1 protein and overall complement activity, as well as impaired clearance of bradykinin. Two predominant varieties of HAE exist: type 1 is characterized by decreased C_1-INH production and type 2 by production of incompletely effective C_1-INH protein. Acquired C_1-INH deficiency (acquired angioedema, AAE) can occur owing to use of ACE inhibitors. Less commonly, conditions that produce anti-C_1-INH antibodies such as malignancy, hepatitis B or C infection, or autoimmune disorders can cause AAE.

APPROACH/THE FOCUSED EXAM

Angioedema patients present with signs of nonpitting edema in the subcutaneous and submucosal regions of the body. Once the patient is deemed to be hemodynamically stable and has an intact airway, a detailed history and physical exam should differentiate angioedema from angioedema-like conditions (see differential diagnosis section) and HMA from BMA. Management of angioedema requires an accurate diagnosis of the form of angioedema.

Assessing Patient Stability

Signs of hemodynamic instability and airway compromise should be first assessed and treated. Clinicians should look for symptoms and signs of hoarseness, stridor, drooling, dysphagia, and odynophagia. An early flexible laryngoscopy should be performed promptly for airway assessment.

Medical History and Physical Exam

History taking should assess for any prodromal symptoms, symptom onset and duration, triggers of attack, trialed medications and their responses, personal or family history of angioedema, medication list (eg, angiotensin converting enzyme inhibitor [ACEI]), allergies, and a complete review of systems to assess all organ systems involved. **Table 15.1** lists clinical features of the angioedema subtypes. Patients with HMA present with pruritic urticaria and typically report other allergic symptoms like flushing, wheezing, vomiting, and abdominal pain. By contrast, patients with BMA generally do not report pruritus, flushing, or wheezing but do frequently have abdominal pain.[3] Patients with HMA develop symptoms within minutes of exposure and usually have rapid resolution with the treatment cocktail of epinephrine, corticosteroids, and antihistamine. BMA, in contrast, typically has a much slower course of onset and resolution.

Family history of angioedema can signify a subset of BMA, HAE. Patients with HAE present with recurrent episodes of cutaneous and submucosal swelling that frequently begin before age 20 years. In contrast, patients with acquired C_1-INH deficiency typically present during or after the fourth decade of life and do not have familial history.[4]

More than half of patients with AAE have an underlying autoimmune or lymphoproliferative disorder. It is therefore important to ask for a history of monoclonal gammopathy of uncertain significance (MGUS), chronic lymphocytic leukemia, non-Hodgkin lymphoma, Waldenstrom macroglobulinemia, splenic marginal zone lymphoma, or autoimmune disorders such as systemic lupus erythematosus.[4]

The physical exam should focus on common sites affected: lips, tongue, pharynx, larynx, periorbital area, extremities, genitalia, and gastrointestinal system. It is important to assess for signs of urticaria to differentiate between HMA and BMA. Clinicians should be aware that mucosal swelling in angioedema can lead to temporary bowel occlusion, which can present as severe tenderness, guarding, and rebound tenderness of the abdomen; this can mislead physicians to seek surgical treatment for an acute abdomen.[3]

Laboratory Testing

Subtypes of angioedema can be diagnosed through laboratory testing of C1-INH and function, C4 levels, and C_1q levels obtained from blood samples (**Table 15.2**). However, in the emergency setting, diagnosis of angioedema is clinical, because laboratory results may take days or weeks to result.

TABLE 15.1 Clinical Features in Angioedema Subtypes

		Demographic	Onset	Symptom Duration	Prodromal Symptoms	Urticaria	Response to Antihistamine Treatment	Triggers of Attack
Histamine-mediated angioedema	Allergic	Any	<1-2 hr	12-24 hr	–	+	+	Food, environmental allergens, drugs or insect venom
Bradykinin-mediated angioedema	HAE	Female, less than 20 yr	Slow onset (hr)	48-72 hr/last up to 5 d	+ fatigue, malaise, mood changes, erythema marginatum, and joint/muscle pain	–	–	Trauma/medical procedures to the face, mouth or upper airway, stress, infection, estrogen (HAE with normal C1-INH)
	AAE caused by ACEi	African-American, Females	Immediate or delayed (up to 6 months since last drug taken)	48-72 hr	–	–	–	ACEi
	AAE caused by C1-INH deficiency	More than 40 yr	Slow onset	Depends on treatment for underlying disease	–	–	–	Associated with underlying lymphoproliferative disorder and autoimmune disease

AAE, acquired angioedema; ACEi, angiotensin-converting enzyme inhibitor; C1-INH, C1-inhibitor; HAE, hereditary angioedema.

TABLE 15.2 Laboratory Evaluations for Angioedema Subtypes

	C1-INH	C1-INH Function	C4	C1
HAE type I	Decrease	Decrease	Decrease	Normal
HAE type II	Normal	Decrease	Decrease	Normal
HAE with normal C1-INH	Normal	Normal	Normal	Normal
AAE with C1-INH deficiency	Decrease	Decrease	Decrease	Decrease
AAE caused by ACEi	Normal	Normal	Normal	Normal
HMA	Normal	Normal	Normal	Normal

AAE, acquired angioedema; ACEi, angiotensin-converting enzyme inhibitor; C1-INH, C1-inhibitor; HAE, hereditary angioedema; HMA, histamine-mediated angioedema.

DIFFERENTIAL DIAGNOSIS

The differential diagnosis for swelling includes all subtypes of angioedema as well as angioedema-like conditions, termed pseudoangioedema. Pseudoangioedema may be caused by anasarca syndromes, hypothyroidism (myxedema), facial lymphedema, superior vena cava syndrome, and acute dermatitis (acute contact dermatitis, dermatomyositis, and systemic capillary leak syndrome [Clarkson disease]).[4]

According to the European Academy of Allergy and Clinical Immunology classification, BMA is classified by its underlying pathophysiology (acquired or hereditary) and by its response to treatment.[5] Four types of AAE and three types of HAE are identified and summarized in **Figure 15.1**.[6]

MANAGEMENT

Airway Management

In patients with angioedema, a difficult airway should be anticipated in all cases. Symptoms of stridor, hoarseness, dysphagia, and drooling should provoke concern. In cases with threatened airway, definitive management requires endotracheal intubation. Constricted oropharyngeal volume complicates direct laryngoscopy, and even video laryngoscopy may become difficult or impossible despite adequate views of the larynx. Vocal cord edema may not permit passage of an endotracheal tube. A respiratory drive-preserving sedative such as ketamine should be used and empiric paralysis avoided. Fiberoptic intubation is preferred if the operator is trained and comfortable with the technique, but video laryngoscopy is an alternative. Providers can consider intubation in the operating room with anesthesia and ENT; however, more urgent situations may not allow this. Early surgical management with cricothyroidotomy is indicated if difficulty is encountered with laryngoscopy.

In patients with upper airway swelling, flexible laryngoscopy can help delineate the extent and degree of upper airway involvement. An initial baseline flexible laryngoscopy, followed by serial scope exams can provide information on the progression or resolution of angioedema.

Medical Management

The first-line medical management in cases of HMA with airway involvement, pulmonary involvement, or shock is administration of intramuscular (IM) epinephrine with a plan to intubate if rapid clinical improvement is not observed. Persistent hypotension should be treated with a crystalloid bolus and epinephrine infusion. Hypoxemia typically resolves rapidly with epinephrine, but should also be treated with supplemental oxygen and bronchodilators. Providers should plan to intubate if rapid resolution is not observed. Patients with HMA should receive steroids, and antihistamines can be considered, although their use is controversial. Patients with HMA who improve following treatment should be observed for a brief period of time in the ED to monitor for biphasic reactions—although the exact duration of such an observation period also remains

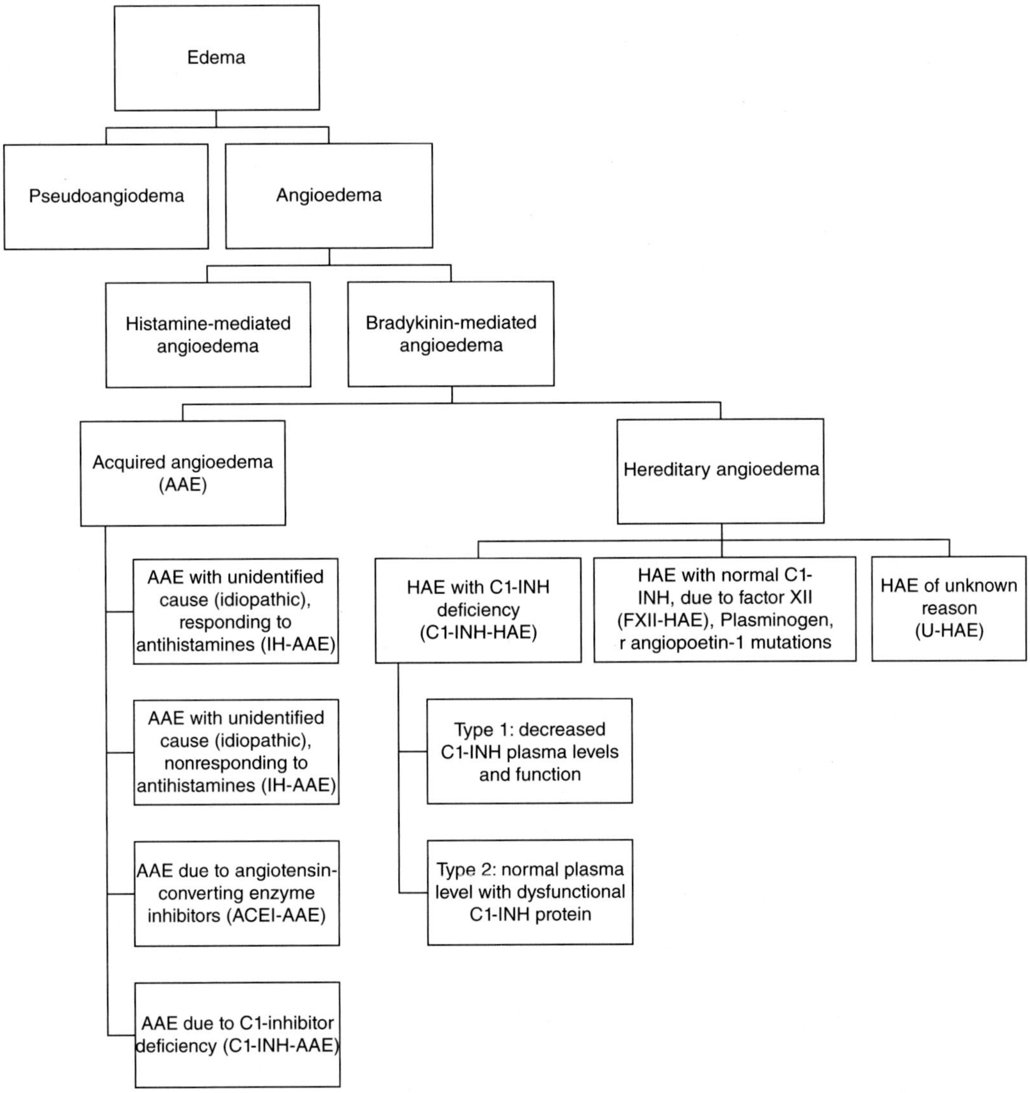

Figure 15.1: Differential diagnosis for edema. AAE, acquired angioedema; ACEi, angiotensin-converting enzyme inhibitor; C1-INH, C1-inhibitor; HAE, Hereditary angioedema.

controversial—and discharged with a course of steroids, potentially antihistamines, and an epinephrine autoinjector with bedside injection training.

For BMA, three bradykinin-specific medical therapies have been developed for use in HAE: (1) concentrated plasma C_1-INH; (2) Icatibant, a B2 receptor antagonist, and (3) Ecallantide, a recombinant kallidin inhibitor. All three therapies reduce the duration of symptoms in HAE and have been extrapolated to have benefit in AAE, but large randomized trials are lacking. If these medications are not available, fresh frozen plasma (FFP), which contains mixed plasma protein including C_1-INH, can be administered. In ACE-inhibitor-induced angioedema, cessation of the provoking medication is key.

Evidence is lacking regarding the duration of observation for cases of BMA with isolated involvement not including vital structures; however, it is the author's practice to observe such patients until swelling is no longer worsening and appears stable. Patients with bowel involvement resulting in partial or complete obstruction should receive bradykinin-reducing therapy along with emergent surgical consultation. Many cases of isolated swelling without involvement of oropharyngeal and laryngeal structures can be simply observed after discontinuing provoking medications. Patients with BMA and involvement of vital structures—particularly structures involving the airway, pertinent to alimentation, or with concern for threatened vision or extremity perfusion—who do no not require immediate intubation should be observed closely in the intensive care setting. Both HMA and BMA patients should be given referral to a specialist trained in allergy and immunology.

TIPS AND PEARLS

- Angioedema is mediated through two main pathways: HMA and BMA. An understanding of the pathophysiology and differences in clinical presentation aids in diagnosis and precise management.
- Pruritic urticaria is a useful clinical sign to differentiate HMA and BMA.
- Signs of hemodynamic instability and airway compromise should be first assessed and treated. Symptoms of upper airway edema should prompt early flexible laryngoscopy by a trained provider or ENT consultant.
- In BMA, epinephrine, antihistamine, and corticosteroid treatments are not effective. Instead, Icatibant, concentrated C1-inhibitor, or Ecallantide are the treatments of choice. When these are not available, FFP should be administered.

EVIDENCE

Is epinephrine effective in BMA?

Patients presenting with BMA often receive epinephrine, antihistamines, and steroids during their initial empiric therapy.[7] There is no mechanism by which these medications would influence bradykinin pathways, and there is no clinical evidence of efficacy.[8] In fact, rare cases exist of morbidity and mortality attributable to epinephrine administration in BMA.[7] In cases of undifferentiated angioedema, rapid onset of airway symptoms, or if the clinical presentation is not completely consistent with BMA, epinephrine should be given in order to ensure that a subtle case of HMA does not go untreated.

What is the optimal laryngoscopy technique for intubation in angioedema?

Fiberoptic intubation has classically been considered the traditional preferred approach in airway management of patients with angioedema when available. A small retrospective study performed in the operative setting recently demonstrated equivalent success rates with both video laryngoscopy and fiberoptic laryngoscopy with a mildly shorter procedural duration with the video technique.[9] This study supports the practice of using the intubation technique with which the airway operator has the greatest degree of comfort. The intubation should still be performed by the most skilled airway operator present in the most closely monitored setting available without delaying care.

Is administration of antihistamines effective in HMA?

Antihistamines are often administered as a component of the therapeutic cocktail—along with epinephrine and steroids—for cases of anaphylaxis with HMA both for the purpose of relieving symptoms for the initial reaction and for prevention of a biphasic reaction. However, the evidence regarding this practice is sparse. A 2007 Cochrane review found no high-quality studies evaluating the therapeutic use of H_1-antihistamines for HMA.[10] There is no clinical mechanism by which H_2-antihistamines would affect angioedema or other life-threatening sequelae of anaphylaxis; however, a small study did demonstrate potential effect on the duration of pruritis and urticaria and other mild nonemergent symptoms.[11] Potential harms to the administration of H_1-antihistamines include hypotension, sedation, and respiratory depression.[10] In this context, practices will vary at the local, departmental, and individual physician level, and there is insufficient evidence to recommend for or against H_1-antihistamines for treatment of emergent features of anaphylaxis or for prevention of biphasic reactions.

What is the correct duration of observation in HMA?

Although the existence of a biphasic reaction in a subset of patients with anaphylaxis—including those with this HMA—is known, it is unclear how frequently this occurs and how often a patient must be observed to monitor for such a reaction. A meta-analysis conducted in 2019 examining the risk of biphasic reactions in adult patients treated for anaphylaxis found that absence of a secondary reaction at 1 hour carried a negative predictive value (NPV) of 95%, whereas observation until 8 hours carried an NPV of 97.3%, and observation until 12 hours 98.2%.[12] The NPV remain unimproved at 98.2% at 24 hours, and improved to 99.9% at 48 hours.[12] Although these data did not evaluate patients with HMA separately from other presentations of anaphylaxis, these data can likely be extrapolated to apply to presentations of HMA. A 1-hour period of observation is likely reasonable in generic cases of HMA with complete resolution of symptoms following treatment with longer periods of observations for cases in which the physician has particular concerns such as cases at increased risk for biphasic reactions or those with a past history of biphasic reactions. Risk factors for biphasic reactions include a personal history of drug-related anaphylaxis, prolonged time of onset to administration of epinephrine, and cases requiring administration of more than one dose of epinephrine.[13]

Is administration of FFP effective in treating BMA?

FFP has been used as an alternative therapy in cases of BMA where bradykinin-specific therapies are not available. No prospective randomized controlled trials have been conducted, but a retrospective cohort study comparing FFP with observation demonstrated a substantial reduction of the need for intubation in the FFP group.[14] Although evidence is limited, the authors believe that this study supports the use of FFP for cases of HMA with airway or bowel obstruction where specific therapies are not available given the balance of potential risks and benefits.

Is Icatibant effective for treatment of non-HAE BMA?

Icatibant has been demonstrated to be rapidly effective in cases of HAE but remains expensive, and its utility in other forms of BMA is unclear.[15] A recent small randomized controlled trial compared Icatibant with observation for ACE-induced angioedema and found a substantial reduction in the duration of symptoms.[16] The trial was not powered to determine a mortality difference, and no patients in either arm required endotracheal intubation, but a likely benefit in cases with severe airway edema can be inferred.

References

1. Kelly M, Donnelly JP, McAnnally JR, Wang HE. National estimates of emergency department visits for angioedema and allergic reactions in the United States. *Allergy Asthma Proc.* 2013;34(2):150-154.
2. Kim S, Brooks JC, Sheikh J, Kaplan MS, Goldberg BJ. Angioedema deaths in the United States, 1979-2010. *Ann Allergy Asthma Immunol.* 2014;113(6):630-634.
3. Depetri F, Tedeschi A, Cugno M. Angioedema and emergency medicine: from pathophysiology to diagnosis and treatment. *Eur J Intern Med.* 2019;59:8-13.
4. Cicardi M, Zuraw BL. Angioedema due to bradykinin dysregulation. *J Allergy Clin Immunol Pract.* 2018;6(4):1132-1141.
5. Cicardi M, Aberer W, Banerji A, et al. Classification, diagnosis, and approach to treatment for angioedema: consensus report from the Hereditary Angioedema International Working Group. *Allergy.* 2014;69(5):602-616.
6. Kazandjieva J, Christoff G. Angioedema as a systemic disease. *Clin Dermatol.* 2019;37(6):636-643. doi:10.1016/j.clindermatol.2019.07.035
7. Curtis RM, Felder S, Borici-Mazi R, Ball I. ACE-I angioedema: accurate clinical diagnosis may prevent epinephrine-induced harm. *West J Emerg Med.* 2016;17(3):283-289.

8. Richman MJ, Talan DA, Lumry WR. Treatment of laryngeal hereditary angioedema. *J Emerg Med.* 2012;42(1):44-47.
9. Wood A, Choromanski D, Orlewics M. Intubation of patients with angioedema: a retrospective study of different methods over three year period. *Int J Crit Illn Inj Sci.* 2013;3(2):108-112.
10. Sheikh A, Broek VT, Brown SGA, Simons FER. H_1-antihistamines for the treatment of anaphylaxis: cochrane systemic review. *Eur J Allergy Clin Immunol.* 2007;62(8):830-837.
11. Lin RY, Curry A, Pesola GR, et al. Improved outcomes in patients with acute allergic syndromes who are treated with combined H_1 and H_2 antagonists. *Ann Emerg Med.* 2000;36(5):462-468.
12. Kim TH, Yoon SH, Hong H, Kang H, Cho S, Lee S. Duration of observation for detecting biphasic reaction in anaphylaxis: a meta-analysis. *Int Arch Allergy Immunol.* 2019;179:31-36.
13. Pourmand A, Robinson C, Syed W, Mazer-Amirshahi M. Biphasic anaphylaxis: a review of the literature and implications for emergency management. *Am J Emerg Med.* 2018;36:1480-1485.
14. Saeb A, Hagglund KH, Cigolle CT. Using fresh frozen plasma for acute airway angioedema to prevent intubation in the emergency department: a retrospective cohort study. *Emerg Med Int.* 2016;2016:1-6.
15. Cicardi M, Banerji A, Bracho F, et al. Icatibant, a new bradykinin-receptor antagonist, in hereditary angioedema. *N Engl J Med.* 2010;363:532-541.
16. Bas M, Greve J, Stelter K, et al. A randomized trial of icatibant in ACE-inhibitor-induced angioedema. *N Engl J Med.* 2015; 372:418-425.

CHAPTER 16

Epiglottitis

Mona Gangar
Emmagene Worley

THE CLINICAL CHALLENGE

Epiglottitis is an acute inflammatory condition of the epiglottis and supraglottic structures that can quickly progress to fatal airway obstruction. Although initially a pediatric condition, the advent and widespread use of the *Haemophilus influenzae* type B (Hib) vaccine in the 1990s has led to demographic shifts. By 1995, Hib disease levels had declined by more than 95%.[1] Because this decrease was mostly caused by the significant decline in pediatric disease, adults now have the higher incidence and mortality. The most recent analysis found a mortality rate of 0.006 per 100 000 in adults and 0.001 per 100 000 in children, the majority in children ages 0 to 3 years. Of the 1187 US deaths from epiglottitis over 39 years, adults accounted for 63.5%.[1] Hospital admissions show a similar pattern, with the mean admission age of a patient with epiglottitis of 45 years.[2]

Whereas children often have dramatic presentations with sudden onset sore throat, drooling, fever, respiratory distress, and tripoding, adults have a slightly more insidious onset, developing symptoms over the prior 24 hours. The most common presenting complaints are sore throat, dysphagia and odynophagia, along with muffled voice, hoarseness, and drooling. Because there is much overlap with common, unobstructive viral upper respiratory infections, the diagnosis of epiglottitis in adults remains challenging. In addition to timely diagnosis, airway management remains a central clinical challenge. Because of the infectious process and edema, the airway is tenuous and has distorted anatomy. This makes intervention more difficult, and even minor interventions can precipitate airway decompensation and laryngospasm.

PATHOPHYSIOLOGY

Acute inflammation and infection of the epiglottis and supraglottic structures lead to the clinical condition of epiglottitis. The microbiology of causative agents has shifted since the *Hib* vaccine, resulting in more similar adult and pediatric profiles. *Streptococcus* was the most common pathogen in a recent meta-analysis, found in 22.1% of swab cultures and 10.5% of blood cultures.[3] *Staphylococcus*, other strains of *Haemophilus*, and *Neisseria* are also encountered. Most blood cultures do not grow a causative organism, and surface cultures from endoscopy are usually negative.

Of note, caustic or thermal injuries to the epiglottis present identically to infectious epiglottitis. Thermal injury can occur after ingestion of hot foods or beverages, and direct traumatic injury can occur after ingestion of a foreign body or retrieval of that foreign body with blind finger sweeps. Epiglottitis has even been reported owing to traumatic placement of a laryngeal mask airway.[4]

APPROACH/THE FOCUSED EXAM

When epiglottitis is suspected, great care should be taken with all physical exam maneuvers while maintaining a calm environment. Because the airway is precarious, patients should be evaluated in an environment suitable for managing a difficult airway, and ENT and anesthesia consults should be called immediately for airway support.

In adults, special attention should be paid to sore throat complaints that are disproportionate to physical exam findings. Stridor, voice change, and dyspnea are often later signs and are concerning for impending airway compromise. Tachycardia and tachypnea should be taken seriously as signs of respiratory distress and sepsis. Complications of epiglottitis include abscess formation, sepsis, and exacerbations of other underlying chronic diseases, such as asthma, chronic obstructive pulmonary disease (COPD), or diabetes.

The diagnosis of epiglottitis is clinical, and direct inspection on endoscopy is the gold standard for definitive diagnosis. Edema and erythema of the epiglottis, arytenoids, and aryepiglottic fold are the most common findings (**Figure 16.1**).

If flexible laryngoscopy is not readily available, imaging studies can aid in making the diagnosis and determining the need for airway intervention. Lateral neck films are low-cost and easily obtained. Radiographic features suggestive of epiglottitis include the thumb sign (**Figure 16.2**), vallecula sign, thickened aryepiglottic folds, and hypopharyngeal distention. According to two studies, an epiglottic width greater than 5 mm, especially when measured at the base of epiglottis, is the most accurate objective parameter.[5,6] It is important to note that lateral neck films are dependent on positioning, and reporting of results is variable, leading to a false-negative rate of approximately 30%.[5] Ultrasound has been investigated as a potential diagnostic modality for epiglottitis. In transverse views of the neck, an increase in the anterior-posterior width of the epiglottis and a "P-sign" in longitudinal view at the thyrohyoid membrane have been described.[7] Ultrasound, however, suffers from being both operator-dependent for image acquisition and subjective in result interpretation. Computed tomography (CT) and magnetic resonance imaging (MRI) have also been used in this context and can be helpful for identifying associated deep neck space involvement or abscesses (**Figure 16.3**). However, these should be obtained judiciously—maintaining the airway is of utmost importance, and having the patient lie flat on an imaging table can precipitate further obstruction.

DIFFERENTIAL DIAGNOSIS

The differential diagnosis for epiglottitis includes other conditions affecting the upper airway structures. In adults, it is most often confused with either viral pharyngitis or strep throat. In comparison, epiglottitis is more abrupt in onset and the pain of the sore throat more severe. In children, the differential includes croup, bacterial tracheitis, and foreign body ingestion (**Table 16.1**).

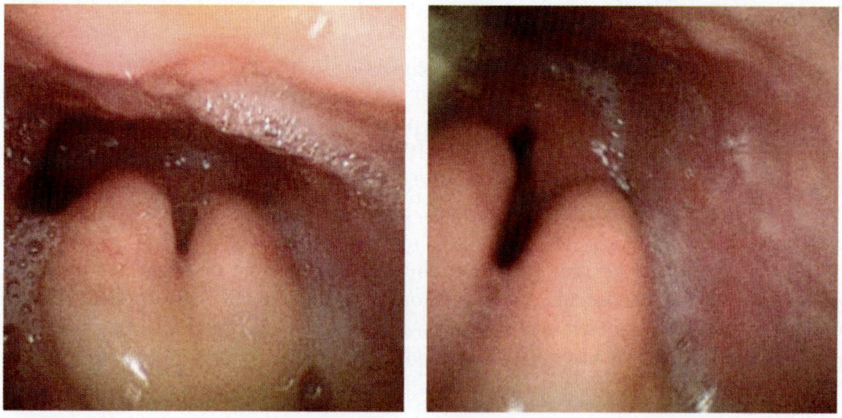

Figure 16.1: Epiglottitis on laryngoscopy.

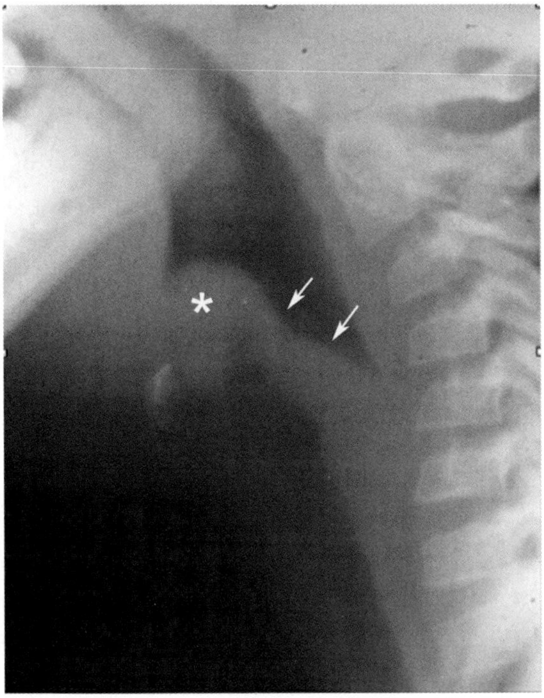

Figure 16.2: Thumb sign as seen on lateral neck X-ray. Asterisk indicates thickened epiglottis or thumb sign and arrows indicate thickened aryepiglottic fold. (Courtesy of Stephen L. Done, MD, Seattle, Washington and from Iyer R. Upper airway obstruction. In: Iyer R, Chapman T, eds. *Pediatric Imaging: The Essentials*. 1st ed. Wolters Kluwer; 2016:1-8. Figure 1.5A.)

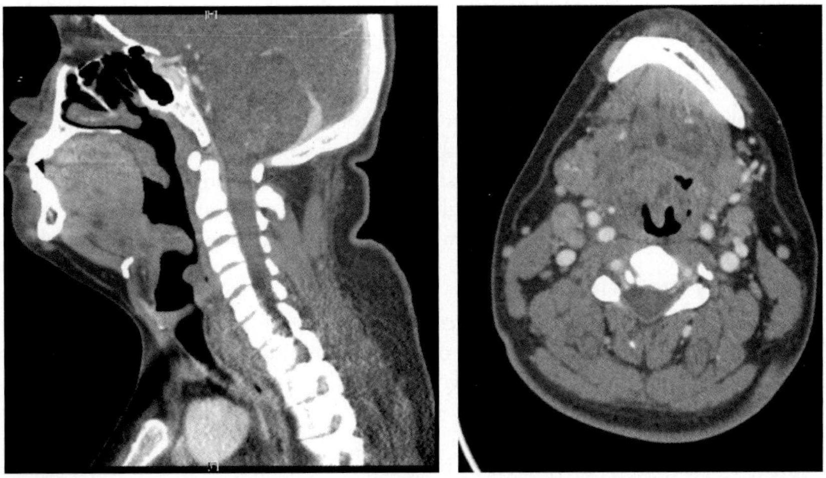

Figure 16.3: Epiglottitis as seen on CT imaging.

TABLE 16.1 Differential Diagnosis Table

	Viral Prodrome	Tonsillar Erythema	Airway Compromise	Distinguishing Characteristic
Viral pharyngitis	✔	✔	✖	Nontoxic appearing
Strep throat	✖	✔	✖	Tonsillar exudates
Croup	✔	✖	✖	Barking cough Steeple sign on X-ray
Bacterial tracheitis	✔	✖	✔	Tracheal tenderness Irregular tracheal margins on X-ray
Retropharyngeal abscess	✔	✔	✖	Posterior oropharyngeal bulging Limited neck ROM/ unusual neck position
Peritonsillar abscess	✖	✔	✖	Unilateral tonsillar bulging Uvular deviation Trismus
Foreign Body aspiration	✖	✖	+/−	Acute onset Often with clear history
Epiglottitis	✖	✖	✔	*Sniffing or tripod position* *Thumb sign on X-ray*

Croup

An infection of the upper airway usually viral in etiology. The classic barking cough of croup is not associated with epiglottitis. Croup generally has a 3- to 4-day prodrome of viral upper respiratory symptoms, such as nasal congestion, cough, and fever, before patients develop stridor or difficulty breathing. It is also associated with the "steeple sign" on X-ray, rather than the "thumb sign."

Bacterial Tracheitis

A rare complication of a preceding upper respiratory viral infection, where after a viral illness, patients develop worsening symptoms with high fevers, cough and stridor. Airway obstruction is caused by thick mucopurulent discharge, and tenderness exists along the trachea. While X-ray can show irregular tracheal margins and subglottic narrowing, the diagnosis is made with bronchoscopy. Bacterial tracheitis is treated very similarly to epiglottitis, often requiring intubation.

Foreign Body Ingestion

More common in pediatrics but can be present in all age groups. Foreign body ingestion is associated with dyspnea and stridor depending on the level of obstruction and shape or material of the foreign body. There is often a clear history.

Thermal or Chemical Injury

Less common than infectious epiglottitis but present identically to infectious epiglottitis and are managed similarly.[4] With the increased use of electronic cigarettes in adolescents, case reports of vaping resulting in supraglottic edema have been cited in the literature and should be considered.[8]

Retropharyngeal Abscess (RPA)

Classically found in children younger than 4 years, an RPA develops over several days as an infection of the potential space between the posterior pharyngeal wall and the prevertebral fascia.

Symptoms include neck pain, fever, dysphagia, and children may hold their neck in unusual positions. Limited neck range of motion is frequently associated with RPA. There is often bulging of the posterior oropharynx on exam.

Peritonsillar Abscess (PTA)

A deep oropharyngeal infection, a PTA presents with sore throat, fever, trismus, and voice change and can include unilateral ear pain. Exam shows unilateral swelling and deviation of the uvula away from the affected side.

MANAGEMENT

The immediate consideration in the management of patients with epiglottitis is evaluation of the airway. Because the disease process affects the supraglottic structures, rapid deterioration and airway collapse may result if a serious case is not recognized early. Diagnostic workup should *not* precede airway management in patients with impending respiratory decompensation.

Direct visualization of the airway is the gold standard for evaluating involvement of supraglottic structures (Figure 16.1 and **Video 16.1**). ENT consult for flexible laryngoscopy should be requested as soon as possible, especially in cases exhibiting stridor, drooling, voice changes, and increased work of breathing. Anesthesia and critical care teams should be alerted as well. If visualization of the supraglottis is attempted, it should be performed in a location where the airway can be secured immediately if required. Careful consideration for bedside laryngoscopy should be given to pediatric patients where the risk of upsetting the child, possibly resulting in respiratory collapse, should be balanced with the benefit of airway visualization (see Pediatric Issues section).

Approximately 10% of patients with epiglottitis require a secure airway via either intubation or tracheotomy. Indications for airway intervention include severe respiratory distress, significant supraglottic edema found on exam, inability to maintain oxygen saturation, as well as increasing anxiety, unmanageable secretions, muffled voice, tripod positioning, or severe stridor. One study found that a history of diabetes, presence of an abscess, and bacteremia were associated with a higher likelihood of airway intervention.[2] If the patient is stable for transfer, the operating room is the most ideal location for airway intervention. Intubation may be accomplished by awake fiberoptic nasotracheal intubation or via direct laryngoscopy. Video laryngoscopy can aid during intubation. Supraglottic airways such as laryngeal mask airway should *not* be used, because these are ineffective in upper airway obstruction and distorted anatomy. Tracheotomy/cricothyrotomy equipment should be available in the rare event that intubation is unsuccessful (**Figure 16.4**). Ideally, patients should be stably transferred to the operating room, where after airway management epiglottic cultures should be obtained.

All patients with epiglottitis, regardless of airway status, should be admitted to a monitored setting initially. Humidified supplemental oxygen should be readily available and utilized. Heliox may also be helpful in nonintubated patients because it decreases the work of breathing by improving laminar flow.[10]

Treatment consists of antibiotic therapy, most commonly with a third-generation cephalosporin and an anti-MRSA agent. Therapy may subsequently be tailored based on results of blood and epiglottic cultures, although these are often negative. Transition to an oral antibiotic regimen can be considered once the edema has sufficiently improved; a 7- to 10-day total course is generally acceptable. Steroids are also often administered as an adjunct to hasten edema resolution, although data regarding effectiveness is limited. Please see a summary in **Table 16.2**.

PEDIATRIC ISSUES

Before immunization, children ages 2 to 6 years were most commonly affected, but since the introduction of the *Hib* vaccine, older children and adolescents are more likely to be affected. A recent increase in antivaccination sentiment should remind providers to specifically obtain vaccination status in the history. Additionally, immunocompromised children are at higher risk for supraglottitis.

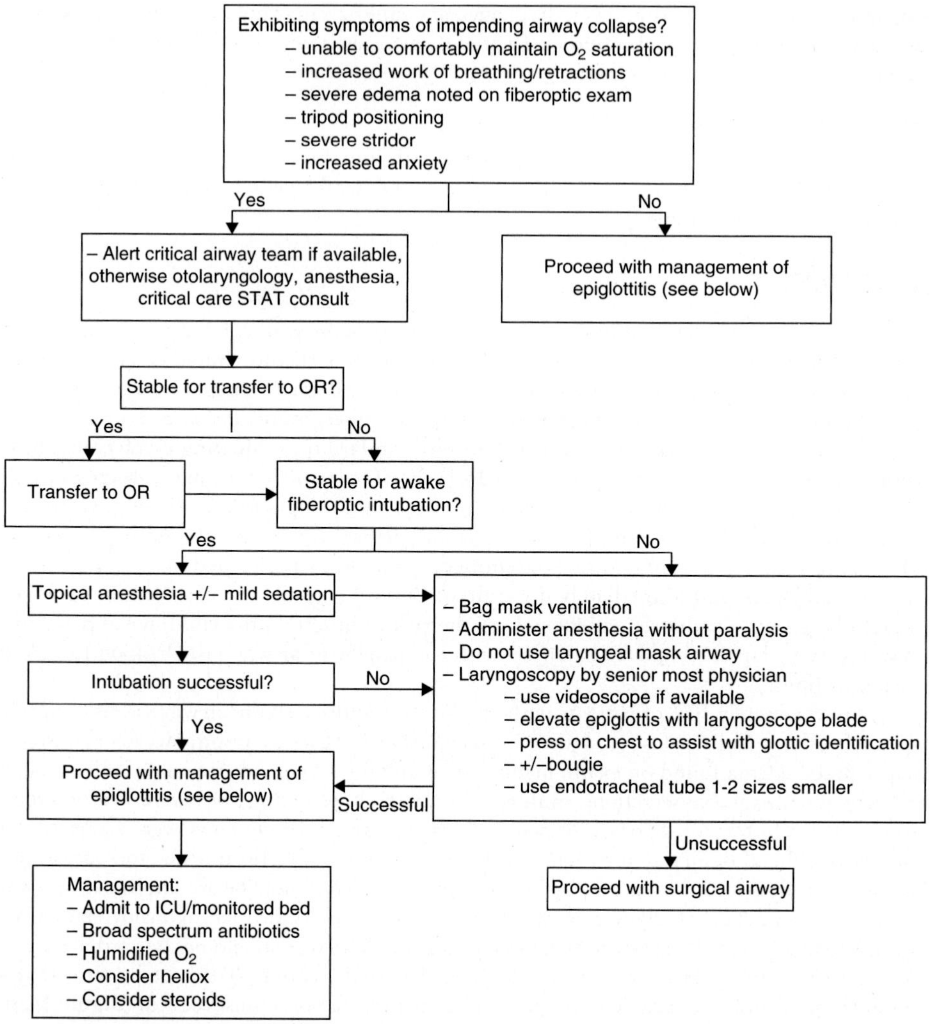

Figure 16.4: Airway management.

Compared with adults, children often have more rapid progression with symptom onset in less than 24 hours, often within 12 hours. Young children are more likely to present with classic symptoms of drooling and tripod positioning, whereas adolescents tend to present similarly to adults.

In pediatric patients, tongue blade examination of the oral cavity, placement of IVs, blood draws, examination of the larynx, and radiographs need to wait until the airway is deemed stable. The patient should be kept with the parent, preferably seated in their lap, to minimize agitation and anxiety. Although bedside laryngoscopy can be performed in stable adolescent and adult patients, pediatric laryngeal exam in the emergency department (ED) should be carefully considered on a case-by-case basis. The small size of the larynx in young patients makes it prone to quick decompensation. Younger children and those patients with signs of impending airway obstruction such as stridor, tripod positioning, and retractions should be immediately evaluated by anesthesia, critical care, and ENT to determine whether intubation or tracheotomy is indicated.

TABLE 16.2 Summary Table

Signs/ Symptoms	Pathophysiology	DDx	Workup	Management	Pediatric Issues
• Sore throat out of proportion to exam • Fever • Odynophagia • Drooling • Tripod positioning • Stridor • Muffled/ hoarse voice • Tachycardia • Tachypnea	• Streptococcus • Staphylococcus • H. flu • Neisseria • Caustic injury • Thermal injury • Traumatic injury	• Strep throat • Viral pharyngitis • Peritonsillar abscess • Retropharyngeal abscess • Croup • Bacterial tracheitis • Foreign body ingestion/ aspiration	• Airway evaluation (laryngoscopy preferred over imaging) • Lateral neck film • U/S • CT • MRI • Blood/ epiglottic cultures • CBC	• Evaluate and secure airway if necessary • ICU admission • Broad spectrum antibiotics (third generation cephalosporin and antistaph agent) • Humidified O_2 • Consider heliox • Consider steroids • Extubate when edema resolves/ air leak present	• Symptom onset usually <24 hr • Obtain vaccination history • Proceed with caution for any airway evaluation • Avoid aggravating maneuvers (instrumented oral exam, placement of IV, blood draws, etc.) • Keep child with parent

TIPS AND PEARLS

- Anesthesia, critical care, and ENT consults should be sought promptly, even if airway intervention is eventually deemed unnecessary.
- If a secure airway is required, transfer to a controlled setting such as the operating room whenever possible.
- Bag mask ventilation should be attempted initially in the event of decompensation.
- If a definite airway is required in the ED setting, consider alternative techniques such as rapid sequence intubation with avoidance of paralytics, with preparations in place for a surgical airway.[9]
- If intubating, the most experienced physician should attempt intubation. Video laryngoscopy can greatly assist with visualization. The laryngoscope blade should not be placed in the vallecula for indirect elevation of the epiglottis but should rather directly elevate the epiglottis to expose the glottis.
- Do not use laryngeal mask airways.

- If supraglottic edema is severe and the glottis cannot be visualized, pushing on the patient's chest can produce air bubbles at the glottic opening to assist in identification.
- Attempt intubation using a tube one to two sizes smaller than predicted or place a bougie to assist in passing the endotracheal tube.
- Pediatric airway evaluation should be approached with caution. Avoid upsetting and agitating the child. Keeping the child with their parent and refraining from instrumenting the oral cavity or placing intravenous lines/obtaining bloodwork can assist with keeping the patient calm.
- Stridor is a consequence of turbulent flow in the airway, which increases the work of breathing. Heliox may be used a temporizing measure because it produces more laminar flow, thus reducing the work of breathing.[10]

EVIDENCE

How accurate are lateral films at diagnosing epiglottitis?

Lateral neck films are inexpensive, rapid, and readily available. However, criteria for diagnosing epiglottis are subjective, and in mild or early cases, radiographic findings may not be seen. Approximately 79% of epiglottitis cases are positively identified on plain films using subjective criteria.[6]

A recent case-control study from South Korea attempted to identify the accuracy of objective radiographic criteria and to establish values for diagnosing epiglottitis.[6] They found that most patients had findings visible on radiographs. The most reliable measurement in this study appeared to be epiglottic width at the base. Using a cutoff value of 5.02 mm for epiglottic base width, epiglottitis could be diagnosed with a sensitivity of 96.2% and a specificity of 98.2%.

Are steroids useful in the management of epiglottitis?

Steroids are often utilized to hasten edema resolution. The use of steroids in epiglottitis is controversial because, to date, studies have not shown reduced length of stay or shorter intubation times with use of glucocorticoids.[6] The downside of administering steroids is low, with minimal side effects, so they may be considered on an individualized basis. If used, treatment is generally initiated with dexamethasone or methylprednisolone, tapering off after 2 to 3 days when symptoms are resolving. Further studies are needed to determine the efficacy of steroids in this disease process.

Video 16.1 Laryngoscope. Laryngoscopy of epiglottitis patient.

References

1. Allen M, Meraj TS, Oska S, et al. Acute epiglottitis: analysis of U.S. mortality trends from 1979 to 2017. *Am J Otolaryngol*. 2021;42(2):102882.
2. Shah RK, Stocks C. Epiglottitis in the United States: national trends, variances, prognosis, and management. *Laryngoscope*. 2010;120(6):1256-1262.
3. Sideris A, Holmes TR, Cumming B, et al. A systematic review and meta-analysis of predictors of airway intervention in adult epiglottitis. *Laryngoscope*. 2020;130(2):465-473.
4. Dowdy RAE, Cornelius BW. Medical management of epiglottitis. *Anesth Prog*. 2020;67(2):90-97.
5. Lee SH, Yun SJ, Kim DH, et al. Do we need a change in ED diagnostic strategy for adult acute epiglottitis? *Am J Emerg Med*. 2017;35(10):1519-1524.
6. Kim KH, Kim YH, Lee JH, et al. Accuracy of objective parameters in acute epiglottitis diagnosis: a case-control study. *Medicine (Baltimore)*. 2018;97(37):e12256.
7. Jain K, Yadav M, Gupta N, et al. Ultrasonographic assessment of airway. *J Anaesthesiol Clin Pharmacol*. 2020;36(1):5-12.
8. Bozella M, Magyar M, DeBiasi R, et al. Epiglottitis associated with intermittent e-cigarette use: the vagaries of vaping toxicity. *Pediatrics*. 2020;145(3):e20192399.
9. Tintinalli JE, Stephan Stapczynski J, John Ma O, et al. *Tintinalli's Emergency Medicine: A Comprehensive Study Guide*. 8th ed. McGraw-Hill Education; 2016.
10. Charles R, Fadden M, Brook J. Acute epiglottitis. *BMJ*. 2013;347:f5235.

CHAPTER 17

Tracheostomy Emergencies

Christina Chien

Anne Kane

INTRODUCTION

Tracheostomies are placed for a variety of reasons, including prolonged respiratory failure, management of upper airway obstruction, and airway protection.[1] Emergent tracheostomies are life-saving procedures for patients in whom oral and nasal intubations cannot be successfully performed, such as airway obstruction, penetrating laryngeal injury, or LeFort III fractures with craniofacial dislocation.[2] Elective tracheostomies, which are performed in patients already orally or nasally intubated, can be used to facilitate weaning from mechanical ventilation and provide easier access for pulmonary toilet.[2] Tracheostomies are typically more comfortable and tolerable for patients than endotracheal tubes, allowing for decreased sedation needs and increased patient mobility.[2] The number of tracheostomies performed in the United States was over 100 000 annually in 2014 and continues to increase.[3] It is vitally important for emergency providers to know about the management of tracheostomy emergencies, from bleeding to obstruction to infection.

Tracheostomies can be performed via an open surgical approach or percutaneous dilational technique (PDT). Surgical tracheostomies are safer to perform in patients with limited anatomic landmarks, history of prior tracheostomy, and coagulopathies.[4,6] PDT involves a modified Seldinger technique, usually under bronchoscopic or sonographic guidance.[4,5] It is associated with decreased procedural time, less bleeding, and a trend toward lower infection rates.[4] PDT complications include tracheal laceration, arterial injury, and esophageal perforation. Multiple meta-analyses have shown that PDT can be performed at the bedside as safely as the open surgical approach.[5,6]

Tracheostomy complications can arise because of the close proximity of the trachea with surrounding structures (**Figure 17.1**). The trachea is composed of 18 to 22 C-shaped cartilaginous rings anterolaterally and a membranous portion posteriorly.[3] The cricoid cartilage is the top of the trachea; it is a complete ring, whereas the remaining tracheal rings are incomplete. The thyroid gland typically overlies the second to sixth tracheal rings. The recurrent laryngeal nerves are immediately lateral to the cervical trachea. The anterior jugular veins run vertically and close to midline, whereas the internal jugular veins and the carotid arteries are more lateral. The innominate artery crosses over the trachea between the sixth and ninth tracheal rings. Tracheostomies are placed most often between the second and third tracheal rings.[3]

It is also important to be familiar with the tracheostomy equipment (**Figure 17.2**). The outer cannula is the main body of the tracheostomy tube; if present, the inner cannula fits inside the tube and acts as a liner that can be removed and cleaned. The obturator, which is used only when placing a tracheostomy tube, acts as a guide; it has a smooth tip, which prevents airway damage during

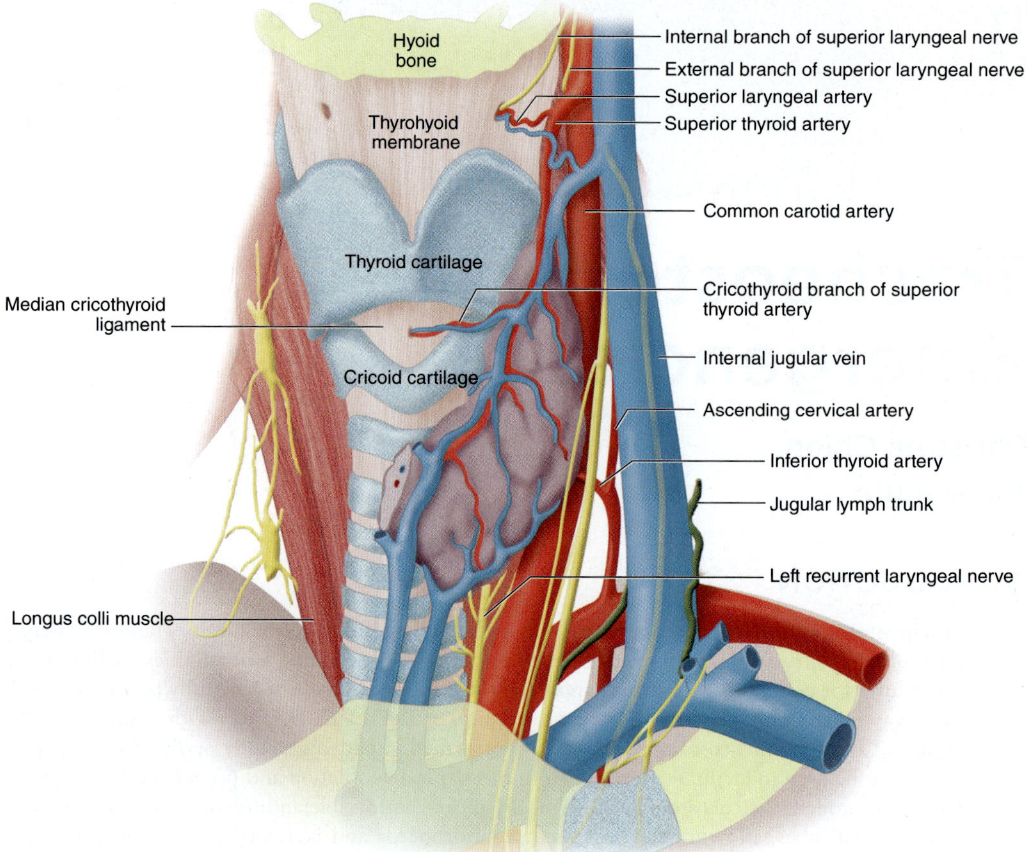

Figure 17.1: Tracheal anatomy. Anatomic diagram showing the relationship of the trachea to the thoracic inlet and surrounding associated anatomic structures. Note that the trachea begins below the cricoid cartilage and that the membranous intervals between the tracheal rings may vary in size, being greater in the upper portion of the trachea. (From Mancuso AA. Trachea: Introduction. In: Mancuso AA, ed. *Head and Neck Radiology.* 2nd ed. Wolters Kluwer; 2011:2058-2064. Figure 209.1a)

insertion. Tracheostomy tubes can be cuffed or uncuffed. Cuffed tubes allow for positive pressure ventilation when inflated and can protect against aspiration.[7] When a patient no longer requires mechanical ventilation, the cuffed tube can be exchanged for an uncuffed tube. Uncuffed and deflated tubes allow patients to speak. Cuffed tubes can lead to tracheal necrosis and stenosis if the tube is malpositioned or if prolonged use of high cuff pressures is needed to maintain an adequate seal. Tubes with foam cuffs exist for patients who have developed tracheal stenosis.[7]

There are a variety of sizes and styles of tracheostomy tubes, but the notable details of the tracheostomy tube are always located on the flange of the tube. The dimensions of the tubes are provided by the internal diameter, external diameter, length, and curvature.[7] The internal diameter is the functional inner diameter, and the external diameter is the largest diameter of the outer cannula. Sizing systems differ between models and manufacturers.

If the tracheostomy tube is too short, the distal end of the tube may not reach the airway; extra length tubes can be used to mediate this problem.[7] The tracheostomy tube shape should also follow

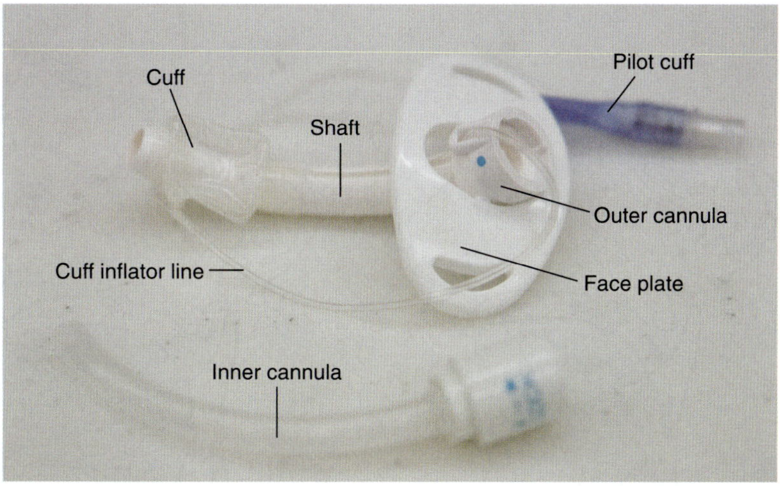

Figure 17.2: Basic tracheostomy equipment. (From Rosdah CB, Kowalski MT. *Textbook of Basic Nursing*. 11th ed. Wolters Kluwer; 2017. Figure 87.5.)

the airway anatomy as much as possible.[7] Proximal extended length tracheostomy tubes, which have extra horizontal length, may be required in patients with thick or obese necks, whereas distal extension tracheostomy tubes, which have extra vertical length, may be required in patients with long tracheas, tracheal obstruction, or tracheomalacia.[3,7] Fenestrated tubes have additional openings in the posterior portion of the tube, allowing for air movement and better phonation; these tubes can be used in preparation for decannulation.[7]

A special population to discuss is the laryngectomy patient. A total laryngectomy involves the removal of the entire larynx and creation of a permanent tracheal stoma, which is sutured to the neck skin; these patients are considered "neck breathers," as there is no connection between the trachea and the upper airway. Often, these patients have "neck breather" armbands to help identify them. Laryngectomy tubes are shorter and differ in appearance from tracheostomy tubes; when removed, a mature laryngectomy stoma is revealed.

Recognizing the differences between tracheostomy and laryngectomy stomas is critical to airway management (**Figure 17.3**). Whereas many tracheostomy patients can be intubated orally or nasally, this is not possible in patients who have undergone laryngectomies. It is critical in laryngectomy patients to intubate them through their stoma and not attempt oral intubation, which will fail and can lead to catastrophic results.

RAPID ASSESSMENT OF THE CRASHING TRACHEOSTOMY PATIENT

The American College of Chest Physicians recommends that patients with tracheostomy tubes presenting to the emergency department (ED) be managed in a resuscitation area. Key information should be obtained immediately:

1. What was the reason for tracheostomy placement?
2. When was the tracheostomy placed?
3. Identify the tracheostomy tube details, such as the size of the tube (internal and external diameters, length, and curvature), cuffed or uncuffed.
4. Determine whether the patient can be intubated orally.

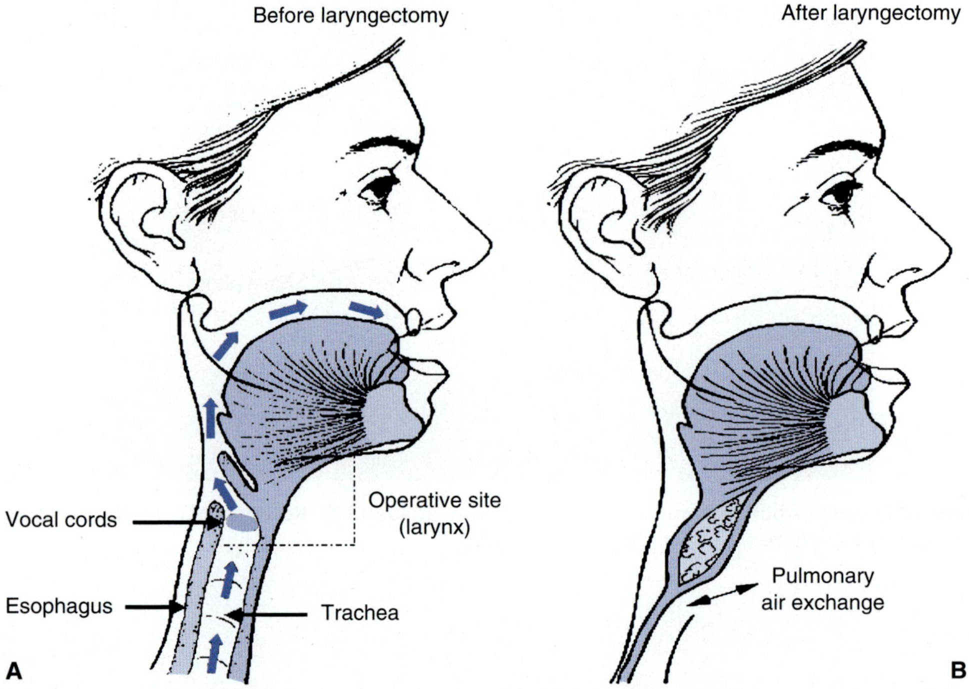

Figure 17.3: Laryngectomy. A, Normal anatomy and air exchange. B, anatomy after laryngectomy and the changes in air exchange. (From Lewin JS, Hutcheson KA. Evaluation and rehabilitation of speech, voice, and swallowing functions after treatment of head and neck cancer. In: Harrison LB, Sessions RB, Kies MS, eds. *Head and Neck Cancer*. 4th ed. Wolters Kluwer; 2014:225-235. Figure 11.8.)

TRACHEOSTOMY COMPLICATIONS

Tracheostomy complications can be divided into 3-time frames: immediate, early, and late[3] (**Table 17.1**). Several of these are discussed in detail in what follows.

TRACHEOSTOMY TUBE DISLODGEMENT

Tube dislodgement is a common complication. Factors that predispose to tube dislodgement include loose neckties, excessive coughing, and agitation.[8] A fresh stoma may reduce in size by half within 12 hours of dislodgement.[8] If a tube becomes dislodged and the stoma has contracted, a temporary catheter, such as a gum-elastic bougie or rubber suction catheter, needs to be placed to ensure that the tract remains open.

A stoma tract is considered mature after 7 days, and the emergency provider can replace tracheostomy tubes in these situations. However, if the tract is immature, the provider cannot blindly replace the tracheostomy tube because this can create a false lumen.[8] Under these circumstances, fiber optic guidance with the assistance of an ENT physician is preferred. If the airway needs to be resecured immediately in these situations, consider oral intubation, if possible, and cover the stoma to prevent air leak.

When replacing tracheostomy tubes, always ensure you have two tracheostomy tubes (one the same size as the current tube and the other a size smaller) as well as a 6.0 cuffed endotracheal tube.[8] A gum-elastic bougie or tube exchanger should be placed first and the replacement tube placed over the bougie or exchanger using the Seldinger technique. The replacement tube should be inserted perpendicularly to the stoma and then directed gently downward, following the curvature of the neck.[9] If using an endotracheal tube for replacement, advance the tube only a few centimeters past the balloon to prevent mainstem bronchial intubation.[8]

TABLE 17.1 Immediate, Early, and Late Tracheostomy Complications

Immediate (Peri-procedure to 24 hr After Procedure)	Early (Less Than 1 Week After Procedure)	Late (Greater Than 1 Week After Procedure)
Bleeding	Bleeding	Tracheal stenosis
Damage to the trachea and surrounding structures	Pneumothorax, pneumomediastinum	Tracheomalacia
Hypoxemia, hypercarbia	Stomal infection	Tracheoinnominate fistula
Air embolism	Stomal ulceration	Tracheoesophageal fistula
Unsuccessful procedure	Accidental decannulation/ creation of a false tract	Accidental decannulation/creation of a false tract

TRACHEOSTOMY BLEEDING

The likely cause of tracheostomy bleeding differs depending on timing after placement. It is imperative to obtain a pertinent history related to the bleeding episodes in order to help determine etiology and necessary next steps for evaluation. Important aspects of the history are as listed as follows:

1. When did the bleeding start? Quantify the amount of bleeding.
2. Was the blood in secretions, or was there bleeding emanating from the tracheostomy tube or around the tracheostomy tube?
3. Has this occurred previously?
4. Is the patient on anticoagulation?
5. Does the patient use humidification?

The inner cannula should be suctioned and cleared of any dried blood to prevent obstruction. The tracheostomy tube site should be evaluated for any acute bleeding. A flexible tracheoscopy or bronchoscopy may often be needed as well.

Differential Diagnosis

1. Acute surgery-related bleeding
2. Lack of humidification/dryness
3. Suction trauma
4. Granulation tissue
5. Tracheoinnominate fistula

Management

Acute Surgery-Related Bleeding

Postoperative bleeding typically occurs within the first 24 to 48 hours after tracheostomy, but it can also occur after (re)starting anticoagulation. For small amounts of "oozing," absorbable hemostatic materials can be placed into the wound. For more significant bleeding, visualization at the bedside may be difficult, and the patient may need to return to the OR for wound exploration and control of hemostasis. Any coagulopathies should be identified and corrected.[10]

Lack of Humidification/Dryness

This is a common problem, particularly in winter months. Tracheoscopy should be performed, which typically reveals excoriated tracheal mucosa with no active specific point of bleeding. Home humidification and saline nebulizer treatments should be utilized, and aggressive suctioning should be avoided.

Granulation Tissue

The prolonged presence of the tracheostomy tube may elicit an inflammatory response that favors the growth of granulation tissue in the tracheal lumen. This is typically a late complication that occurs more commonly in children. Topical treatments include steroid creams, antibiotic ointments, and silver nitrate. For larger amounts of granulation tissue, surgical excision in the operating room is appropriate. Regular tube changes have been shown to reduce the incidence of this problem.[9]

Tracheoinnominate Fistula

Rupture of the innominate artery typically occurs within 3 weeks of surgery but can occur at any time.[10] This emergency complication may be related to several factors, including placing the tracheostomy too low (below the third tracheal ring), an aberrant or abnormally high innominate artery, use of an excessively long tube, prolonged pressure on the tracheal wall by an inflated cuff, or tracheal infection.[9] Rupture of the innominate artery is typically heralded by a "sentinel bleed," a large volume bleed that resolves on its own and that is typically followed hours to days later by a catastrophic bleed. The tracheostomy tube may be seen to pulsate with the patient's heartbeat.[10] If this condition is suspected, ENT and potentially thoracic surgery should be consulted immediately. Imaging studies, including traditional angiography or computed tomography (CT) angiography, can be entertained, but sensitivity is low.[11] High clinical suspicion is critical for any patient with a recent tracheostomy who comes in with a large volume bleed. If catastrophic bleeding occurs, the tracheostomy tube cuff should be overinflated immediately and suprasternal pressure applied. The tracheostomy tube can be exchanged for an endotracheal tube if there is inadequate pressure to stop the bleeding. The patient should be typed and crossmatched and transported to the operating room or to the interventional radiology suite immediately. Surgical options typically require sternotomy with ligation of the innominate artery.[9,10]

TRACHEOSTOMY OBSTRUCTION

Tube obstruction is typically an early complication but can occur at any time. It may be caused by thick mucus and is largely preventable with attentive nursing care, proper humidification, and frequent suctioning. Additionally, the use of an inner cannula allows regular inspection, cleaning, and suctioning.

Differential Diagnosis

1. Mucus plugging
2. Inner cannula obstruction
3. False tract
4. Tracheoesophageal fistula

Management

A flexible suction catheter can be used both for diagnostic (identifying a patent pathway into the airway) and treatment (clearing mucus plugging) purposes. Saline bullets can thin the plug and help remove it. If an obstructing plug cannot be removed, the tracheostomy tube should be removed with the plug and then replaced.

Inability to pass suction catheter may indicate that the tube is sitting in a false tract. Obese patients are particularly vulnerable to this. If a false tract is suspected, ENT should be consulted immediately. The tracheostomy tube should be removed and the tract examined. If necessary for maintenance of the airway, the patient should be intubated from above. It is helpful to have smaller tracheostomy tubes or endotracheal tubes available. Ideally, a flexible laryngoscope or bronchoscope is used with a Seldinger technique to replace the tracheostomy tube.

TRACHEOSTOMY INFECTION

The tracheal wound is typically colonized within 24 to 48 hours following surgery. Tracheostomy wound care, including cleaning, suctioning, and regular tube changes help to decrease bacterial colonization. Tracheobronchitis may be attributable to underlying disease, aspiration, or both. This is treated with suctioning, pulmonary exercise, and antibiotics. It is vital to obtain cultures, as tracheobronchitis often involves multiorganism colonization, most commonly *Staphylococcus aureus*, *Pseudomonas,* and *S pneumoniae*.[12]

TRACHEOMALACIA

Tracheomalacia is a late complication typically occurring in patients who are on prolonged ventilation. Maintaining cuff pressures less than 25mmHg can help to prevent this complication. Tracheomalacia patients typically present with air leaks that recur after cuff reinflation owing to a "megatrachea." These patients can be difficult to manage and ventilate, and management should involve coordination between the pulmonary and ENT specialties.

TIPS AND PEARLS

- When managing tracheostomy complications, always consider intubation from above if the patient has no anatomic contraindications, such as subglottic stenosis or obstructive malignancy.
- Always ensure proper equipment is available in case of tracheostomy emergencies, including smaller tracheostomy tubes and 6.0 or smaller endotracheal tubes.
- A flexible laryngoscope or bronchoscope can be used with a Seldinger technique to help replace the tracheostomy tube.
- Providers should have high clinical suspicion for tracheoinnominate fistula in patients with recent tracheostomy and large volume bleed. Appropriate consultants should be notified on patient arrival.

References

1. McGrath BA, Bates L, Atkinson D, Moore JA. Multidisciplinary guidelines for the management of tracheostomy and laryngectomy airway emergencies. *Anaesthesia*. 2012;67(9):1025-1041. PMID: 22731935.
2. Freeman BD. Tracheostomy update: when and how. *Crit Care Clin*. 2017;33(2):311-322. PMID: 28284297.
3. Cheung NH, Napolitano LM. Tracheostomy: epidemiology, indications, timing, technique, and outcomes. *Respir Care*. 2014;59(6):895-919. PMID: 24891198.
4. Mehta C, Mehta Y. Percutaneous tracheostomy. *Ann Card Anaesth*. 2017;20(Suppl 1):S19-S25. PMID: 28074819.
5. Engels PT, Bagshaw SM, Meier M, Brindley PG. Tracheostomy: from insertion to decannulation. *Can J Surg*. 2009;52(5):427-433. PMID: 19865580.
6. Ifikhar IH, Teng S, Schimmel M, et al. A network comparative meta-analysis of percutaneous dilatational tracheostomies using anatomic landmarks, bronchoscopic, and ultrasound guidance versus open surgical tracheostomy. *Lung*. 2019;197(3):267-275. PMID: 31020401.
7. Hess DR, Altobelli NP. Tracheostomy tubes. *Respir Care*. 2014;59(6):956-973. PMID: 24891201.
8. Long B, Koyfman A. Resuscitating the tracheostomy patient in the ED. *Am J Emerg Med*. 2016;34(6):1148-1155. PMDID: 27073134.
9. Johnson JT, Rosen CA. *Bailey's Head and Neck Surgery: Otolaryngology*. 5th ed. Lippincott Williams & Wilkins, 2013.
10. Ridley RW, Zwischenberger JB. Tracheoinnominate fistula: surgical management of an iatrogenic disaster. *J Laryngol Otol*. 2006;120(8):676-680. PMID: 16709270.
11. Ferber L, Ferber M, Soares RR, et al. Endovascular treatment of tracheoinnominate artery fistula. *J Vasc Surg*. 2018;68(5):E149-E150.
12. Blot M, Bobiaud-Blot P, Favrolt N, et al. Update on childhood and adult infectious tracheitis. *Med Mal Infect*. 2017;47(7):443-452. PMID: 28757125.

CHAPTER 18

Posttonsillectomy Hemorrhage/Pain

Kei U. Wong
Benjamin Tweel

THE CLINICAL CHALLENGE

One of the most commonly performed surgical procedures in the United States is tonsillectomy, with or without adenoidectomy, the two most common indications being recurrent tonsillitis and sleep-related breathing disorders (eg, obstructive sleep apnea).[1,2] Complications associated with tonsillectomy include bleeding, pain, infection, adverse effects of anesthesia, dehydration, and postoperative respiratory complications (especially in patients with obstructive sleep apnea).[2,3]

Recent database studies demonstrate that approximately 6% to 7% of pediatric patients return to the emergency department (ED) or unscheduled outpatient ambulatory settings following tonsillectomy, of whom approximately 16% require inpatient readmission.[1,4] The most common reasons for return visits were bleeding (2%), throat pain (1.2%-1.4%), nausea and vomiting (1%), and dehydration (2.3%-28.2%).[1,4] In a retrospective analysis of 36 210 adult patients who underwent tonsillectomy, 1.5% were readmitted within 14 days postsurgery, 10% of patients had postoperative ED revisits, 6% of whom were treated for hemorrhage, and 11% for pain management.[3]

Posttonsillectomy Hemorrhage

Postoperative hemorrhage is a potentially life-threatening complication associated with tonsillectomy, with an incidence of up to 6% of cases following tonsillectomy.[3] Estimated rates of postoperative bleeding may vary depending on how hemorrhage is defined, and more inclusive criteria have approximated posttonsillectomy hemorrhage in up to 21.8%.[5] In a prospective, multicenter cohort study with 9405 adult and pediatric patients, patients over age 15 years were more than twice as likely to experience hemorrhage after tonsillectomy compared with those under age 6 years.[6] The challenge comes in managing two life-threatening processes simultaneously: hemorrhage and possible subsequent hemodynamic instability as well as maintenance of an intact airway.

Posttonsillectomy Pain

Although postoperative throat pain is an expected outcome rather than a complication, it is also an important cause of morbidity after tonsillectomy. Throat pain can lead to dysphagia, reduced oral intake of liquids, dehydration, weight loss, and, potentially, admission to the hospital.[2] Referred otalgia, throat swelling, excess phlegm, and difficulty swallowing are also common postoperative complaints, which can compound the challenges of appropriate pain control.[2]

PATHOPHYSIOLOGY

The palatine tonsils are highly vascular structures, receiving blood through both the internal (ophthalmic) and external (lingual, ascending pharyngeal, facial arteries) carotid systems. A venous plexus drains the tonsils to the internal jugular vein via the lingual and pharyngeal veins.

Sensation from the tonsil is mediated through the glossopharyngeal nerve (CN IX) and through the lesser palatine nerve, a branch of the maxillary division of the trigeminal nerve (CN V2). Because the glossopharyngeal nerve runs just deep to the tonsillar fossa, tonsillar pain is frequently referred to the ear through the tympanic division of CN IX (Jacobson nerve).

Posttonsillectomy, a fibrinous eschar forms within the first day, then sloughs off around postoperative day 5 to 7. At that time, patients typically note an increase in pain, because loss of the protective eschar causes exposure of the underlying tissue once again. Notably, the first day and days 5 to 7 are also the most common times for postoperative bleeding.[7]

APPROACH/THE FOCUSED EXAM

Posttonsillectomy Hemorrhage

Posttonsillectomy hemorrhage is a common reason for presentation to the ED, but uncommonly life threatening. A cross-sectional data analysis on tonsillectomies in 2010 found a mortality rate of 0.006 percent (two deaths among 36 221 pediatric tonsillectomies).[1]

The management of significant posttonsillectomy bleeding is challenging owing to limited evidence-based practice guidelines and wide variation of practice patterns. Furthermore, management strategies in the adult population have not been extensively studied.

A focused ED assessment is crucial to identify patients at higher risk of severe posttonsillectomy hemorrhage. More importantly, in many community EDs without ENT physicians on call or surgical capabilities, these cases present a greater challenge. The initial ED assessment should focus on active bleeding control and hemodynamic stability. The presence of active bleeding, oozing, or fibrin clot in the oropharynx requires surgical management, and the ED provider should alert the otolaryngologist and anesthesiologist as soon as possible.[7,8]

History

A focused history should include date of surgery, duration, frequency, amount of bleeding, and time of last oral intake. The patient's medical history, difficulties in surgery, and family or personal history of bleeding are also helpful.[7]

Examination

The initial assessment should focus on the airway and hemodynamic stability. In particular, tachycardia is often the first sign of hemodynamic instability.[7] Most patients presenting in the ED will be alert, with intact airway reflexes. A complete visualization of the tonsillar fossa may be challenging owing to patient age, cooperation, and level of discomfort. Careful inspection with adequate light is warranted and the patient positioned upright to avoid airway obstruction.[7] A headlamp is an ideal source of lighting, because it allows both hands of the clinician to be free.

The fibrin clot appearance is dependent on the technique and time following surgery. This will begin to form within the first day, and by day 5 the fibrin clot propagates into a thick cake with a characteristic gray-white appearance (**Figure 18.1**).[8] The separation of protective eschar from underlying granulation tissues coincides with the high-risk period for delayed hemorrhage.[7,8]

Posttonsillectomy Pain

The biggest source of posttonsillectomy morbidity is oropharyngeal pain, which can cause dysphagia, decreased oral hydration intake, dehydration, and weight loss.[2,8] The emergency provider should assess for clinical signs of dehydration (ie, decreased urine output, tachycardia, dry mucous membranes, decreased skin turgor) and address this as indicated. The provider should also inquire about the pain-control regimen at home and if reasonable augment it.[7]

Postoperative nausea and vomiting is another major source of morbidity and can enhance overall pain perception.[2] A single dose of intraoperative dexamethasone during tonsillectomy has been shown to decrease nausea and vomiting and improve postoperative throat pain and swelling.[2,7]

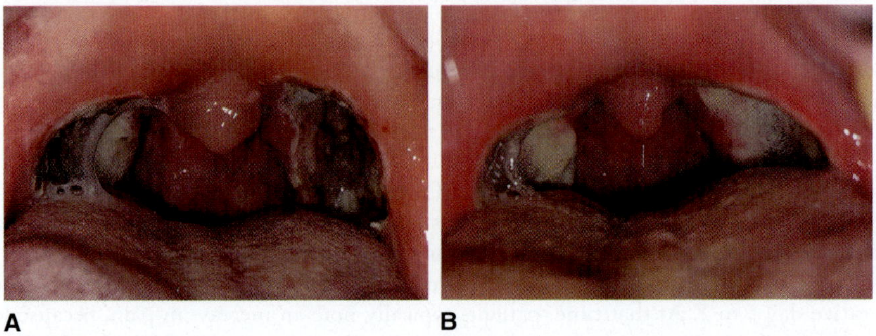

Figure 18.1: A, Stages of posttonsillectomy healing: postoperative day 0. B, Stages of posttonsillectomy healing: postoperative day 6. (Courtesy of Drs. Kei U. Wong and Benjamin Tweel.)

For those who fail outpatient pain control with oral analgesics or who are unable to maintain adequate oral hydration, hospital admission for parenteral pain medication and fluid rehydration should be considered.

DIFFERENTIAL DIAGNOSIS

Posttonsillectomy Hemorrhage

Posttonsillectomy hemorrhage can be classified as either primary (in the first 24 hours) or secondary (after the first postoperative day) following surgery.[7,8] Primary bleeding is often attributed to the surgical procedure itself, such as inadequately addressing bleeding vessels during the course of the operation, whereas secondary hemorrhage results from separation of the eschar from the tonsillar fossa, exposing small surface vessels to local trauma—which may be precipitated by dehydration, vomiting, or, rarely, infection.[7] Reported rates of posttonsillectomy hemorrhage vary, estimated primary and secondary hemorrhage rates occur at 0.2% to 2.2% and 0.1% to 3%, respectively.[2] Secondary hemorrhage is more common and accounts for nearly all who present to an ED. Although the peak incidence of posttonsillectomy bleeding occurs between 5 to 7 days following surgery, patients can experience significant bleeding at any point during the postoperative period.

In published studies, age is the most well-documented risk factor for posttonsillectomy bleeding. Higher rates of hemorrhage are associated with patients over 11 years old.[4,7] As mentioned earlier, Sarny et al. reported that patients over age 15 undergoing a tonsillectomy were more than twice as likely to experience hemorrhage as were children under age 6.[6] One possible explanation is that parents may seek surgical treatment on a young child at an early age to prevent the sequelae of obstructive sleep apnea. Another possible reasoning is the age when physiologic adenotonsillar hypertrophy occurs (peak presentation between ages 6 and 10 years). Children with both treated and undiagnosed coagulopathies (ie, von Willebrand disease) are also at increased risk for bleeding complications, including delayed bleeding (>24 hours postoperatively).[7,8] Lastly, patients undergoing surgery for chronic tonsillitis have been shown to suffer hemorrhage more often than those undergoing tonsillectomy for other indications.[7,9] This is likely because of the lack of a distinct tonsillar dissection plane during removal from chronically scarred tissues.

Posttonsillectomy Pain

Posttonsillectomy pain can be predictably localized to the tonsillar fossae; however, other causes of postoperative pain should not be overlooked. Otalgia is typically attributable to referred pain from the pharynx, but middle ear effusion or otitis media may follow surgery, particularly if adenoidectomy has been performed, so an otoscopic exam is required.

Temporomandibular joint arthralgia is another potential cause of posttonsillectomy pain and otalgia. As retractors are used to hold the mouth open for a prolonged period of time during the procedure, the patient may experience excessive strain in the joint, manifesting as ear pain or fullness.

Tongue pain, particularly if accompanied by taste alterations or paresthesia, may suggest damage to the glossopharyngeal nerve. This nerve runs immediately deep to the tonsillar fossa and can easily be affected by electrocautery. This discomfort will typically resolve within several weeks.

The patient undergoing tonsillectomy is also subject to the typical risks and sequelae of endotracheal intubation, including vocal cord injury, granuloma formation, and uvula edema or injury. These conditions are also largely self-limited and require only supportive care.

MANAGEMENT

Posttonsillectomy Hemorrhage

Sarny et al. reported that 41% of severe bleeding episodes were preceded by a light bleeding episode and that 10.2% of all minor bleeding patients developed severe bleeding.[6] As such, there is a low threshold for immediate ENT consultation, observation in the ED, and/or admission for monitoring for any patient with tonsillar bleeding, oozing, or clot formation.

Minor bleeding is often managed conservatively with instructions to gargle cold water. In the ED setting, the application of pressure to the tonsillar fossa or bedside cauterization with silver nitrate may stop the bleeding. If conservative measures fail to control bleeding, the patient should then be taken to the operating room by the ENT service.[7]

Immediate Surgical Consultation

While in the ED, the patient should remain NPO. Active tonsillar bleeding should be considered as a surgical emergency and requires prompt surgical consultation. Children may need to be transferred to a center with pediatric otolaryngology and operative capabilities. The decision to sedate or intubate prior to transfer remains multifactorial. Factors affecting this decision include provider skill level, condition of the patient, access to rescue airway equipment, in-house anesthesia/surgical backup, transfusion requirement, travel time, and capabilities of the transporting agency.[7]

Airway Assessment

Assessment of airway patency and consideration of sedation or intubation in patients with posttonsillectomy hemorrhage is complicated by risk of aspiration, hypoxia, hypovolemia, and the potential for a difficult airway.[7] For a stable and awake patient, an upright, forward-leaning position will minimize airway obstruction from blood in the oropharynx. Cold water gargle may be helpful in clearing out blood clots by causing vasoconstriction of the bleeding vessel.

If a patient requires intubation, specific precautions must be taken. A highly experienced emergency provider should develop a clear plan to minimize the risk of blood aspiration. In addition, multiple large bore suction apparatuses and forceps should be readily available to clear any active blood or clot. Surgical airway setup should be available in case a dislodged clot or active bleeding prevents traditional intubation.

Assess Hemodynamic Stability

Because severe hemorrhage can rapidly lead to hypovolemia and decompensated shock, initial management includes immediate intravenous access and volume resuscitation with isotonic saline. Laboratory workup includes a complete blood count, coagulation panel, and type and screen. Patients with severe or life-threatening bleeding may warrant blood transfusion, especially younger children with low reserve.[7] In cases of hemodynamic instability, ED providers should also consider activation of the institution's massive transfusion protocol, and any known coagulopathies should be reversed.[7]

Apply Direct Pressure

Depending on the degree of bleeding, patient stability and patient cooperation, control of hemorrhage may be performed at the bedside or in the operating room. The choice of bedside management should not be made lightly, because manipulation of a clot could turn a relatively stable situation into an unstable one. An optimal patient for awake, bedside management of hemorrhage would have a relatively small amount of bleeding or a small clot, an easily visualized tonsillar fossae, hemodynamic stability, and the ability to cooperate with prolonged instrumentation of the oropharynx.

The side and site of bleeding should be identified. In cases of profuse hemorrhage, this is difficult owing to pooling of blood and the gag reflex, so patient cooperation is paramount. Topical decongestants such as epinephrine, oxymetazoline, or phenylephrine may be applied by soaked gauze in order to induce vasoconstriction. Topical hemostatic agents such as tranexamic acid and thrombin may also be helpful. Because of the risk of foreign body aspiration, any soaked gauze should be securely clamped in a forceps when applied. In many cases, a clot may be seen filling all or some of the fossa, and careful consideration should be exercised to decide whether to dislodge the clot in an attempt to localize the source vessel or whether to proceed directly to the operating room.

Posttonsillectomy Pain

Although posttonsillectomy patients are commonly discharged home with opioid oral analgesics (eg, oxycodone or acetaminophen-oxycodone) for pain management, nonopioid pain medication has been shown to be effective in treating posttonsillectomy pain in children.[2,7]

The first-line therapy recommended for postoperative nonopioid analgesia in children includes acetaminophen and/or nonsteroidal anti-inflammatory drugs (NSAIDs), such as ibuprofen. Postoperative use of ibuprofen in children can provide adequate analgesia, and current data do not suggest an increased risk of hemorrhage.[2,7] Furthermore, postoperative nausea with vomiting and constipation are both avoided with ibuprofen, providing an advantage over opioids.[8] Topical lidocaine has also been shown to improve postoperative pain, although the effect of duration is limited and therefore requires repeated dosing.[10]

If postoperative pain is inadequately managed with oral analgesics in the ED setting, consider placement of an intravenous catheter for the administration of intravenous fluids, parenteral analgesics, or glucocorticoid.[7] Although ketorolac is not associated with common opioid side effects (ie, respiratory depression, urinary retention, sedation, nausea and/or vomiting), its use in posttonsillectomy patients remains limited and dependent on provider preference owing to concerns of increased bleeding risk.[2]

For adult patients with severe pain, opioids can be used carefully. For patients with sleep apnea and all pediatric patients, opioids should be minimized or entirely avoided if possible. There is a strong recommendation against codeine for pain control in pediatric patients (<12 years) after tonsillectomy given its variable metabolism and efficacy and higher risk of complications.[2,7]

PEDIATRIC ISSUES

The pediatric posttonsillectomy recovery differs significantly from that of the adult patient. As mentioned previously, studies have consistently shown that the rate of posttonsillectomy hemorrhage is higher in adults and adolescents than in young children.[6,11]

Postoperative pain management also differs between children and adults. For children, NSAIDs will form the basis for posttonsillectomy pain management without increased risk of bleeding, whereas most adults should avoid the use of NSAIDs. In contrast, opioids can be used with discretion in adults but will generally be avoided in children.

TIPS AND PEARLS

- If intubation is required for management of a posttonsillectomy hemorrhage, rapid sequence intubation should be performed. Cricothyroidotomy or tracheotomy equipment should be available in the event that the airway cannot be secured.
- In children, ibuprofen is safe after tonsillectomy and provides good pain relief with fewer side effects than opioids.
- Codeine is no longer recommended for pain control in pediatric patients because of variability of metabolism that can result in fatal overdoses.

EVIDENCE

Are NSAIDs contraindicated in the posttonsillectomy recovery period?

In children, ibuprofen is now a standard part of the postoperative pain control, typically in conjunction with acetaminophen.[2] A number of studies have shown that postoperative bleeding rates are not increased in children taking ibuprofen following tonsillectomy; however, some studies have also suggested a trend toward increased bleeding in this population.[12] Considering the substantial benefits of ibuprofen in pediatric pain control and considering the relatively low rate of postoperative hemorrhage in children, current guidelines recommend ibuprofen for children up to 18 years of age.[2]

In contrast, in adults, NSAIDs have been associated with bleeding in the posttonsillectomy patient.[5,9,13] One study showed that bleeding rates were 5 times higher in adults treated with ketorolac.[13] This continues to be a topic of active debate, however, and some studies have shown no increase in bleeding among adult posttonsillectomy patients treated with NSAIDs.[14]

Should opioids be administered as part of a posttonsillectomy pain management regimen?

Opioids should be avoided in pediatric patients undergoing tonsillectomy except in select circumstances. There have been documented cases of opioid-induced respiratory failure and death in children receiving codeine following tonsillectomy.[15] Obstructive sleep apnea is the leading indication for tonsillectomy in small children, and because sleep apnea is an independent risk factor for opioid-induced respiratory failure, this provides further rationale for avoiding this class of medication in children.[16]

For adults undergoing tonsillectomy, opioids may be administered with caution, as part of a multimodal pain control regimen. However, it is important to consider the negative consequences of opioid prescription, including the role of prescribed opioids in the development of addiction and in the increased risk of postoperative respiratory complications, particularly in patients with sleep apnea recovering from tonsillectomy.[17]

Are there alternative or nontraditional methods of pain control that are effective in the posttonsillectomy setting?

Acupuncture and aromatherapy have shown mixed results in clinical trials and are not widely employed. Studies have consistently shown oral administration of honey to have limited but significant effects on pain control in children following tonsillectomy, as measured by visual analogue scale pain scores or a reduction in the use of pain medication.[18] Finally, there is evidence that cooling agents such as ice or popsicles can lead to a short-term reduction in pain.[18] Popsicles have the added benefit of providing hydration, maintenance of which can be challenging for many young patients.

References

1. Shay S, Shapiro NL, Bhattacharyya N. Revisit rates and diagnoses following pediatric tonsillectomy in a large multistate population. *Laryngoscope*. 2015;125(2):457-461.
2. Mitchell RB, Archer SM, Ishman SL, et al. Clinical practice guideline: tonsillectomy in children (update). *Otolaryngol Head Neck Surg*. 2019;160(1_suppl):S1-S42.
3. Seshamani M, Vogtmann E, Gatwood J, et al. Prevalence of complications from adult tonsillectomy and impact on health care expenditures. *Otolaryngol Head Neck Surg*. 2014;150(4):574-581.
4. Duval M, Wilkes J, Korgenski K, et al. Causes, costs, and risk factors for unplanned return visits after adenotonsillectomy in children. *Int J Pediatr Otorhinolaryngol*. 2015;79(10):1640-1646.
5. Inuzuka Y, Mizutari K, Kamide D, et al. Risk factors of post-tonsillectomy hemorrhage in adults. *Laryngoscope Investig Otolaryngol*. 2020;5(6):1056-1062.
6. Sarny S, Ossimitz G, Habermann W, et al. Hemorrhage following tonsil surgery: a multicenter prospective study. *Laryngoscope*. 2011;121(12):2553-2560.
7. Wall JJ, Tay K-Y. Postoperative tonsillectomy hemorrhage. *Emerg Med Clin*. 2018;36(2):415-426.
8. Isaacson G. Tonsillectomy care for the pediatrician. *Pediatrics*. 2012;130(2):324-334.

9. Mudd PA, Thottathil P, Giordano T, et al. Association between ibuprofen use and severity of surgically managed posttonsillectomy hemorrhage. *JAMA Otolaryngol Head Neck Surg*. 2017;143(7):712-717.
10. Kaygusuz İ, Susaman N. The effects of dexamethasone, bupivacaine and topical lidocaine spray on pain after tonsillectomy. *Int J Pediatr Otorhinolaryngol*. 2003;67(7):737-742.
11. Pfaff JA, Hsu K, Chennupati SK. The use of ibuprofen in posttonsillectomy analgesia and its effect on posttonsillectomy hemorrhage rate. *Otolaryngol Head Neck Surg*. 2016;155(3):508-513.
12. Lewis SR, Nicholson A, Cardwell ME, et al. Nonsteroidal anti-inflammatory drugs and perioperative bleeding in paediatric tonsillectomy. *Cochrane Database Syst Rev*. 2013(7):CD003591.
13. Chan DK, Parikh SR. Perioperative ketorolac increases post-tonsillectomy hemorrhage in adults but not children. *Laryngoscope*. 2014;124(8):1789-1793.
14. McClain K, Williams AM, Yaremchuk K. Ketorolac usage in tonsillectomy and uvulopalatopharyngoplasty patients. *Laryngoscope*. 2020;130(4):876-879.
15. Chidambaran V, Senthilkumar Sadhasivam MM. Codeine and opioid metabolism–implications and alternatives for pediatric pain management. *Curr Opin Anaesthesiol*. 2017;30(3):349.
16. Kelly LE, Sommer DD, Ramakrishna J, et al. Morphine or ibuprofen for post-tonsillectomy analgesia: a randomized trial. *Pediatrics*. 2015;135(2):307-313.
17. Kharasch ED, Brunt LM. Perioperative opioids and public health. *Anesthesiology*. 2016;124(4):960-965.
18. Keefe KR, Byrne KJ, Levi JR. Treating pediatric post-tonsillectomy pain and nausea with complementary and alternative medicine. *Laryngoscope*. 2018;128(11):2625-2634.

CHAPTER 19

Nasal Trauma: Fractures, Septal Hematoma

Chen He
Shirley Hu

INTRODUCTION

In addition to functional impairment, facial injuries pose potential psychological and social consequences, because the face is vital to human appearance, emotion, and identity. Thus, although treatment of facial injuries in the emergency department (ED) and urgent care setting must focus first on life-threatening issues, important secondary considerations are preservation of function and long-term cosmesis. The nose is a defining facial feature that also provides important physiologic function. Nasal fractures are the most frequently isolated facial fracture, likely owing to the physical prominence of the nose.

PATHOPHYSIOLOGY/EPIDEMIOLOGY

Nasal Fractures

The nose is composed of very thin bone that can be fractured with minimal force. The bony structure of the nose is formed by the maxilla, frontal bone, and a number of smaller bones. The bony prominence of the nose, located between the brows, is formed by the nasal part of the frontal bone, which ends in a serrated nasal notch. From here, the left and right nasal bones emanate, bridging the frontal bone to the frontal process of the maxilla. Internally, the roof of the nasal cavity is the ethmoid bone's cribriform plate, through which the sensory fibers of the olfactory nerve pass. As such, damage to this region can result in anosmia. The nasal septum separates the two nares and is composed of bone proximally and cartilage toward the nasal tip. Finally, the floor of the nose is formed from the incisive bone and the horizontal plates of the palatine bones, which join at the midline to form the posterior nasal spine.

Nasal bone fractures most commonly occur from blunt trauma.[1] In adults, the most frequent causes are fights and traffic accidents. Young males are most likely to sustain nasal injuries, with peak incidence occurring at age 20 to 30 years. In children, the most frequent cause is sports.

Patients present with swelling, pain, ecchymosis, and/or bleeding, with symptoms dependent on time from injury. No specific classification system exists for nasal bone fractures, but severity of injury is defined by number and complexity of fractures, degree of displacement, and open versus closed injuries. Low-velocity injuries (eg, falling from a standing position or walking into a wall) often lead to simple fractures, whereas high-velocity injuries (eg, motor vehicle accidents) tend to be associated with multiple or complex fractures. Understanding the mechanism of injury not only helps to predict the severity of the facial injury but can also assess the risk of associated brain or cervical injuries.

Septal Hematoma

The nasal septum separates the left and right nares of the nasal cavity; it contains bone and cartilage and is normally about 2 mm thick. Proximally, the perpendicular plate of the ethmoid and the vomer combine to form the bony structure of the septum. Distally, the septum is composed of septal cartilage, ending in a fleshy external end known as the columella. At the base, a narrow strip of bone, called the maxillary crest, runs the length of the septum.

A nasal septal hematoma can occur when blood collects in the space between the septal cartilage and its overlying perichondrium (**Figure 19.1**). This condition requires emergent diagnosis because the septal cartilage does not have its own blood supply, so pressure from the hematoma can lead to ischemia and destruction of the septum. This condition is more common in children (**Figure 19.2**).

APPROACH/THE FOCUSED EXAM

The initial evaluation of nasal trauma should focus on threats to the airway and on stopping active bleeding. Within the first few hours of the injury, full evaluation of the anatomy at the site is still possible. However, usually by the time of presentation to an ED or urgent care setting, significant edema has developed, distorting the shape of the nose and limiting detailed examination. Patients often have some degree of nasal airway obstruction, which is not concerning unless concomitant oral airway compromise exists. Other common presenting symptoms are pain and tenderness, visible deformity, or epistaxis.

Externally, the nose should be visually inspected for swelling, deformity, or bleeding. It should be palpated for tenderness, crepitus, and abnormal movement. Each nare should be held closed to make sure that the other is patent for breathing. The patient should also be asked to identify whether there is any change to their sense of smell. A muffled or hyponasal voice may suggest occlusion of the nose or nasopharynx. Evaluation for the presence of a nasal septal hematoma should be done urgently to allow for timely drainage.

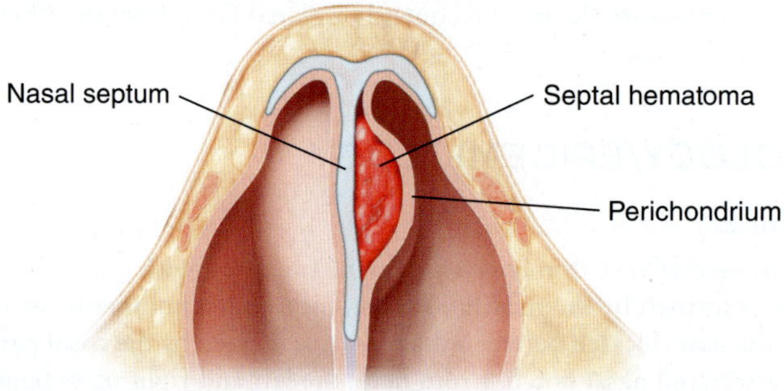

Figure 19.1: A septal hematoma forms when blood accumulates in the potential space between the perichondrium and nasal septum. (From Chung KC, Gosain A. *Operative Techniques in Pediatric Plastic and Reconstructive Surgery*. 1st ed. Wolters Kluwer; 2020. Figure 45.2)

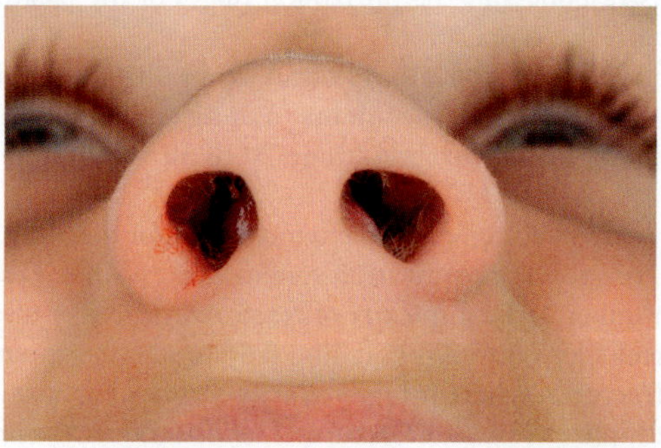

Figure 19.2: Nasal septal hematoma visible on inspection 1 week after trauma. (From Larrabee WF, Ridgway J, Patel S. *Master Techniques in Otolaryngology - Head and Neck Surgery: Facial Plastic Surgery*. 1st ed. Wolters Kluwer; 2018. Figure 22.1)

Septal Hematoma

Internal examination of the nose with a nasal speculum or lighted otoscope is facilitated by use of an inhaled vasoconstrictor such as oxymetazoline. A septal hematoma appears as a purple mass extending from the septum, and, on palpation, feels like a soft, fluctuant mass. Persistent clear fluid from the nose in the setting of trauma should raise the possibility of a cerebrospinal fluid (CSF) leak. A quick bedside filter test (a drop of the fluid on filter paper will result in a rapidly advancing halo of clear fluid around red blood) has a sensitivity of greater than 86%, but a beta transferrin level on the fluid is more objective.

DIAGNOSIS

Nasal bone fractures and septal hematomas are diagnosed primarily by detailed physical examination. Suspicion for nasal bone fracture is raised when the patient has swelling, bruising, epistaxis, infraorbital ecchymosis, and/or pain. Typical imaging for facial fractures are plain X-rays and computed tomography (CT). Magnetic resonance imaging (MRI) is not an optimal choice, as fractures are better visualized on CT than on MRI. Patients with tenderness and swelling isolated to the nasal bridge without septal hematoma, can breathe through each nare, and lack a significant deformity do not require an X-ray in the ED, because the results would not alter management. However, suspicion for other facial injuries should prompt CT imaging.

MANAGEMENT

Nasal Bone Fractures

Acute management of nasal bone fractures often involves controlling epistaxis. Comprehensive management of epistaxis is discussed in Chapter 10, but, generally, the patient should apply ice to the nose and elevate the head to reduce edema. Nasal decongestants reduce swelling and mucosal congestion in the acute period. Not all nasal fractures require treatment; if the fractured bones remain symmetric, and the nasal airway is not significantly obstructed, observation alone is appropriate. If edema is significant at the time the patient is evaluated, patients should be informed that any external deformity may manifest only once the edema recedes. In the case of an obvious nasal deformity, consultation with an ENT, maxillofacial surgeon, or plastic surgeon is warranted.

Displaced nasal fractures can be treated by closed or open reduction. The timing of repair is nuanced and depends on the severity of injury and soft tissue edema. If patients present within a few hours of the injury and significant edema has not yet developed, closed reduction can be performed immediately. However, patients more commonly present once edema has set in, and reduction that is attempted amid substantial swelling can be inaccurate because bony contours and position are obscured. Therefore, reevaluation should occur as soon as the swelling has improved and before the fractures consolidate, within 1 to 2 weeks. This timeline allows for successful closed reduction if indicated. With severe comminution of the nasal bones, closed reduction may still be effective up to 3 weeks after the initial trauma, because multiple bony fragments often take longer to stabilize. After 2 weeks, however, the provider and the patient should be prepared for an open technique such as formal septorhinoplasty. In some cases, closed reduction may be inadequate, and if nasal obstruction persists after healing, open reduction is indicated.

Simple closed reduction can be performed at the bedside in the acute setting under local and topical anesthesia, typically by an ENT specialist. An infraorbital nerve block and oxymetazoline-soaked cottonoids often provide adequate anesthesia for the procedure. A variety of instruments may be employed during closed reduction of nasal bone fractures. Typically, a set will include a nasal speculum, bayonet forceps, suction tips, and an elevator (eg, Goldman). The bone on the side that is depressed is first elevated using the Goldman elevator. External pressure is then placed on the protruding or convex side. During this maneuver, a bimanual technique is paramount for the tactile feedback of an accurate reduction. An external splint of adhesive strips and rigid material such as a cast must be applied at the conclusion of the reduction. The patient should be advised to avoid further trauma for at least 1 month after reduction. More involved procedures, if necessary, will require general anesthesia and should be performed by a surgical service.

Complications related to nasal bone fractures include injury to the nasolacrimal complex, or fracture of the cribriform plate. Consultation with an ophthalmologist is required for the former, whereas the latter can predispose to leakage of CSF, risking rare but extremely serious complications such as meningitis, encephalitis, or brain abscess. Drainage of clear rhinorrhea immediately after trauma to the midface and up to several days later should raise the possibility of a CSF leak. These patients should have urgent consultation with an otolaryngologist and/or neurosurgeon and CT of the face with fine cuts to evaluate the skull base. They should also be placed on strict precautions to minimize intracranial pressure (bed rest, stool softeners, head elevation, etc.).

Septal Hematoma

Septal hematomas must be addressed immediately, usually with local and topical anesthetic, although young or uncooperative patients may require sedative such as intranasal midazolam or ketamine. Cotton pledgets soaked in oxymetazoline and topical lidocaine are placed in the nares to accomplish topical anesthesia and decongestion. A scalpel incision is then made through the fluctuant area of septal mucosa to allow drainage. In the case of a bilateral hematoma, incisions are made in an offset manner on each side to decrease the risk of septal perforation. The clot is suctioned, and the space is irrigated copiously with sterile saline. Hemostat forceps are used to disrupt any septations or abscess pockets that may have formed. To prevent reaccumulation, a small Penrose-type drain can be placed and sutured to the mucosa, and compressive packing is placed in both nares. Alternatively, resorbable transseptal mattress sutures can be placed, in which case intranasal packing is not necessary. The patient should be started on oral antibiotics with antistaphylococcal coverage and have follow-up within 2 to 3 days. The drain and packing are removed once drainage has stopped for 24 hours.

PEDIATRIC ISSUES

The pediatric nose is relatively protected from fractures because the dorsum is less projected, and the skeleton is more cartilaginous and less prone to comminution. However, the pediatric nasal septum is vulnerable to dislocation, and septal hematomas are more common in children than in adults.[2] Thus, the septum must be evaluated especially carefully in pediatric nasal trauma. Prior to adolescence, the nasal septum acts as a growth center for both the nose and the midface. Thus, to minimize effects on facial development, nasal fractures in the pediatric population are more often managed conservatively with closed reduction. Open reduction of bony injuries with osteotomies or septal reconstruction is rarely indicated, except in cases of severe trauma that often involve the orbit or midface simultaneously. Pediatric nasal fractures should be addressed faster, within 7 to 10 days, given their tendency to heal more rapidly. It is important to advise parents that nasal trauma may result in functional obstruction or aesthetic concerns later in life.

TIPS AND PEARLS

- Isolated nasal bone fractures do not frequently warrant immediate intervention aside from control of epistaxis and drainage of any nasal septal hematoma. It is paramount to wait 1 to 2 weeks for initial edema to abate before closed reduction is attempted in order to maximize success. However, the time window for treatment is tight while bones are still mobile enough for closed reduction, so it is important to refer to an appropriate surgeon expeditiously.
- Nasal septal hematomas must be incised and drained urgently to prevent septal destruction, perforation, and potential dorsal collapse. They are more common in pediatric patients, who are also more prone to develop disruptions in nasal and midface development as a result of nasal bone fractures.
- Nasal bone fractures may be accompanied by more severe injuries, such as cribriform plate fractures, nasoethmoid complex fractures, and orbital fractures. Consultations with otolaryngology, plastic surgery, maxillofacial surgery, neurosurgery, and/or ophthalmology should be sought as necessary.

EVIDENCE

Most studies on treatment of nasal bone fractures are retrospective and not of high quality; randomized controlled trials are lacking. No clear consensus exists on the best treatment algorithm in an acute trauma setting, despite various attempts at streamlining the approach to management.[3]

Is imaging necessary for diagnosis of presumed isolated nasal bone fractures?

Whereas radiographic imaging is recommended in the setting of high-energy facial trauma with concern for multiple injuries, plain film radiographs for diagnosis of isolated nasal trauma has been repeatedly shown to be noncontributory. CT scans provide high-resolution imaging of isolated nasal fractures but also do not improve patient management.[4]

What is the best treatment algorithm of nasal bone fractures in the ED?

In the ED, options for management of acute nasal fractures primarily include: (1) observation and (2) closed nasal reduction. If the fractured bones remain well aligned and the nasal airway is patent, observation alone is adequate. If the patient is seen within hours of the injury and the edema is mild, closed reduction of unilateral or bilateral displaced fractures with only mild septal deviation on examination can be performed safely. When fractures are comminuted or septal deviation is severe, attempts at closed reduction should be delayed and the patient referred to a specialist. If significant edema has already set in that precludes an accurate examination and diagnosis of nasal bone fracture, intervention should be delayed and the patient reevaluated on an outpatient basis once the swelling subsides.[3]

References

1. Hwang K, Ki SJ, Ko SH. Etiology of nasal bone fractures. *J Craniofac Surg*. 2017;28(3):785-788.
2. Alcaraz N, Lawson W. Trauma of the nose and nasoethmoid complex in children and adolescents. *Facial Plast Surg Clin North Am*. 1999;7:175-183.
3. Hoffmann JF. An algorithm for the initial management of nasal trauma. *Facial Plast Surg*. 2015;31(3):183-193.
4. Westfall E, Nelson B, Vernon D, Saltagi M, et al. Nasal bone fractures and the use of radiographic imaging: an otolaryngologist perspective. *Am J Otolaryngol*. 2019;40(6):102295.

CHAPTER 20

Facial Trauma: Frontal Sinus, Maxillary and Mandibular Fractures, Dental Injuries

Benjamin Wyler
Benjamin D. Malkin

THE CLINICAL CHALLENGE

Maxillofacial injuries may be blunt or penetrating and may involve soft tissue, bone, and/or neurovascular structures. Knowledge of the underlying anatomy is key in being able to identify which structures have been affected. Careful physical examination, along with appropriate use of imaging, can provide details of the nature and extent of the injury and guide management.

PATHOPHYSIOLOGY

The facial skeleton consists of 14 bones—six paired and two unpaired (**Figure 20.1A**). They form a system of buttresses that provides support and structure to the face and allows dispersion of oncoming forces away from the cranium. The vertical buttresses consist of paired nasomaxillary, zygomaticomaxillary, and pterygomaxillary midfacial buttresses, and the rami of the mandible. The four horizontal buttresses are the frontal bar, zygoma-inferior orbital rim, hard palate, and mandible.

The 20 primary teeth consist of two types of incisors (four central and four lateral), four canines and two types of molars (four first and four second). The 32 permanent teeth, which begin erupting at age 6 to 7 years, have an additional 8 premolars and 4 third molars (see Chapter 2 for the Universal Numbering System). Each tooth sits in a socket of alveolar bone and receives a neurovascular input at the root.

A 2007 review of 407,167 emergency department (ED) visits for facial fractures found that the most common fracture sites were nasal bones (58.6%), mandible (16.2%), and zygoma/maxilla (13.9%). Twenty-one percent of visits resulted in hospital admission. Males accounted for 68% of cases, and the most common mechanisms of injury were assault (37%), falls (24.6%), and motor vehicle accidents (12.1%).[1]

APPROACH/THE FOCUSED EXAM

The approach to the patient with facial trauma begins with an assessment for any life-threatening injury. Additionally, owing to relatively high rates of concurrent cervical spine injury, all patients should have their necks immobilized until an injury can be ruled out.

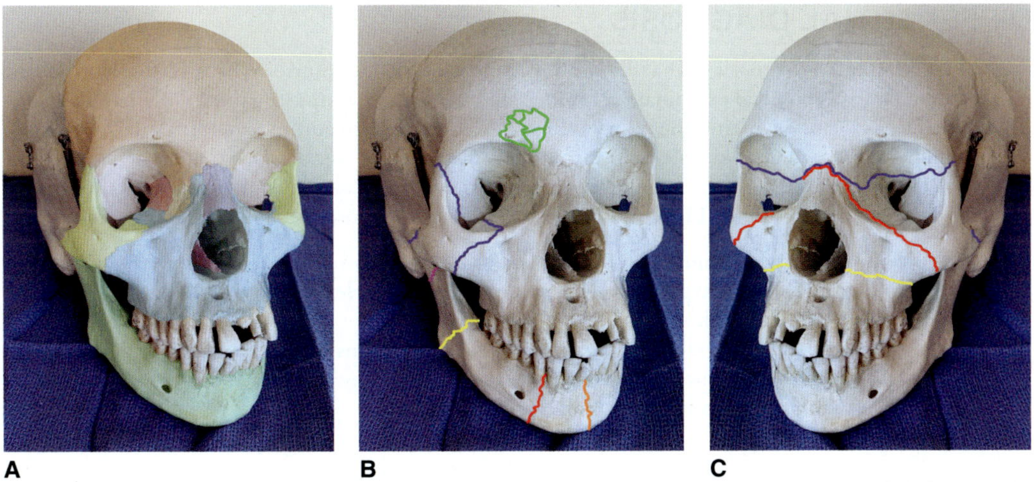

Figure 20.1: A, Skull with facial bones shaded. Paired—inferior turbinate (not seen), lacrimal (light yellow), maxilla (turquoise), nasal (indigo), palatine (aqua), zygoma (lime); unpaired—mandible (green), vomer (purple); additionally seen are the frontal (orange), sphenoid (rose), and ethmoid (red) bones. Skulls with common fracture patterns indicated- B, frontal sinus (green), zygomaticomaxillary complex (blue), mandibular symphysis (orange), parasymphysis (red), angle (yellow), and subcondylar (purple). C, Le Fort I (yellow), II (red), and III (blue).

Maxillofacial examination should begin with initial visual inspection to identify any obvious soft tissue injuries, bony deformities, or functional deficits such as cranial nerve weakness. Next, the head and neck should be palpated for step-offs, bony mobility, crepitus, and tenderness. A complete eye exam should be performed (see Chapters 25 and 28). Anterior rhinoscopy can be used to identify sources of epistaxis and septal fractures or hematoma; significant clear rhinorrhea may be an indication of cerebrospinal fluid (CSF) leak. Midface fractures can be assessed by manipulating the central maxillary alveolar ridge while having the other hand on the patient's nasal bridge or forehead. The extent of the mobile bony segment can suggest one of the three Le Fort fracture patterns. Malar flattening from a zygoma fracture can be assessed by looking from the top of the patient's head, although this is sometimes obscured by edema. In the presence of prezygomatic soft tissue swelling, the zygomatic arch can be palpated for tenderness through the buccal vestibule.

A careful intraoral exam is essential. Dental evaluation involves examining for missing teeth and occlusal disturbances and evaluating each tooth for injury, mobility, percussion tenderness, and loss of sensation. If a tooth is avulsed and cannot be accounted for, the possibility of aspiration must be considered. Multiple teeth moving together but separate from the adjacent teeth suggests an alveolar fracture. Gingival lacerations, floor of mouth ecchymosis, and displacement of an entire segment are suggestive of a mandibular fracture. It is important to note areas of malocclusion, trismus, and open bite deformities; patients can often report whether their bite feels different from usual and in what way. The tongue blade test is useful in screening for mandibular fractures. While the patient bites down on a tongue blade placed between the molars, the blade is twisted along its long axis. Inability to break the blade is 95% sensitive for mandibular fracture.[2]

Although conventional X-rays can identify many fractures, computed tomography (CT) imaging is the cornerstone of evaluating facial fractures and is employed as the imaging modality of choice. Axial, coronal, and sagittal cuts should be reviewed to identify the fracture pattern(s). In complicated fractures, three-dimensional (3D) reconstruction can be helpful in visualizing fracture planes and for surgical planning. Cone beam CT is one alternative that can provide favorable bony imaging; soft tissue detail is sacrificed in exchange for a lower dose of radiation. Mandible fractures and dental injuries may also be imaged with panoramic radiographs.

DIFFERENTIAL DIAGNOSIS

The differential diagnosis of maxillofacial fractures and dental injuries is usually narrowed based on the patient's physical examination findings and confirmed with subsequent CT imaging. Considerations include whether the injury is limited to the soft tissue or involves the underlying bone, whether the fracture is simple or comminuted, displaced or nondisplaced, open or closed, and whether there is associated nerve or ocular injury. Fractures are usually characterized based on their location and pattern (**Figure 20.1B and C**). A commonly used scheme includes the following:

- Skull base/cranial vault—Frontal sinus, skull base, and cranium.
- Midface—Le Fort, zygoma (zygomaticomaxillary complex or isolated arch), orbit, nasal, naso-orbito-ethmoid.
- Mandible—Symphysis/parasymphysis, body, angle/ramus, condylar/subcondylar.
- Dentoalveolar—Enamel infraction, fracture (crown, crown-root, root, alveolus), concussion, subluxation, luxation (extrusive, lateral, intrusive), avulsion.

MANAGEMENT

Management of facial fractures should be approached in the context of a stepwise trauma protocol, because many result from high-energy mechanisms that can cause associated intracranial, cervical spine, or multisystem injury. Patients can also present with extensive hemorrhage or airway compromise. After life-threatening or potentially disabling injuries have been excluded or stabilized, definitive treatment of fractures can usually be performed electively. Early consultation with a facial trauma specialist (ENT, plastic surgeon, or oral maxillofacial surgeon) is warranted if there are complex, unstable or open fractures, significant trismus, difficulty swallowing, or uncontrolled pain. The focus of definitive treatment is to restore form, function, and stability. Many nondisplaced or minimally displaced fractures do not require operative management. Antibiotics and tetanus vaccine should be considered in the setting of open fractures or dental fractures.

Frontal and Maxillary Sinus Fractures

Fractures of the frontal sinus are characterized by involvement of the anterior and posterior tables and/or nasofrontal outflow tract and the amount of displacement. Isolated anterior frontal sinus fractures can be referred for outpatient management and have largely moved from an open-intervention to a minimally-invasive/observational approach, with endoscopic (endonasal and transcutaneous) techniques becoming increasingly common.[3] Posterior frontal sinus fractures risk violation of cranial integrity and should prompt neurosurgery and ENT consultation. Maxillary sinus fractures can involve any wall of the sinus and often occur in the setting of multiple facial bone fractures. Most isolated anterior wall fractures are managed conservatively. Isolated posterior wall fractures are rare, often occurring in association with a mandible fracture.[4] Fractures of the maxillary sinus floor often involve the dentition and may lead to oroantral fistula. They require repair if there is communication with the oral cavity. Maxillary sinus roof (orbital floor) fractures will be discussed separately (Chapter 28).

Le Fort Fractures

Le Fort fractures comprise three general patterns of complex midfacial fractures that can result from high-energy trauma. The patterns of injury depend largely on the vector of force applied to the face. Bilateral symmetry of fracture planes does not always apply, so unilateral or combined patterns can occur. All Le Fort fractures involve fracture of the pterygoid plates of the sphenoid bone.

Le Fort I fractures result from an impact to the upper teeth or anterior maxilla with a downwardly directed force (**Figure 20.2**). This force results in a transverse fracture along the maxilla above the level of the dental roots, separating the floor of the nasal cavity and the maxillary sinus from the rest of the midface and resulting in a "floating palate." Le Fort II fractures, the most common of the Le Fort fractures, result from traumatic force directed at the nasal bones. They are pyramidal fractures that separate the entire maxilla and nasal bones from the zygomatic and cranial bones. Le Fort III fractures result from a high-energy force directed slightly inferiorly at

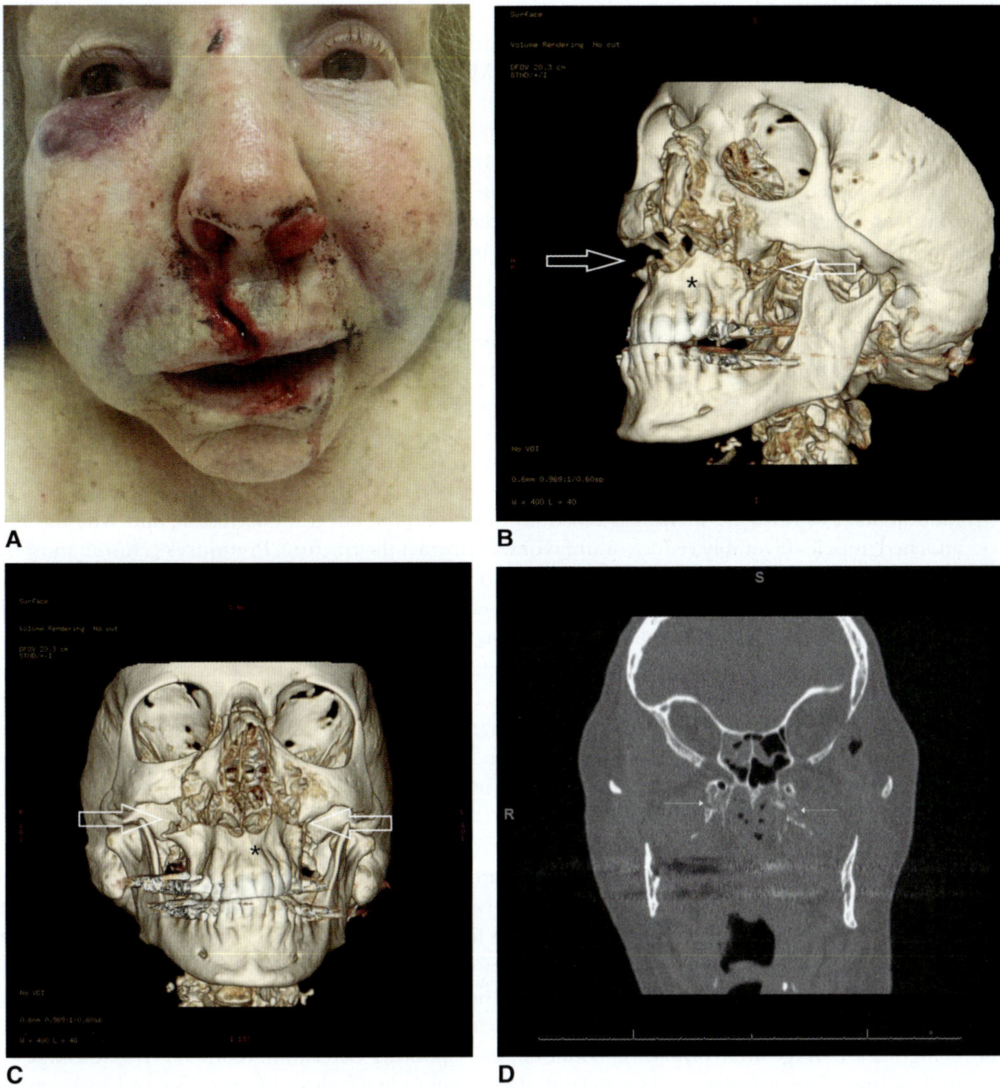

Figure 20.2: A 79-year-old woman fell and hit the center of her face on a concrete planter. A, Clinical photograph on presentation to the emergency department; B and C, three-dimensional computed tomography (CT) reconstructions showing a LeFort I fracture (*white arrows*). Note the separation of the inferior maxilla (*) from the rest of the facial skeleton; D, CT scan, coronal cut, demonstrating the fracture line extending posteriorly through the pterygoid processes (white arrows).

the level of the orbits, causing craniofacial disjunction and completely separating the facial bones from the cranial base. Associated cranial injuries can lead to CSF leak, and oropharyngeal or nasal hemorrhage can be present. Le Fort III fractures carry a high risk of injury to the globe and cranial nerves (optic, oculomotor, abducens, trochlear) and are often associated with basilar skull fractures, brain injury, and shock.

Le Fort fractures can lead to airway compromise or life-threatening hemorrhage and are associated with intracranial and/or cervical spine injury in 15% or more of cases.[5,6] It is important to take a stepwise approach to their management, beginning with securing the airway, supporting respiration, performing hemorrhage control and resuscitation in the setting of shock, and assessing for and protecting against neurologic injury. A retrospective review of 64 patients with Le Fort fractures identified a need for an emergency advanced airway in 34%, of whom 72% were intubated orotracheally, whereas 19% required a surgical airway.[7] Management of the fractures themselves is typically elective, requiring reduction of the displaced segments, followed by stabilization with plates and often maxillomandibular fixation (MMF).

Zygomaticomaxillary Fractures

Repair of zygomaticomaxillary complex (ZMC) fractures is often performed for cosmetic purposes, although sometimes functional deficits necessitate intervention. Indications for repair include concomitant orbital fractures, severely inwardly displaced zygomatic arches resulting in coronoid process impingement and trismus, and infraorbital nerve impingement with persistent pain or hypesthesia. An isolated displaced zygomatic arch fracture is usually reduced via either open or closed approach but not fixated. Displaced ZMC fractures, sometimes referred to as tripod or tetrapod fractures, often disrupt the integrity of the orbit, can cause impingement of the temporalis muscle and/or infraorbital nerve, and are managed operatively. Often, surgery is delayed for a week after the injury to allow resolution of soft tissue edema and easier visual assessment of fracture reduction.

Mandibular Fractures

Mandibular fractures are identified based on their location, effect on occlusion, and whether the attached muscles favorably reduce or unfavorably distract the fracture. Preinjury occlusion must be reestablished, which can be challenging owing to mobility of the mandible relative to the midface. Some nondisplaced fractures with no change in occlusion can be treated conservatively with a soft diet, but most will need operative repair. Treatment decisions are guided by the patient's age, location of fracture, degree of displacement, dental status, and impact on occlusion. Bilateral parasymphyseal fractures of the mandible, although rare, can lead to airway compromise through posterior displacement of the fracture fragment and tongue. This may be temporized by positioning the patient upright and/or through anterior traction on the fracture fragment. If intubation is necessary, orotracheal intubation is usually facilitated by the mobility of the fractured anterior mandible.

Traumatic Dental Injuries

Tooth avulsion accounts for 0.5% to 3.0% of dentoalveolar trauma, and up to 79% of avulsed teeth are maxillary central incisors. A tooth may also be displaced laterally (lateral luxation), into or out of the alveolar bone (extrusion or intrusion), or may be loose in the socket without displacement (subluxation). All cases involve injury to the periodontal ligament and potential disruption of vascular supply to the pulpal tissue. Complete avulsion of a tooth from its socket caries a high risk of tooth loss if it is not replanted in a timely manner, with 73% to 96% of replanted teeth eventually being lost.[8] Storage after injury, replantation, and splinting determine tooth survival. Storage in milk, saline, Hank solution, and saliva from the patient or in the cheek of an awake and cooperative patient prevents periodontal ligament desiccation and death.

Repositioning and/or splinting may improve tooth survival and can be attempted in the ED or urgently in a dental office. Replantation should occur as soon as possible after injury, ideally within 90 minutes. The tooth should be grasped by the crown and gently rinsed in saline before being placed into the socket and splinted. Splinting of avulsed, luxated, or fractured teeth can be accomplished with a variety of materials. Options include using a patient's own mouthguard or clear orthodontic retainer and forming a molding around the dental arch with Blu-Tack or a double layer of aluminum foil covered with thermoplastic acrylic.[9] Another option is to bond a semirigid bridging material (0.4 mm wire, bondable ribbon or the metal strip found on the nasal bridge of a Hudson respiratory mask) to the affected tooth and adjacent stable teeth using composite or tissue adhesive.

Dental fractures are classified by whether they involve the crown or root and by the dental tissues they involve. Exposed dentin appears yellow, whereas pulp appears pink or bloody. Both should be gently irrigated with saline and covered with calcium hydroxide paste. Antibiotics are recommended. Fractures involving the root may be difficult to identify clinically but may benefit from splinting in anatomic alignment. Fractures of the alveolar process are rare, estimated to account for less than 3% of traumatic dental injuries. When they do occur, 74% occur in the maxilla, with the incisors and canines being the most affected teeth.[10] Exam findings may include local or segmental mobility, anesthesia of associated teeth, and occlusal disturbances. Radiographs or CT should be performed when there is suspicion for alveolar bone fracture, and consultation with an oral maxillofacial surgeon is advised. Management consists of reduction and splinting of the affected fragment and suturing of gingival lacerations.

PEDIATRIC ISSUES

Facial fractures in children are much less frequent and differ from adults owing to differences in anatomy and age-specific activity exposure (learning to walk, sports activities, etc.). The most common fracture sites are the mandible (32.7%), nasal bone (30.2%), and maxilla and zygoma (28.6%).[11] Treatment needs to minimize disruption of growth potential, and a "less is more" approach is often best.[12] Avulsed primary teeth are not replanted to prevent damage to the underlying permanent tooth bud. Injuries to permanent dentition are managed as in adults. Nonaccidental trauma is a critical consideration, especially when there are metachronous fractures, dentoalveolar injuries, or delayed presentation.

TIPS AND PEARLS

- Do not let dramatic findings of facial injury distract you from performing a systematic trauma assessment focused on life-threatening and disabling injury.
- Perform a thorough physical examination including assessment of the eyes, any associated nerve injury, and intraoral structures to identify potential complications of facial fracture.
- Obtain a CT scan of the facial bones if physical exam findings or mechanism of injury suggest the possibility of a maxillofacial fracture.
- Most fractures do not need operative repair, and those that do can often be repaired on an elective basis. However, early consultation is recommended in the setting of complex or unstable fractures, open fractures, and fractures associated with nerve injury, uncontrolled hemorrhage, visual disturbance, or significant trismus.

EVIDENCE

Is antibiotic prophylaxis indicated for traumatic facial injuries?

Antibiotic prophylaxis for facial fractures and dental injuries is controversial. Despite traditional recommendations in favor of antibiotics, there are limited data available to suggest a benefit. Based on mostly expert consensus, mandible fractures with gingival lacerations should be treated with antibiotics.[13,14] Preferred antibiotics are penicillins, doxycycline in children older than 12 years, and clindamycin.

When should facial fracture repair be performed?

The ideal timing for treatment of facial fractures has not been well established. A systematic review of the effects of treatment delay on facial fracture outcomes included 30 studies, but almost all were retrospective case series. The authors argued that definitive conclusions could not be drawn from the current literature.[15] In practice, definitive repair of midface fractures is often delayed for up to 1 week to allow resolution of associated edema. Further delay risks making reduction more difficult owing to initiation of fibrous healing of the fractured bone.

References

1. Allareddy V, Allareddy V, Nalliah RP. Epidemiology of facial fracture injuries. *J Oral Maxillofac Surg*. 2011;69(10):2613-2618.
2. Caputo ND, Raja A, Shields C, Menke N. Re-evaluating the diagnostic accuracy of the tongue blade test: still useful as a screening tool for mandibular fractures? *J Emerg Med*. 2013;45:8-12.
3. Banks C, Grayson J, Cho DY, Woodworth BA. Frontal sinus fractures and cerebrospinal fluid leaks: a change in surgical paradigm. *Curr Opin Otolaryngol Head Neck Surg*. 2020;28:52-60.

4. Simmonds JS, Whitlow CT, Chen MYM, Williams DW. Isolated fractures of the posterior maxillary sinus: CT appearance and proposed mechanism. *Am J Neuroradiol*. 2011;32:468-470.
5. Farkkila EM, Peacock ZS, Tannyhill RJ, et al. Frequency of cervical spine injuries in patients with midface fractures. *Int J Oral Maxillofac Surg*. 2020;49:75-81.
6. Bellamy JL, Mundinger GS, Reddy SK, et al. Le Fort II fractures are associated with death: A comparison of simple and complex midface fractures. *J Oral Maxillofac Surg*. 2013;71:1556-1562.
7. Ng M, Saadat D, Sinha UK. Managing the emergency airway in Le Fort fractures. *J Craniomaxillofacial Trauma*. 1998;4(4):38-43.
8. Day PF, Duggal M, Nazzal H. Interventions for treating traumatized permanent front teeth: avulsed (knocked out) and replanted (Review). *Cochrane Database Syst Rev*. 2019;2:1-55.
9. DeAngelis AF, Barrowman RA, Harrod R, Nastri AL. Maxillofacial emergencies: maxillofacial trauma. *Emerg Med Australas*. 2014;26:530-537.
10. Andreasen JO, Lauridsen E. Alveolar process fractures in the permanent dentition. Part 1. Etiology and clinical characteristics. A retrospective analysis of 299 cases involving 815 teeth. *Dent Traumatol*. 2015;31:442-447.
11. Imahara SD, Hopper RA, Wang J, Rivara FP, Klein MB. Patterns and outcomes of pediatric facial fractures in the United States: a survey of the National Trauma Data Bank. *J Am Coll Surg*. 2008;207:710-716.
12. Chandra SR, Zemplenyi KS. Issues in pediatric craniofacial trauma. *Facial Plast Surg Clin N Am*. 2017;25:581-591.
13. Malekpour M, Bridgham K, Wild J, et al. Utility of prophylactic antibiotics in non-operative facial fractures. *J Craniofacial Surg*. 2016;27:1677-1680.
14. Morris LM, Kellman RM. Are prophylactic antibiotics useful in the management of facial fractures? *Laryngoscope*. 2014;124:1282-1284.
15. Hurrell MJL, Batstone MD. The effect of treatment timing on the management of facial fractures: a systematic review. *Int J Oral Maxillofac Surg*. 2014;43:944-950.

CHAPTER 21

Cerebrospinal Fluid Otorrhea, Rhinorrhea, and Temporal Bone Fractures

Todd Spock
Christopher P. Hogrefe

THE CLINICAL CHALLENGE

Recognition of cerebrospinal fluid (CSF) leaks from the anterior or lateral skull base requires a high level of suspicion and a thorough examination to prevent potentially life-threatening sequelae. Blunt skull trauma, which disrupts the dural integrity and allows for CSF fistulization, accounts for 80% to 90% of CSF leaks. Patients with persistent CSF leaks have a 10% to 37% risk of developing meningitis, which carries a mortality rate of nearly 10%.[1] In cases of basilar skull fracture, epistaxis or hemotympanum may obscure the presence of clear fluid drainage from the nose or ear, making the diagnosis challenging. The temporal bone is involved in 18% to 40% of all skull fractures and may also contribute to a CSF leak.[2,3] Despite this noteworthy incidence, concomitant injuries usually associated with this diagnosis may distract providers' attention. A thorough examination to identify injuries to nearby neurovascular structures (eg, facial nerve, internal carotid artery, internal jugular vein) and potential CSF leak is critical. In addition to trauma, CSF leaks may occur iatrogenically from surgeries of the sinus, skull base, or ear. Finally, although less common in the emergency setting, approximately 10% of patients suffer nontraumatic etiologies of CSF leaks, including those resulting from increased intracranial hypertension or sinonasal neoplasms.

PATHOPHYSIOLOGY

Cerebrospinal Fluid

Approximately 400 to 600 mL of CSF is produced per day, allowing complete renewal three to five times per day. CSF is confined to the subarachnoid space by dura mater. At the interface with the nasal cavity, the dura is further bound by the bone of the ethmoid roof and the paranasal sinus mucosa.

Disruption of the barriers separating the subarachnoid space from the nasal cavity or middle ear space allows for bidirectional transmission of CSF, air (pneumocephalus), and microbes (meningitis). The magnitude or flow of CSF is a function of the location and size of dural disruption, as well as the pressure differential between the subarachnoid and extracranial spaces. When the efflux of CSF outpaces the rate of production, intracranial hypotension may result, leading to headaches, nausea, and vomiting.

In rare cases of dural disruption in conjunction with CSF leak, tension pneumocephalus can occur. In this scenario, air accumulates within the subdural space, leading to displacement of the brain parenchyma by mass effect. Ball-valving obstruction of the subdural space or application of positive pressure ventilation often exacerbates the development of tension pneumocephalus. This may lead to altered mental status, focal neurologic deficits, and even cardiac arrest if not emergently addressed.

Elevated Intracranial Pressure (ICP) and Spontaneous CSF Leaks

Idiopathic intracranial hypertension (IIH), also known as pseudotumor cerebri, is a syndrome of elevated ICP without identifiable cause, such as hydrocephalus, cerebral venous sinus thrombosis, or intracranial masses.[4] Clinical manifestations of IIH include headaches, visual disturbances (eg, papilledema, sixth cranial nerve palsy), and pulsatile tinnitus. The elevated ICP and constant pulsations from the dura may cause thinning of the skull base and eventual bony dehiscence, allowing encephaloceles and CSF fistulas to form. Locations of the skull base that are naturally thin, such as the lateral lamella of the cribriform plate, are particularly vulnerable. The resulting spontaneous CSF leakage often provides significant ICP diversion, which masks the common symptoms of IIH and inhibits the development of papilledema.[5] Therefore, unilateral, clear rhinorrhea may be the only presenting symptom in patients with IIH and is often confused with allergic rhinitis.

The demographic common to patients with IIH and spontaneous CSF leaks is that of an overweight female of childbearing age. The rising epidemic of obesity in western culture has mirrored the increased incidence of IIH. Obesity is thought to increase intra-abdominal and intrapleural pressures, leading to decreased cardiac filling. As a result, decreased venous return from the brain leads to a sustained elevation of ICP and subsequent IIH. In addition to obesity, patients with obstructive sleep apnea (OSA) have 4.7 times greater odds of developing spontaneous CSF fistula because hypoxia and hypercapnia precipitate increased cerebral blood flow and elevated ICP.[6]

Traumatic CSF Leaks, Anterior Skull Base, and Temporal Bone Fractures

The anterior skull base and temporal bone are both sites that are highly susceptible to CSF leak with blunt trauma. The anterior skull case has thin bone at the ethmoid roof and tight adherence of the dura in this region; a defect in this area causes CSF rhinorrhea. Similarly thin bone exists at the roof of the middle cranial fossa formed by the temporal bone and greater wing of the sphenoid. Fractures along the tegmen of the temporal bone with CSF leak permit fluid to accumulate within the air cells of the mastoid and petrous bone or middle ear space. Fluid may transgress a ruptured tympanic membrane to produce otorrhea or travel through the eustachian tube to cause clear rhinorrhea or postnasal drip.

The paired temporal bones articulate with the sphenoid bones anteriorly, occipital bones posteriorly, and parietal bones superiorly. The temporal bone is a complex structure housing numerous structures, including the internal carotid artery, posterior meningeal artery, internal jugular vein, greater petrosal nerve, and portions of cranial nerves VII through XI as well as the middle and inner ear components. Consequently, a great deal of potential pathology can arise from temporal bone injury. As the thickest bone in the body, it requires up to 1875 pounds (850 kg) of force to fracture the temporal bone. Such fractures are typically the result of lateral, high-energy force such as motor vehicle collisions, falls, and assaults. Approximately 90% of temporal bone fractures are accompanied by concomitant intracranial injuries, whereas 9% of the time a cervical spine injury will also be present.[7]

Although several classification systems exist to describe these fractures, the historically most utilized characterizes the fracture as longitudinal, transverse, or mixed in reference to the long axis of the petrous ridge of the temporal bone (**Figure 21.1**). Longitudinal fractures (paralleling the long axis of the petrous temporal bone) constitute approximately 80% of all temporal bone fractures and are more likely to result in CSF otorrhea, tympanic membrane perforation, and conductive hearing loss. Conversely, transverse temporal bone fractures are less common but more likely to result in violation of the otic capsule or injury to the facial nerve.[3,8] The modern classification describes involvement or violation of the otic capsule, which is the dense bony labyrinth that contains the components of the inner ear (ie, cochlea, semicircular canals, and vestibule). Fractures that violate the otic capsule are more likely to result in hearing loss (both sensorineural and conductive), facial nerve weakness, and CSF leakage.[9] Overall, most temporal bone fractures are unilateral, with only 8% to 29% occurring bilaterally.

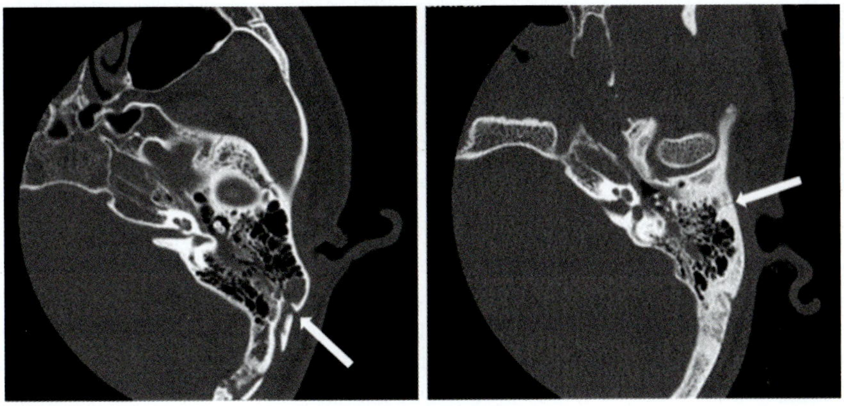

Figure 21.1: Axial CT of left temporal fractures (A) longitudinal fracture (white arrow) without violation of the otic capsule and (B) transverse fracture (white arrow) without violation of the otic capsule.

APPROACH/THE FOCUSED EXAM

A meticulous history often provides the key to elucidating the diagnosis and etiology of a CSF leak. Commonly, a patient with a CSF leak describes unilateral, clear rhinorrhea that worsens with bending forward or straining. This fluid is often described as being watery rather than having the consistency of mucus. Salty or metallic tasting nasopharyngeal drainage often accompanies these symptoms and persists despite topical steroid management, differentiating a CSF leak from chronic rhinitis or sinus disease. Iatrogenic CSF leaks are a rare but well-documented complication of endoscopic sinus surgery caused by occult skull base injuries. Iatrogenic leaks may present in a delayed fashion, so any historical account of sinus surgery, skull base surgery, or septoplasty should be considered a risk factor. Recurrent epistaxis, nasal obstruction, or constitutional symptoms (eg, fevers, night sweats, weight loss) may suggest a neoplasm involving the skull base. IIH may be considered in patients with known risk factors (eg, overweight females of childbearing age) and should be screened for by inquiring about headaches or vision changes prior to the onset of rhinorrhea.

It is imperative to consider a temporal bone fracture in any trauma to the head, particularly those with significant force, such as direct blows to the head from motor vehicle collisions, falls, and/or assaults. Studies suggest an increased proportion of temporal bone fractures caused by assaults versus motor vehicle collisions.[3,7] The force of the injury may be temporal or parietal (causing longitudinal fractures) versus frontal or occipital (resulting in transverse fractures). Hypacusis (total or significant hearing loss), tinnitus, balance problems, and vertigo are common complaints.[10] In cases of blunt head trauma, altered patients may not be able to describe symptoms, which can lead to delay in the recognition of a CSF leak. In addition, epistaxis or hemotympanum from skull base fractures may obscure clear rhinorrhea or otorrhea (**Table 21.1**). In these instances, a high index of suspicion and radiographic imaging will be necessary to unmask a CSF fistula.

Otologic and Temporal Bone Examination

For patients with blunt head trauma and suspected temporal bone fractures, examination of the pinna, external auditory canal, and tympanic membrane is important. Debridement of impacted cerumen or coagulated blood may be necessary for a detailed examination of the tympanic membrane. Bloody otorrhea or hemotympanum is highly suggestive of a temporal bone fracture. Additional physical examination findings suggestive of a temporal bone fracture include nystagmus and facial nerve damage (present immediately in 50% of transverse fractures and 20% of longitudinal fractures, though often delayed). A serous middle ear effusion in the setting of trauma may herald a CSF fistula. CSF trapped within the middle ear space may travel through the eustachian tube into the nasopharynx, resulting in salty or metallic tasting postnasal drainage.

TABLE 21.1 Signs and Symptoms Associated With Temporal Bone Fractures

Hypacusis	Vertigo
Tinnitus	Balance problems
Epistaxis	Hemotympanum
Nystagmus	Facial paralysis

Rhinologic Examination

Anterior rhinoscopy is performed at the bedside with a nasal speculum or otoscope to evaluate the nasal vestibule and anterior nasal cavity. In a patient with suspected basilar skull fracture or CSF leak, a more detailed endoscopic evaluation will provide important diagnostic information, including the presence of chronic inflammation, meningocele, encephalocele, sinonasal tumors, or a stream of clear rhinorrhea suggestive of a CSF leak.

Historically, the "halo sign" has been used to screen for CSF fluid mixed with bloody rhinorrhea in patients with head trauma (**Figure 21.2**). This sign is based on principles of chromatography, wherein CSF or other fluid components will separate from higher-density components of blood on filter paper. Bloody rhinorrhea that contains at least 30% concentration of CSF forms a characteristic double ring or "halo" on tissue paper or other filtering medium. However, this nonspecific test is confounded by the presence of inflammatory rhinorrhea, tears, or saline, all of which may produce a double ring. Therefore, if the nasal or otologic drainage can be collected, laboratory tests provide more reliability in confirming the presence of CSF.

Biochemical Markers

Although biochemical markers cannot localize the source of CSF leak, they can reliably confirm the presence of CSF. The current laboratory gold standard for identifying CSF in a fluid sample is β-2 transferrin, which is exclusively found in CSF, perilymph, and ocular vitreous fluid. This test carries a 100% sensitivity and a 71% specificity for detecting CSF.[11] The clinical utility of β-2 transferrin is limited by the difficulty of collecting a sufficient volume of fluid, particularly with low-flow, intermittent discharge, immobile individuals, and/or uncooperative patients. Some authors suggest that diluting a sample by up to 8-fold to obtain sufficient volume may still yield highly sensitive data, although this is lab specific. Additionally, testing is often processed off-site, leading to delays in results. β-2 transferrin is stable only at room temperature for 4 hours and cannot be frozen, so it must be refrigerated for transport and is subject to degradation.

Before the identification of β-2 transferrin, the presence of glucose was often considered as the most reliable marker for CSF mixed with nasal secretions or blood, confirmed by applying a

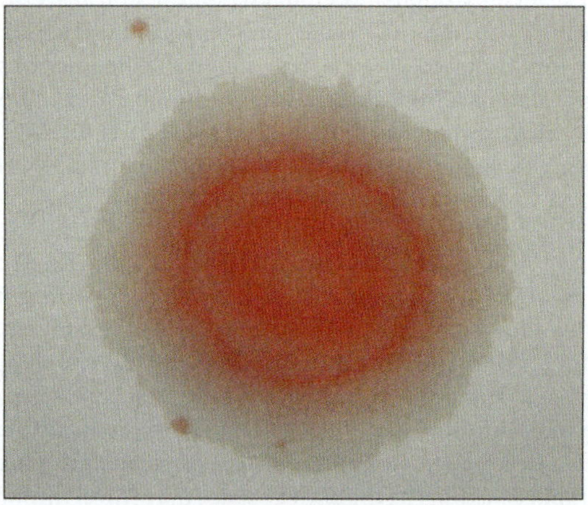

Figure 21.2: The "halo sign" indicative of a cerebrospinal fluid (CSF) leak.

sample of fluid to a glucose-oxidase test strip. This method is rapid and easily performed but, unfortunately, highly unreliable, with high false-positive rates caused by the glucose-reducing capability of nasal secretions and tears. Conversely, patients with active bacterial meningitis have reduced concentrations of glucose in CSF, and this may lead to falsely negative results. Owing to these factors and the wider availability of β-2 transferrin assay, glucose testing is no longer recommended.

Imaging

In patients with suspected or biochemically confirmed CSF rhinorrhea or otorrhea, high resolution CT (HRCT) imaging with 1 mm cuts is indicated for detailed anatomic evaluation of the skull base. HRCT localizes bony fractures or dehiscences of the skull base but cannot adequately distinguish a CSF leak from meningocele, meningoencephalocele, or neoplasm. In patients with CSF otorrhea, evaluation of the middle fossa tegmen is performed with coronal HRCT. In rare cases, posterior fossa defects may manifest as lateral skull base CSF leaks and can be found on axial HRCT.

Magnetic resonance imaging (MRI) complements HRCT for evaluating associated soft tissue pathology. In patients with IIH, an empty sella may be found on MRI, with a CSF-filled sella turcica displacing the pituitary gland from its anatomic location. These patients may have multiple sites of skull base thinning or dehiscence owing to the diffuse nature of the elevated ICP.

Temporal Bone Fracture Imaging

HRCT is the image of choice for identifying fractures of the temporal bone along with their possible sequelae (eg, CSF leak, facial paralysis, and/or vascular injuries). Although HRCT scans with dedicated fine cuts through the temporal bone are often ordered, it has been found that standard HRCT scan ordered for routine trauma evaluation has a sensitivity of 99% for temporal bone fractures.[12] As such, some authors now argue that a dedicated temporal bone HRCT scan may not be necessary as a separate study.[13] Even if a temporal bone fracture is not directly appreciated, secondary findings may suggest occult fracture, such as air around the temporal bone or opacification of mastoid air cells or the middle ear cavity.[14] CT angiography can be secured in cases of suspected associated vascular injury. Of note, MRI has poor sensitivity and specificity for identifying temporal bone fractures and should be reserved for assessing intracranial contents, a cranial nerve palsy without a clear etiology on HRCT, and/or surgical planning.

DIFFERENTIAL DIAGNOSIS

CSF otorrhea represents a minority of patients who present with ear drainage. Inflammatory or infectious processes, such as otitis externa or serous otitis media with tympanic membrane perforation, are far more common. Similarly, chronic rhinosinusitis or vasomotor rhinitis much more commonly present with watery rhinorrhea than do patients with CSF fistula. Traumatic etiologies of skull base CSF leaks, including accidental and iatrogenic injuries, represent 90% of all cases.[15] Atraumatic causes are separated into patients with increased ICP (eg, IIH-associated or "spontaneous" CSF leaks) and those with normal ICP (eg, tumor-related or congenital). While evaluating temporal bone fractures, other concomitant injuries (eg, epidural hematomas) often associated with the high-energy mechanisms of injury should be explored.

MANAGEMENT

CSF Rhinorrhea

Most CSF leaks from blunt trauma resolve spontaneously and can be managed conservatively with the aim of reducing ICP and allowing spontaneous dural healing. Conservative management typically consists of a 7- to 14-day period of strict bed rest, head elevation, stool softeners, nasal precautions (eg, no nose blowing or nasal positive pressure ventilation), and immunization against *Streptococcus pneumoniae, Hemophilus influenzae*, and meningococcus. The use of prophylactic antibiotics and lumbar drains (LD) is controversial (see *"Evidence"* section). Conservative management may also be employed for low-flow or intermittent CSF leaks, but penetrating injuries, high-flow or iatrogenic leaks, and spontaneous leaks rarely heal on their own and often require surgical intervention. Anterior skull base defects may be able to be repaired with a variety of endoscopic techniques.

CSF Otorrhea

The management paradigms for patients with lateral skull base defects overlap significantly with those with anterior skull base defects, albeit with a few notable differences. The surgical approach to these defects is often an open approach via middle fossa craniotomy, transmastoid, or combined middle fossa-transmastoid.

Temporal Bone Fractures

Except for open temporal bone fractures, which warrant consideration of intravenous antibiotics and/or surgical debridement, treatment should be dictated by the sequelae of these fractures. Immediate paralysis and/or significant degeneration of the facial nerve is an indication for surgical exploration and/or decompression. Acute facial nerve palsies rarely respond to glucocorticoid treatment and carry a poor prognosis for nerve recovery. If the onset of facial nerve palsy is delayed, a hematoma or neural edema is likely. In these cases, glucocorticoids for one to 3 weeks can be considered as a component of treatment. Other associated injuries such as hypacusis and vertigo are generally evaluated in further depth and treated on an outpatient basis.

TIPS AND PEARLS

- Confirmation of CSF in patients with equivocal exam findings or fluid mixed with mucus or blood is aided by the presence of β-2 transferrin and further localized with HRCT.
- Conservative management of CSF leaks may be considered as first-line treatment in patients with early recognition (ie, <7 days) of CSF leak after blunt trauma (without major intracranial injury) or delayed recognition after iatrogenic injury.
- Temporal bone fractures are frequently the result of high-energy mechanisms of injury, so the initial focus should be on evaluating for intracranial and/or cervical spine pathology.
- When assessing for a temporal bone fracture, a dedicated HRCT of the temporal bones is typically not necessary. Assess for signs suggestive of this injury, including air around the temporal bone or opacity in a mastoid air cell or the middle ear cavity.

EVIDENCE

Is chemoprophylaxis against meningitis indicated for patients presenting with basilar skull fractures?

Owing to the creation of a direct communication between the central nervous system and the nasal cavity or middle ear, the risk of developing meningitis with persistent (>7 days) CSF leak without surgical intervention ranges from 10% to 37%.[16] Therefore, empiric antibiotic administration against the most common pathogens (ie, *Streptococcus pneumoniae* and *Hemophilus influenza*) has historically been advocated to reduce the risk of this life-threatening complication. These antibiotics often include IV ceftriaxone or ampicillin/sulbactam. Yet chemoprophylaxis has been shown to increase the emergence of resistant organisms in the nasopharynx,[1] risks causing allergic reactions, and has been reported to conversely increase the risk of meningitis in certain studies.[17] A Cochrane Systematic Review of five randomized clinical trials including 208 total participants concluded that in patients with basilar skull fractures, the risk of meningitis was not significantly different in patients receiving intravenous antibiotics compared with placebo.[17] Therefore, unless there is gross wound contamination, the evidence does not support antibiotic prophylaxis.

Does the use of CSF diversion by lumbar drain improve outcomes in traumatic, spontaneous, or idiopathic CSF leaks?

CSF diversion via LD is often employed as an adjunct to conservative and postoperative management to reduce ICP and facilitate dural closure. However, placement of a lumbar drain requires close monitoring to avoid dangerous decreases in ICP and in certain cases may cause pneumocephalus (by aspirating air through a patent skull base defect), meningitis, persistent lumbar CSF leak, and even death. Several studies, including a meta-analysis of 289 patients undergoing surgical intervention, found a high rate of successful repair regardless of the use of lumbar drainage.[18] In traumatic CSF leaks managed conservatively, sparse evidence suggests a more rapid resolution of

CSF leak with LD (4.83 +/− 1.88 days vs 7.03 +/− 2.02 days) but with no difference in overall rates of resolution.[19]

In patients with IIH, surgical repair of spontaneous CSF leaks may lead to reelevation in ICP that was previously lowered by the constant egress of CSF. This pressure reelevation places a patient at increased risk of treatment failure, so LD diversion is often employed adjunctively. In the short-term, an LD is often used to measure opening pressure and decrease ICP during the immediate postoperative period. Elevated opening pressures may also be used to risk stratify patients who may require acetazolamide or a ventriculoperitoneal shunt in the long term.

References

1. Choi D, Spann R. Traumatic cerebrospinal fluid leakage: risk factors and the use of prophylactic antibiotics. *Br J Neurosurg*. 1996;10(6):571-575.
2. Brodie HA, Thompson TC. Management of complications from 820 temporal bone fractures. *Am J Otol*. 1997;18(2):188-197.
3. Johnson F, Semaan MT, Megerian CA. Temporal bone fracture: evaluation and management in the modern era. *Otolaryngol Clin North Am*. 2008;41(3):597-618
4. Kutz JW, Jr., Tolisano AM. Diagnosis and management of spontaneous cerebrospinal fluid fistula and encephaloceles. *Curr Opin Otolaryngol Head Neck Surg*. 2019;27(5):369-375.
5. Aaron G, Doyle J, Vaphiades MS, Riley KO, Woodworth BA. Increased intracranial pressure in spontaneous CSF leak patients is not associated with papilledema. *Otolaryngol Head Neck Surg*. 2014;151(6):1061-1066.
6. Bakhsheshian J, Hwang MS, Friedman M. Association between obstructive sleep apnea and spontaneous cerebrospinal fluid leaks: a systematic review and meta-analysis. *JAMA Otolaryngol Head Neck Surg*. 2015;141(8):733-738.
7. Sun GH, Shoman NM, Samy RN, Cornelius RS, Koch BL, Pensak ML. Do contemporary temporal bone fracture classification systems reflect concurrent intracranial and cervical spine injuries? *Laryngoscope*. 2011;121(5):929-932.
8. Alvi A, Bereliani A. Acute intracranial complications of temporal bone trauma. *Otolaryngol Head Neck Surg*. 1998;119(6):609-613.
9. Little SC, Kesser BW. Radiographic classification of temporal bone fractures: clinical predictability using a new system. *Arch Otolaryngol Head Neck Surg*. 2006;132(12):1300-1304.
10. Montava M, Mancini J, Masson C, Collin M, Chaumoitre K, Lavieille JP. Temporal bone fractures: sequelae and their impact on quality of life. *Am J Otolaryngol*. 2015;36(3):364-370.
11. McCudden CR, Senior BA, Hainsworth S, et al. Evaluation of high resolution gel beta(2)-transferrin for detection of cerebrospinal fluid leak. *Clin Chem Lab Med*. 2013;51(2):311-315.
12. Schubl SD, Klein TR, Robitsek RJ, et al. Temporal bone fracture: evaluation in the era of modern computed tomography. *Injury*. 2016;47(9):1893-1897.
13. Szczupak M, Kravietz A, Patel J, Grobman A, Sidani C, Hoffer ME. Utilization of computed tomography in temporal bone fractures at a large level I trauma center. *Laryngoscope*. 2021;131(1):E278-E282.
14. Ulano AC, Vedantham S, Takhtani D. Revisiting the indirect signs of a temporal bone fracture: air, air, everywhere. *Emerg Radiol*. 2017;24(5):497-503.
15. Citardi M, Fakhri S. Cerebrospinal fluid rhinorrhea. In: Flint P, ed. *Cummings Otolaryngology: Head and Neck Surgery*. 7th ed. Elsevier; 2020:745-758.
16. Oakley GM, Orlandi RR, Woodworth BA, Batra PS, Alt JA. Management of cerebrospinal fluid rhinorrhea: an evidence-based review with recommendations. *Int Forum Allergy Rhinol*. 2016;6(1):17-24.
17. Ratilal BO, Costa J, Pappamikail L, Sampaio C. Antibiotic prophylaxis for preventing meningitis in patients with basilar skull fractures. *Cochrane Database Syst Rev*. 2015;(4):CD004884.
18. Hegazy HM, Carrau RL, Snyderman CH, Kassam A, Zweig J. Transnasal endoscopic repair of cerebrospinal fluid rhinorrhea: a meta-analysis. *Laryngoscope*. 2000;110(7):1166-1172.
19. Albu S, Florian IS, Bolboaca SD. The benefit of early lumbar drain insertion in reducing the length of CSF leak in traumatic rhinorrhea. *Clin Neurol Neurosurg*. 2016;142:43-47.

CHAPTER 22

Penetrating Neck Injuries

Erica Mayland
Joshua Gauger

THE CLINICAL CHALLENGE

The human neck is a highly complex anatomic region containing vital vascular, neurologic, and aerodigestive structures within a relatively small space. The structures of the neck are also relatively unprotected and therefore susceptible to traumatic injury. As a result, evaluation and management of trauma to this region is challenging.

Penetrating neck trauma is relatively rare, with 5% to 10% of traumas presenting with injury to the neck and representing only 1% of all trauma admissions in the United States.[1] Although penetrating neck trauma has a low incidence, the mortality rate can be as high as 10%.[2] A comprehensive understanding of the anatomy of the neck, injury patterns of the region, and current recommendations on management is critical for clinicians to adequately manage these patients.

Anatomy

By definition, a penetrating trauma to the neck is any injury that violates the platysma muscle,[2] which is a broad thin sheet of muscle covering most of the anterior and lateral neck and extending from below the clavicle to above the angle of the jaw. The depth of the neck wound is an important part of the initial evaluation. Wounds superficial to the platysma muscle do not warrant further investigation, but wounds penetrating the platysma are at high risk for violating deeper vital structures (**Figure 22.1**).

The anterior and posterior neck are defined by the sternocleidomastoid muscle, which originates at the clavicle/manubrium and inserts at the mastoid tip. The triangle anterior to the sternocleidomastoid muscle contains anatomically critical structures, including the larynx, pharynx, trachea, esophagus, carotid artery, and jugular vein. The triangle posterior to the sternocleidomastoid muscle contains the spinal accessory nerve and the spinal column.

The neck has classically been divided into three zones to aid in the evaluation and management of traumatic injury[3,4] (**Figure 22.2**). Zone I encompasses the area between the clavicle and sternum inferiorly to the cricoid superiorly. Zone II transverses the space from the cricoid cartilage to the angle of the mandible. Zone III is the area of the neck ranging from the angle of the mandible, extending superiorly to the skull base. Zone classification can be useful to determine which structures are at risk for injury (**Table 22.1** and **Figure 22.3**), but caution should be taken when relying solely on these zones, because penetrating injuries can traverse zones.[5,6]

APPROACH/THE FOCUSED EXAM

Patients with penetrating neck injuries have the potential to rapidly decompensate. Therefore, evaluation should be prompt and follow a systematic approach to cover all critical aspects of care, immediately assessing airway, breathing, and circulation.

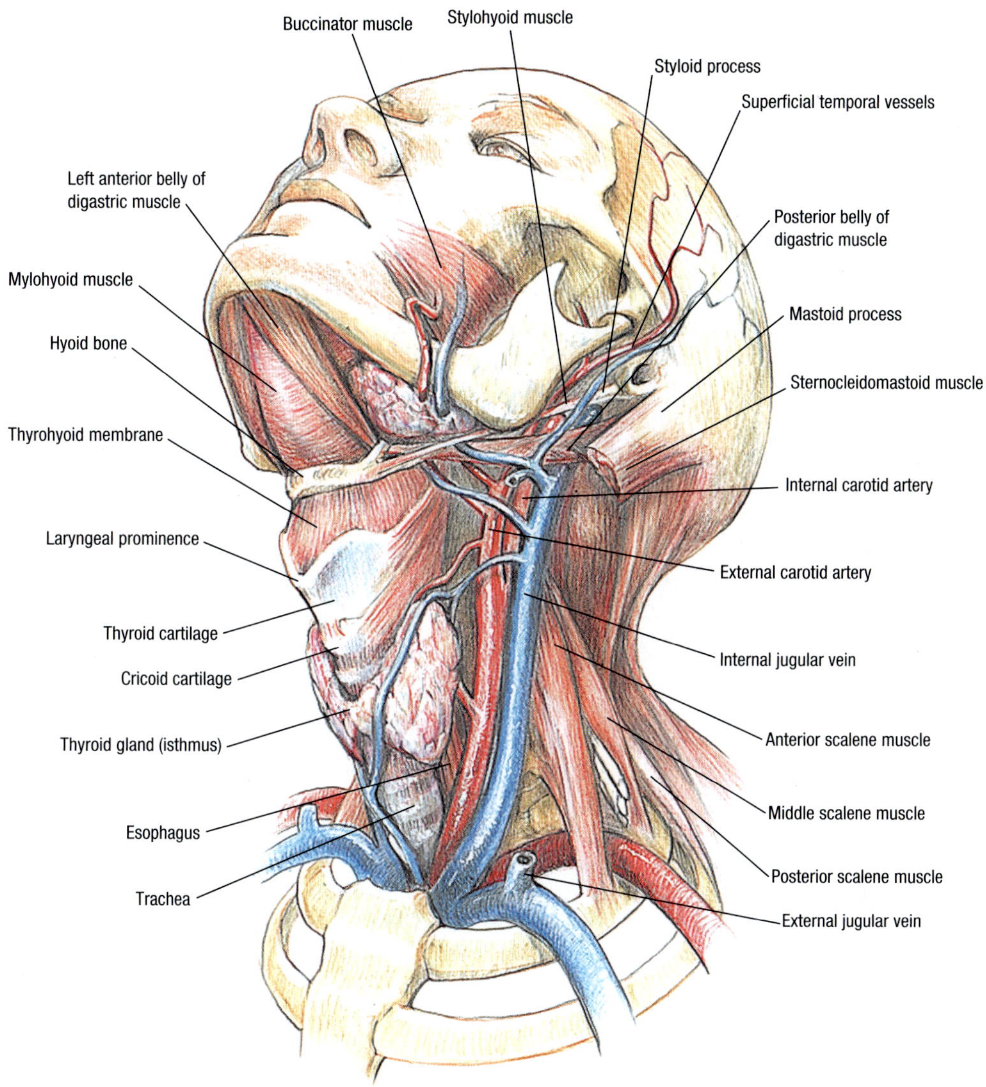

Figure 22.1: Deep structures of the neck. (From The Anatomical Chart Company. *ACC Atlas of Human Anatomy.* Wolters Kluwer; 2002.)

Regardless of the zone of injury, unstable patients exhibiting "hard signs" indicate the need for emergent surgical management. These signs include airway compromise, expanding or pulsatile hematoma, active brisk bleeding, hemorrhagic shock, hematemesis, signs of stroke or cerebral ischemia, massive subcutaneous emphysema, unilateral pulse deficit, and air bubbling through the wound.[7] Presence of at least one hard sign is associated with a 90% rate of major injury.[1] However, absence of hard signs does not exclude injury to the underlying structures of the neck, so in their absence, clinical assessment should guide decisions for further testing.

Airway

In penetrating neck wounds, evaluation and management of the airway is particularly critical. The provider should first assess whether the airway is protected or whether the patient requires immediate airway intervention. A careful evaluation of the oral, pharyngeal, laryngeal, and tracheal structures will usually reveal whether airway intervention is needed. Some clinical signs that

Orientation

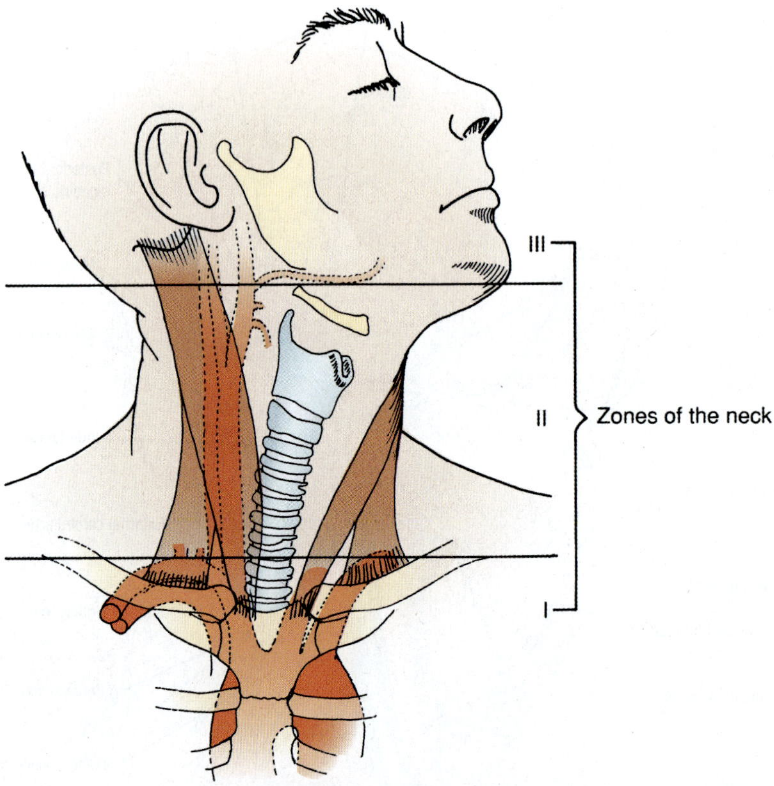

Figure 22.2: Zones of the neck as defined for purposes of trauma. (From Helling KD, Pelaez CA. Neck Exploration for Trauma. In: Scott-Conner CE, ed. *Scott-Conner & Dawson: Essential Operative Techniques and Anatomy*. 4th ed. Wolters Kluwer; 2014:98-104. Figure 13.1.)

TABLE 22.1 Critical Structures by Zone

	Zone I	Zone II	Zone III
Anatomic landmarks	Clavicle/sternum to cricoid cartilage	Cricoid cartilage to angle of mandible	Angle of the mandible to base of skull
Critical anatomic structures	Carotid arteries Subclavian arteries Vertebral arteries Lung apices Trachea Esophagus Thoracic duct Spinal cord	Carotid arteries Vertebral arteries Jugular veins Pharynx Trachea Esophagus Larynx Vagus nerve Spinal cord	Carotid arteries Vertebral arteries Jugular veins Cranial nerves Spinal cord

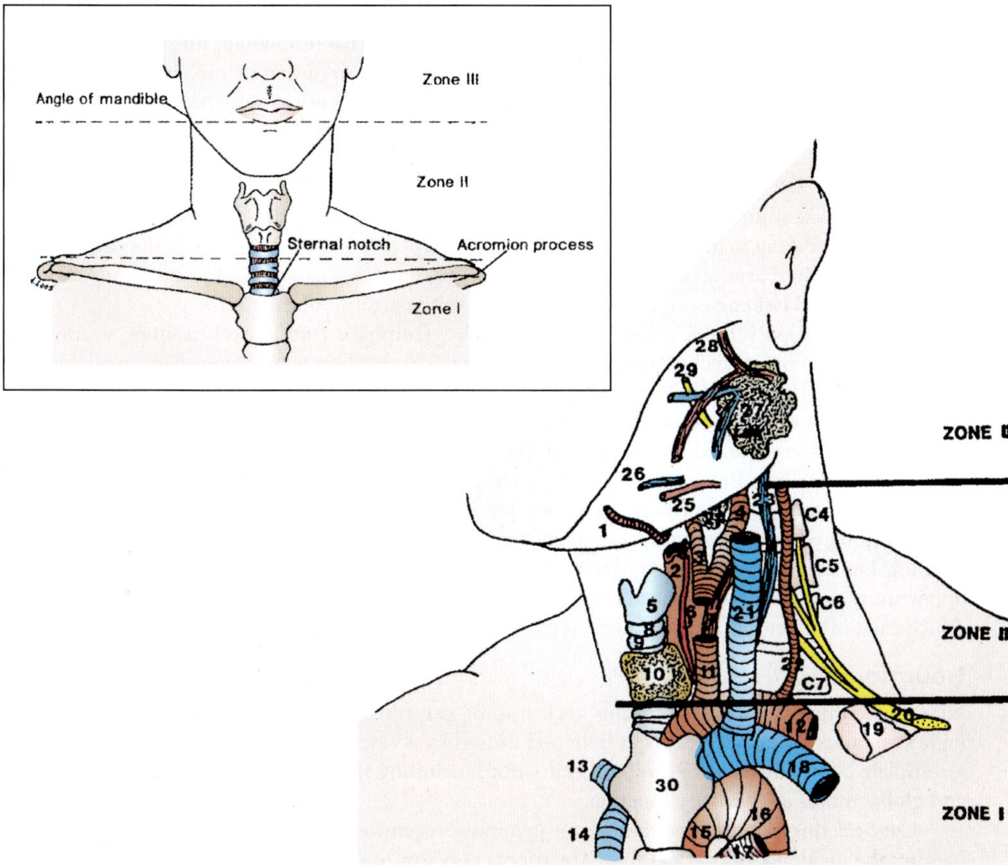

Figure 22.3: Cervical structures contained in Zones I, II, and III: (1) facial artery; (2) esophagus; (3) internal carotid artery; (4) external carotid artery; (5) thyroid cartilage; (6) sympathetic trunk; (7) vagus nerve; (8) cricothyroid membrane; (9) cricoid cartilage; (10) thyroid cartilage; (11) common carotid artery; (12) subclavian artery; (13) right innominate vein; (14) superior vena cava; (15) ascending aorta; (16) descending aorta; (17) pulmonary artery; (18) subclavian vein; (19) clavicle; (20) brachial plexus; (21) internal jugular vein; (22) vertebral artery; (23) phrenic nerve; (24) submandibular gland; (25) lingual artery; (26) hypoglossal nerve; (27) parotid gland and duct; (28) facial nerve and its branches; (29) maxillary artery; (30) sternal manubrium. The thoracic duct is not shown in this figure. (Adapted from Ordog GJ, Albin D, Wasserberger J, et al. 110 bullet wounds to the neck. *J Trauma* 1985; 25:238–46; inset reproduced with permission from Baker RJ, Fischer JE. *Mastery of Surgery*. 4th ed. Lippincott Williams & Wilkins; 2001.)

suggest an airway injury include vocal hoarseness, stridor, dysphonia, subcutaneous emphysema, bubbling from the wound, and large volume hematemesis.[6]

If indicated, the method of airway intervention depends on the clinical setting, resource availability, and provider skill and experience. Methods that allow direct visualization of the airway are preferred, because blind techniques can exacerbate injuries. The team should prepare with multiple backup options, double suction, and supplies for surgical airway. Bag valve mask ventilation should be performed with caution owing to risk of air dissection into injured tissue planes.

For patients with intact anatomy, rapid sequence intubation has been shown to be safe and effective as a method for securing the airway. If there is a large amount of blood in the oral cavity, then direct laryngoscopy may be advantageous over video laryngoscopy. If anatomic difficulties are suspected, "awake" (while the patient maintains spontaneous respiration) fiber-optic laryngoscopy and intubation may be the preferred method. Fiber-optic and video-assisted intubation have the added benefit of allowing the care team to examine the internal pharyngeal and laryngeal structures for injury. Finally, surgical airway management should be used when orotracheal intubation has been unsuccessful or is otherwise contraindicated. Indications for immediate surgical airway management include massive anatomic distortion of the upper airway or inability to visualize the glottis secondary to anatomic injury or heavy bleeding. Cricothyrotomy or emergency tracheostomy are both options that are chosen based on provider experience.

Vascular

Penetrating neck injuries to any of the three anatomic zones have the potential to cause severe vascular injury owing to the high density of critical vascular structures. Injuries to the carotid, subclavian, or vertebral arteries or to the subclavian or jugular veins can all lead to exsanguination. In addition, cerebral ischemia can result from trauma to the arteries of the neck.

Exsanguination is the leading cause of mortality from penetrating neck trauma, so immediate hemorrhage control techniques can be lifesaving. Various hemostatic agents are available, but direct pressure will usually be sufficient to stabilize an injury until the need for surgical repair can be evaluated. If an injury cannot be controlled with external pressure, Foley balloon catheter tamponade is a well-recognized technique that may temporize bleeding (**Figure 22.4**). This technique involves introducing a Foley catheter along the track of the wound, then inflating the balloon with 10 to 15 mL of saline or water until resistance is met. The Foley catheter is then clamped to prevent back-bleeding through the catheter, and sutures are used to close the wound around the catheter. Gaining hemorrhage control may facilitate hemodynamic stabilization and may even allow the opportunity to obtain imaging, such as helical computed tomography (CT) scans or angiography, which can aid in determining the next steps.

Neurologic

Neurologic injuries from penetrating neck trauma can result from either direct injury to neurologic structures in the neck or from ischemia caused by a vascular injury. Patients should undergo a complete comprehensive neurologic evaluation, including mental status, cranial nerve function, and global motor and sensory function.

Cervical spine immobilization is not generally recommended for penetrating neck trauma, because the incidence of cervical spine fracture is very low and cervical collars can obstruct clinical

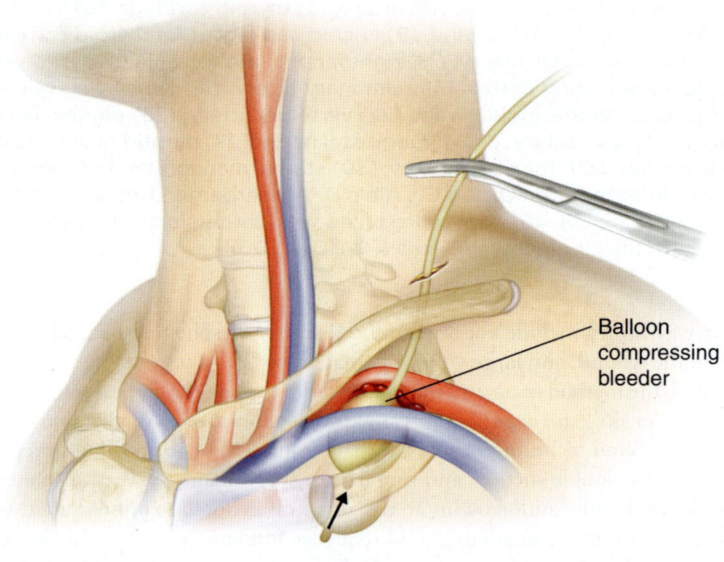

Figure 22.4: Balloon tamponade for bleeding control from the subclavian vessels. It can also be used for bleeding control from other zones in the neck. (From Corcos A, Peitzman AB. Penetrating neck injuries. In: Fischer JE, ed. *Fischer's Mastery of Surgery*. 7th ed. Wolters Kluwer; 2019:462-474. Figure 35.7.)

evaluation and make airway management more difficult. However, cervical collars should be applied in cases of focal neurologic deficit with high clinical suspicion for a spinal injury in a patient with significant altered consciousness.

DIFFERENTIAL DIAGNOSIS OF INJURY BY ZONE

Zone I

Zone I injuries may affect the great vessels of the neck and mediastinum, as well as the cervical and thoracic trachea and esophagus. These structures should be evaluated regardless of symptoms, because a missed injury in this zone could be fatal.

Diagnosis of esophageal injury is crucial, because an untreated esophageal leak into the chest could lead to mediastinitis and sepsis. Evaluation typically begins with an esophogram, using one of two contrast agents, barium and diatrizoate meglumine/diatrizoate sodium. Barium, a thicker contrast agent, allows for a higher sensitivity when detecting esophageal leaks, but if a leak is present, there is a higher risk of infection and inflammation caused by the barium itself. By contrast, diatrizoate meglumine/diatrizoate sodium is water soluble and less toxic to the chest if a leak is present. Often, a diatrizoate meglumine/diatrizoate sodium study is used initially, but if clinical concern for a leak continues despite a negative test, providers may obtain a thinned barium study.[8] Of note, diatrizoate meglumine/diatrizoate sodium has been shown to cause severe pneumonitis and should be withheld if a concomitant tracheal injury is suspected.[9] Flexible or rigid esophagoscopy are alternatives to upper gastrointestinal (GI) radiography. Esophagoscopy is the most sensitive diagnostic test but is more invasive, requiring general anesthesia.[10] A CT scan of the neck and chest may also be useful in determining the path of the injury to either increase or decrease clinical suspicion of an esophageal injury.

Vascular injuries can be evaluated through multiple modalities, including CT angiography (CTA), MR angiography, color Doppler ultrasound, and angiogram. Many practitioners use CTA as first line to evaluate vascular injury with 90% to 100% sensitivity and 94% to 100% specificity in picking up even the smallest intimal injuries.[11] Catheter angiography allows for concomitant diagnosis and intervention but is a more invasive initial diagnostic study. In cases of high suspicion of vascular injury, consider going straight to formal angiogram so that intervention is possible at the time of the study (see **Table 22.2**).

TABLE 22.2 Physical Exam Findings and Diagnostic Testing in Penetrating Neck Trauma

Examination of Penetrating Neck Injuries		
Injury	**Physical Exam**	**Diagnostic Testing**
Esophageal	Crepitus Hematemesis Dysphagia Odynophagia	Esophagram (barium or gastrografin) Esophagoscopy (flexible or rigid)
Laryngeal	Crepitus Shortness of breath Stridor Hemoptysis Hoarseness Pneumomediastinum Bubbling neck wound	Bedside flexible laryngoscopy CT scan Operative direct laryngoscopy
Vascular	Hemodynamic instability Neck hematoma Active hemorrhage Neurologic changes Paralysis	CT Angiogram Formal Angiography

Zone II

Zone II is the largest and most commonly injured. Patients with Zone II injuries who exhibit symptoms of hematoma, crepitus, active hemorrhage, or airway compromise should undergo immediate neck exploration. In patients who do not exhibit hard signs, awake flexible laryngoscopy by the ENT service can evaluate for laryngeal or pharyngeal abrasions, lacerations, or hematomas and provides visualization of the glottic and subglottic airway. If laryngeal trauma is suspected, a direct laryngoscopy in the operating room can provide a more thorough evaluation of the larynx. A CT scan, preferably with 1 mm thin slices, evaluates for fractures of the cricoid and thyroid cartilages, helping surgeons to determine whether repair is necessary. In addition, the esophagus and neck vasculature should be evaluated in a similar manner to Zone I.

Zone III

Penetrating injuries to Zone III can potentially violate major blood vessels and cranial nerves in a difficult-to-access area near the skull base. These injuries are often best treated by interventional radiology owing to the difficult surgical approach to this area. Regardless, a vascular evaluation should be performed through CT angiogram or angiography.

Face and Parotid Region

For penetrating injuries to the face and parotid region, a thorough facial nerve exam should be performed. Stable patients with penetrating injury and immediate facial paralysis should undergo exploration with nerve repair or grafting. In injuries medial to the lateral canthus of the eye, surgical exploration is not necessary, because spontaneous nerve regeneration is typically adequate. Additionally, parotid duct injury should be considered for wounds below the zygomatic arch involving the buccal branch of the facial nerve. Clear saliva may be seen in the wound, and surgical exploration with stent placement or ligation should be performed (see **Figure 22.5**).

MANAGEMENT

Esophageal Injury

Clinical signs of pharyngeal and esophageal injury include crepitus, pharyngeal bleeding, hemoptysis, and hematemesis. A history of penetrating neck trauma followed by fever, tachycardia, and chest pain may indicate a missed perforation resulting in mediastinitis, a devastating complication. Once identified, a patient with an esophageal injury should be made nothing per os (NPO) and taken to the operating room for surgical repair to correct dangerous leakage of saliva into the neck or chest.

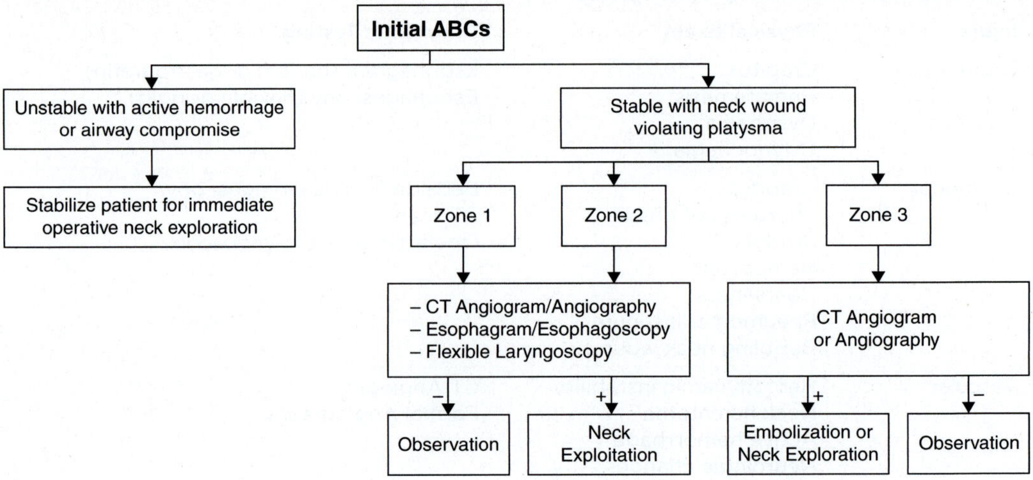

Figure 22.5: Initial assessment of penetrating neck injury.

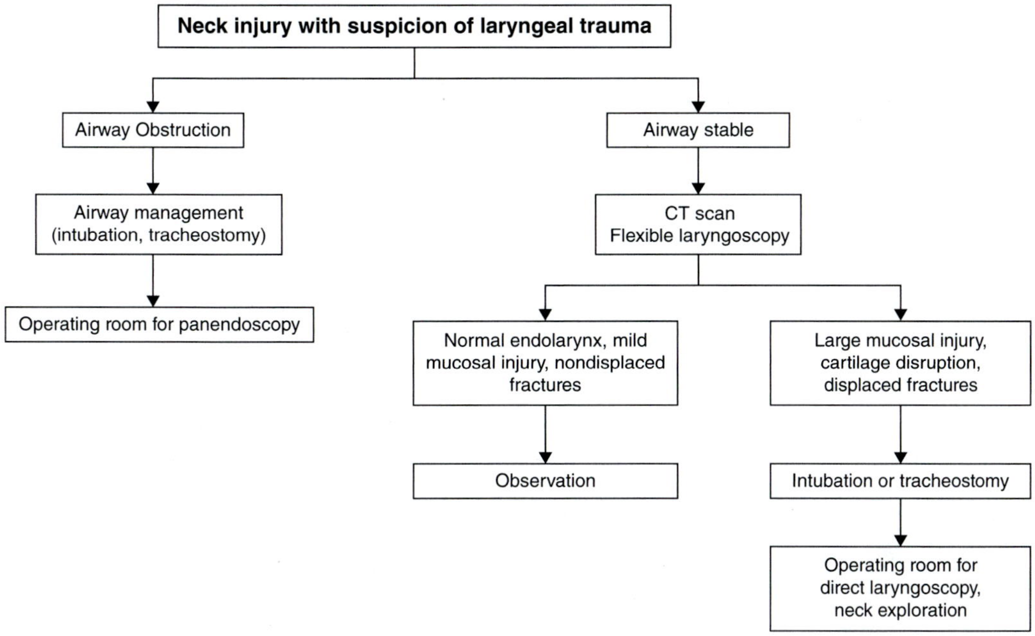

Figure 22.6: Evaluation of laryngotracheal injury in penetrating neck trauma. CT, computed tomography.

Laryngeal Injury

Tracheobronchial injury occurs in up to 20% of penetrating neck injuries.[12] Minor laryngeal injuries causing edema, small hematomas, lacerations without exposed cartilage, or nondisplaced thyroid fractures may be managed conservatively. Laryngeal trauma patients are often admitted for observation to ensure stability of airway. The head of the bed should be elevated, and cool humidified air prevents crust formation. Systemic corticosteroids may be used to reduce edema following laryngeal trauma. Proton pump inhibitors are often utilized to prevent gastric reflux onto the damaged larynx. In cases with mucosal disruption, antibiotics may also be started. Patients with large mucosal defects, exposed cartilage, vocal cord paralysis, displaced thyroid or cricoid fractures, or avulsed arytenoid cartilage often require surgical intervention (**Figure 22.6**).

TIPS AND PEARLS

- Airway management in cases of penetrating neck trauma can be a complicated and daunting task. If an airway needs to be secured, one should have all necessary supplies available, including a range of endotracheal tube sizes, multiple direct laryngoscopy tools (Macintosh/Miller blades, video laryngoscope), intubating flexible bronchoscope, and tracheostomy set.
- When evaluating for esophageal injuries, a nasogastric tube should never be placed without first knowing the status of a potential perforation. Blind placement of a nasogastric tube through an esophageal perforation can inadvertently cause it to end up in the mediastinum.
- Nasogastric tubes should not be placed in patients with Zone III injuries, and a possible skull base fracture as inadvertent intracranial placement can have lethal complications. If esophageal perforation or skull base fracture is identified after trauma, nasogastric tubes should be placed under direct visualization.

TABLE 22.3 Hard and Soft Signs of Penetrating Neck Injury

Hard and Soft Signs	
Hard Signs	**Soft Signs**
Hemodynamic instability	Venous bleeding/oozing
Shock	Crepitus
Active hemorrhage	Dysphagia
Expanding neck hematoma	Dysphonia
Air bubbling wound	Paresthesia
Airway instability	Nonexpanding hematoma
Neurologic changes	

EVIDENCE

Can a "no zone" approach be used to accurately predict vascular injury?

Several authors have noted that the traumatic entry site does not always correlate with internal injury,[5,6] leading to the development of a "no zone" approach, which focuses instead on clinical assessment. This system classifies the clinical assessment by "hard and soft signs" (**Table 22.3**). Patients with hard signs require immediate neck exploration, whereas asymptomatic patients or those with soft signs may undergo observation with associated diagnostic testing.

In an 8-year retrospective review, Ibraheem et al. investigated 337 patients with penetrating neck injury, dividing them into hard signs, soft signs, and asymptomatic.[13] Of the 99 asymptomatic patients, no missed vascular injuries occurred with the use of CTA. Patients with hard signs underwent immediate neck exploration with a high rate of therapeutic neck exploration (76%). The study also found that patients with hard and soft signs had similar rates of therapeutic neck exploration regardless of zone. The group theorized that the "no zone" approach may reduce unnecessary negative neck explorations, but further prospective studies would need to be done to make that conclusion.

Does subcutaneous emphysema predict aerodigestive injury?

Following penetrating neck trauma, it is common to find subcutaneous emphysema on examination or on imaging, raising the question of an underlying aerodigestive injury. When retrospectively evaluating over 300 patients at an Arizona Level 1 trauma center, 80 patients were noted to have subcutaneous emphysema without aerodigestive "hard signs."[14] Sixty-two percent of these patients were managed nonoperatively, and there were no missed injuries or complications. Although further prospective studies would be needed to make a definitive conclusion, this study may encourage providers to monitor patients with subcutaneous emphysema who lack "hard signs" of aerodigestive injury.

References

1. Evans C, Chaplin T, Zelt D. Management of major vascular injuries: neck, extremities, and other things that bleed. *Emerg Med Clin North Am.* 2018;36(1):181-202.
2. Borsetto D, Fussey J, Mavuti J, Colley S, Pracy P. Penetrating neck trauma: radiological predictors of vascular injury. *Eur Arch Otorhinolaryngol.* 2019;276(9):2541-2547.
3. Roon AJ, Christensen N. Evaluation and treatment of penetrating cervical injuries. *J Trauma.* 1979;19(6):391-397.
4. Monson DO, Saletta JD, Freeark RJ. Carotid vertebral trauma. *J Trauma.* 1969;9(12):987-999.
5. Prichayudh S, Choadrachata-anun J, Sriussadaporn S, et al. Selective management of penetrating neck injuries using "no zone" approach. *Injury.* 2015;46(9):1720-1725.

6. Chandrananth ML, Zhang A, Voutier CR, et al. "No zone" approach to the management of stable penetrating neck injuries: a systematic review. *ANZ J Surg.* 2021;91(6):1083-1090.
7. Sperry JL, Moore EE, Coimbra R, et al. Western Trauma Association critical decisions in trauma: penetrating neck trauma. *J Trauma Acute Care Surg.* 2013;75(6):936-940.
8. Tanomkiat W, Galassi W. Barium sulfate as contrast medium for evaluation of postoperative anastomotic leaks. *Acta Radiol.* 2000;41(5):482-485.
9. Trulzsch DV, Penmetsa A, Karim A, Evans DA. Gastrografin-induced aspiration pneumonia: a lethal complication of computed tomography. *South Med J.* 1992;85(12):1255-1256.
10. Schaefer SD. Management of acute blunt and penetrating external laryngeal trauma. *Laryngoscope.* 2014;124(1):233-244.
11. Schroeder JW, Baskaran V, Aygun N. Imaging of traumatic arterial injuries in the neck with an emphasis on CTA. *Emerg Radiol.* 2010;17(2):109-122.
12. Nowicki JL, Stew B, Ooi E. Penetrating neck injuries: a guide to evaluation and management. *Ann R Coll Surg Engl.* 2018;100(1):6-11.
13. Ibraheem K, Khan M, Rhee P, et al. "No zone" approach in penetrating neck trauma reduces unnecessary computed tomography angiography and negative explorations. *J Surg Res.* 2018;221:113-120.
14. Jehan F, Ahmed F, Joseph B, et al. Subcutaneous emphysema in penetrating neck trauma is not significant. *J Surg.* 2017;225:4

CHAPTER 23

Foreign Bodies of the Ears, Nose, and Throat

Alyssa Hackett
Tabitha Ford

THE CLINICAL CHALLENGE

Foreign bodies of the ears, nose, and throat are common. Their incidence, potential for morbidity or mortality, and management algorithms vary greatly depending on patient age, as well as location and physical properties of the foreign object.

EAR FOREIGN BODIES

Approximately 44 000 ED visits are due to ear foreign bodies in the pediatric population alone, most occurring in children ages 3 to 12.[1] The ear canal is the most common site, followed by the earlobe when an earring back becomes embedded under the skin.

Approach and Management

With the appropriate equipment (**Figure 23.1**) and visualization, the removal of an object from the ear canal is often straightforward with a compliant adult, even with concomitant edema or infection. Visualization may be adequate with a conventional otoscope, but, if available, microscopic binocular visualization is preferred.

Small Foreign Bodies

Items such as pencil lead or sand may often be removed simply by flushing the canal with water. However, irrigation should be avoided in cases: (1) where tympanic membrane rupture is suspected or tympanostomy tubes are in place; (2) when organic foreign bodies such as food particles are lodged, as the fluid may cause swelling of the foreign body; (3) a button battery is to be removed.

Larger Graspable Foreign Bodies

In adults, cotton swabs are the most common foreign body. In pediatric patients, paper is also frequently found. These are often easily removed with alligator or Tobey forceps. Caution should be used to avoid grasping a fragile object too firmly and tearing it apart. Organic objects that break apart easily may be removed by gently maneuvering a wax loop or curette behind the foreign body to pull it out.

Nongraspable Foreign Bodies

Objects with smooth surfaces may require a range of instrumentation. A loop or curette may be used to pull the object out from behind. A sharp Rosen pick may also be advantageous to poke into

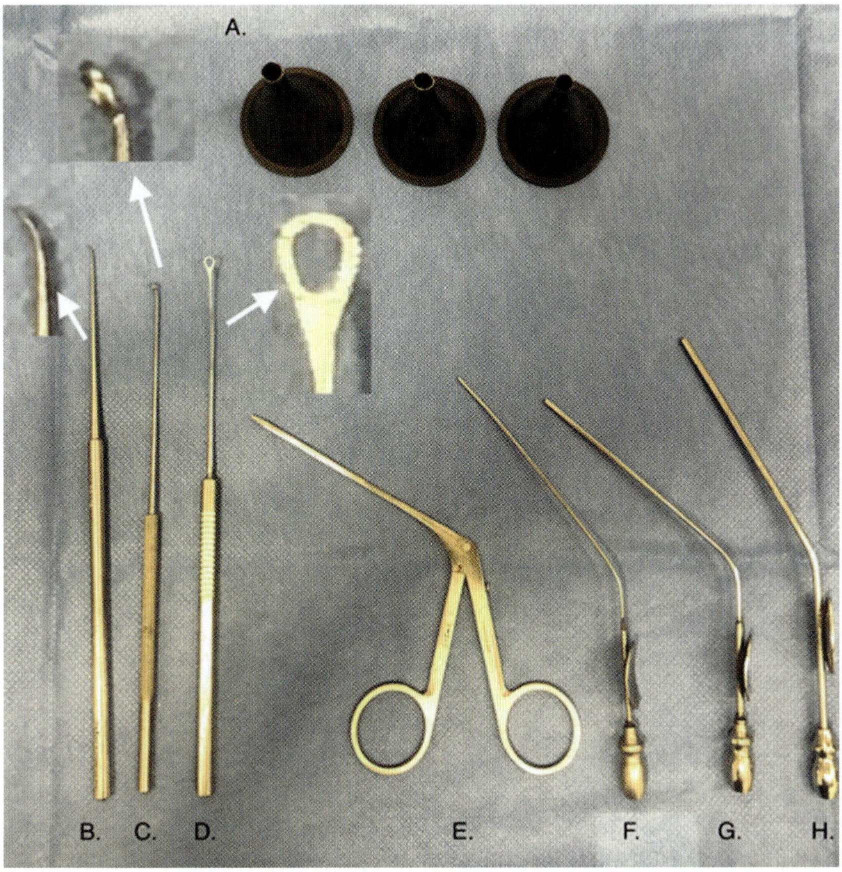

Figure 23.1: Ideal instrumentation for foreign body removal. A, Variety of ear speculum sizes. The ones pictured are designed to be used with the microscope. Speculums for the handheld otoscope are available in 3, 4, and 5 mm sizes. B, Rosen pick. C, Small round Buck curette. These come in a variety of diameters, but a 3 mm or under diameter is advantageous in foreign body removal. D, Weber-Loch curette. Arrows point to a magnified version of each of the three labeled instruments below (B, C, and D). Similar to the Buck curette, these come in a variety of sizes, but the 3 mm size is preferred over large sizes. These tend to be thinner and slightly more flexible than the buck curette, with ridges on one side to help grip wax or foreign objects. E, Alligator forceps. F, 3Fr suction. G, 5Fr suction. H, 7Fr suction.

the side of a semifirm object for removal (eg, an eraser), while avoiding insertion of the pick into the center of the object and pushing it deeper into the canal. Suction may also work if the object is not tightly wedged in the canal.

Live Foreign Bodies

A patient reporting the sensation of movement or abnormal noise may suggest the presence of an insect. A noninvasive removal technique may be attempted by turning off the room lights, then introducing a light source adjacent to the external ear to motivate the insect to extricate itself from the canal.[2] If this fails, application of mineral oil or a lidocaine solution should first be used to euthanize the insect, followed by removal, commonly by alligator forceps or suction.

Summary

After an object is removed from the ear canal, the external auditory canal and the eardrum should be inspected for trauma and for additional foreign bodies. If there is significant trauma and/or edema, ototopical drops with either an antibiotic or antibiotic-steroid combination may be indicated. If tympanic membrane perforation is suspected, neomycin or gentamicin drops should be avoided because of their potential ototoxic effects on the inner ear via absorption through the round window membrane.

Although most ear foreign bodies present a low potential for infection or damage if removal is delayed by days to weeks, a few special circumstances warrant urgent or emergent ENT consult. Although button batteries in the ear do not cause the same tissue damage as in the nose or esophagus, they should still be promptly removed, and ENT should be consulted if emergency department (ED) provider attempts are unsuccessful. Additionally, sharp foreign bodies or those suspected to have penetrated the tympanic membrane should be removed semiurgently by ENT without attempts by an emergency medicine (EM) provider; most small perforations will heal thereafter without the need for surgical intervention. Finally, semiurgent ENT follow-up is indicated in circumstances in which removal attempts by an EM provider are unsuccessful or predicted to be difficult.

Pediatric Issues

Whereas ear foreign body removal in an adult is typically straightforward, the same procedure in a child is often a test of patience and skill. Referral to an outpatient ENT may be the best approach for many young children, because specialized tools exist to increase the chance of success on the first removal attempt, minimizing emotional trauma for the patient. Edema, trauma, or signs of infection can be treated with ototopical drops while waiting for outpatient evaluation.

EARLOBE FOREIGN BODIES

An embedded foreign body of the earlobe is easily removed with local anesthesia. The foreign body may be massaged out of a weak spot in the skin or may require a small incision to facilitate removal. Oral antibiotics are indicated if there is purulence in the wound bed.

NASAL FOREIGN BODIES

Nasal foreign bodies are usually found in children, classically presenting as unilateral rhinorrhea, often with a bad odor or purulence. The presence of the inferior and middle turbinates usually keeps the object firmly wedged in the nasal cavity, limiting migration into more vulnerable portions of the airway.

Approach and Management

Since nasal foreign bodies are almost exclusively a pediatric entity, ENT involvement is frequently advantageous. Decongestion (topical oxymetazoline or neosynephrine) and anesthesia (topical 4% lidocaine spray) facilitates nasal access, and utilization of a papoose or involvement of the parent or second assistant is almost universally necessary. Visualization is preferred with a rigid nasal endoscope, but a handheld otoscope may be adequate. Similar instrumentation is used for extraction of nasal foreign bodies as is used in the ear (Figure 23.1).

Soft Foreign Bodies

Sponges and tissue are typically best removed with alligator forceps.

Firm Foreign Bodies

Beads and other smooth objects can be removed by passing a small ring curette behind the object and moving it forward. Alternatively, the balloon of a device such as a Katz extractor (**Figure 23.2**) or an infant foley catheter may be advanced beyond the foreign body, then pulled out after the balloon is inflated.

It may be appropriate to refer young children to an outpatient ENT office setting for nasal foreign body removal. Because of the potential risk for toxic shock syndrome, oral antibiotic prophylaxis against *Streptococcus pyogenes* and *S aureus* should be prescribed if the object is unknown or is a porous substance (eg, tissue or sponge). Beads and rocks carry less potential for colonization and do not require antibiotic prophylaxis.

Although most nasal foreign bodies are not immediately dangerous, button batteries require removal as quickly as possible to avoid mucosal burns and septal perforation. A small thin, strong magnetic rod or a small ring curette can rapidly extract a button battery. If removal cannot be

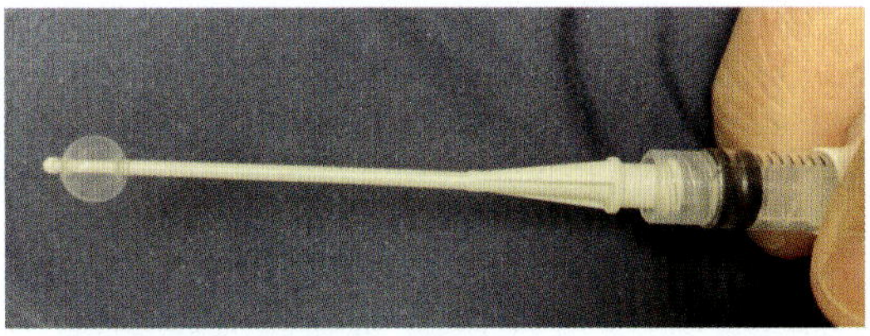

Figure 23.2: Katz extractor with balloon inflated.

achieved quickly in the ED setting, application of honey, carafate, or orange or apple juice to the site may help slow the rate of injury while waiting for the ENT to remove the battery.[3] Irrigation with acetic acid (0.25% or 3%) after removal can help limit evolving tissue damage.[4]

PHARYNGEAL FOREIGN BODIES

Occasionally, foreign bodies may become lodged in the pharyngeal soft tissues, including the tonsils, base of the tongue, vallecula, or the posterior oropharynx. Common objects identified in the posterior oropharynx include fish or other animal bones.

Approach and Management

In these patients, observe for stridor, respiratory distress, or cyanosis. History should include the composition of the foreign body, time of occurrence, and presence and evolution of symptoms.

If the foreign body cannot be identified on direct examination with a tongue depressor, flexible nasopharyngoscopy in the hands of a skilled provider may reveal the location of the object. If no foreign body is identified, and the patient is no longer symptomatic, the object may have spontaneously dislodged. In these cases, patients may be suitable for discharge without imaging, with strict follow-up precautions. However, if the object cannot be identified and the patient continues to have localized symptoms, imaging should be performed. Fishbone foreign bodies are best identified on noncontrast CT of the chest and neck. Other bones and metallic objects are more radiopaque than fishbones and may be identified on plain films alone.

If the foreign body can be adequately visualized in the oropharynx on bedside examination, removal may be attempted with forceps. The rate of complications (retropharyngeal abscess or hematoma, mediastinitis, or soft tissue migration of the foreign body) increases with retention of the foreign body greater than 24 hours.[5,6] In addition, consider the close proximity of the internal carotid artery to the posterior oropharynx in cases involving penetration with larger foreign bodies. These cases should be treated similarly to a stab wound of the neck, necessitating vascular imaging.

AIRWAY FOREIGN BODIES

Airway foreign bodies can occur at any age but are more common in young children and in patients with underlying oropharyngeal swallowing dysfunction. A child typically presents with a severe coughing/choking event, possibly with a color change, that may last for a minute or more before the event quiets down. Even though a child may appear stable at evaluation, these high-risk situations require a full airway evaluation to check for a foreign body. If an event was witnessed and the foreign body is a food likely to dissolve in a moist environment, observation may be appropriate in the stable or asymptomatic patient.

In patients with significant airway compromise, emergent stabilization of the airway is warranted. The Heimlich maneuver should be attempted on conscious patients. In unresponsive patients, laryngoscopy may demonstrate a foreign body in the proximal airway that may be removed with Magill forceps, but in pediatric patients, distal airway foreign bodies are more common.[7] If an obstructing foreign body is suspected but not visualized, and the patient cannot be successfully ventilated after confirmed endotracheal tube (ETT) placement, the provider may attempt to advance the ETT or a Bougie to force the object into the right mainstem bronchus, then pull the ETT back to an appropriate depth and attempt to ventilate the left lung.

When possible, a history should be obtained to determine whether the event was witnessed, the severity of the event, the type of presumed foreign body, when the event happened and current NPO status. PA and lateral X-rays (**Figure 23.3**) can be helpful, understanding that many foreign bodies are not radiopaque and also may not cause radiographically obvious air trapping. Normal

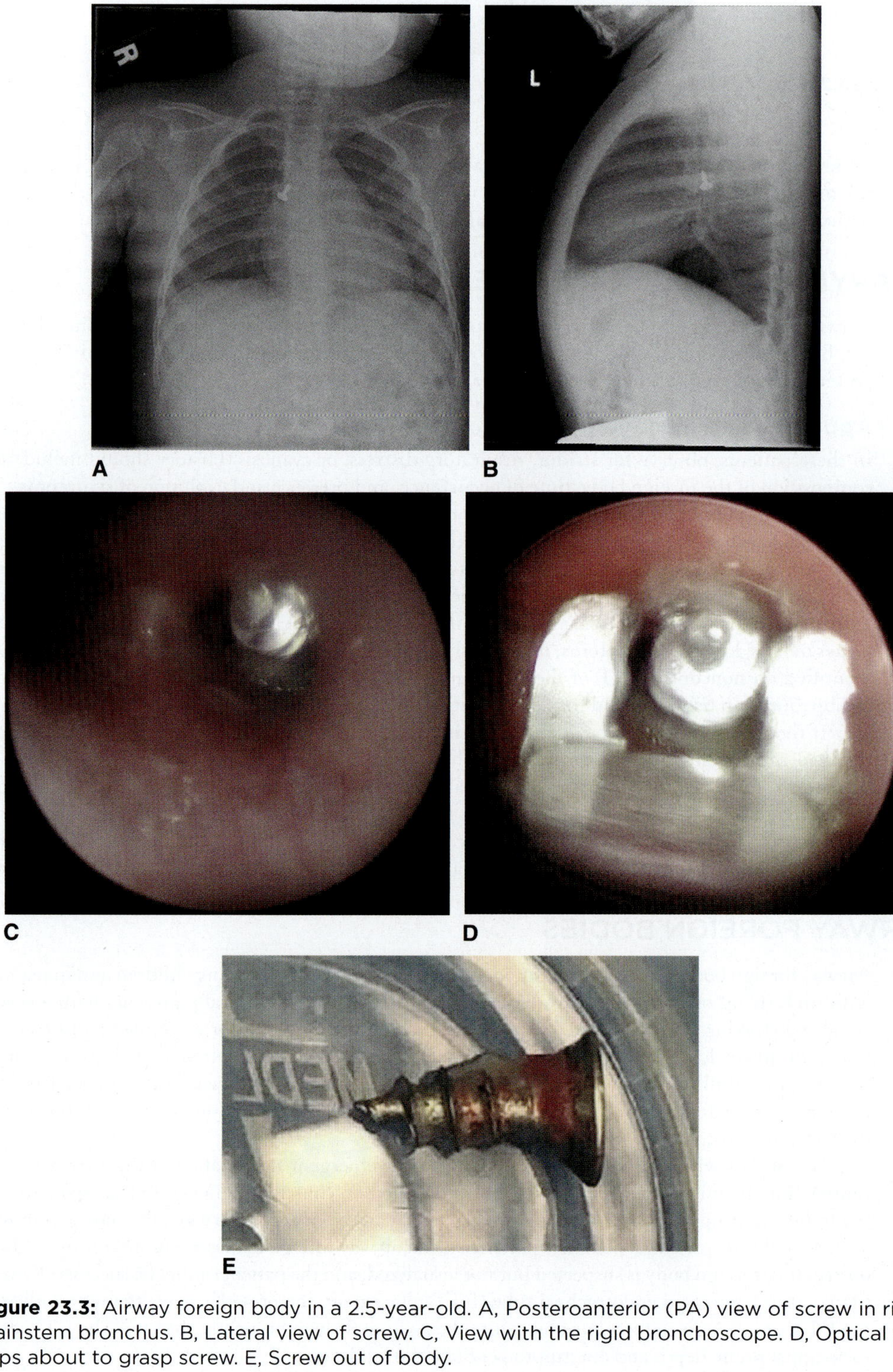

Figure 23.3: Airway foreign body in a 2.5-year-old. A, Posteroanterior (PA) view of screw in right mainstem bronchus. B, Lateral view of screw. C, View with the rigid bronchoscope. D, Optical forceps about to grasp screw. E, Screw out of body.

imaging findings should not dissuade the provider from maintaining a high index of suspicion and involving ENT early for a formal airway evaluation.

Although flexible laryngoscopy can be performed, it is typically not useful for laryngotracheal and bronchial foreign bodies, because the vocal cords are the limit for bedside evaluation (**Figure 23.4**). The gold standard management is rigid laryngoscopy and bronchoscopy in the operating room.

Considerations when planning the timing of transfer to the operating room can be complex. In a patient who is not NPO, there is risk of aspiration of stomach contents with induction of anesthesia, but, on the other hand, organic foreign bodies may swell in the moist environment of the airway, making removal more difficult with passing time. The ENT and anesthesia teams weigh the risks in the context of the patient's clinical picture to determine the safest course of action with respect to timing of the bronchoscopy.

ESOPHAGEAL FOREIGN BODIES

Children are more likely than adults to present with an esophageal foreign body, although there are some medical conditions in adults that may predispose them to food impaction (eg, eosinophilic esophagitis and achalasia).[8] The upper esophageal sphincter is at the cricopharyngeus muscle and is the first choke point for ingested objects. Once an object becomes wedged at or below this muscle, regurgitation is unlikely to resolve the impaction.

In situations concerning for radiopaque foreign body or potential perforation, proper evaluation consists of a careful history, examination, and a chest X-ray (posteroanterior [PA] and lateral). These patients should also be made NPO and have IV hydration initiated until a foreign body is either removed or ruled out. A normal chest X-ray cannot rule out a foreign body, because both food and plastic items are not radiopaque. In adults with a normal chest X-ray, a computed tomography (CT) scan can be a helpful adjunct to confirm and localize the presence of a nonfood foreign body prior to involving ENT or gastroenterology for removal.

The timing of endoscopy depends on several factors, but most objects do not require emergent removal. The important exception is a battery, where immediate removal is vital, as tissue damage can begin as early as 15 minutes after ingestion, with significant injury potential within 2 hours.[4] If the patient is over 12 months old and the ingestion happened fewer than 12 hours prior, swallowing honey or Carafate can mitigate tissue injury while awaiting definitive management.[3] Other indications for emergent endoscopy include complete obstruction, signs of perforation, or significant aspiration risk. In the event of a food bolus, there is some evidence to suggest the efficacy

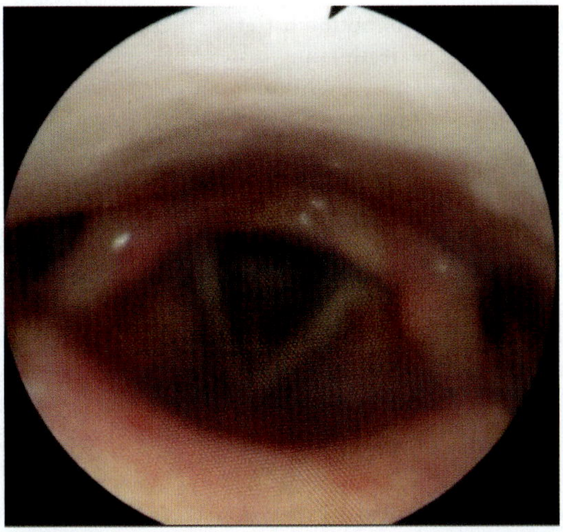

Figure 23.4: View of vocal cords via a bedside flexible fiberoptic laryngoscopy. Note that there are limits to the resolution of a flexible scope and that the vocal cords are the limit of this evaluation with limited, if any, view of the subglottis and more distal airway.

of ingestion of effervescent liquid (eg, soda) and minimal data to support the safety and use of other medications, including glucagon.

Pediatric Issues

Whereas adults and older children usually give a clear history of the food or item that is suspected to be impacted, younger children may present in a delayed fashion with little history. Young children often present with new onset of dysphagia or drooling, refusal to swallow, or new onset of gagging with swallowing. When history suggests a possible esophageal foreign body in a child, esophagoscopy should be considered even without localizing imaging given the risks of radiation and the potential need for sedation when imaging young children.

TIPS AND PEARLS

- It is common for children to have more than one foreign object in the nose. After an object is removed, visualization to the nasopharynx is performed to ensure all objects have been removed.
- In adults over 40, fishbone foreign bodies are more likely to be found in the esophagus rather than the oropharynx.[9]
- A battery lodged in the body is a true emergency. Application of honey or Carafate to the site may reduce tissue injury while preparing for removal.
- Plain films are not sufficient to rule out the presence of a foreign body.

EVIDENCE

Are antibiotics necessary after successful removal of a fishbone foreign body?

The evidence on this topic is quite limited, but case reports exist of retropharyngeal abscess and other infectious complications of fishbone foreign bodies.[5,6] In addition, foreign body impaction (predominantly fishbone) was listed as the most common etiology of retropharyngeal abscess in a large retrospective analysis performed in Spain.[10] Although this is low-quality evidence, it is reasonable to prescribe a short course of prophylactic antibiotics covering oropharyngeal flora after removal of a pharyngeal foreign body.

Are button batteries really that dangerous?

Despite awareness of the dangers of button batteries, these injuries continue to be common, with the incidence of serious injury or death rising instead of declining. Part of the reason for this increase is the popularization of 20 mm 3 V lithium button batteries, which are larger and stronger than the previous generations of button batteries. Contrary to widespread belief, pressure necrosis and leakage of battery contents are not major causes of injury. Rather, the generation of an electric current when the battery is in contact with moist tissues causes a liquefactive necrosis. Tissue in contact with the negative pole is at higher risk for severe damage.[11]

Over the past decade, multiple studies have sought best practices to limit damage from button battery ingestion. A sentinel article examining honey and Carafate as well as apple juice, orange juice, and other juices, found that Carafate and honey had superior efficacy in minimizing the tissue damage of the button battery.[3] However, honey is contraindicated in children under 12 months of age secondary to the risk of botulism. A second study found that a single irrigation of the affected mucosa with sterile acetic acid after battery removal helped reduce the resultant visible eschar.

References

1. Xiao CC, Kshirsagar RS, Rivero A. Pediatric foreign bodies of the ear: a 10-year national analysis. *Int J Pediatr Otorhinolaryngol*. 2020;138:110354.
2. Alfaifi AJ, Khan LA, Mokarbesh HM. Light-assisted removal of ear canal live insect—a noninvasive approach for first level responders. *J Family Med Prim Care*. 2019;8(9):3042-3044.

3. Anfang RR, Jatana KR, Linn RL, Rhoades K, Fry J, Jacobs IN. pH-neutralizing esophageal irrigations as a novel mitigation strategy for button battery injury. *Laryngoscope*. 2019;129(1):49-57.
4. Jatana KR, Rhoades K, Milkovich S, Jacobs IN. Basic mechanism of button battery ingestion injuries and novel mitigation strategies after diagnosis and removal. *Laryngoscope*. 2017;127(6):1276-1282.
5. Kim HU. Oroesophageal fish bone foreign body. *Clin Endosc*. 2016;49(4):318-326.
6. Singh B, Kantu M, Har-El G, Lucente FE. Complications associated with 327 foreign bodies of the pharynx, larynx, and esophagus. *Ann Otol Rhinol Laryngol*. 1997;106(4):301-304.
7. Oyama LC. Foreign bodies of the ear, nose and throat. *Emerg Med Clin North Am*. 2019;37(1):121-130.
8. Long B, Koyfman A, Gottlieb M. Esophageal foreign bodies and obstruction in the emergency department setting: an evidence-based review. *J Emerg Med*. 2019;56(5):499-511.
9. Klein A, Ovnat-Tamir S, Marom T, Gluck O, Rabinovics N, Shemesh S. Fish bone foreign body: the role of imaging. *Int Arch Otorhinolaryngol*. 2019;23(1):110-115.
10. Sanz Sanchez CI, Morales Angulo C. Retropharyngeal abscess. Clinical review of twenty-five years. *Acta Otorrinolaringol Esp (Engl Ed)*. 2021;72(2):71-79.
11. Ing RJ, Hoagland M, Mayes L, Twite M. The anesthetic management of button battery ingestion in children. *Can J Anaesth*. 2018;65(3):309-318.

CHAPTER 24

Anatomy of the Eye

Daniel S. Casper

ORBITAL AND OCULAR ANATOMY

Osteology

The eyes, or globes, are located in bilateral orbital cavities in the anterior, superior skull. These pear-shaped cavities have large anterior openings to permit vision and small apertures posteriorly for communication with the middle cranial fossae. The two bony orbits share three bones equally: the frontal, sphenoid, and ethmoid; four other paired bones—the maxillae, zygomas, lacrimal, and palatines—are duplicated and present individually on each side (**Figure 24.1**).

The boxy ethmoid sits behind the root of the nose, separating the orbits. Its thin, fragile lateral walls make up most of the medial orbital walls. The centrally located sphenoid bone traverses the skull and can be seen externally in each infratemporal fossa. It contains the sella turcica, which houses the pituitary gland. The sphenoid wings make up much of the lateral orbital walls, which are the interface between orbit and middle cranial fossa.

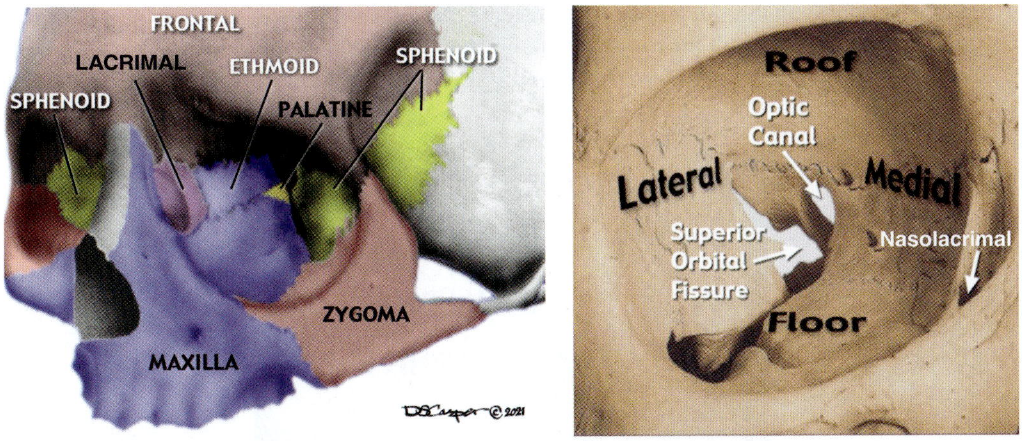

A B

Figure 24.1: A, Seven bones form each orbit, three of which are single bones that cross the midline, and the remaining four contribute separately to each orbit. (Illustration modified from Casper DS, Cioffi GA, eds. *The Columbia Guide to Basic Elements of Eye Care: A Manual for Healthcare Professionals*. Springer; 2019. Reproduced with permission from Springer International Publishing.) B, The orbit is described as having four walls, the superior and lateral being thicker, and the medial and inferior being thinner and more delicate. The medial optic canal and the more lateral superior orbital fissure both connect the orbit with the middle cranial fossa.

The orbits are arbitrarily divided into four walls that have no sharp boundaries. The roof is made up mostly of frontal bone, the medial walls are made of the lateral portion of the ethmoid; the floor is largely maxillary bone and overlies the maxillary sinus, and the lateral wall is mostly sphenoid sinus. The floor and medial walls are the thinnest and fracture more commonly with trauma. The lateral wall, recessed about a centimeter from the orbital opening, affords enhanced peripheral vision but also renders the lateral globe more susceptible to trauma owing to its greater exposure.

The posteriorly located apex houses the two major orbital portals to and from medial fossa. The optic canal carries the optic nerve, most of the orbital arterial supply via the ophthalmic artery, and sympathetic autonomic nerve fibers. Temporal to the optic canal is the superior orbital fissure, which carries all other neurovascular structures of importance, including cranial nerves III (oculomotor), IV (trochlear), V (the first trigeminal division, ophthalmic), and VI (abducens), as well as the superior ophthalmic vein and parasympathetic fibers.

Periorbital sinuses surround the orbits. The ethmoid sinus is located between the orbits; the sphenoid, posterior to the orbits; and the maxillary sinuses lie beneath the orbital floors. The paired frontal sinuses are located above the brows, medially, within the frontal bone (**Figure 24.2**).

The orbits are effectively enclosed spaces, with small posterior apical conveying structures to and from the middle cranial fossae, and anterior apertures (the palpebral fissures), from which the anterior globe protrudes slightly. A space-occupying lesion, such as an abscess, hemorrhage, or tumor located within the orbit will displace orbital structures, and the only outlet to accommodate such an increase in volume is the anterior opening. As orbital tissues are displaced, the eye is forced anteriorly, resulting in a bulging appearance known as proptosis, or exophthalmos (**Figure 24.3**).

Extraocular Muscles

Six extraocular muscles control movement and the position of each eye (**Figure 24.4**). The lateral and medial recti control horizontal movements; the superior and inferior recti primarily control vertical action; the superior and inferior oblique muscles bring about oblique (ie, nonvertical or horizontal) movements.

Horizontal muscles move the eye directly along the horizontal plane, left or right. The vertical recti, however, do not attach to the globe in the visual, anatomical plane, because the orbits deviate outward slightly from the medially located apices. Because of this off-axis alignment, muscle contraction does not simply elevate or depress the eye in the vertical axis; instead, there is a lateral component in addition to the main vertical direction. The oblique muscles similarly attach to the globes of the primary axis. Thus, the vertical recti and obliques must work together to move the eye directly up or down.

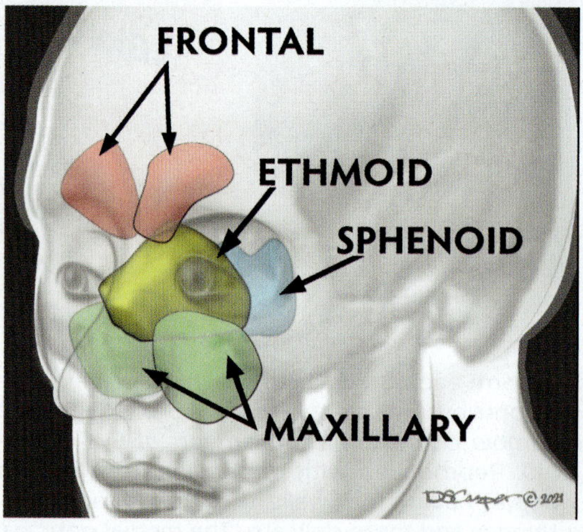

Figure 24.2: Sinuses almost entirely surround the orbits, with frontal above, maxillary below, ethmoid in between, and sphenoid posterior and inferior. (Illustration modified from Casper DS, Cioffi GA, eds. *The Columbia Guide to Basic Elements of Eye Care: A Manual for Healthcare Professionals*. Springer; 2019. Reproduced with permission from Springer International Publishing.)

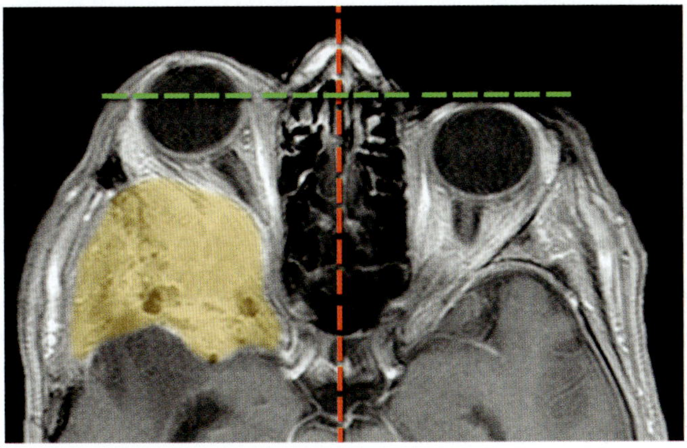

Figure 24.3: Because the orbits are essentially closed posteriorly, space-occupying lesions usually force the eye outward, called proptosis or exophthalmos, as seen in this case of a sphenoid wing meningioma (the tumor has been highlighted in color). A line drawn perpendicular to the anatomic axis across the cornea on the normal side shows the degree of ocular displacement. (Courtesy of Michael Kazim, MD.)

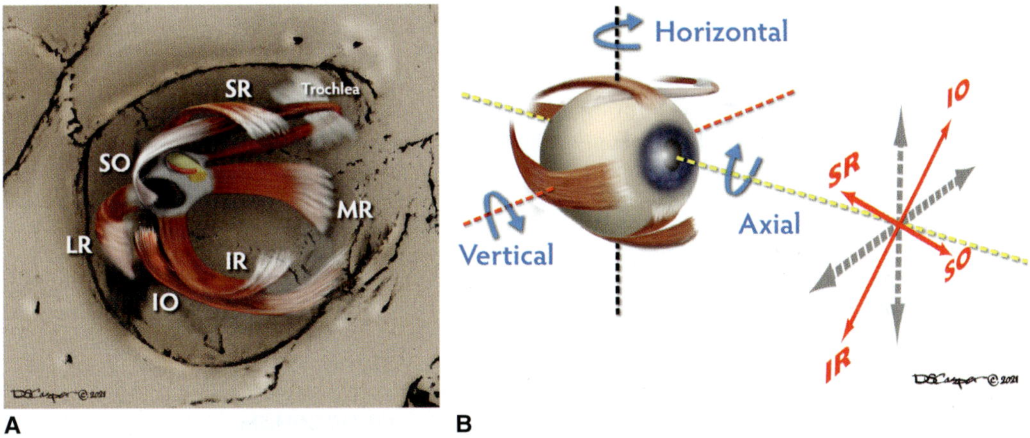

Figure 24.4: A, Six extraocular muscles control movements of the eyes; all originate from the Annulus of Zinn at the apex, except the inferior oblique, which originates from the orbital floor anteriorly. B, Because the superior and inferior rectus muscles are not aligned with the anteroposterior plane, they do not rotate the eye perfectly upward or downward. In order to elevate or depress the eye in the vertical plane, a combined action is required with the oblique muscles. IO, inferior oblique; IR, inferior rectus; LR, lateral rectus; MR, medial rectus; SO, superior oblique; SR, superior rectus. (B, modified from Casper DS, Cioffi GA, eds. *The Columbia Guide to Basic Elements of Eye Care: A Manual for Healthcare Professionals*. Springer; 2019. Reproduced with permission from Springer International Publishing.)

The superior oblique, unlike the other extraocular muscles, does not attach directly to the globe but instead travels through a fascial sling, the trochlea, in the superior medial orbit; the tendonous terminal portion reverses direction to attach to the posterior, superior globe. The inferior oblique, which originates from the orbital floor, follows the same course as the superior oblique tendon and attaches to the posterior, inferior globe. Oblique muscle action is counterintuitive: the superior deviates the eye *downward* and medially, and the inferior deviates the eye *upward* and medially. The consequence of this anatomic configuration is that vertical, upward (90°) eye movement requires the combined action of the superior rectus and inferior oblique and that the inferior rectus and superior oblique move the eye in a straight downward direction.

Innervation

Sensory visual data processed by the retina is transmitted to the brain via cranial nerve II, the optic nerve. This nerve can be visualized with ophthalmoscopy at its origin as the optic disk in the posterior pole of the eye. After exiting the eye, it follows a sinuous course (which allows for free movement of the eye within the orbit) toward the apex of the orbit, where it enters the medially located optic canal and is conveyed into the middle cranial fossa, anterior to the pituitary gland. The right and left optic nerves comingle to form the optic chiasm. Postchiasmal optic tracts, comprised of combined fibers from both eyes, carry information derived from the contralateral visual hemifields to the lateral geniculate nuclei in the thalamus. From there, optic radiations proceed posteriorly to the occipital lobes, where visual perception occurs (**Figure 24.5**).

All other sensory innervation is supplied by cranial nerve V, the trigeminal nerve. The first division of the trigeminal (V_1), the ophthalmic nerve, provides sensory fibers to the forehead, nose, upper lid, lacrimal gland, and the globe. The second division of the nerve (V_2) provides sensation primarily to the lower lid and cheek. As this nerve (the maxillary nerve) travels within the thin orbital floor, it is subject to entrapment or direct injury from floor fractures.

Motor innervation is provided by cranial nerves III, IV, VI, and VII. Cranial nerve III, the oculomotor nerve, supplies all extraocular muscles except the superior oblique and lateral rectus, which are innervated by cranial nerves IV, the trochlear, and VI, the abducens, respectively. These nerves all pass through the superior orbital fissure to enter the orbit posteriorly (**Figure 24.6**). Cranial nerve VII, the facial nerve, innervates the muscles of the eyelids and upper face through its temporal and zygomatic branches.

Orbital autonomic nerve fibers control pupillary muscular action, innervate sympathetic fibers located in the lids, and play a role in the regulation of the lacrimal tear glands.

Vascular System

The common carotid arteries divide in the neck into external and internal carotids, both of which contribute to the circulatory supply of the globe and its surrounding structures. The external remains superficial, continuing upward anterior to the ear, giving off the facial artery, which anastomoses with orbital arteries. The maxillary artery runs through the cheek to exit at the inferior orbital fissure. The

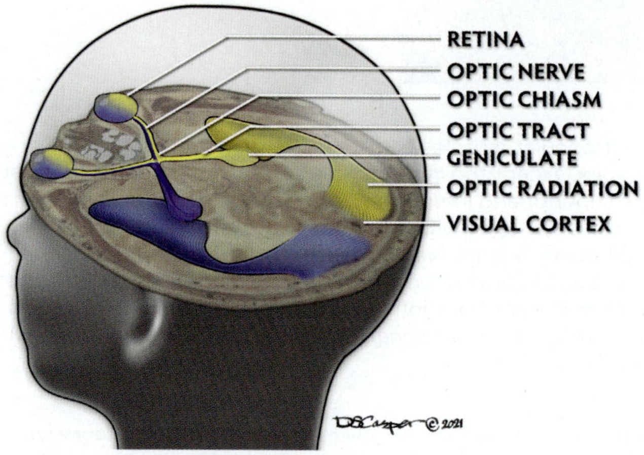

Figure 24.5: A schematic view of the visual pathway from object to the visual cortex. Image projections are separated along the retinal vertical medians and travel together. Combined nasal and temporal nerve fibers enter the middle cranial fossa as the optic nerves but segregate into separate temporal and nasal retinal fibers at the optic chiasm. Segregated right and left information continues in the optic tracts, is further processed in the lateral geniculate nuclei and reaches the posterior visual cortex via the optic radiations. (Illustration modified from Casper DS, Cioffi GA, eds. *The Columbia Guide to Basic Elements of Eye Care: A Manual for Healthcare Professionals*. Springer; 2019. Reproduced with permission from Springer International Publishing.)

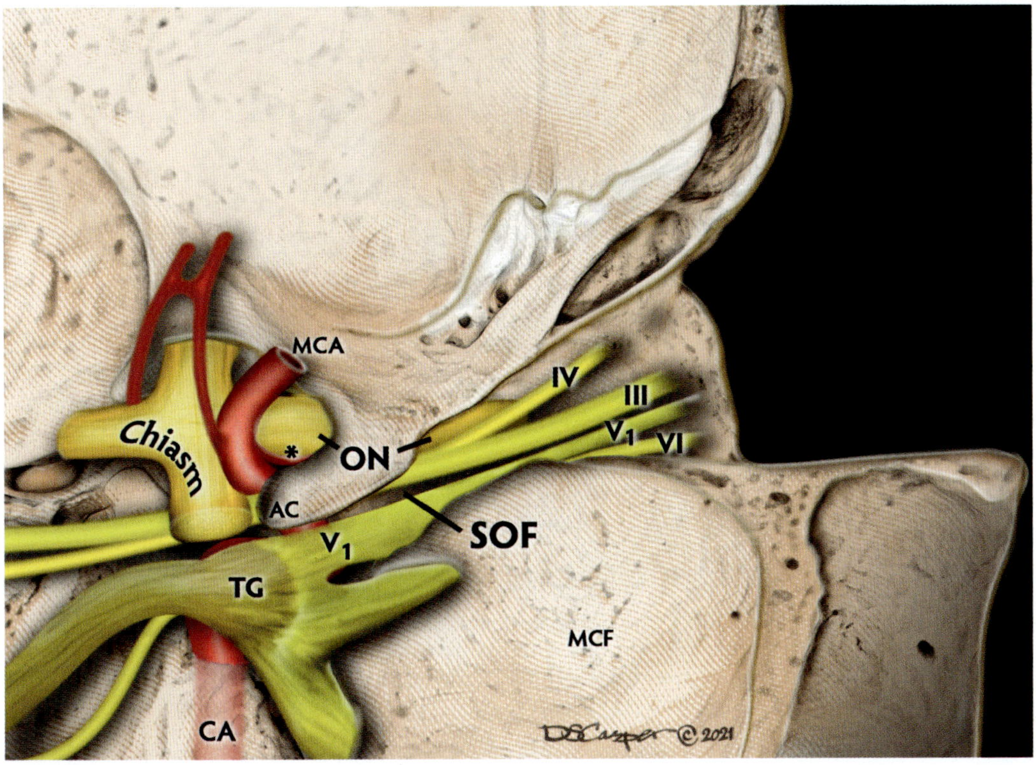

Figure 24.6: Cranial nerves. The skull is viewed from the right, posteriorly; the top of the cranium and the superior temporal quadrant of the right orbit and the globe have been removed. Cranial nerve II passes through the optic canal, and nerves III, IV, V_1, and VI pass through the superior orbital fissure to enter the orbit (anatomic details in the orbit are not shown). AC, anterior clinoid; CA, carotid artery; MCF, middle cranial fossa; ON, optic nerve; SOF, superior orbital fissure; TG, trigeminal ganglion; V_1, ophthalmic nerve; * indicates the ophthalmic artery entering the optic canal beneath the optic nerve. (Illustration modified from Casper DS, Cioffi GA, eds. *The Columbia Guide to Basic Elements of Eye Care: A Manual for Healthcare Professionals*. Springer; 2019. Reproduced with permission from Springer International Publishing.)

external carotid terminates as the superficial temporal artery, which is a common source for biopsy to diagnose giant cell arteritis (temporal arteritis), a potentially blinding condition.

The internal carotid enters the skull and divides into terminal branches in the middle cranial fossa adjacent to the sella turcica. The ophthalmic artery, the main source of arterial blood to the orbit and eye, is a relatively small carotid branch that enters the posterior optic canal beneath the optic nerve. Numerous intraorbital branches are given off, including the central retinal artery, which enters the optic nerve and can be seen with ophthalmoscopy at the optic disk. Smaller branches extend to the extraocular muscles, lacrimal gland, lids, and as ciliary branches to the globe. Terminal branches enter the medial wall and supply superficial tissues of the cheek and forehead as the supraorbital, supratrochlear, and infraorbital vessels and anastomose with external carotid branches (**Figure 24.7**).

Apex and Cavernous Sinus

The orbital apices serve as conduits for all major neurovascular structures that connect orbit and middle cranial fossa. Posterior to the apices, located in the middle cranial fossae, are the bilateral cavernous sinuses, formed by a cleft in the dura, and located on either side of the body of the sphenoid bone. Most orbital neurovascular structures, excepting the optic nerves, pass through these venous sinuses, which also contain the carotid arteries.

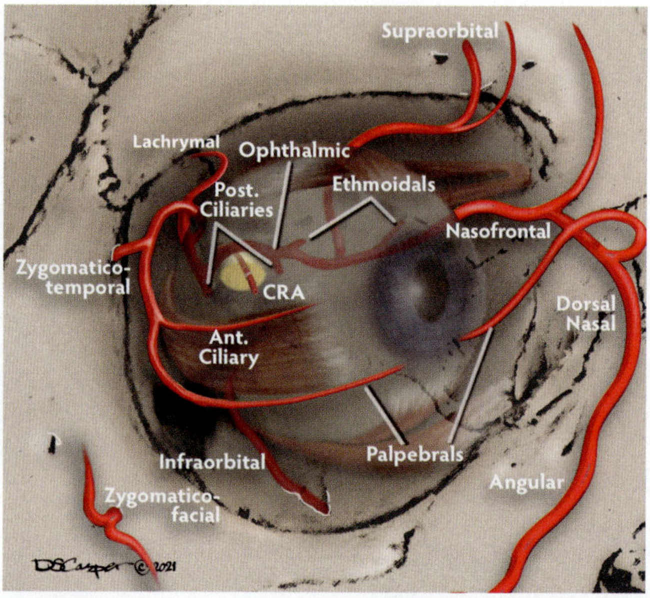

Figure 24.7: Orbital arterial supply. The ophthalmic artery is the main supplier of arterial blood to the eye and orbit; anastomotic connections with extraorbital vascular channels also supplement the orbital circulation. Some of the major orbital branches are schematically shown here. CRA, central retinal artery.

Eyelids

The movable lids regulate palpebral fissure size and protect the underlying eye. The eyelids join nasally at the medial canthus and temporally at the lateral canthus. The normal fissure size, in the adult, is usually about 30 mm wide by 10 mm high.

Deep to the skin layer is the orbicularis muscle, which enables lid closure. Beneath the orbicularis is a fascial sheet, the orbital septum, which originates off the periosteum of the skull at the orbital rim, and acts like a diaphragmatic layer that partitions the orbit into pre- and postseptal compartments. Preseptal pathology is usually more easily treated and less vision-threatening than deeper, postseptal disease (**Figure 24.8**).

The tarsal plates are cartilaginous "skeletons" of the lids and contain vertically arranged Meibomian glands, which open along the lid margins and produce the lipid component in basal tears. Anterior to the tarsi, also along the margin, are the lashes, which filter out debris. In addition to being more mobile than the lower lid, the upper lid is approximately three times as high at the midpoint. The inner surface of the lids is lined with conjunctiva (the palpebral portion), a transparent membrane that reflects back (the bulbar portion) at the upper and lower fornices to blend into the globe at the sclerocorneal border, known as the limbus.

Retractor muscles, the antagonists of the orbicularis, open the lids. Upper lid retractor musculature is anatomically more complex than that in the lower lid. The levator system raises the upper lid approximately 15 mm; for additional opening (or if the normal retractor system is impaired), brow musculature (the frontalis) can further elevate the lid about 2 mm. Sympathetically innervated fibers are also found in the lids and have a role in lid position abnormalities in conditions such as Horner syndrome and Graves' disease.

The lids, anchored at the canthi, are constructed like a hammock and maintain a vertical position by balance of normal external and internal forces. The equilibrium of skin, muscle, septum, and conjunctival forces keeps the lids positioned properly against the globe; should there be a disturbance in this balance, either an inward (entropion) or an outward (ectropion) lid turn results.

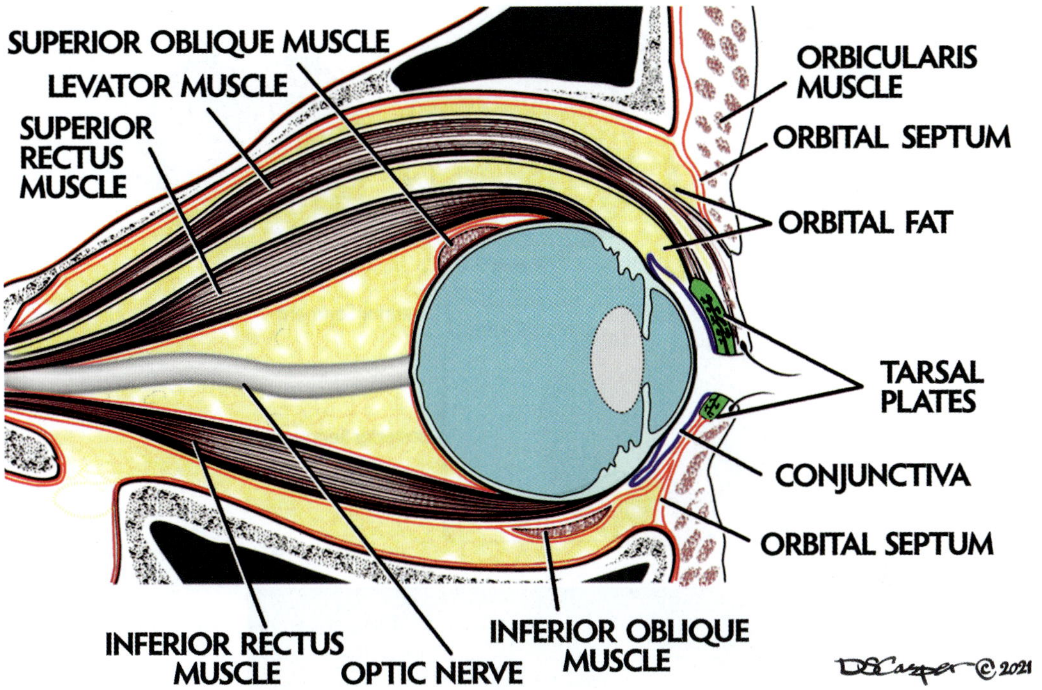

Figure 24.8: A sagittal section through midorbit showing lids and periorbital structures. The diaphragm like orbital septum defines pre- and postseptal compartments. The tarsal plates, and the protractor (orbicularis) and retractor (primarily levator) muscles are shown. (Illustration modified from Casper DS, Cioffi GA, eds. *The Columbia Guide to Basic Elements of Eye Care: A Manual for Healthcare Professionals*. Springer; 2019. Reproduced with permission from Springer International Publishing.)

Lacrimal System

The lacrimal system provides constant lubrication to the cornea and conjunctiva. It is comprised of two separate arms that provide an ocular "tear film." The basal component is produced by glands within the conjunctiva, lids, and the bilobed lacrimal gland, located subconjunctivally in the superolateral orbit. This trilaminar fluid consists of lipid, aqueous, and mucin layers, supplemented with electrolytes, enzymes, antibodies, and immunoglobulins. A separate system produces reflex tears, which, as the name implies, are made as a result of insult (dry eye, foreign body, wind, heat, etc.) or emotional episodes (with associated crying) and are comprised of aqueous fluid made by the lacrimal gland.

The lacrimal system also includes a drainage component. Tears enter the punctae, openings located in the medial upper and lower lids, which lead into canaliculi and are conveyed to the nasolacrimal sac and duct and down the nasolacrimal canal. Ultimately, excess tears enter the nasal cavity beneath the inferior turbinate and drain via the pharynx.

The Globe

The eye wall can be conceptualized as a trilaminar structure. The outermost layer is the opaque sclera, which is contiguous anteriorly with the clear cornea. This tunic is formed primarily of collagen fibers, and it is their architectural arrangement that determines transparency. The sclerocorneal tunic acts as the skeleton of the eye, providing structural support to the globe's spheroid shape. The cornea has a smaller radius than the overall globe, so its smaller curvature bulges out slightly at the front of the eye (**Figure 24.9**).

The innermost layer of the globe is the photosensitive retina, which receives light information focused at the posterior pole of the eye. The multilayered retina processes and refines image signals before they depart via the optic nerve.

Sandwiched between the outer and inner layers is the uvea, the vascular tunic of the eye. The uvea has three contiguous components: the anteriorly placed iris, visible through the cornea;

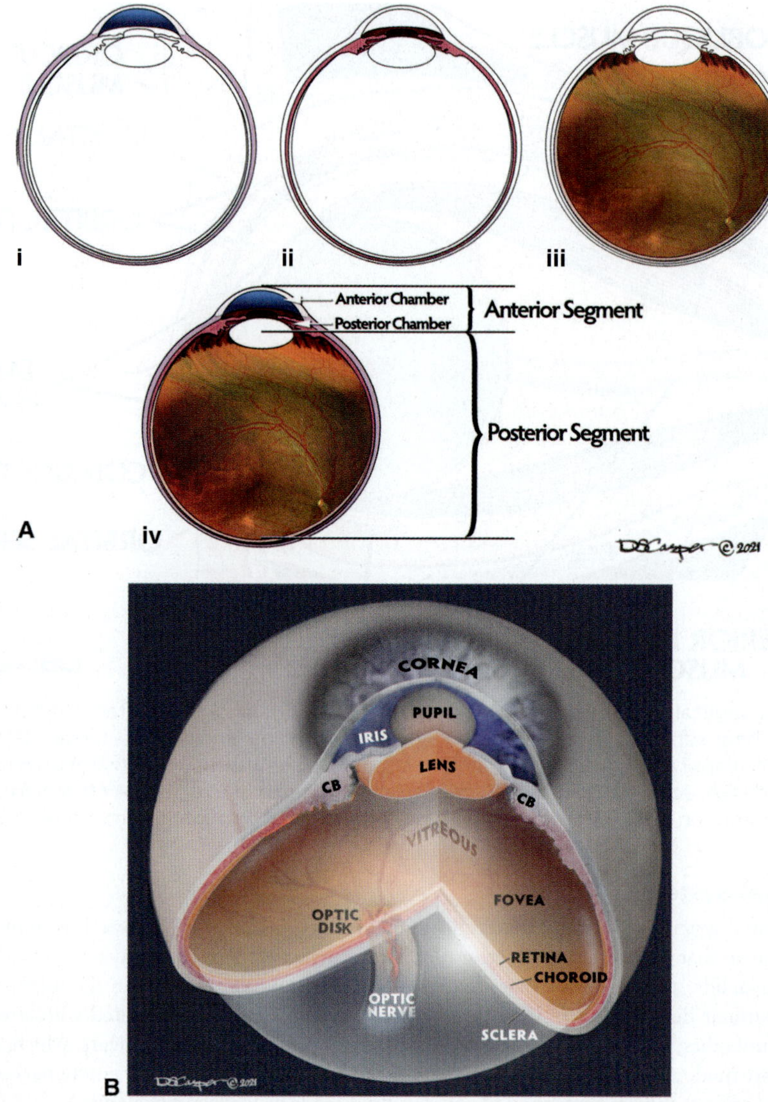

Figure 24.9: A, The globe has three main layers, or tunics: (i) the outer sclerocorneal tunic; (ii) the middle, vascular uvea; (iii) and the innermost retina, the photosensitive layer of the eye; (iv) the anterior (containing anterior and posterior chambers) and posterior segments of the globe. B, A representation of the major structures of the globe. CB, ciliary body. (Illustration modified from Casper DS, Cioffi GA, eds. *The Columbia Guide to Basic Elements of Eye Care: A Manual for Healthcare Professionals*. Springer; 2019. Reproduced with permission from Springer International Publishing.)

posterior to the iris is the ciliary body; and behind the ciliary body, beneath the retina, is the choroid. The uvea's primary function is ocular nourishment, although these structures also have secondary functions (the iris's central opening is the mobile pupillary aperture; the ciliary body produces aqueous fluid and contains muscles that control the intraocular lens shape; the choroid controls thermoregulation and may participate in image focusing).

The front portion of the eye is the anterior segment (**Figures** 24.9 and **24.10**). This consists of the clear cornea, the main focusing element of the eye, which fuses with the sclera and overlying conjunctiva at the limbus. Beneath the cornea is the anterior chamber, which is defined anteriorly by the inner (endothelial) surface of the cornea and posteriorly by the anterior iris surface. The anterior chamber is filled with aqueous fluid produced by the ciliary body, located posterior to the iris root. Behind the iris is the crystalline lens, which attaches to the ciliary body by thin zonular

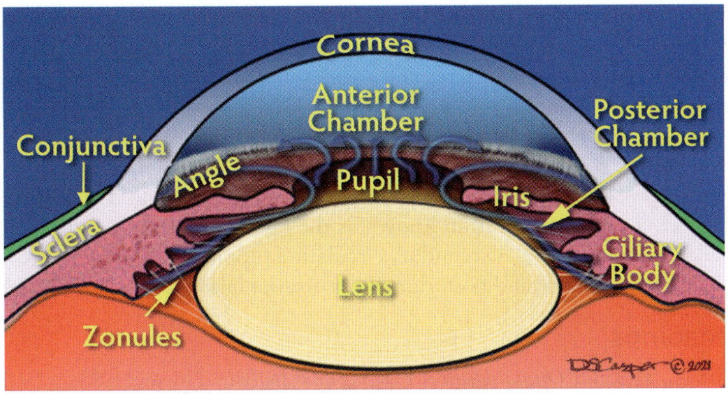

Figure 24.10: The anterior segment, consisting of the cornea, anterior chamber, iris, posterior chamber, and lens. The opaque sclera, confluent with the clear cornea at the limbus, overlies the ciliary body, which controls lens shape via zonular fibers. Aqueous fluid (dark blue arrows) also produced by the ciliary body, drains via the angle. (Illustration modified from Casper DS, Cioffi GA, eds. *The Columbia Guide to Basic Elements of Eye Care: A Manual for Healthcare Professionals*. Springer; 2019. Reproduced with permission from Springer International Publishing.)

fibers; changes in ciliary muscle fiber tension result in lens shape alterations, which enable focusing of near objects (part of the process known as accommodation).

Aqueous fluid, produced continuously by the ciliary body, flows forward over the anterior lens, through the pupil, and into the anterior chamber. Prior to entering the anterior chamber, aqueous passes through a small recess behind the iris, anterior to the zonular fibers and ciliary processes, which is the posterior chamber. After traversing the pupillary aperture, aqueous flows peripherally toward the iris-scleral junction, known as the chamber angle; this area houses the sievelike trabecular meshwork, through which aqueous fluid exits the globe before entering the venous system.

The anterior and posterior chambers together form the anterior segment. The remaining portion of the eye is known as the posterior segment, comprised of sclera, underlying choroid and retina, and the optic nerve (**Figure 24.11**). Within the posterior segment, the globe is filled with vitreous, a clear and gelatinous substance, encased within a clear membrane.

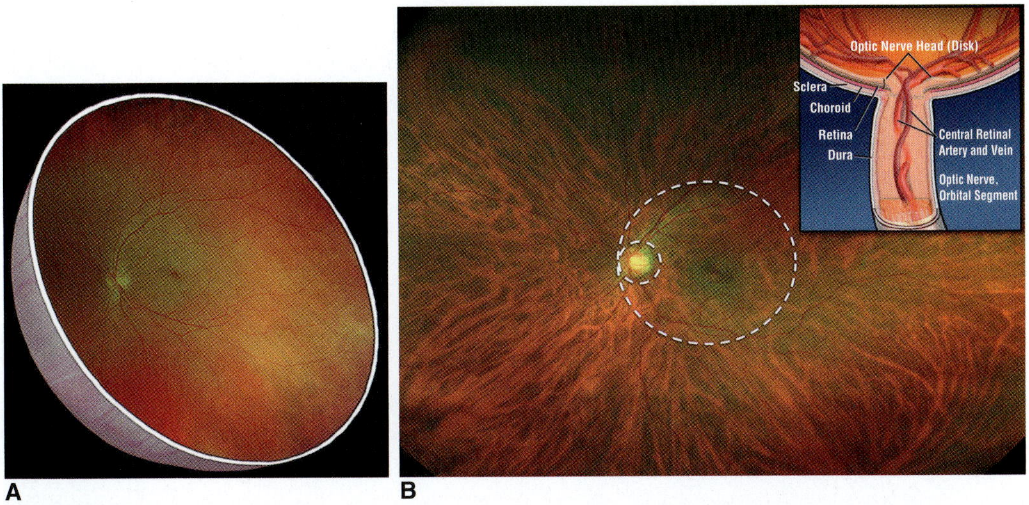

Figure 24.11: A, An illustration of the posterior half of a sectioned eye showing how the retina follows the curvature of the globe. B, A wide-field fundus image shows how the retina appears "flattened" in a two-dimensional image. The large white dashed circle outlines the posterior pole, including the optic disc (smaller dashed circle) and the macula. The fovea is in the central macula. An illustration showing the structure of the optic nerve in cross section (inset).

The central retinal artery, the first branch of the ophthalmic artery, enters the globe by traveling within the optic nerve and splits into four main branches at the disk: two large temporal arcades and two smaller nasal arcades. The temporal arcades surround and define the central retina, known as the macula, where, owing to the high density of cone photoreceptor cells, the eye has its most acute vision and color perception. The retina peripheral to the macular region has predominantly rod photoreceptor cells, which have less distinct acuity, and monochromatic vision predominates.

The optic nerve head, or disk, can be viewed at the posterior pole. The nerve is circular or oval in shape and has a central depression known as the optic cup, through which the central retinal vessels enter and exit the globe. A secondary circulation supplies the photoreceptors via the choroid, which is made up of anterior and posterior ciliary arteries (also branches of the ophthalmic artery).

Suggested Readings

Casper D, Chi L, Trokel S. *Orbital Disease: Imaging and Analysis*. Thieme; 1993.

Casper DS and Cioffi GA, eds. *The Columbia Guide to Basic Elements of Eye Care: A Manual for Healthcare Professionals*. Springer; 2019.

Dutton JJ. *Atlas of Clinical and Surgical Orbital Anatomy*. Saunders; 1994.

Doxanas M, Anderson R. *Clinical Orbital Anatomy*. Williams & Wilkins; 1984.

Oyster C. *The Human Eye: Structure and Function*. Sinauer Associates; 1999.

Warwick R. *Wolff's Anatomy of the Eye and Orbit*. Saunders; 1976.

CHAPTER 25

Evaluation of Ocular Emergencies

David J. Harris, III
Bradley D. Gordon

THE CLINICAL CHALLENGE

A significant percentage of patients who present to emergency departments (EDs) or urgent care centers seek care for an eye complaint.[1,2] Although complete evaluation of the eye may require an ophthalmologist's in-depth knowledge of ophthalmic disease and familiarity with specialized ophthalmologic equipment, on-site ophthalmology consultation is not always available. Knowledge of the ophthalmologic examination and key components of a relevant history allow the ED or urgent care provider to diagnose and manage some conditions and to determine whether patients require immediate or nonurgent ophthalmologic consultation. This chapter will review the steps and skills necessary to evaluate a patient presenting with ocular symptoms.

Patient History

As is the case in the medical evaluation of any patient, obtaining a history is an important step in the evaluation of the eye. Questions should be directed in much the same fashion as when evaluating non-eye-related patient complaints, albeit with a focus on the chief complaint and its relation to the vision system.

Chief Complaint

Eye complaints generally fall into three groups: visual disturbance, eye pain, and change in the appearance of the eye. Visual disturbances involve either difficulty seeing what is there (blurred vision, foggy vision, dim vision, wavy vision, blind spots, double vision, or total loss of vision) or seeing things that are not there (flashing lights, shimmering lights, floaters, scintillating scotomata, or formed hallucinations).

Eye pain may be characterized as foreign-body sensation, burning, aching, photophobia, or periorbital pain. Patient-reported changes in the appearance of the eye may include redness of the eye or periocular structures, discharge from the eye, white spots on the eye, unequal pupils, bulging of the eye, droopy or retracted eyelids, and swelling or discoloration of the tissues around the eye.

History of Present Illness

After establishing the chief complaint, further details surrounding the presenting symptoms should be obtained. The causative factor for an eye complaint may be obvious, as in the case of recent mechanical or chemical injury. When an eye injury is reported, ask when the injury occurred and by what mechanism. Ask if the patient was wearing protective glasses. The clinician should also be aware of patient activities such as grinding or hammering metal objects, mowing the grass, or using a line-trimmer that can produce small high-velocity projectiles. These objects can result in a penetrating eye injury that is easily missed on examination. The resultant retained intraocular foreign object, if untreated, puts the eye at markedly increased risk for endophthalmitis and profound vision loss.

The quality, duration, severity, location, associated symptoms, and any alleviating or exacerbating factors should be noted. Ask the patient if they have had recent eye surgery or have ever experienced similar symptoms in the past. Sometimes, a patient will give misleading information about causation, reinforcing the importance of a careful organized history. Examples include the contact lens wearer who reports having scratched their eye because they are experiencing foreign-body sensation, when in reality the problem is a bacterial ulcer, or the postoperative cataract patient who reports pain and vision loss after bumping their eye, when the real cause is postoperative endophthalmitis.

Medications and Allergies

Ask the patient about all the medications they use and if they have any allergies to medications. This includes eye drops and homeopathic medications. It is important to note whether any medications have been recently started. Many systemic medications, including antihistamines, anticholinergics, cholinergics, adrenergics, antiepileptics, glucocorticoids, antibiotics, and antirheumatics can result in acute or chronic ocular side effects.

Past Ocular History

Ask the patient if they have established care with an ophthalmologist or optometrist. Ask if they wear eyeglasses or contact lenses, have been diagnosed with any eye diseases, have had eye surgery, or have a history of significant eye injury.

Nonocular History

Obtain a history of the patient's medical problems and past surgeries. It is common for systemic medical conditions to have secondary eye findings. Examples include diabetes (diabetic retinopathy), hypertension (hypertensive retinopathy), rheumatoid arthritis (dry eye, peripheral ulcerative keratitis), cancer (choroidal metastasis), idiopathic intracranial hypertension (papilledema), and autoimmune disease (uveitis).

Gather the patient's general family history, but also ask the patient specifically whether any eye diseases are prevalent in their family. Glaucoma, congenital cataract, retinal detachment, and numerous retinal and corneal dystrophies run in families.

The social and occupational history may reveal important information concerning risk of eye injury and exposure to caustic compounds. Tobacco, alcohol, and illicit drug use should also be documented. Intravenous drug abuse can produce endocarditis, with endophthalmitis secondary to septic emboli as the initial clinical manifestation. Crack cocaine use can result in corneal perforation from chronic denervation. Prescribed and illicit opioids are known to produce pupillary abnormalities.

A focused review of systems should always be completed, because it may produce important information that can lead the clinician to the correct diagnosis. For example, many patients with acute angle closure glaucoma complain of headache, nausea, and vomiting in addition to their primary complaints of unilateral eye pain and decreased vision.

EXAMINATION OF THE EYE

Visual Acuity

A patient's presenting visual acuity is the most important part of the eye exam diagnostically, prognostically, and medicolegally. Visual acuity should be assessed for each eye individually by having the patient or an assistant cover the eye not being tested. Vision is best assessed using a Snellen chart or a near acuity card. Having the patient wear their own glasses, contacts, or readers for the assessment of visual acuity is preferred. Either the examiner or the patient can hold the near acuity card. If a Snellen chart or near acuity card is not available, the clinician can still assess the patient's vision by having them read print in a magazine or a book or on a smartphone application. It is important to document how the visual acuity was measured and to adhere to the distance calibration for the eye chart or card used.

If the patient is unable to read any print, the examiner should then assess whether the patient can count fingers and record at what distance they are able to do so. For example, the patient may be able to count fingers held 2 feet from their face, in which case the visual acuity should be recorded as "count fingers (CF) at 2 feet." If the patient is unable to count fingers, the clinician should note whether the patient can see hand movements, and, if so, the visual acuity should be recorded as "hand movements (HM)." If the patient cannot perceive hand movements with a given eye, the eye should be tested for the ability to perceive light; if they can, visual acuity is recorded as "light perception (LP)." For an eye unable to see any light, record "no light perception (NLP)." The fellow eye should be covered to make sure the unaffected eye is not seeing the test image.

It should be noted that light perception vision can sometimes be determined with a bright light even when a patient is unable or unwilling to open the eye. An aversive maneuver by an uncooperative or noncommunicative patient to avoid a bright light shone on an eye may be good evidence of light perception. Pupillary reaction alone is not adequate evidence of light perception.

External Eye Examination

The external examination refers to the part of the eye examination that a clinician can do in room light or with a flashlight. First, the examiner should assess the patient's face with attention directed to the periocular areas. A general assessment of whether there is facial paralysis, head injury, or other abnormality should be documented. The skin surrounding the eyes and the eyelids should be evaluated for lesions, rashes, lacerations, edema, erythema, and bony malformations. When the patient reports foreign body sensation, the upper and lower eyelids should be everted and inspected for foreign objects. Special attention should be given to any lacerations near the medial canthus because there is a higher probability of canalicular lacerations. The presence of preauricular or cervical adenopathy should be noted when assessing for infections. Ocular signs such as conjunctival redness, corneal haze, layered blood (hyphema), or layered pus (hypopyon) in the anterior chamber can be seen on external exam and should be recorded. These findings should then be further investigated with a slit-lamp microscope.

Ocular Motility

The best way to evaluate eye movement is to hold the patient's head still with one hand and ask the patient to track a light or other object as it is moved through the cardinal fields of gaze. Any eye movement limitations or restrictions should be noted.

If diplopia is part of the patient's complaint, a critical job of the examiner is to determine whether the diplopia is monocular or binocular. Simply stated, if the diplopia goes away when either eye is occluded, the diplopia is binocular, and the differential diagnosis includes disorders of eye movement. If the diplopia persists after occlusion of one eye, the diplopia is monocular, and the diagnostic possibilities shift to refractive, corneal, and lens abnormalities, most of which are not eye emergencies.

Visual Fields

A confrontation visual field exam should be completed for each eye to assess the patient's peripheral vision. The examiner tests the patient's right visual field by facing the patient at a distance of 20 inches. The examiner closes their right eye and covers the patient's left eye so that the patient's right eye is looking at the examiner's left eye. The examiner then holds up a given number of fingers in the right superior, right inferior, left superior, and left inferior quadrants, taking care to ensure that the hand is equidistant from the examiner's left eye and the patient's right eye. The patient is asked how many fingers they see at each point, while the examiner assures that the patient is staring straight ahead. If the examiner can distinguish the fingers at any point in the visual field, the patient should be able to also, and inability to do so may suggest a scotoma. The visual field of the patient's left eye is then evaluated analogously.

Pupils

Assessment of the pupils can be performed with any handheld light source in a dimly lit room. The right and left pupils should be assessed for size in millimeters, shape (round or irregular), and reactivity to light (brisk, sluggish, nonreactive). In the setting of a reported eye injury, an irregular shaped or peaked pupil should raise suspicion of a penetrating globe injury. Anisocoria is evaluated by measuring any difference in the pupils' sizes in room light and again in dim light. The swinging flashlight test can be performed to determine whether a relative afferent pupillary defect (RAPD), also known as a Marcus-Gunn pupil, is present. The details of the swinging flashlight test can be found in Chapter 48.

In room light, pupils are normally black in color. If they appear white (leukocoria), the most common cause is a mature, end-stage cataract, but other causes are possible. If the pupils are examined while looking through a direct ophthalmoscope, an orange color reflecting from the choroid and retina is normally seen. If there are dark obstructions to this "red reflex," media opacities such as corneal scars, cataracts, or vitreous hemorrhage are possible etiologies. If the reflex is white, retinal scars or an intraocular tumor such as retinoblastoma may be present.

Intraocular Pressure

The intraocular pressure (IOP) in a normal eye is between 10 and 21 mm Hg. In an ED or urgent care setting, this is usually measured with a Tono-Pen® or iCare® tonometer. The use of these devices is relatively straightforward, but they do require proper operation, which is detailed in their respective owner's manuals. It is important to note that use of the Tono-Pen® requires prior application of a topical anesthetic drop, such as tetracaine or proparacaine. If IOP measuring equipment is unavailable, the clinician can gently palpate over the patient's closed upper eyelid of each eye to assess for any significant differences in firmness between the eyes. If there is any possibility of a ruptured globe, do not attempt to palpate over the eye.

Slit-Lamp Biomicroscopy

Examination of the conjunctiva, cornea, anterior chamber, iris, and lens is best performed using a slit-lamp microscope (**Figure 25.1**).

The cornea is clear, highly innervated, and covered by a thin epithelium. Staining the cornea with fluorescein highlights any defect in the corneal epithelium, including those caused by abrasions, bacterial ulcers, and herpes simplex keratitis. Fluorescein staining can be performed by moistening a fluorescein impregnated strip with water, saline, or topical anesthetic and then gently tapping it on the inner side of the everted lower eyelid. The cornea is then viewed with a blue light source. If there is an epithelial defect, the affected area will appear fluorescent yellow. This test does not require the slit-lamp microscope as long as there is a blue light source such as a Woods lamp or a blue light filter on an ophthalmoscope.

If there is a poor view of the iris and pupil through the slit-lamp microscope, there is either a cloudy cornea or a cloudy anterior chamber. There are several reasons why the cornea may not be clear, such as edema, scars, vascularization, foreign bodies, white blood cell infiltrates in response to

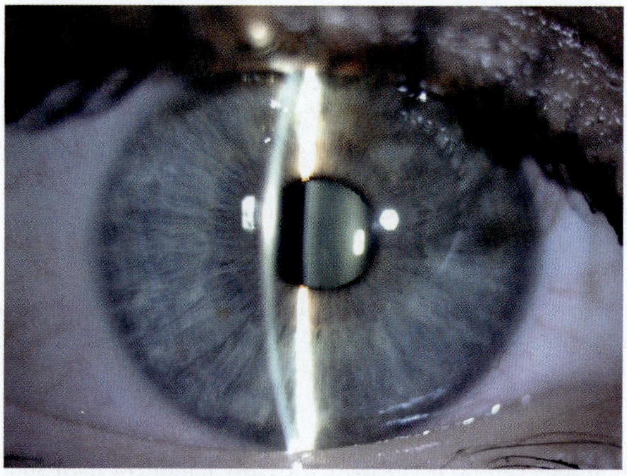

Figure 25.1: High-magnification view of a normal eye using a slit-lamp microscope. The external structures of the eye are clearly visible for examination.

infection, and inherited dystrophies and degenerations. The anterior chamber, normally filled with clear aqueous humor, can be cloudy owing to red or white blood cells that have not layered out into a hyphema or hypopyon, respectively.

The anterior chamber should be a few millimeters deep. Its depth is best visualized using the slit-lamp microscope, but it can also be evaluated by viewing the eye from the side while shining a light obliquely onto the eye. There are several reasons why the anterior chamber might be shallow, such as penetrating trauma or acute angle closure glaucoma. Full thickness corneal lacerations can have the iris pulled anteriorly into the defect causing the anterior chamber to be shallow.

The iris is easily examined with the slit-lamp microscope. Neovascularization of the iris (rubeosis iridis), iris defects, and pupillary membranes should be noted. Part of the iris may protrude anteriorly through a corneal laceration, confirming a penetrating injury to the eye.

Posterior to the iris is the lens. The lens is crystal clear at birth and becomes less clear throughout life, eventually developing into a cataract. It is difficult to fully assess the lens without pharmacologic dilation of the pupil. Slit-lamp examination of the lens may show cataractous opacities that vary in color from white to red, brown, and black. If the lens has been traumatized, it may show gross dislocation or rupture of its capsule with extruding white cortex filling the anterior chamber.

TIPS AND PEARLS

Slit-Lamp Microscope

There are many slit-lamp microscope designs, but most are operated in a similar fashion. If available, the examiner can use these tips for proper operation.

- Position the patient with their chin on the chin rest and their forehead touching the forehead band. Their eye level should be adjusted by raising or lowering the chin rest so that their eyes are in line with the black mark on the two support posts. A height-adjustable chair can be helpful when trying to position the patient. **Figure 25.2** shows a patient properly positioned at the slit-lamp microscope.
- Enable maximal depth perception for the examiner by moving the right and left oculars together or apart, confirming that each eye independently has a view of the patient's eye.
- The examiner should turn on the light source. The brightness, width, and height of the light beam can be adjusted by dials located on the microscope or the table/base. The angle of the beam (direct, oblique, etc.) that is shined on the eye can be changed to highlight various ocular structures. In general, the brightness of the light should be kept on a lower setting to minimize patient discomfort.
- Each of the patient's eyes can be viewed by moving the microscope in front of the eye of interest. This is accomplished by moving the joystick laterally toward the patient's left or right eye. The joystick can also be rotated clockwise or counterclockwise to raise or lower the light beam, respectively.
- The slit-lamp microscope can be used to view the structures of the anterior part of the eye. This can be completed by guiding the microscope forward or backward using the joystick to adjust the plane of focus. The slit lamp can focus only as far posteriorly as the anterior vitreous.

Ophthalmoscopy

In the presence of a clear ocular media, dilation and direct ophthalmoscopy by an experienced clinician may give a view of the posterior ocular segment adequate to diagnose disorders of the optic nerve or retina. Some clinicians may have access to a PanOptic™ ophthalmoscope, which provides a larger viewing area than a direct ophthalmoscope. The optic nerve should be examined for edema, hemorrhages, and pallor. The retina should be assessed for hemorrhages, exudates, edema, vessels abnormalities, and tears or detachments. Additional methods to evaluate the posterior segment include ultrasound, radiologic imaging, and fundus photography, which are discussed in the next chapter.

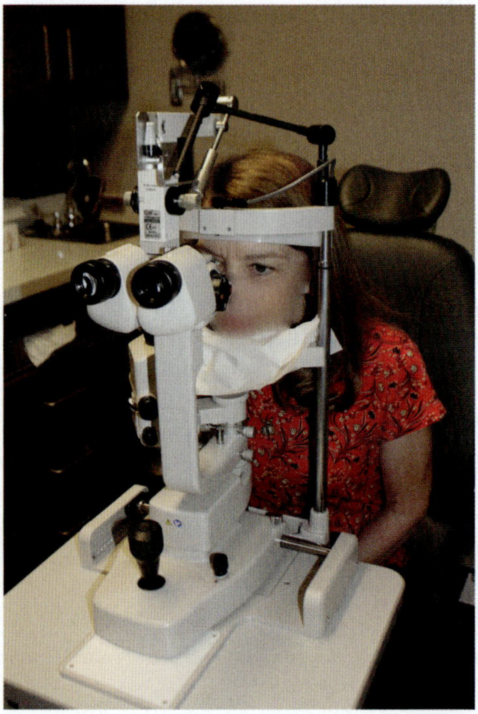

Figure 25.2: A patient properly positioned at the slit-lamp microscope.

Pediatric Patient Considerations

Pediatric patients can present additional challenges to the clinician trying to perform an eye exam. Children can be averse to an examination when they are afraid, sick, or injured. Nonetheless, the physical exam is critical in children because they are often unreliable historians.

The examiner may be unable to perform a formal visual acuity measurement, but should, at a minimum, assess whether the child can follow an object such as their finger or an interesting toy. If the child can fixate on and follow the object when it is moved, the vision can be documented as "fix and follow." This is optimally completed with each eye independently but still has value if performed binocularly. If the child can participate more, but is unable to read, the examiner can ask the child if they can see specific pictures or objects at varying distances (this technique may also be used with illiterate adults).

Depending on the child's age and size, it may be possible to complete portions of the eye examination with the help of parents or other medical staff restraining the child. However, the examiner should be cautious to avoid inadvertent injury to the child's eye or face if they are combative or uncooperative. When it is deemed unsafe to continue with an eye examination, it may be necessary for the child to be sedated to allow for a thorough examination of the eyes and surrounding structures. If this is the case, the patient may need to be transferred to a facility where sedation can be performed and ophthalmology consultation is available.

TIPS AND PEARLS

- If a patient is complaining of severe sharp eye pain and it resolves after the application of a topical anesthetic, this implies corneal pathology such as a corneal abrasion, ulcer, erosion, or laceration.
- If the patient wears contact lenses, any complaint of pain, redness, or decreased vision should be assumed to result from a bacterial corneal ulcer, until deemed otherwise by an ophthalmologist.

- If a patient reports a chemical injury, especially alkali, copiously irrigate the eyes before commencing your eye examination.
- If an open-globe injury is suspected, do not apply any pressure to the globe as it could expel the intraocular contents. Apply a rigid shield without a patch pending evaluation by the ophthalmologist.
- If a patient has eye pain within the first few days after ocular surgery, they are at high risk for acute endophthalmitis, and an ophthalmologist should be consulted.
- Infants who are being evaluated for nonaccidental trauma or shaken baby syndrome must have a dilated eye examination by an ophthalmologist.

EVIDENCE

Are dilating eye drops safe?

Pupillary dilation is routinely performed in ophthalmology practices but rarely done by other medical professionals owing to concern of inducing angle closure glaucoma. In fact, this complication is exceedingly rare. In a large diabetic screening program involving over 95 000 instances of dilation, there were only three cases of angle closure glaucoma, equating to a rate of 1 in 31 755.[3] When considering dilation, it may be helpful to determine whether the patient is far-sighted (hyperopic) by observing whether their distance glasses appear to magnify images. If they do, dilation should be deferred because these patients are at greater risk for angle closure glaucoma.[4] Emergency physicians infrequently feel compelled to dilate a patient's eyes, and we recommend against routinely performing a dilated exam in the emergency setting.

References

1. Channa R, Zafar SN, Canner JK, et al. Epidemiology of eye-related emergency department visits. *JAMA Ophthalmol*. 2016;134(3):312-319. doi:10.1001/jamaophthalmol.2015.5778. PMID: 26821577.
2. Stagg BC, Shah MM, Talwar N, et al. Factors affecting visits to the emergency department for urgent and nonurgent ocular conditions. *Ophthalmology*. 2017;124(5):720-729. doi:10.1016/j.ophtha.2016.12.039. Epub 2017 Jan 31. PMID: 28159379; PMCID: PMC5668138.
3. Lagan MA, O'Gallagher MK, Johnston SE, et al. Angle closure glaucoma in the Northern Ireland Diabetic Retinopathy Screening Programme. *Eye (Lond)*. 2016;30(8):1091-1093. doi:10.1038/eye.2016.98. Epub 2016 May 27. PMID: 27229706; PMCID: PMC4985689.
4. Shen L, Melles RB, Metlapally R, et al. The association of refractive error with glaucoma in a multiethnic population. *Ophthalmology*. 2016;123(1):92-101. doi:10.1016/j.ophtha.2015.07.002. Epub 2015 Aug 8. PMID: 26260281; PMCID: PMC4695304.

CHAPTER 26

Ocular Imaging

Gareth M. C. Lema
Penelope C. Lema

THE CLINICAL CHALLENGE

A primary challenge for the emergency provider is choosing the appropriate diagnostic imaging test in evaluation of the eye. Some radiologic studies can unnecessarily expose patients to ionizing radiation or may be time-consuming and costly. Diminished access to the ideal test may be another limitation. Computed tomography (CT) and MRI are not always readily available, and waiting for testing could cause delays in patient care or diagnosis. Point-of care ultrasound (POCUS) is accessible in most emergency departments (EDs) but requires specialized training to perform and interpret the test. Ocular imaging, such as fundus photography, requires a trained photographer.

Developing a differential diagnosis from a focused history and physical exam is critical to choosing the optimal test. Familiarity with the imaging modalities available at your institution will also inform your decision. In this chapter, we will describe the tests that you may need to diagnose ocular conditions and describe their limitations and contraindications to help you choose the optimal imaging modality. Our discussion will be limited to ophthalmic applications of imaging tests available in the ED or urgent care center.

RADIOGRAPHY (X-RAY)

A plain X-ray has limited use for ocular disorders. Its primary use is to detect radiopaque foreign bodies within the globe or orbit. In most instances, a CT is preferable owing to greater sensitivity and better characterization of orbital pathology, including fractures. X-ray may be used to rule out a metallic foreign body prior to ordering an MRI.

ULTRASOUND (B-SCAN)

Ocular ultrasound is a readily available point-of-care imaging modality that is portable, performed at the patient's bedside, and without ionizing radiation. It is often referred to as "B-scan" by ophthalmologists because they use both the A-mode and the B-mode in clinical practice. Only the B-mode ultrasound is used in emergency situations (**Figure 26.1**).

In the acute setting, a high-resolution linear ultrasound transducer is used to image the eye in two planes. An endocavitary transducer can be used, specifically to evaluate the diameter of the optic nerve sheath from the lateral canthus in the coronal plane.[1] Ocular ultrasound should adhere to the principle of ALARA (as low as reasonably achievable) because the eye is potentially sensitive to the mechanical and thermal effects of ultrasound. Ocular presets should be used, or settings can be adjusted, with the mechanical index (MI) $\leq$0.23 and the thermal index limited to $\leq$1.[2] The scan should be performed over a closed eyelid. The use

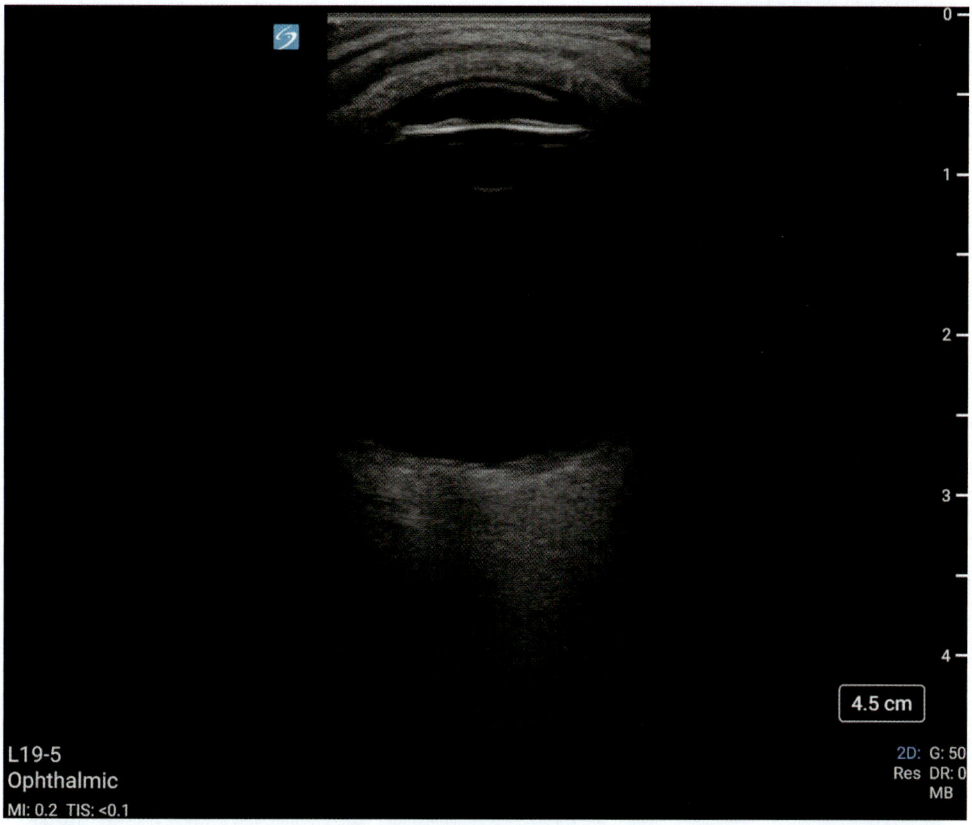

Figure 26.1: Ocular ultrasound. Transorbital ocular ultrasound obtained with a linear high-frequency transducer.

of an individually packaged, single use lubricant is recommended as an acoustic medium to decrease the risk of infection from contaminated gel.

One of the primary uses of ultrasound is to distinguish between a retinal detachment, posterior vitreous detachment, and vitreous hemorrhage, because all three can present with flashes, floaters, and vision loss of varying degrees.[3] However, several other types of pathology can be identified that may lead to a diagnosis. These include intraocular tumors, endophthalmitis, lens dislocation, mature cataracts, choroidal detachment, or posterior scleritis.

Optic nerve disorders, such as severe cupping in glaucoma or disc swelling in optic neuritis, can also be seen in some cases. The identification of an enlarged optic nerve sheath diameter (ONSD) can assist in the diagnosis of elevated intracranial pressure or pathology such as idiopathic intracranial hypertension. Finally, intraocular foreign bodies may be identified, and sometimes ultrasound is more accurate at determining whether a foreign body has perforated the posterior sclera and entered the orbit.

Ultrasound should be avoided or used with extreme caution in cases of suspected or known open globe. This is especially important in cases of blunt trauma or large lacerating injuries. Pressure from the transducer can expel ocular contents, and gel may get into the eye and increase the risk of infection. If ultrasound is used in trauma when the presence of an open globe is unknown, the probe should be held over the lid and coupled to the surface with a copious amount of gel so that the probe does not touch the lid.

In eyes that have had recent retinal detachment surgery, gas or silicone oil used as a tamponade will scatter the ultrasound waves and distort the image. A scleral buckle may indent the natural curvature of the globe and create a shadow on ultrasound. Similarly, in eyes that have had glaucoma surgery, extraocular implant(s) may be noted.

COMPUTED TOMOGRAPHY (CT)

CT is widely used as an initial imaging study owing to its efficiency, availability, and variety of applications (**Figure 26.2**). The key advantages of CT include the ability to obtain the exam and interpretation relatively quickly and its near universal availability. The greatest disadvantage is radiation exposure, especially in pediatric populations. Its use should therefore be limited to cases in which it will contribute to the diagnosis or affect the patient's treatment plan.

A typical head CT is not adequate to assess the globe or facial bones owing to insufficient resolution. Whenever CT is used to evaluate the globe, an orbital or facial bones protocol should be ordered. This will produce 1 to 3 mm cuts and should include direct axial and direct coronal views. If a foreign body is suspected or the optic nerve is being evaluated, 1 mm cuts are required.

Head or facial trauma is one of the most common indications for CT. The orbital bones, sinuses, globe, skull, and brain can all be assessed in a single study. CT without intravenous contrast is the imaging modality of choice for fractures. It can also be used to identify intraocular or orbital

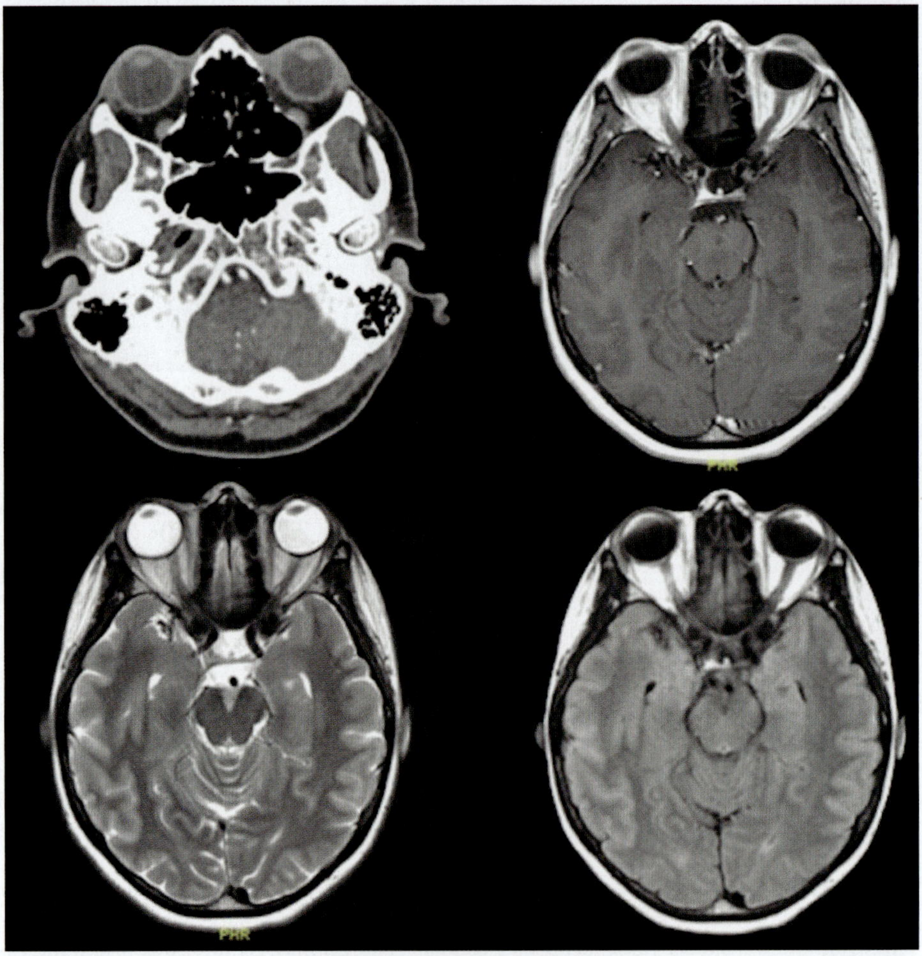

Figure 26.2: Computed tomography (CT) and magnetic resonance imaging (MRI) images of the globes and orbits. All images were acquired from the same patient. Upper left, Normal CT scan of both globes. There is a normal contour of the globes, and the lens can be seen anteriorly. Upper right, T1-weighted MRI with contrast. Lower left, T2-weighted MRI. Lower right, T2/FLAIR images.

foreign bodies. The integrity of the globe can also be assessed by comparing both eyes. A misshapen contour of the eye wall may indicate the presence of an open globe, but CT is not a suitable substitute for a complete eye exam or surgical exploration.

Proptosis is another important indication for CT. CT can be critical for the diagnosis and evaluation of orbital compartment syndrome by demonstrating stretching of the optic nerve and tenting of the posterior hemisphere of the globe. It is also helpful to identify masses or a retrobulbar hemorrhage.

CT with iodinated contrast is useful for differentiating preseptal from orbital cellulitis. It may be used to identify orbital inflammation, abscesses, and tumors. In cases of suspected orbital inflammation or infection, contrast will better differentiate soft tissue, such as an orbital abscess. In most cases, MRI will better characterize soft tissue abnormalities even if they are identifiable by CT.

MAGNETIC RESONANCE IMAGING (MRI)

MRI has specific indications compared to CT. Its major advantages as an imaging modality are improved contrast in soft tissue and multiple sequences that allow for better characterization of orbital and intracranial lesions (Figure 26.2). Additionally, it does not require the use of radiation or iodinated contrast dye.

MRI is not readily available and takes longer than CT, so relying on MRI may delay a critical ocular diagnosis. It is also a very expensive test. There are several contraindications, because any ferromagnetic foreign body precludes its use. Specific to ophthalmology, MRI should never be used if there is the possibility of a metallic intraocular or intraorbital foreign body.

Depending on the acuity and severity of the patient's symptoms, MRI may be warranted in cases of unexplained proptosis, papilledema, or inflammatory disorders such as optic neuritis. Similar to CT, the resolution depends on the spacing between slices. You may need to carefully consider the anatomic region to target when choosing the particular MRI study. When concerned about the optic nerve, obtain an orbital scan with 1 mm cuts. If the presence of papilledema raises concern for a cavernous sinus thrombosis, then magnetic resonance venography (MRV) should be added.

In T1-weighted sequences, the vitreous is dark and the orbital fat is bright. Orbital structures can be resolved because they appear relatively dark. If gadolinium is used, fat suppression must also be ordered, or else the enhancement may get lost in the bright fat signal.

In T2-weighted sequences, the vitreous, orbital fat, and cerebrospinal fluid (CSF) are bright, making orbital structures and intraocular lesions difficult to distinguish. However, the T2-weighted FLAIR (fluid attenuated inversion recovery) sequence suppresses CSF, making this an optimal choice when evaluating patients with optic neuritis.

It is also notable that some ophthalmic implants may be visible radiographically but are not contraindications to MRI. For instance, scleral buckles can be radiopaque, but they contain no metal components. Some older buckles are secured with tantalum clips, but these are also not magnetic.[4] Intraocular lenses do not contain metallic components. Almost all modern ocular implants are nonmetallic or made of nonmagnetic metals, like titanium. Only in rare instances should the presence of a ferromagnetic metal be a concern. A good medical and surgical history should identify the patient's risk. If there is any doubt, CT or X-ray can identify whether a component is potentially metallic. Further information can then be obtained prior to completing the MRI study.

ANGIOGRAPHY

Angiography plays an important role in identifying vascular anomalies, such as carotid-cavernous fistula, arteriovenous malformations, carotid dissection, and, most importantly, intracranial aneurysms. There are three forms of angiography: digital subtraction angiography (DSA), computed tomography angiography (CTA), and magnetic resonance angiography (MRA). All of these can be used to identify vascular anomalies, but each has distinct advantages.

DSA remains the gold standard for identifying intracranial lesions and aneurysms. One advantage is that it can accomplish both diagnosis and treatment depending on the pathology identified. However, it is invasive and requires radiation exposure. CTA is a fast, high-resolution modality that has become the study of choice in many cases. It requires much higher levels of radiation than a typical CT and should be avoided in children unless essential. MRA is slower than CTA. It carries distinct advantages in that it lacks radiation and an iodinated dye is not used. In cases of gadolinium intolerance, a lower resolution scan can be done without dye.

Your institution may have a protocol and/or preferred modality for angiography. CTA is becoming an initial test of choice owing to its efficiency and diagnostic sensitivity. In some situations, such as in the case of a suspected aneurysm, clinical suspicion may guide the decision to order DSA in lieu of a pure imaging modality or despite an initial negative CTA or MRA scan.

FUNDUS PHOTOGRAPHY

Fundus photography uses an autofocusing nonmydriatic camera to acquire a color image of the posterior pole (the optic nerve and central retina). Because these cameras do not require dilation, they can serve as a rapid substitute for a dilated fundus exam in a teleophthalmology consultation model. This can offer a distinct advantage in hospitals that do not have ophthalmology coverage. The images can be interpreted remotely to develop a plan for point-of-care treatment and referral to a tertiary center when needed.[5]

Most cameras take a 30° to 50° photo, which includes the optic nerve and macula (**Figure 26.3**). This is ideal for documenting vast vision threatening conditions such as papilledema, diabetic retinopathy, retinal artery occlusion, glaucoma, and macular degeneration, to name just a few. Indirectly, media opacities can be identified. A cataract may cause a blurred, yellowed image. A vitreous hemorrhage or vitritis can obscure part of the photo or completely prevent image acquisition.

Fundus photographs cannot replace a full dilated exam. Any lesions that are confined to the peripheral retina will be outside the view of the camera. Not all etiologies of vision loss can be diagnosed by photos alone. Finally, a trained operator is required to use the camera, so availability can be a limitation. Nonetheless, fundus imaging in the ED has the potential to substantially enhance access to ophthalmic care.

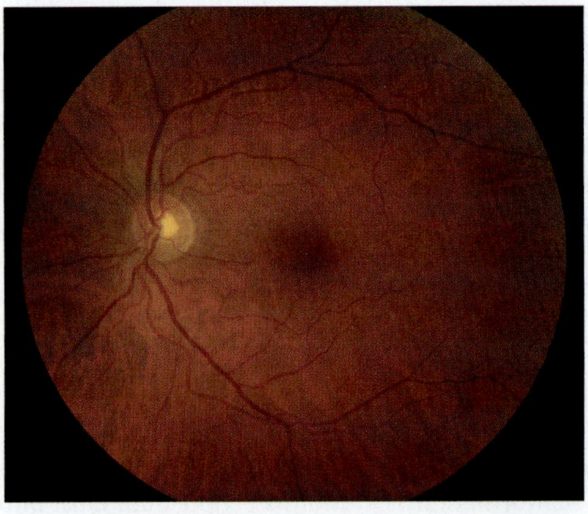

Figure 26.3: Fundus photography. Normal 50° fundus photo of the left eye.

TIPS AND PEARLS

- Obtain a CT or X-ray of the orbit if there is any suspicion of a retained metallic foreign body prior to a MRI.
- Avoid pressure on the eyelid when an open globe is suspected.
- Individually packaged gel is recommended for ocular ultrasound to decrease the risk of infection from contaminated ultrasound gel. Surgical lubricant may be readily available and can be used instead of ultrasound gel. Surgical lubricant is also less irritating than ultrasound gel if it gets into the eye.
- CT and MRI evaluation of the orbit may require that small slice intervals are ordered. An orbital imaging study should have 1 to 3 mm slice intervals. To image a foreign body or optic neuritis, request 1 mm slice intervals.

SUMMARY

Ocular imaging is invaluable for diagnosing ophthalmic disorders and characterizing the extent of traumatic injury. A good history and physical exam, sound clinical judgment, and awareness of the capabilities and limitations of your institution will all help guide your choice of the optimal studies to order. In some cases, consulting a radiologist or ophthalmologist may help choose the optimal test for your patient.

EVIDENCE

What is the best imaging modality for nonmetallic intraocular or intraorbital foreign bodies?

Although MRI is better at resolving all types of nonmetallic foreign bodies, noncontrast CT is the most practical and effective initial test. On MRI, nonmetallic foreign bodies will universally appear as very low intensity (a black void) with a ring of variable hyperintensity at the border of the foreign body.[6,7] CT is a quick test that will identify most nonmetallic foreign bodies very well. The attenuation of the foreign body depends on the material, so some are more easily identified than others.[8] Plastics and organic matter like wood can be low intensity or undetectable on CT but can be identified on ultrasound. Glass, stone, and metals are generally of moderate or high intensity. Thus, when CT identifies a foreign body, it may also help indicate the type of material.

It is critical to determine whether or not the material is potentially magnetic before ordering an MRI.[9] If the trauma history affirms with certainty that any possible foreign body is nonmagnetic, then MRI can be done as a primary test. Usually, MRI will be done secondarily if the foreign body is not identified with CT or needs to be better characterized. It is important to request 1 mm slices and remember that very small foreign bodies could be missed.

Ultrasound can be useful for diagnosing small intraocular foreign bodies. However, noncontact imaging is safer in patients with an open globe. CT and MRI can also better localize the foreign body and identify orbital foreign bodies. No imaging modality is perfect, and patients at risk for an intraocular foreign body (IOFB) should be evaluated by ophthalmology in the ED or referred for a dilated fundus exam within 24 hours.

Can sonographic measurement of the optic nerve sheath diameter (ONSD) serve as a proxy finding for elevated intracranial pressure?

Transorbital sonographic measurement of the ONSD with a linear transducer has been shown to correlate with intracranial pressure (ICP).[10] Generally, an ONSD greater than 5mm in diameter measured 3mm posterior to its attached to the globe suggests elevated ICP. However, limitations of this measurement include interrater variability as well as disagreement regarding the optimal transducer and technique to obtain an accurate measurement.

Traditionally, the linear transducer is used to obtain an axial transorbital measurement of the ONSD. Coronal axis views from the lateral canthus with an endocavitary transducer have been considered an alternate technique and may be a more accurate measurement when compared with MRI.[11] The transorbital visual axis measurements are noted to be artifactually larger owing to optical artifacts produced by the cornea and lens. The transorbital measurement of the ONSD may also represent shadowing from the optic disc or other structures.[1,11] Although this technique potentially has great value for emergent diagnosis, more studies are needed to standardize the measurement and interpretation of this data.

References

1. Shah S, Kimberly H, Marill K, et al. Ultrasound techniques to measure the optic nerve sheath: is a specialized probe necessary? *Med Sci Monit*. 2009;15(5):MT63-MT68.
2. American Institute of Ultrasound in Medicine Official Statements. Safety in diagnostic ultrasound educational activities using nonpregnant participants. https://www.aium.org/officialStatements/76. Approved May 19, 2020. Accessed May 24, 2021.
3. Baker N, Amini R, Situ-LaCasse EH, et al. Can emergency physicians accurately distinguish retinal detachment from posterior vitreous detachment with point-of-care ocular ultrasound? *Am J Emerg Med*. 2018;36(5):774-776.
4. Lane JI, Watson RE Jr, Witte RJ, et al. Retinal detachment: imaging of surgical treatments and complications. *Radiographics*. 2003;23(4):983-994.
5. Vasseneix C, Bruce BB, Bidot S, et al. Nonmydriatic fundus photography in patients with acute vision loss. *Telemed J E Health*. 2019;25(10):911-916.
6. Modjtahedi BS, Rong A, Bobinski M, et al. Imaging characteristics of intraocular foreign bodies: a comparative study of plain film X-ray, computed tomography, ultrasound, and magnetic resonance imaging. *Retina*. 2015;35:95-104.
7. Moisseiev E, Last, D, Goez D, et al. Magnetic resonance imaging and computed tomography for the detection and characterization of nonmetallic intraocular foreign bodies. *Retina*. 2015;35:82-94.
8. Rong AJ, Fan KC, Golshani B, et al. Multimodal imaging features of intraocular foreign bodies. *Semin Ophthalmol*. 2019;34(7-8):518-532.
9. Moisseiev E, Barequet D, Zunz E, et al. Validation of an algorithm for nonmetallic intraocular foreign bodies' composition identification based on computed tomography and magnetic resonance imaging. *Retina*. 2015;35:1898-1904.
10. Kimberly HH, Shah S, Marill K, et al. Correlation of optic nerve sheath diameter with direct measurement of intracranial pressure. *Acad Emerg Med*. 2008;15(2):201-204.
11. Blehar DJ, Gaspari RJ, Montoya A, et al. Correlation of visual axis and coronal axis measurements of the optic nerve sheath diameter. *J Ultrasound Med*. 2008;27(3):407-411.

CHAPTER 27

Communication with Ophthalmology Consultants and Telehealth

Sophia Mirza Saleem

Emergency providers request specialty consultation to seek opinions and expertise to provide high-quality care for patients. This request is made with expectations of minimal or no delay in care, but, increasingly, seeking a consulting physician prolongs lengths of stay and exacerbates volume dilemmas.

Similarly to most emergency providers, covering consultants also face higher patient volumes and several global and specialty-specific disincentives to cover call. The Emergency Medical Treatment and Active Labor Act (EMTALA) guidelines, established to protect uninsured patients who need acute care, have also increased nonreimbursed and nonurgent care being delivered in emergency departments (EDs). Increasing malpractice insurance costs and low or nonexistent compensation for taking call further deters specialists from participating in call pools.[1] This creates an even larger burden for surgical specialists who might need to perform emergency procedures that are not reimbursed.[2] Related to these reasons, surgical specialty coverage is demonstrating a well-documented decline across the country.[2] The lack of specialists available to EDs may result in negative outcomes for patients owing to delays in definitive care or increased number of transfers to tertiary centers.[3]

The limited literature suggests serious gaps in ophthalmology coverage for EDs.[4] An analysis in Florida indicates that ophthalmologists take less call than other surgical subspecialists.[5] The American Academy of Ophthalmology also published an editorial to describe the reasons why the ophthalmology coverage gap exists and why they speculate it will continue to expand. The article suggests the growth of ambulatory surgery centers, which reduces private practice surgeons' dependence on hospitals, outdated ED equipment, and growth of specialization, which reduces the number of ophthalmologists who feel clinically comfortable taking call.[6] This same update indicated that consultants rarely need to physically come in because most calls are for advice or follow-up.

Many ophthalmologists who take call will often remotely discuss a patient and make a recommendation. A conversation between two physicians about a patient without examination, review of the chart, or consultant documentation of their findings and recommendation is defined as a curbside consult. There are several perils in performing curbside consults. First, providing an opinion about a patient without knowing the individual details of the case can lead to unsafe decisions by the care team and may result in delay of appropriate care or patient harm. This can also lead to wasted resources to correct the care plan or manage complications. There is also liability that the consultant incurs during a curbside consult. Often, the requesting physician will document the consulting physician's name and whether a curbside or formal consult was performed. This puts the consultant at risk for recommendations that they might not have made after examining the patient or reviewing diagnostic testing. Additionally, without a documented request and written recommendation, the consult is generally not billed and reimbursed, reducing revenue for the hospital that is potentially paying the physicians to take call. Although ophthalmologists are accustomed to giving opinions over the phone as an alternative to coming to the ED, this method of practicing medicine can be unsafe and lead to poor quality yet more costly care.

Specialty coverage inconsistencies, especially when there is no physician to take call, are particularly problematic, resulting in delays, potential errors, or excessive and costly transfers. The poor availability results in significant clinical, financial, and operational impact for patients, providers, and health systems.

Background on Tele-ophthalmology

Several strategies are being employed to help increase the attractiveness for specialists to take call. Taking call was previously required and uncompensated when affiliated with a hospital. Over the last two decades, physicians are expecting remuneration for call, whether they are employed by the hospital or not. The acquiescence of hospitals to reimburse providers for call has given rise to many models of call compensation, which often depends on the specialty, the regional availability of that specialty, payer mixes and facility types, and the use of telemedicine at reduced physician payment to cover call.

Several cost-reduction methodologies have been shown to improve the gap[7]; however, it has been difficult to demonstrate how these changes immediately make it easier for specialists to deliver care quickly and handle volume more efficiently. Leaders in health care policy believe that crowded EDs have been a long-standing issue and look to innovative solutions such as telemedicine to expedite care.[8]

The COVID-19 pandemic exacerbated existing ED specialty coverage gaps, while also creating new gaps related to social distancing and initial scarcity of personal protective equipment. Solutions were quickly needed to continue to provide basic and specialty care to patients in all care settings, especially in the ED. Telemedicine, in all its forms, was quickly implemented to fill these gaps. After the emergence of SARS-CoV-2, relaxations in telemedicine regulations, improved reimbursement, as well as the need to reduce exposure to health care workers prompted increased usage of telemedicine across all care settings.[9] What might have taken 5 to 10 years to accomplish to advance telemedicine was implemented in a mere 9 to 12 months. By integrating telemedicine into ED workflows, hospitals are poised to improve access to specialists, increase throughput, reduce wait times and transfers, standardize care quality and access, and maneuver future pandemics. The final memorialization of current regulations and reimbursement structures will dictate the extent to which telemedicine may become more ubiquitous.

The concept of telemedicine use in the ED is not new. It is used to expedite specialty care access, including burn and trauma transfer decisions, acute stroke management, psychiatric evaluation, and even tele-ultrasound support. A meta-analysis of telemedicine use in the ED reported positive findings for services like triage, treatment of minor illness or injury, and connecting providers to specialists. Telemedicine also added value in terms of productivity for the EDs.[10] These studies were reported prior to the COVID-19 pandemic, and since 2020, telemedicine has expanded and grown exponentially, with thousands of articles describing the value-add of telemedicine to support ED clinical operations.

Telemedicine in ophthalmology has evolved over several decades, yet its use in the ED has been fairly basic and unstructured. Prior to the COVID-19 pandemic, the use of telemedicine in ophthalmology was mostly described in the ambulatory care settings. Opinion surveys of telehealth prior to 2020 indicate that most ophthalmologists already practice store-and-forward telemedicine, meaning they received photos of patients and were asked to provide a clinical opinion. Additionally, the survey indicated that most of them are amenable to using telemedicine for consultations.[11]

Rudimentary forms of acute care telemedicine currently employed by ophthalmologists and emergency providers help close the ED coverage gap. Although many eye physicians do not consider themselves telehealth providers, ophthalmologists taking ED call over the last few decades often practice telephone-based telemedicine (a curbside consult). The use of the curbside consult in ophthalmology demonstrates that triage can occur remotely. In fact, most ocular-related visits to the ED are nonacute and unrelated to trauma.[12] Of patients who present to the ED for ophthalmic complaints, 97% are treated and released. **Table 27.1** lists the most typical reasons for ocular complaints in the ED.

TABLE 27.1 Most Common Ocular Diagnoses in ED

Ocular Diagnoses	Frequency of ED Presentation
Conjunctivitis	33.8%
Corneal injury without foreign body	13.1%
Corneal foreign body	7.8%
Eye pain	4.2%
Hordeolum (stye)	4%

ED, emergency department.

Adapted from Vaziri K, Schwartz SG, Flynn HW, Kishor KS, Moshfeghi AA. Eye-related emergency department visits in the United States, 2010. *Ophthalmology*. 2016;123(4);917-919. doi:10.1016/j.ophtha.2015.10.032

Many of these conditions can be triaged or diagnosed and managed successfully via telemedicine examination, which allows the ophthalmologist to remotely begin management of the patient. Clinically visible findings for certain emergencies can be directed by initiation of further testing, starting medication, arranging for next day follow-up, and expediting care. Certainly, performing tele-ophthalmology for triage requires examination of the whole patient, their demeanor, their medical history, their symptoms, reviewing testing, prior ocular history if available, and the quantitative data as collected by the emergency provider.

Tele-ophthalmology ostensibly lends itself to particular subspecialties such as oculo-plastics and neuro-ophthalmology, both of which were successfully accomplished and published during 2020.[13,14] Many of the top 10 acute eye diseases can be triaged via the same techniques used for oculoplastics and neuro-ophthalmology telemedicine because there is significant overlap.

Communicating With Your Ophthalmology Consultant on the Telemedicine Platform

Performing a tele-ophthalmology consult should always start with a request or order for the consultation. This not only serves to document the query for the consult for compliance and billing purposes but can also function as a trigger to start the process. An electronic request may flow to supporting staff who can monitor the consult's progress as well as the ophthalmologist who is made aware of the consult. An order can contain specific instructions and/or questions for the ordering physician, including a reminder to obtain consent for telemedicine, call-back or video visit session information to inform the consultant how to connect with the ED, and clinical questions.

Communication of essential clinical elements to your consultant from the initial ED history and physical exam provides excellent context for the consulting eye physician. Guiding questions for ophthalmology include the following:

Which eye is affected?
Does the patient have blurry vision? If yes, is this binocular or monocular?
Does the patient have eye pain?
Does the patient have light sensitivity?
Is that patient reporting flashing lights or new floaters?
Measured visual acuity for right eye and left eye? Corrective lenses used?
Does the patient wear corrective lenses at baseline?
What does the eye look like? Describe the gross appearance of the upper and lower eyelids, conjunctiva, iris, pupillary reaction.
Does that patient have any extraocular movement deficit?
Is a photo of the affected eye uploaded in the electronic medical record/via secure texting?
If available, what is the measured intraocular pressure of the affected and unaffected eye?
Is there fluorescein uptake?

The visual acuity is the most important initial vital sign of the eye and is required for successful triage. Once the consulting provider is engaged and given basic exam information, the eye physician should be able to decide whether more information is needed.

The ophthalmologist may ask for additional information via further diagnostic imaging such as computed tomography (CT) or ultrasound, or a simple in-focus picture of the affected eye. Often, these additional pieces of data are instrumental in either triaging or diagnosing the patient. The ophthalmologist may also ask an ED team member to facilitate an examination over video.

Anterior segment examination may be completed by photo or video, although this requires the presence of appropriate equipment in the ED, the ability to store images in the medical record and transmission over a secure platform. The photo may be a slit-lamp photo or otherwise high magnification and should be stored as part of the medical record; the still image may be enough to make a diagnosis and should be documented. For ophthalmology, a gross, no-zoom, video stream is helpful to complete a dynamic exam. There is also technology available that supports high-resolution video with remote pan, tilt, and zoom control capacity. If the patient's head is stabilized, for instance while sitting in a chair with the back of the patient's head resting against the wall, high magnification is possible without degradation of the image. In fact, an ophthalmologist would easily be able to identify common acute issues such as hyphema, subconjunctival hemorrhage, eyelid disease, eyelid laceration, and corneal disease with appropriate corneal staining.[15] Proper lighting is key for maintaining good image quality, and it is recommended to keep a light source near the patient, especially for higher magnification zoom. Additionally, some examination calls for the light to be off in order to use cobalt blue light. It is important to have a strong light source to perform corneal staining examinations with cobalt blue light.

Posterior segment examination is more difficult to complete over telemedicine. Point-of-care ultrasound can rule in or out several ocular pathologies, including retinal detachment, vitreous hemorrhage, and open globes. Nonmydriatic fundus cameras are also available in smaller handheld and larger table top forms. Generally speaking, the smaller cameras often require more dexterity and skill to capture a well-focused and clinically useful picture or video to transmit to a remote ophthalmologist. In fact, the best use case for a handheld retina camera may be employed by either ophthalmology trainees who practice vitreoretinal examinations daily or well-trained emergency providers who may require regular optimization training sessions.

Tabletop cameras are much easier to use by nonophthalmic clinical teams. These machines can obtain posterior segment photos with higher fidelity but can only be used if the patient is able to sit at the machine and open their eyes and their pupils are 2.5 to 3 mm or larger. Their best use case may be to rule in a central retinal vessel occlusion or evaluate for optic nerve head disease. The use of this camera may not be cost-effective in a small ED given the limited clinical scenarios seen on fundus photo. There are cameras that can also obtain a nonmydriatic optical coherence tomography (OCT) that provides images of retinal and nerve fiber layers quickly. Although OCT technology is generally used to diagnose chronic conditions, newer, nonmydriatic devices allow for its use in nonophthalmic clinical areas such as ED mainly to diagnose acute conditions such as central retinal artery occlusions or optic nerve head edema. **Table 27.2** provides a list of commonly evaluated emergent ocular conditions and the respective workup that can be performed in the ED and communicated via telemedicine.

Once the ophthalmologist obtains as complete an exam as possible, they may be able to make suggestions regarding intervention, further testing, additional consults to request, need for transfer, or prompt outpatient follow-up. Sometimes, the telemedicine-based examination is either not satisfactory for any assessment or indicates a need for an in-person examination. A transfer may be proposed for further examination or if an immediate intervention such as surgery is needed. The most common recommendation, however, is for next day outpatient follow-up to confirm the assessment made on telemedicine using proper examination equipment and diagnostic testing at the outpatient office. For this reason, it is recommended that any ED tele-ophthalmology program establish a standing scheduled morning outpatient appointment slot at nearby ophthalmology practices for ED follow-ups.

Although telemedicine can never replace an in-person full ophthalmic examination, it can extend a specialist to take call and triage patients for treatment stabilization, initiation of medication, or necessary transfer for further evaluation or intervention. There are some obvious concerns about using telemedicine. The first is patient safety and patient expectations. Recognizing that telemedicine is utilized in this instance as an alternative to the absence of any specialty ophthalmology care immediately increases its value. However, the patient should be made aware that the telemedicine delivered does not replace a comprehensive eye exam by an ophthalmologist. For this reason, each

TABLE 27.2 Emergent Ocular Conditions and How to Triage via Telemedicine

Emergent Ocular Conditions	Methods to Triage via Telemedicine
Endophthalmitis	HPI, Video, Still photos
Carotid-cavernous fistula	HPI, Video, Still photo, CT with contrast
Retinal detachment	HPI, Ultrasound performed by onsite ED team, may use video to help direct bedside team member
Bacterial keratitis	HPI, Video, Still photos
Open globe	HPI Still photo, CT scan
Angle closure glaucoma	HPI, ED team checking IOP, Video with penlight exam to illuminate anterior chamber
Retrobulbar hemorrhage	HPI, imaging (CT, ultrasound)
Uveitis	HPI, Video Visit
Third nerve palsy	HPI, Video Visit, CTA/MRA
Ischemic optic neuropathy	HPI, Ultrasound performed by onsite ED team, Fundus Photo (if available), ESR/CRP
Central vessel occlusion	HPI, Ultrasound performed by onsite ED team, Fundus photo/OCT (if available), ESR/CRP

CRP, c-reactive protein; CT, computed tomography; CTA, computed tomography angiography; ED, emergency department; ESR, erythrocyte sedimentation rate; HPI, history of present illness; MRA, magnetic resonance angiography; OCT, optical coherence tomography.

patient should receive a follow-up appointment with an eye physician shortly after discharge if they are not transferred or admitted.

Another obvious concern is the medical liability an ophthalmologist may incur practicing telemedicine versus in-person examination. Ultimately, the patient is in the care of the emergency provider, and they should obtain from the consulting ophthalmologist if there are any pathologies that might warrant more immediate in-person evaluation. There should be a lower than usual threshold to transfer if the ophthalmologist is concerned that something may be missed. Many ophthalmologists practice triage by telephone currently, and adding the ability to perform a limited exam via telemedicine improves patient care.

It is important to remember that the value proposition is to provide triage and stabilization for patients seeking acute ophthalmic care, and telemedicine can be used to create cost-effective access to an ophthalmologist when this was previously not available. The combination of added value and previously successful models of remote triage for urgent eye care indicates that telemedicine for ED ophthalmology consultation is feasible and scalable.[16] Understanding its place in medicine will allow health systems and providers to improve care quality that is cost effective rather than using it as an addition to status quo care models.

TIPS AND PEARLS

- Curbside consults often result in lower quality care, delayed care, and higher care costs.
- Basic history and exam findings—including visual acuity, intraocular pressures, and pupillary exam—are essential data. Having accurate information available improves the efficiency of the consult.
- Remote exams require bedside support from skilled personnel who can operate the imaging equipment and acquire additional exam data, which requires a collaborative agreement between the ED and ophthalmology.
- Establishing follow-up is essential. Prearranged appointments at an affiliated or local eye clinic can help prevent lapses in care.

References

1. Krueger KJ, Halperin EC. Perspective: paying physicians to be on call: a challenge for academic medicine. *Acad Med*. 2010;85(12):1840-1844.
2. Rao MB, Lerro C, Gross CP. The shortage of on-call surgical specialist coverage: a national survey of emergency department directors. *Acad Emerg Med*. 2010;17(12):1374-1382.
3. Menchine MD, Baraff LJ. On-call specialists and higher level of care transfers in California emergency departments. *Acad Emerg Med*. 2008;15(4):329-336.
4. Wedekind L, Sainani K, Pershing S. Supply and perceived demand for teleophthalmology in triage and consultations in California emergency departments. *JAMA Ophthalmol*. 2016;134(5):537-543.
5. Witmer MT, Margo CE. Analysis of ophthalmology workforce and delivery of emergency department eye care in Florida. *Arch Ophthalmol*. 2009;127(11):1522-1527.
6. Mott M. Who's on call? Emergency care crisis looms. 2019. Accessed June 2, 2021. https://www.aao.org/eyenet/article/whos-on-call-emergency-care-crisis-looms
7. Simonet D. Cost reduction strategies for emergency services: insurance role, practice changes and patients accountability. *Health Care Anal*. 2009;17(1):1-19.
8. Dress J. Viewpoint: how telemedicine may reshape emergency medicine. 2020. Accessed June 2, 2021. https://www.beckershospitalreview.com/telehealth/viewpoint-how-telemedicine-may-reshape-emergency-medicine.html
9. Centers for Medicare and Medicaid Services. COVID-19 emergency declaration blanket waivers for health care providers. 2020. Accessed: May 25, 2021. https://www.cms.gov/files/document/summary-covid-19-emergency-declaration-waivers.pdf
10. Ward MM, Jaana M, Natafgi N. Systematic review of telemedicine applications in emergency rooms. *Int J Med Inform*. 2015;84(9):601-616.
11. Woodward MA Ple-Plakon P, Blachey T, et al. Eye care providers' attitudes towards teleophthalmology. *Telemed J E Health*. 2015;21(4):271-273.
12. Vaziri K, Schwartz SG, Flynn HW, Kishor KS, Moshfegi AA. Eye-related Emergency Department Visits in the United States, 2010. *Ophthalmology*. 2016;123(4):917-919.
13. Kang S, Thomas BPM, Sim DA, Parker RT, Daniel C, Uddin JM. Oculoplastic video-based telemedicine consultations: Covid-19 and beyond. *Eye (Lond)*. 2020;34(7):1193-1195.
14. Ko MW, Busis NA. Tele-neuro-ophthalmology: vision for 20/20 and beyond. *J Neuroophthalmol*. 2020;40(3):378-384.
15. Woodward MA, Musch DC, Hood CT, et al. Teleophthalmic approach for detection of corneal diseases: accuracy and reliability. *Cornea*. 2017;36(10):1159-1165.
16. Ribeiro AG, Rodrigues RA, Guerreiro AM, Regatieri CV. A teleophthalmology system for the diagnosis of ocular urgency in remote areas of Brazil. *Arq Bras Oftalmol*. 2014;77(4):214-218.

CHAPTER 28

Orbital Trauma

Joshua Gentges
Douglas Marx

THE CLINICAL CHALLENGE

The orbit is defined by the bony structures that form the orbital floor and wall. It contains and protects many important soft tissue structures, including the eye, extraocular muscles, blood vessels, fascia, ligaments, and cranial nerves (CN) to the orbital structures and face.[1] It also contains the eyelids, tear glands, and lacrimal glands (**Figure 28.1**). Because of the complex bony and soft tissue anatomy, trauma can lead to significant intraocular and extraocular pathology. Careful attention to a focused history and physical examination is important, because missed orbital trauma may lead to loss of vision, intracranial infection, or death in the setting of penetrating orbital injuries.[2]

The diagnosis of orbital injuries is not always apparent because trauma patients may have distracting injuries, have altered mental status, or be unable to participate in a complete examination. Injuries to the orbit can cause orbital fractures, which can lead to organ threatening pathology, including orbital compartment syndrome (OCS), entrapment of extraocular muscles and other intraorbital tissue, globe rupture, vascular injury, optic neuropathy, or nerve avulsion. Evaluation for entrapment of orbital contents is particularly challenging in trauma patients. External signs of injury may not be present in all cases. OCS is clinically challenging because it is both rare (0.088% of craniomaxillofacial [CMF] injuries) and devastating, leading to vision loss that is progressive with increased time to intervention.[2-4]

PATHOPHYSIOLOGY

Assaults cause most orbital fractures (~40%), followed by falls (~25%), recreational or sports related injuries (~16%), and motor vehicle incidents (~13%).[2] The mechanism for orbital fractures can be either direct trauma to the bone or increased intraorbital pressure, causing a "blowout" fracture.[5] Orbital fractures account for half of all facial fractures, and nearly half of these (47.9%) involve the orbital floor, which can lead to entrapment of intraocular tissues, extraocular musculature, or orbital infection.[2] More extensive fractures can lead to loss of support of the eye, causing inferior displacement of the eye (hypophthalmos) and diplopia.[6]

The medial orbital wall is the thinnest part of the orbit, but fractures less commonly owing to reinforcement by the ethmoid. Medial orbital wall fractures can lead to orbital emphysema, tear outflow obstruction, injury to the ethmoidal arteries, and medial rectus entrapment.[6] Lateral wall fractures are also less common because of the relative thickness of the lateral wall and its association with the zygomatic bone and the orbital rim. A lateral wall fracture is usually caused by direct force to the cheek and fracture to the zygomatic arch. Orbital roof fractures occur in the setting of high-impact injuries to the head and face. An orbital roof fracture is usually associated with additional facial fractures and neurologic injury.[2]

An orbital fracture can cause entrapment of intraocular fat, extraocular musculature, or direct damage to the globe. Intraocular fat can herniate through a medial or inferior wall fracture, causing pain with extraocular muscle movement and inflammation. Extraocular muscles can also herniate through an orbital fracture. If the fractured bone "rebounds" from the fracture faster than the muscle, the muscle will become entrapped in the fracture, causing reduced ocular motility and

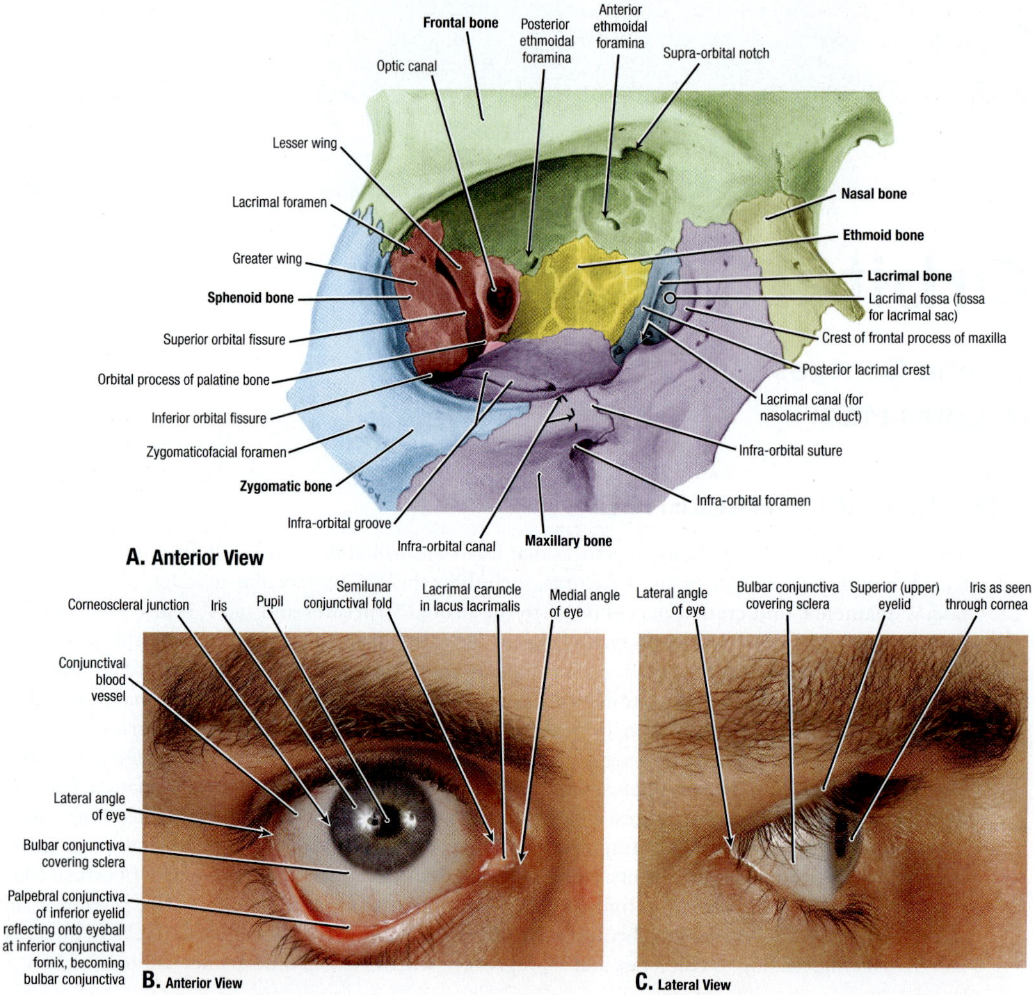

Figure 28.1: Orbital Cavity and Surface Anatomy of Eye A. Bones and features of orbital cavity. B. and C. Surface anatomy of eye. (From Agur AMR, Dalley AF II. *Grant's Atlas of Anatomy*. 15th ed. Wolters Kluwer; 2021. Figure 7.36.)

diplopia. This is more common in children and young adults because the bone in these populations is more elastic.[7] Clinicians should be aware of the oculocardiac reflex, vagally mediated bradycardia with nausea, vomiting, and vertigo caused by extraocular muscle entrapment most commonly in the orbital floor. This finding in isolated facial trauma should prompt rapid evaluation for orbital fracture with entrapment and increase the urgency of primary repair of a facial fracture.[8,9]

Orbital fractures, or even an orbital contusion without fracture, can lead to increased intraorbital pressure from orbital emphysema, hemorrhage, inflammatory changes, or infection when presentation is delayed. Increasing pressures can lead to OCS with multiple downstream effects, including ischemia; damage to the optic nerve and retina; and rapid, progressive vision loss.[3] As intraorbital pressure increases, the orbital contents move toward the area of least resistance, in most cases the front of the orbit, causing exophthalmos.

Direct trauma to intraorbital components can result in globe penetration or rupture, which are ophthalmologic emergencies. Optic nerve transection or neuropathy, hyphema, foreign body, traumatic cataract, and retinal detachment can also occur. In general, these injuries require urgent but not necessarily emergent ophthalmologic referral and intervention.[2] Intraorbital trauma often occurs concomitantly with orbital fractures,[7] so emergency clinicians must maintain a high level of suspicion for intraorbital injury when diagnosing an orbital fracture.

APPROACH/THE FOCUSED EXAM

Orbital injuries can be isolated but more commonly occur in conjunction with other traumatic injury, prompting a complete trauma evaluation. A focused examination should be performed noting lacerations or swelling or tenseness of the eyelids, exophthalmos, active bleeding, tear leakage, penetrating lesions, and extraocular movements. The periorbital regions should be palpated for any bony instability and crepitus. Malar flattening or malocclusion of the teeth should be identified.

For lucid patients, ask them to open their eyes. If the patient cannot open their eye easily owing to eyelid swelling, it is appropriate to attempt gentle assistance. Resistance to eyelid opening, or, conversely, severe proptosis pushing the lids open with difficulty closing them, may suggest increased intraorbital pressure.

Test visual acuity one eye at a time, ideally, with the patient wearing their usual corrective lenses. Perform visual field testing with confrontation. Clinicians should perform a penlight examination, noting patient ability to see light and movement, complaints of pain or diplopia with extraocular muscle movement, a "teardrop" pupil indicating ciliary muscle injury or globe rupture, and pupillary reaction to light. A light source shining in one eye should cause consensual constriction of both pupils, and when removed both pupils should enlarge; this is the basis of a negative swinging flashlight test. A positive test means a relative afferent pupillary defect (RAPD)[10] and indicates damage to the optic nerve or tract.

Subconjunctival hemorrhage (**Figure 28.2**) may be present and when severe may be indicative of hidden globe rupture or significant contusion. If feasible, stain the affected eye with fluorescein dye to look for corneal abrasions, ulcerations, lacerations, and the Seidel sign (a stream of fluid washing away the fluorescein, indicating a ruptured globe). Intraocular pressure testing can be challenging in the setting of trauma but should be performed if evaluation for ruptured globe is negative.

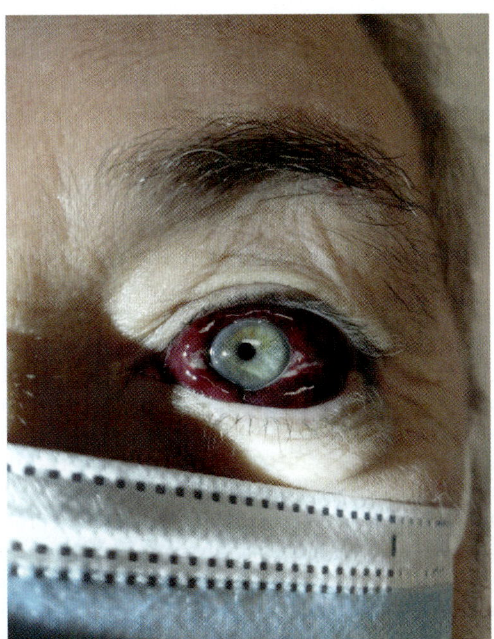

Figure 28.2: Chemosis of the eye. (Courtesy of Lori Whelan, MD, Vice Chair, University of Oklahoma Department of Emergency Medicine, Used by permission.)

Computed tomography (CT) examination of the orbit, including thin slices taken through the orbital wall, has high sensitivity and specificity for orbital fracture, orbital emphysema, or hemorrhage. A bedside ultrasound of the orbit can find retinal detachment, irregularities in the globe suggesting globe rupture, intraocular hemorrhage, or lens detachment. Please refer to chapter 26 on Ocular Imaging for further details.

As an ophthalmic emergency, OCS should be considered in all patients even though it can often be quickly ruled out. Positive signs to suggest OCS include decreased vision, RAPD, resistance to retropulsion, and a tented contour of the posterior globe on ultrasound or CT scan.

DIFFERENTIAL DIAGNOSIS

The orbit is a complex structure, and trauma to it can involve multiple systems. These systems include the following:

- Bony injuries: Fractures to the orbital walls and floor, the orbital rim, and the zygoma.
- Soft tissue injuries: Direct damage to soft tissues includes injury to the extraocular muscles, intraorbital fat and connective tissue, lacerations to the lids, and injuries to the lacrimal glands and ducts. Indirect injuries resulting from bony injuries include herniation of orbital contents through the fracture line.
- Injuries to nervous tissue, including the optic, trigeminal, and facial nerves.
- Vascular injuries can include damage to the ophthalmic vein and artery, the retinal artery, or to the arterioles and capillaries supplying the intraorbital contents. This can lead to conjunctival ecchymosis or chemosis, hyphema, or OCS.
- Globe injuries include globe rupture, retinal detachment, dislocation or evisceration of the lens, vitreous hemorrhage from the anterior or posterior chambers, iritis, and conjunctival or corneal lacerations.

MANAGEMENT

For most traumatic orbital injuries, treatment and referral are urgent but should not delay care of other emergent injuries. The clear exception is OCS, which requires rapid intervention to avoid permanent vision loss. Patients will ultimately need ophthalmology consultation for definitive surgical decompression and repair. However, many emergency providers do not have immediate access to ophthalmology or the ability to transfer without unacceptable delays. Emergency providers must be familiar with and willing to perform an urgent lateral canthotomy with cantholysis, which can be vision saving. Patients treated within 2 hours have an 85% probability of achieving a final Snellen visual acuity of 6/12 or greater, whereas patients treated after 2 hours have only a 25% probability of 6/12 or greater final visual acuity.[3]

The anatomy involved in a lateral canthotomy is represented in **Figure 28.3**. The lateral canthal tendon lies posterior to the lateral canthus. It attaches to the lateral canthal tubercule, which is a projection of the lateral zygomatic portion of the orbital rim. The tendon has both superior and inferior arms and attaches the tarsal plates to the orbital rim, providing anterior support to the globe. Cutting through the lateral canthus and ligating the lateral canthal tendon removes this support, allowing the globe to move anteriorly more freely and reducing pressure on the optic nerve. The procedure for lateral canthotomy is detailed in **Table 28.1** and graphically represented in **Figure 28.4**. Providers should be aware that the anatomy may be distorted owing to edema or obscured by bleeding and that local anesthetic may be relatively less effective in damaged, partially anoxic tissue.

Most orbital fractures do not need to be repaired. Traditionally, orbital fractures requiring emergent or urgent repair have muscle entrapment. This entrapment can lead to significant ischemia of the muscle and resultant permanent diplopia. Larger fractures are usually repaired after the acute swelling of the orbital and periorbital regions has improved. Operative fractures include orbital floor or medial wall fractures that involve more than 50% of the wall, result in more than 2 mm of

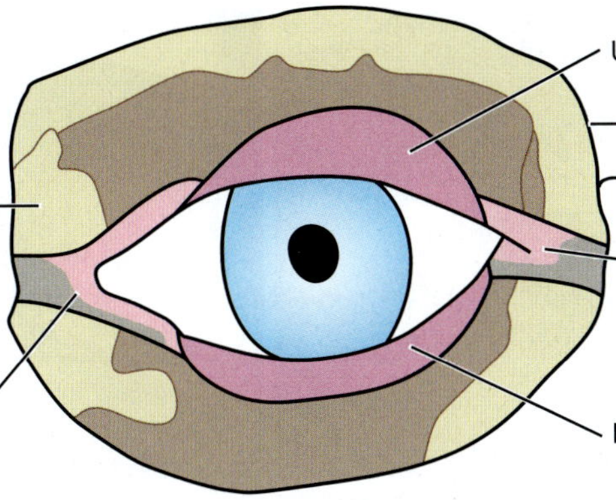

Figure 28.3: Canthal anatomy. (From Amer E, El-Rahman Abbas A. Ocular compartment syndrome and lateral canthotomy procedure. *J Emerg Med*. 2019;56(3):294-297. Figure 1.)

TABLE 28.1 Lateral Canthotomy

Equipment

- Small forceps (Paufique)
- Small hemostats
- Small scissor (Stevens scissor)
- Local anesthetic
- 4 × 4 gauze
- Disposable high-temp cautery

Procedure

- Have the patient lie in a supine position
- Inject local anesthetic into the region of the lateral canthus, with the needle pointing away from the globe
- Prep the lateral canthal region with betadine or chlorhexidine
- Using the hemostats, crush the tissues of the lateral canthus from the lateral margin to the lateral bony orbital rim for 30 s to 1 min
- Place the posterior blade of the scissors along the conjunctival side of the lateral canthus
- Cut across the lateral canthus in a full-thickness fashion
- Hold the cut edge of the lateral lower eyelid with the forceps, and pull the lid superiorly and away from the globe
- Insert the scissors into the wound with the tip pointed toward the nasal region
- Make a subcutaneous incision across the eyelid just below the tarsal plate (approximately 5 mm inferior to the eyelid margin)
- Continue the incision until the lower eyelid is very mobile
- Provide hemostasis with pressure and a disposable high-temp handheld cautery if needed.

Findings

- Pain
- Reduced eye movements
- Loss of vision or reducing vision
- Tight eyelids

Cautions

- Local anesthetic should always be injected with the needle pointing away from the globe
- Despite local anesthetic, patients will often still experience some degree of discomfort during the procedure and should be cautioned accordingly beforehand.

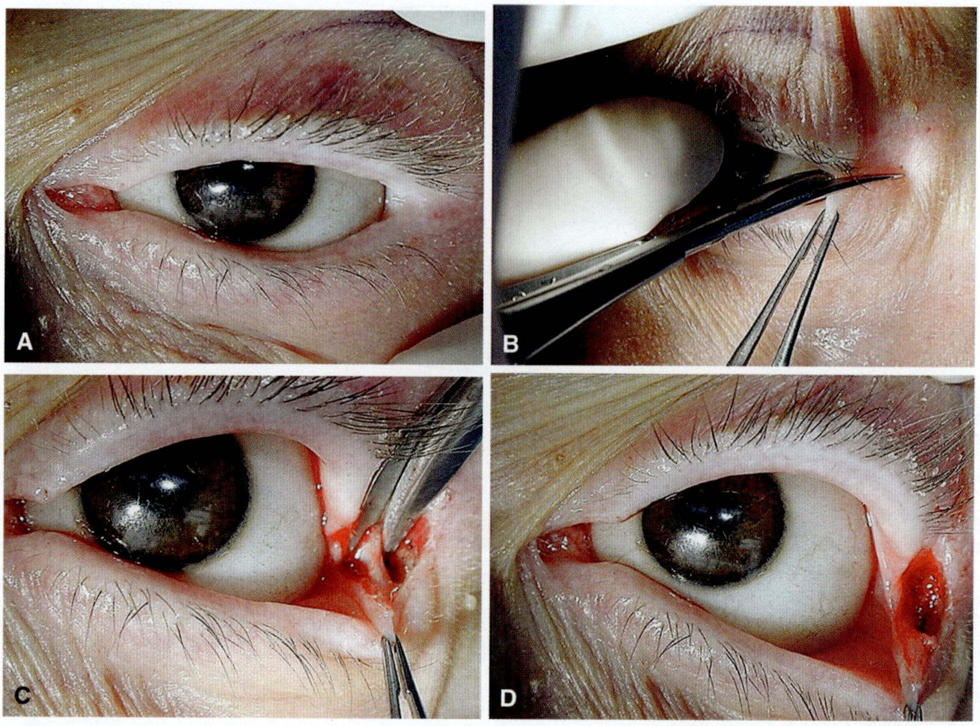

Figure 28.4: A-D, Lateral canthotomy procedure. (From Amer E, El-Rahman Abbas A. Ocular compartment syndrome and lateral canthotomy procedure. *J Emerg Med*. 2019;56(3):294-297. Figure 2.)

enophthalmos, or where nonresolving diplopia is present.[3,5] Lateral wall fractures, including zygomaticomaxillary complex fractures, typically benefit from repair if malocclusion or trismus is present and in cases of malar flattening. Orbital roof fractures rarely require repair, even when quite large, unless optic nerve compromise is present, visual acuity is worsening, or if there is pulsatile proptosis.

PEDIATRIC CONCERNS

The main difference between pediatric and adult patients in orbital trauma is the increased incidence of extraocular muscle entrapment. The bones of the orbit are more elastic and resilient in children than in adults, and, therefore, when a fracture occurs it may rebound into a nondisplaced position, taking and trapping extraocular musculature into the fracture line. This injury can be challenging to diagnose in young children, who may not be able to comply with examination requirements. It is also possible for such an injury not to cause pain or diplopia immediately, leading to delayed diagnosis. Clinicians should have a high index of suspicion for entrapment of extraocular muscles in children and a low threshold for CT imaging if orbital fracture is suspected.

TIPS AND PEARLS

- Lateral canthotomy with inferior cantholysis can be vision saving in cases of OCS and must not be delayed for ophthalmology consultation unless immediately available.
- The threshold for orbital imaging should be low. Orbital fracture and other injuries are common in multisystem trauma and may not be initially apparent on examination.
- Except for OCS, most orbital injuries can be repaired after initial patient stabilization and surgical care for other traumatic injuries. Surgical timing is controversial but in studies is measured in days or weeks rather than hours. Consultation with ophthalmology can help the emergency provider and the patient decide the appropriate timing of definitive care.

EVIDENCE

What is the threshold for imaging the orbit in patients presenting with orbital trauma?

Forty-three percent of pediatric patients and 5% of adults with orbital fractures do not have external visible signs on examination.[2] Clinicians should image (with CT) pediatric patients with a mechanism suggesting orbital trauma. In adults, pursue imaging in obtunded patients or in patients with chemosis, a Seidel sign, exophthalmos, bony tenderness to the orbital rim, or visual field or acuity changes. Do not discount pain with extraocular muscle movement, diplopia, or orbital contusion—they are all closely associated with orbital fracture even if there are no visible signs suggesting fracture.

How emergently do lateral canthotomies need to be performed?

Delaying the procedure of lateral canthotomy with cantholysis leads to adverse patient outcomes. These can include reduced vision or blindness. The sooner this can be performed, the better, and within 2 hours from the time of development of OCS is necessary to prevent vision loss.[5] Although there is a time-associated increased loss of vision with delay in addressing OCS, there does not appear to be a strict "cutoff" time after which lateral canthotomy becomes futile, so a delay in patient presentation is not an indication to omit this procedure.[11] There does not appear to be an association between the specialty of the performing clinician and visual outcomes after lateral canthotomy, so emergency providers should not delay lateral canthotomy owing to fears of procedural competence or iatrogenic complications.[11]

What is the recommended timeline for ophthalmology evaluation of entrapped soft tissue in orbital fractures?

Most orbital fractures do not appear to require immediate repair, although the literature is conflicting on appropriate surgical timing. A meta-analysis[12] of studies analyzing the timing of surgical repair found more persistent diplopia in patients repaired more than 14 days post injury but was weakened by inclusion of studies with differing definitions of diplopia and based on studies that came to heterogeneous conclusions on the timing of surgical repair. Consultation with an ophthalmologist can help the emergency provider to determine the timing of follow-up and repair. In general, if there is no evidence of OCS, referral can be urgent rather than emergent.[2,5]

References

1. Turvey TA, Golden BA. Orbital anatomy for the surgeon. *Oral Maxillofac Surg Clin North Am*. 2012;24(4)525-536.
2. Roth FS, Koshy JC, Goldberg JS, Soparkar CN. Pearls of orbital trauma management. *Semin Plast Surg*. 2010;24(4):398-410.
3. Voss JO, Hartwig S, Doll C, Hoffmeister B, Raguse JD, Adolphs N. The "tight orbit": incidence and management of the orbital compartment syndrome. *J Craniomaxillofac Surg*. 2016;44(8):1008-1014.
4. McCallum E, Keren S, Lapira M, Norris JH. Orbital compartment syndrome: an update with review of the literature. *Clin Ophthalmol*. 2019;13:2189-2194.
5. Yamanaka Y, Watanabe A, Sotozono C, Kinoshita S. Impact of surgical timing of postoperative ocular motility in orbital blowout fractures. *Br J Ophthalmol*. 2018;102(3):398-403.
6. Lozada KN, Cleveland PW, Smith JE. Orbital trauma. *Semin Plast Surg*. 2019;33(2):106-113.
7. Park J, Yang SC, Choi HY. Epidemiology and clinical patterns of ocular trauma at a level 1 trauma center in Korea. *J Korean Med Sci*. 2021;36(1):e5.
8. Kim BB, Qaqish C, Frangos J, Caccamese JF Jr. Oculocardiac reflex induced by an orbital floor fracture: report of a case and review of the literature. *J Oral Maxillofac Surg*. 2012;70(11):2614-2619.
9. Worthington JP. Isolated posterior orbital floor fractures, diplopia and oculocardiac reflexes: a 10-year review. *Br J Oral Maxillofac Surg*. 2010;48(2):127-130.
10. Broadway DC. How to test for a relative afferent pupillary defect (RAPD). *Community Eye Health*. 2016;29(96):68-69.
11. Dixon JL, Beams OK, Levine BJ, Papas MA, Passarello BA. Visual outcomes after traumatic retrobulbar hemorrhage are not related to time or intraocular pressure. *Am J Emerg Med*. 2020;38(11):2308-2312.
12. Damgaard OE, Larsen CG, Felding UA, Toft PB, von Buchwald C. Surgical timing of the orbital "blowout" fracture: a systematic review and meta-analysis. *Otolaryngol Head Neck Surg*. 2016;155(3):387-390.

CHAPTER 29

Orbital Tumors

Alison V. Crum

Samantha F. Bordonaro

THE CLINICAL CHALLENGE

There are many types of orbital tumors or masses that can occur in and around the orbit. The diagnosis and management can vary greatly depending on the cause. Owing to the potentially slow progression of this type of orbital disease, diagnosis can be difficult, and exam findings may be extremely subtle. The urgency required in terms of identification and treatment may also vary, making it important for any type of provider to have some baseline knowledge about orbital tumors and their identification and early management.

PATHOPHYSIOLOGY

When considering the pathophysiology of orbital tumors, there are several main categories to consider. These can be broken down into several groups: inflammatory lesions, orbital cystic lesions, orbital vascular and hemorrhagic lesions, orbital peripheral nerve and other neural tumors, lacrimal gland primary epithelial tumors, orbital histiocytic tumors/pseudotumors, and neoplastic tumors (**Table 29.1, Figures 29.1-29.5**).[1-3] Neoplastic tumors include lymphoid tumors and leukemia, which may be primary or secondary or represent metastases.

APPROACH/THE FOCUSED EXAM

Findings related to orbital tumors on exam may be subtle and may have developed over time, making it difficult for the patient to have noticed much change. On exam, looking at the position of the eyeballs within the face and determining whether the face appears completely symmetric is an important place to start (**Figure 29.6**).

In the emergency department (ED) or urgent care center, providers may have access only to rulers. However, more sophisticated devices for a more objective symmetry assessment may be available with the McCoy facial trisquare or Hertels exophthalmometer (**Figure 29.7**).

Assessing the patient with a "worm's eye view" may also be helpful. This is when you have the patient look up to the ceiling and view the face from the chin looking upward (**Figure 29.8**).

When approaching the exam, consider "the P's" of orbital lesions.[4]

Proptosis

Proptosis describes one eye being farther forward in the eye socket than normal. There are two types of proptosis to recognize. Axial proptosis occurs owing to thyroid orbitopathy or thyroid eye disease. You can assess firmness of proptosis with "resistance to retropulsion." Have the patient close their eyes, and with equal pressure from your two thumbs, press gently onto their upper eyelid. The globe will move posteriorly into the eye socket. This can be described as "soft" or "no resistance to retropulsion," like compressing a grape or cherry tomato. Patients' upper lids with orbital

TABLE 29.1 Pathophysiology of Common Orbital Tumors

Orbital Tumor	Pathophysiology
Inflammatory lesions (61%)	• Inflammatory lesions can often masquerade as orbital tumors and include diagnoses such as preseptal and orbital cellulitis, conjunctivitis, uveitis, and episcleritis.

Orbital cystic lesions (10%)	• Orbital dermoid cysts are the most common (37%).
	  • This is a congenital lesion that forms from epithelial cells that are entrapped during embryogenesis beneath the surface epithelium, often near bony sutures.
	• Mucoceles usually arise from frontal or ethmoid sinuses owing to chronic inflammation that invades the orbit.
	  • If pus filled, this is called mucopyocele.
	  • If children, may be from cystic fibrosis.

Orbital vascular and hemorrhagic lesions (5%)	• Cavernous hemangioma:
	  • Most common benign adult vascular orbital tumor. A congenital abnormality resulting in slow growth of endothelial cell-lined vessels surrounded by a fibrous capsule. Usually become apparent during middle age and may not exhibit swelling or external signs (Figure 29.1).
	• Arteriovenous fistulas:
	  • Occur from abnormal communications between previously normal arteries and veins. 75% occur owing to trauma, often in younger patients. 25% can occur spontaneously and are more likely in the elderly.
	  • Two forms:
	    • Carotid cavernous fistulas are considered high flow (Figure 29.2).
	    • Dural cavernous fistulas are considered low flow and often caused by systemic hypertension and atherosclerosis.

Orbital peripheral nerve tumors/ other neural tumors	• Orbital neurofibroma (Figure 29.3):
	  • Benign peripheral nerve tumor
	  • Often presents with proptosis, globe displacement, diplopia
	  • May be localized or plexiform. The plexiform type is always associated with Neurofibromatosis Type 1 (NF-1)

Lacrimal gland primary epithelial tumors	• Lacrimal gland duct epithelial cyst (dacryops):
	  • Inclusion cyst develops secondary to occlusion of one or more of the ducts that drains from the lacrimal gland to the conjunctival fornix.
	  • Usually arises from the palpebral lobe, may be unilateral or bilateral, will often be painless and nontender.

Orbital histiocytic tumors/ pseudotumors	• Langerhans cell histiocytosis (eosinophilic granuloma and formerly known as Histiocytosis X) (Figure 29.4):
	  • Pathologic Langerhans cells proliferate, often with inflammatory cells (primarily eosinophils) causing local, often bony, destruction.
	  • Typically occur in the 1st decade of life and often present as swelling in the superotemporal aspect of the orbit and often accompanied by pain, redness, tenderness, rarely bilateral.

Neoplasms	• Primary orbital neoplasms:
	  • Lymphoma is the most common in the orbit (Figure 29.5).
	  • Malignant proliferation of abnormal lymphocytic cells (often B-cell origin) and include the following:
	    • Extranodal marginal cell lymphoma (EMZL) a.k.a. mucosal associated lymphoid tissues (MALT)
	      • Follicular lymphoma
	      • Diffuse large B-cell lymphoma (DLBCL)
	      • Mantle cell lymphoma (MCL)
	  • Most common presenting symptoms include swelling (48%), mass (49%), and proptosis (37%).
	  • Primary intra*orbital* lymphomas are often associated with autoimmune disease.
	• Orbital metastatic neoplasms:
	  • The most frequent adult metastatic cancers include breast, lung, renal cell, thyroid, and prostate cancer.

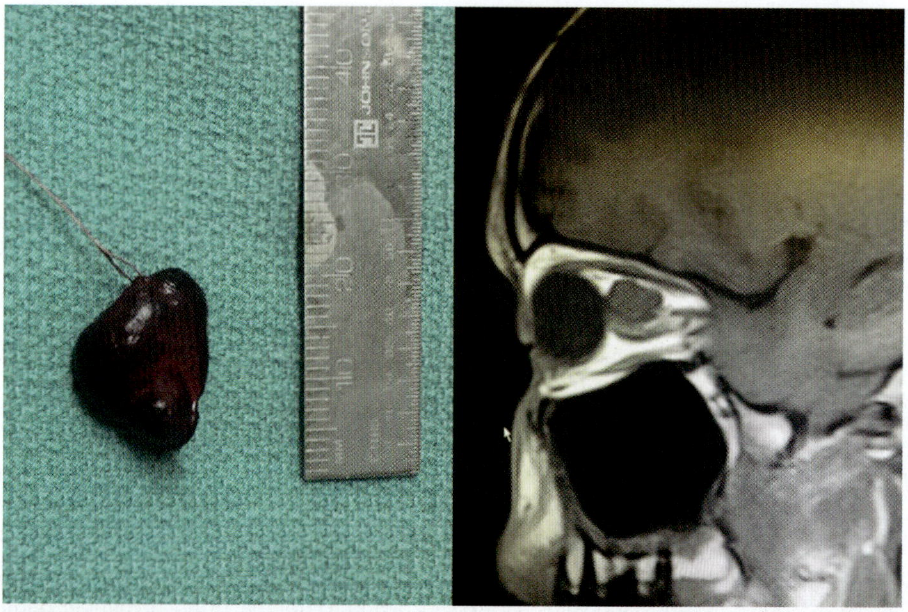

Figure 29.1: Left: Cavernous hemangioma seen as an encapsulated mass with homogeneous enhancement. Right: Cavernous hemangioma as seen on magnetic resonance imaging (MRI). (Courtesy of Alison V. Crum, MD, John A. Moran Eye Center, University of Utah.)

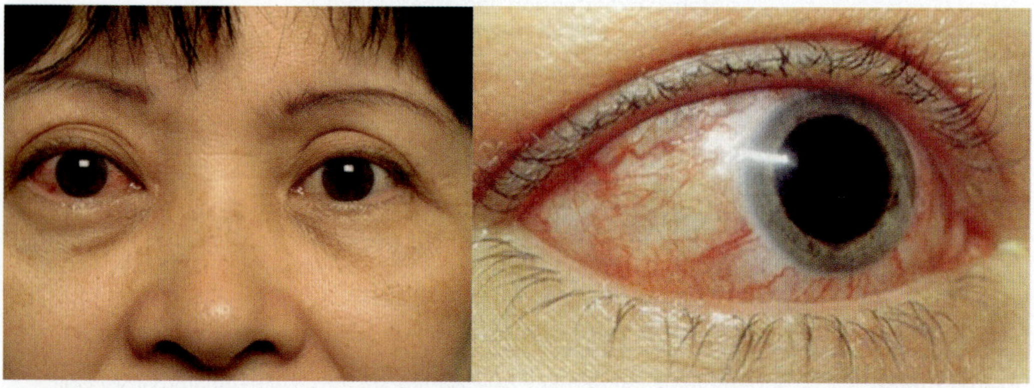

Figure 29.2: Left: Patient with carotid cavernous fistula of right eye. Right: dilated conjunctival "corkscrew" vessels and appearance of congestion of the ocular tissues of the upper and lower eyelids.

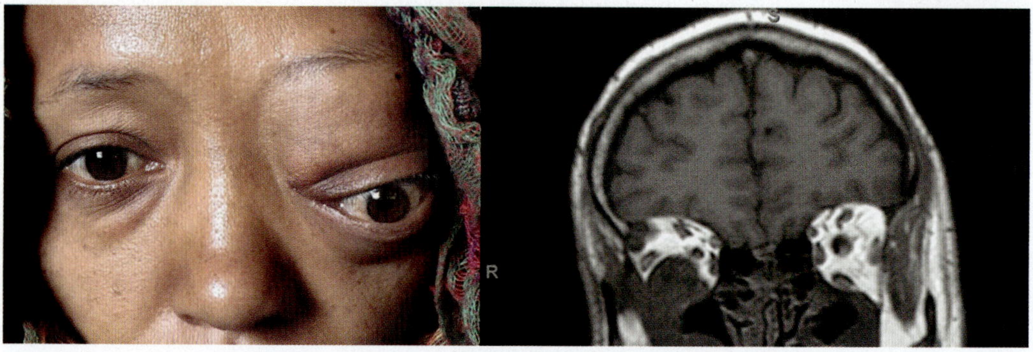

Figure 29.3: Left: Orbital neurofibroma in a patient with Neurofibromatosis Type 1 (NF1) of right orbit. Right: MRI of a different patient with NF1 causing inferior displacement of the globe. (Courtesy of Alison V. Crum, MD, John A. Moran Eye Center, University of Utah.)

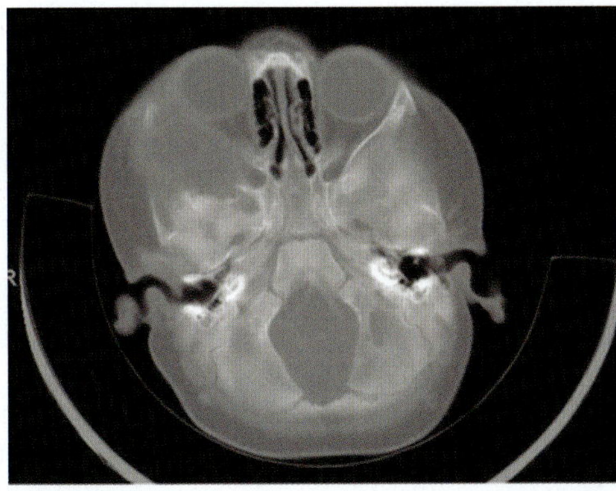

Figure 29.4: Langerhan cell histiocytosis on magnetic resonance imaging (MRI) demonstrating bony erosion of the sphenoid bone of the right lateral orbit. (Courtesy of Alison V. Crum, MD, John A. Moran Eye Center, University of Utah.)

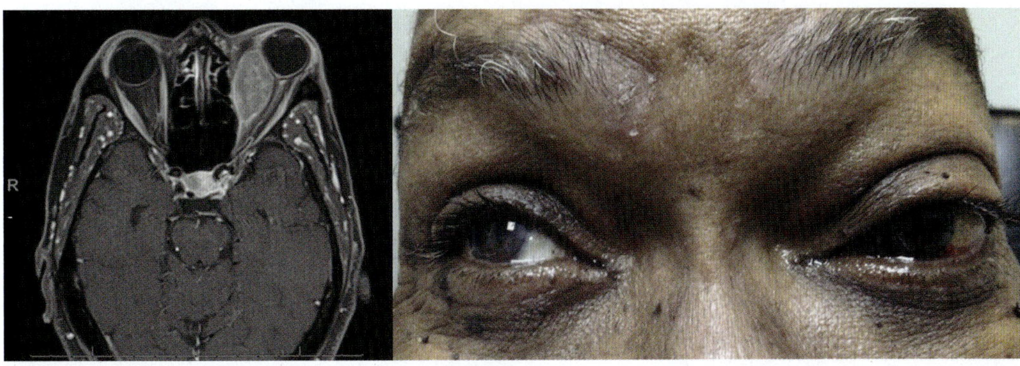

Figure 29.5: Large B-cell lymphoma. Left: Magnetic resonance imaging (MRI) showing tumor in the patient's medial left orbit. Right: Same patient with clinical signs of left-sided proptosis and difficulty adducting their left eye. (Courtesy of Alison V. Crum, MD, John A. Moran Eye Center, University of Utah.)

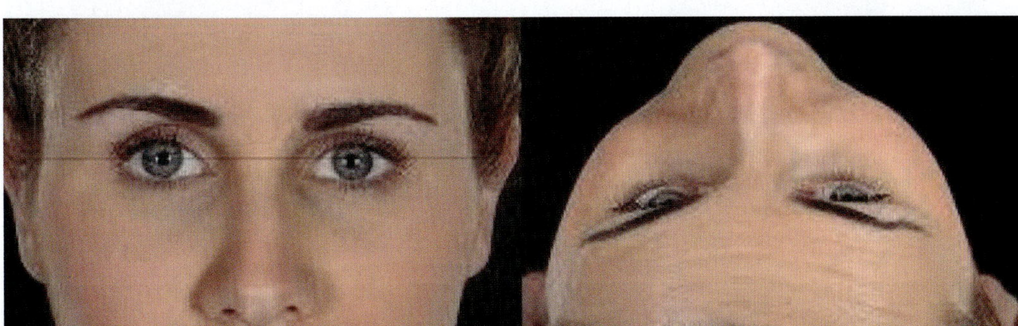

Figure 29.6: Silent sinus syndrome. The images show hypoglobus and enopthalmos of the patient's left eye in the anterior project (left image) and from above (right image). (From Ferro A, Basyuni S, Santhanam V. Not so silent sinus syndrome: a case report. *Int J Surg Case Rep.* 2016;23:1-3.)

masses or thyroid orbitopathy will resist your thumb's pressure and will feel harder, like pressing on your chin/on a bone. This can be described as "moderate to severe resistance to retropulsion."

Nonaxial proptosis occurs when tumors infiltrate from around the "orbital bony box," pushing the orbital contents forward (**Figure 29.9**). Interpupillary distance is one way to assess nonaxial proptosis. Orbital tumors can arise from the medial wall of the orbit, for example tumors that arise

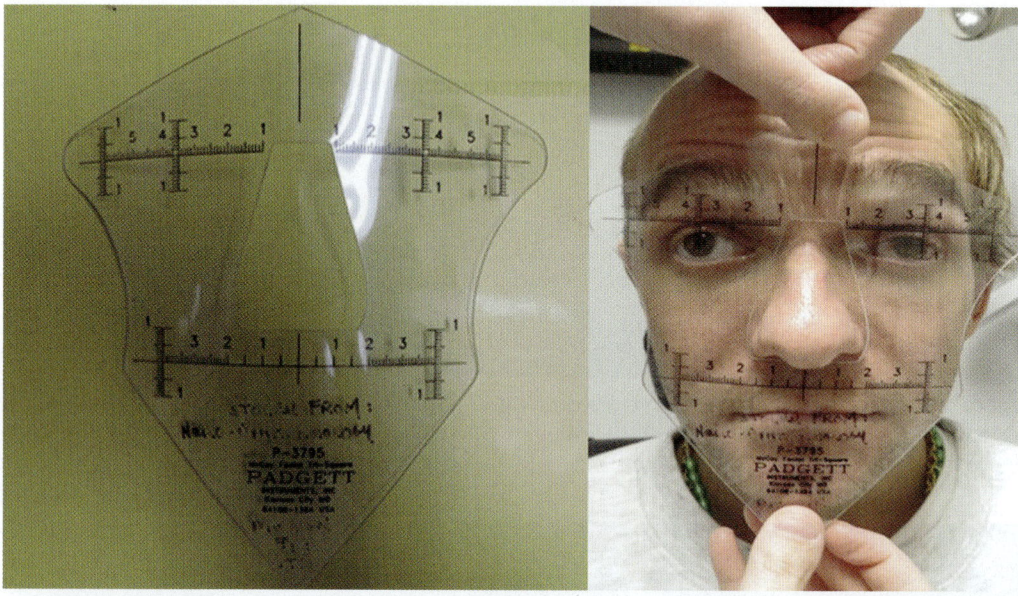

Figure 29.7: The trisquare tool shown by itself and then with correct placement on a patient's face to measure asymmetry. (From Goldberg RA, Shorr N. The McCoy Facial Trisquare: A useful instrument for measuring dystopia of the globe and canthi. *Ophthalmic Surg; Pitman*. 1993;24(5):355-356.)

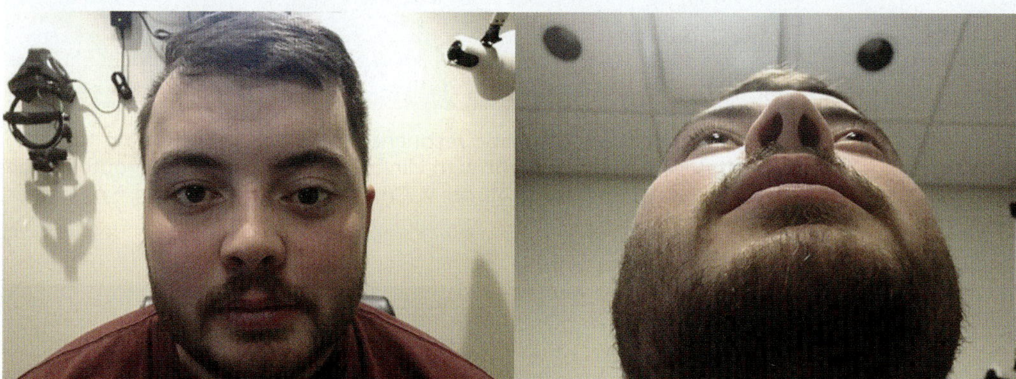

Figure 29.8: Right: Patient with inferior displacement of the left eyeball (hypoglobus). Left: Same patient with a "worm's eye view" revealing mild proptosis. (Courtesy of Alison V. Crum, MD, John A. Moran Eye Center, University of Utah.)

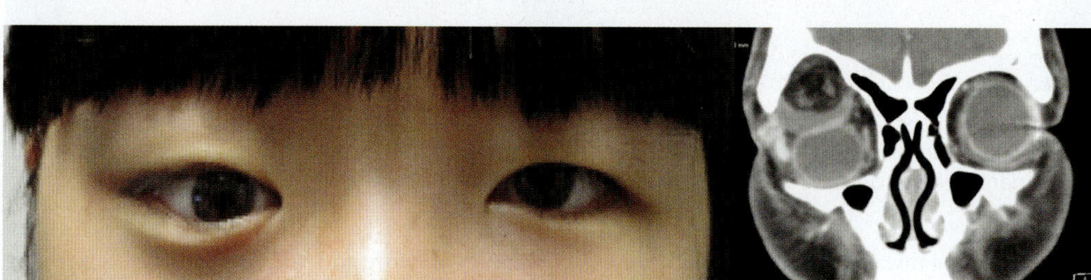

Figure 29.9: Left: Proptosis and hypoglobus of right eye. Right: Intraorbital dermoid lesion in the same patient. (Courtesy of Alison V. Crum, MD, John A. Moran Eye Center, University of Utah.)

within the nasal cavity or abscesses that arise owing to a subperiosteal abscess collection from sinus disease. Interpupillary distance can be thought of as the distance between eyeballs. Enlarged interpupillary distance is often a difference in genetics or facial mechanics and is not caused by an acute change, such as an injury or trauma; however, in some rare cases, subperiosteal abscesses or fluid collections can cause globe movement laterally.

Hypoglobus refers to one eye being lower than the other. This may be attributable to negative pressure in the maxillary sinus, pulling the orbital floor downward, causing the floor to bow and orbital tissue to sink back and cause the appearance of the eye to be smaller (enophthalmos) as in silent sinus syndrome, from maxillary sinusitis (Figure 29.8).

Pain

More invasive, rapidly progressive tumors are commonly associated with pain owing to destruction of bone or compression of orbital tissue or orbital vessels leading to congestion. On exam, congestion can be indicated by redness of conjunctival vessels, which become tortuous and may appear twisted like a corkscrew (Figure 29.2). This can be seen all over the globe (common with a carotid cavernous fistula), or it can be segmental (just medially and laterally), as in thyroid eye disease. Edema of eyelids also suggests decreased venous outflow or obstruction.

Progression

Rapid progression is more likely to be malignant. When examining the patient, it can be helpful to compare their current appearance to that on their driver's license to get a sense of the degree of change.

Pulsatility

This occurs with erosion of the bony walls of the orbit and can be seen with carotid cavernous fistula, neurofibromatosis, or orbital cephalocoele.

DIFFERENTIAL DIAGNOSIS

The differential diagnosis for orbital tumors can be broad and is often dependent on the location of the tumor. If you consider the orbit to be like a box or a shot glass with the open top looking out at you, the displacement of the eye can guide your differential. Considering what anatomic structures surround the orbit can help one identify what might be invading it. Potential orbital tumors may push the globe in from the frontal area of the orbit, up from the maxillary sinus/area, in from the ethmoids, or lateral from the sphenoid wing (**Table 29.2**).

TABLE 29.2 Differential Diagnosis of Common Orbital Disorders Based on Globe Displacement

Displacement of the Globe	Differential Diagnosis
Superior displacement	• Maxillary sinus tumor
Superonasal displacement	• Mucocele • Mucopyocele • Encephalocele • Neurofibroma • Lymphoma
Inferomedial displacement	• Frontozygomatic suture-line dermoid • Lacrimal gland tumor • Lymphoma
Inferior displacement	• Frontal sinus tumor • Meningocele
Inward displacement (enophthalmos)	• Sclerosing tumors (ie, scirrhous breast cancer)
Outward displacement (exophthalmos)	• Thyroid orbitopathy (grave)[a] • Lymphoma • Idiopathic orbital inflammation

[a]Often bilateral.

TABLE 29.3 Differential Diagnosis of Orbital Tumors Based on Age

Most Common Pediatric Tumors/Masqueraders	Most Common Adult Tumors/Masqueraders
• Orbital cellulitis • Pseudotumor • Dermoid cysts • Capillary hemangioma • Lymphangioma • Rhabdomyosarcoma • Glioma • Neurofibroma • Metastases • Neuroblastoma • Leukemia	• Thyroid orbitopathy (50%) • Inflammatory lesions (11%) • Cystic lesions (10%) • Vascular neoplasms (4%) • Vascular, structural (1%) • Lymphoproliferative lesions (5%) • Lacrimal gland lesions (2%) • Secondary tumors (4%) • Mesenchymal lesions (4%) • Metastatic lesions (2%) • Optic nerve tumors (3%)

The differential diagnosis can also be approached based on the age of the patient. Different orbital tumors or entities masquerading as tumors may vary based on age (**Table 29.3**).[5]

MANAGEMENT

Management will vary based on the cause, location, and extent of the orbital tumor and can vary greatly (**Table 29.4**).[6]

TABLE 29.4 Management of Most Common Orbital Tumors

Orbital Tumors	Management
Inflammatory lesions (61%)	• Discussed elsewhere
Orbital cystic lesions (10%)	• May observe but most are removed with care to avoid rupture to prevent postoperative inflammation. • Rupture causes an inflammatory reaction that may resemble cellulitis or dacryoadenitis.
Orbital vascular and hemorrhagic lesions (5%)	• Cavernous hemangioma • Small asymptomatic hemangiomas can be observed but require surgical excision once they become symptomatic. Those occurring at the apex may require a transcranial approach.

Orbital peripheral nerve tumors/other neural tumors	• Orbital neurofibroma
	  • Diffuse plexiform type is unresectable and would be managed conservatively with debulking if needed.
	  • Localized orbital neurofibroma would be managed similar to other tumors with resection when indicated.

Lacrimal gland primary epithelial tumors	• Lacrimal gland ductal epithelial cyst (dacryops)
	  • Asymptomatic dacryops are observed.
	  • Symptomatic are resected.

Orbital histiocytic tumors/ pseudotumors	• Orbital Langerhans cell histiocytosis (eosinophilic granuloma) (formerly known as Histiocytosis X)
	• May spontaneously heal without treatment
	  • Open biopsy may be performed.
	  • Surgical curettage and steroid injection

Neoplasms	• Lymphoma
	  • Treatment is stage dependent.
	  • Early stage is treated with external beam radiation therapy (EBRT).
	  • Later stage is treated with chemotherapy such as rituximab and often combined with EBRT.

TIPS AND PEARLS

- When checking for resistance to retropulsion, assess the patient by comparing the test eye to your own eyes and/or the patient's unaffected eye.
- When assessing enophthalmos, the patient's eyelid position can be deceptive. An enophthalmic eye can create the appearance of ptosis if the eyelid falls against the eye at a lower position. Likewise, ptosis may make the eye appear small in some cases.

EVIDENCE

Is radiographic imaging so advanced that diagnosis of orbital lesions can be made with imaging only?

According to authors Koukkoulli et al. in the UK, who evaluated over 100 orbital lesions, diagnosis cannot be made with imaging alone, and surgical biopsy should be the gold standard.

A total of 112 orbital biopsies were carried out over a 12-year period, and the correct diagnosis was only reached by ophthalmologists and radiologists in just over 50% of the cases shown to them. Orbital lesions that were of a vascular etiology were usually accurately identified; however, lesions that were inflammatory or hematologic lesions were more difficult to identify radiologically without a pathologic sample. Surgical biopsy is still the gold standard for orbital lesion diagnosis.[7]

References

1. Calandriello, L. Cavernous venous malformation (cavernous hemangioma) of the orbit: current concepts and a review of the literature. *Surv Ophthalmol*. 2017;62(4):393-403.
2. Gunduz, AK. Overview of benign and malignant lacrimal gland tumors. *Curr Opin Ophthalmol*. 2018;29(5):458-468.
3. Heegaard, S. Orbital lymphoma—an interventional multicenter retrospective study. *Am J Ophthalmol*. 2019;199:44-57.
4. Alkatan, HM. Demographics of pediatric orbital lesions: a tertiary eye center experience in Saudi Arabia. *J Epidemiol Glob Health*. 2019;9(1):3-10.
5. Patel, SR. Interventions for orbital lymphangioma. *Cochrane Database Syst Rev*. 2019;5:CD013000.
6. Parker, RT. Optic nerve sheath meningiomas: prevalence, impact, and management strategies. *Eye Brain*. 2018;10:85-99.
7. Koukkoulli, A. How accurate is the clinical and radiological evaluation of orbital lesions in comparison to surgical orbital biopsy? *Eye*. 2018;32:1329-1333.

CHAPTER 30

Preseptal and Orbital Cellulitis

Jamie Lea Schaefer
Jimmy Truong

CLINICAL CHALLENGE

Periorbital infections are a relatively common presenting complaint in the emergency and urgent care settings, especially for children.[1] The extent of infection is what distinguishes preseptal from orbital cellulitis, and differentiation between the two is important because morbidity and treatment can vary greatly.[2] Preseptal cellulitis is an infection that has not extended posterior to the orbital septum with vision and eye movements typically unaffected, whereas orbital cellulitis extends deep into the tissues of the orbital socket and is often marked by changes to ocular function.[2,3] Furthermore, noninfectious or associated etiologies, such as idiopathic orbital inflammation, complicate the differential diagnosis and must be considered.

PATHOPHYSIOLOGY

The orbital septum is a fibrous connective tissue barrier that separates the preseptal eyelid skin and orbicularis muscle from the orbital tissues—the globe, extraocular muscles, orbital fat, and neurovascular tissues.

Common portals through which pathogens enter the periocular tissues include the mucosal surfaces of the eye, respiratory and digestive tracts, as well as the skin.[3-5] Ingress from the skin may result from insect bites, trauma, and other inflammatory conditions of the Meibomian glands and hair follicles along the eyelid margin. Sinusitis, dental abscesses, infections of the lacrimal sac (dacryocystitis) (**Figure 30.1**), or other adjacent infections can extend into the periorbital region as well. The ethmoid sinuses are often the source of orbital cellulitis—the thin bone of the lamina papyracea, bordering the medial side of the orbit, is perforated by numerous vessels and nerves and can allow extension of sinusitis.[2,6]

Most periorbital infections are secondary to the *Staphylococcus*, *Streptococcus,* and *Haemophilus* species.[2,5] Importantly, there has been a rise in the occurrence of methicillin-resistant *Staphylococcal* infections, whereas the incidence of infection in children by *Haemophilus* has decreased significantly with the advent of immunization against *H influenza* type B. This reduction secondary to immunization, however, has not been seen with PCV7 vaccination against *Streptococcus* pneumonia. *Moraxella catarrhalis*, in addition to anaerobic organisms of the upper respiratory tract, has also been implicated in periorbital infections. *Peptococcus, Peptostreptococcus,* and *Bacteroides* are organisms known to cause cellulitis after human or animal bites. In patients who are pregnant or otherwise immunocompromised, fungal organisms of *Mucormycosis* and *Aspergillosis* should be considered. Following trauma, *S aureus* and *S pyogenes* are the most common pathogens.

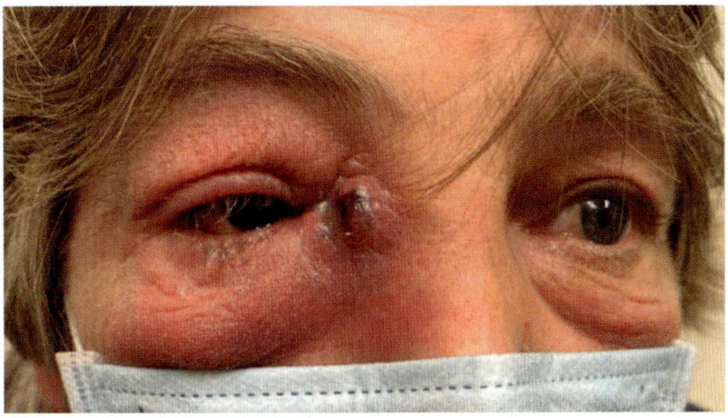

Figure 30.1: Right dacryocystitis with preseptal cellulitis.

Preseptal Cellulitis

Preseptal cellulitis occurs approximately 4 times more often than orbital cellulitis and is more frequent in children, particularly those younger than 5 years of age (**Figure 30.2**). Clinical features include swelling, erythema, and pain of the eyelid with the area of maximal inflammation indicating the likely source of infection. Inflammation may induce ptosis of the upper eyelid and may also be associated with tearing, conjunctival injection, and therefore accompanying blurred vision. This disease is often preceded by an upper respiratory infection, sinusitis, dental pathology, insect bite, trauma or surgery, or other infections in the surrounding area. Conjunctivitis may also develop into preseptal cellulitis. Preseptal cellulitis is often distinguished from deeper orbital infections clinically by the absence of globe displacement, restrictions in ocular motility, or raised ocular or orbital pressure. In uncertain cases, orbital or sinus computed tomography (CT) scans are obtained to rule out orbital cellulitis.

Orbital Cellulitis

Orbital cellulitis (**Figure 30.3**) most commonly extends from infections of the ethmoid sinus, although it may also be acquired from other adjacent structures.[5,7] Less common causes include endophthalmitis, implants, retained foreign materials, or orbital tumors. Hematogenous spread is relatively rare. Orbital cellulitis occurs in all ages, but mostly in children 7 to 12 years old (older age than preseptal cellulitis) and has similar prevalence in males and females except in causes of trauma

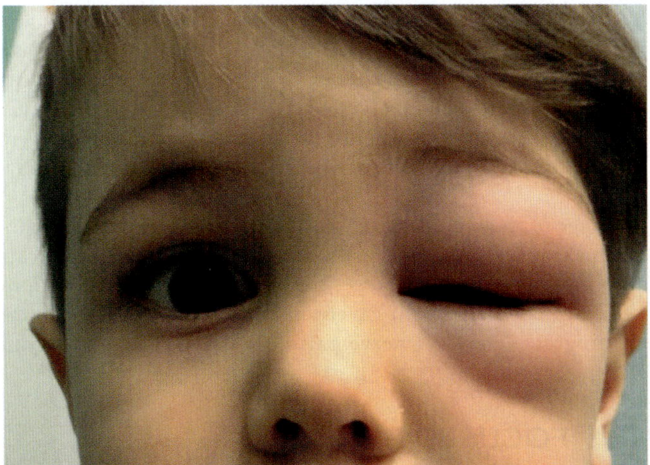

Figure 30.2: Left preseptal cellulitis.

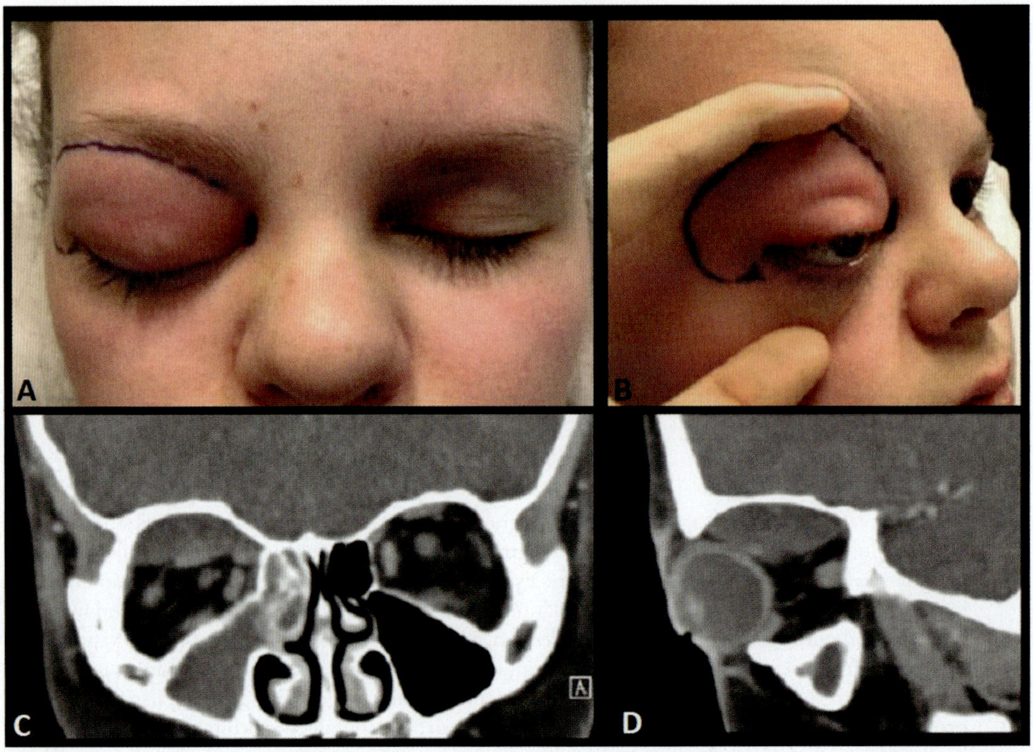

Figure 30.3: External photographs (A and B) of right orbital cellulitis with erythema and swelling confined within the orbital rims associated with proptosis and ophthalmoplegia. Coronal (C) and sagittal (D) orbital computed tomography images of a large right superior and small medial subperiosteal abscess with inferior displacement of the rectus musculature and globe with associated multifocal sinus disease.

where there is a male predominance. Children younger than 10 years are usually infected by a single aerobic pathogen, whereas older children and adults have more complex infections involving aerobic and anaerobic pathogens and are more likely to be polymicrobial.

Clinical features include pain, swelling, and erythema of the conjunctiva and eyelids, usually confined within the orbital rims. Between the bony orbital walls and the periorbita, or periosteum of the orbit, the potential subperiosteal space provides an area for potential accumulation and may lead to a subperiosteal abscess with mass effect similar to a tumor. Proptosis is usually present, and the globe may be displaced with the presence of an abscess. Abscesses larger than 10 mm and those that are in a nonmedial location should be evaluated for surgical drainage. Orbital inflammation may lead to raised intraocular pressure and restricted and painful eye movements with diplopia. Compressive optic neuropathy from orbital compartment syndrome can lead to severe permanent vision loss.

Venous drainage of the orbit through the cavernous sinus connects the orbit to the central nervous system, making severe intracranial infections a possible complication. Cranial nerves III, IV, V_1, and VI traverse the cavernous sinus and can be affected with the spread of orbital cellulitis. Intracranial extension with cavernous sinus thrombosis should be suspected when the patient has progressive cranial nerve palsies, fever, headache, and altered consciousness (see **Table 30.1**).

APPROACH/THE FOCUSED EXAM

Important elements of the history include age, medical history (eg, chronic sinusitis, diabetes, human immunodeficiency virus [HIV], leukemia, and other immunosuppressive disorders), vaccination

TABLE 30.1 Clinical Features of Preseptal Versus Orbital Cellulitis

	Preseptal Cellulitis	Orbital Cellulitis
Eyelid erythema	Erythema of eyelids and/or periorbital area	Erythema of eyelids usually confined to orbital rims
Eyelid swelling	Swelling with ability to sufficiently lift for examination of the globe	If swelling inhibits the ability to lift lid sufficiently to examine suspect orbital cellulitis
Vision	Normal	Impaired (eg, reduced acuity, loss of red color perception)
Pupils	Normal (equal, round, and reactive to light and accommodation)	Normal or relative afferent pupillary defect (RAPD)
Conjunctiva/sclera	White, but can have injection	Injection and/or chemosis
Extraocular movements	Normal and painless	Impaired and/or painful
Globe position	Normal	Possible globe displacement (eg, proptosis)
General/systemic	Well appearing	Possibly toxic appearing

status, and ocular history (eg, stye/chalazion, trauma, surgery, dacryocystitis). Eliciting the history of a recent illness such as upper respiratory infections, sinusitis, or dental infections may provide context for a risk of these infections. It is important to assess eye-specific complaints like pain with extraocular movement or at rest and changes to visual acuity. Specific elements of the ocular examination also include general appearance; visual acuity (use corrective lenses); confrontational visual fields (lift the eyelid if ptosis is present); pupils including the presence of a relative afferent pupillary defect; globe displacement (eg, proptosis); eye movements; eyelid inspection for edema, erythema, and lesions; conjunctiva/sclera inspection for redness or chemosis; fundoscopy for optic nerve swelling or pallor and venous tortuosity. If any discharge is present, cultures should be obtained.

DIFFERENTIAL DIAGNOSIS

For additional details see **Table 30.2**.

TABLE 30.2 Differential Diagnosis of Eyelid Swelling

Disease	Pathophysiology	Signs and Symptoms
Preseptal cellulitis	Infection of the superficial eyelid and soft tissues, anterior to the orbital septum.	Swelling, erythema, and pain of the eyelid; vision and eye movements typically unaffected
Orbital cellulitis	Infection of the soft tissues within the orbit, posterior to the orbital septum	Erythematous, edematous, painful eyelid; extraocular movements limited from pain or muscle involvement; chemosis; vision changes
Autoimmune orbital inflammation (eg, thyroid eye disease)	Noninfectious edema and inflammation of ocular muscles and orbital soft tissues	Bilateral (can be asymmetric) subacute erythema and swelling with possible limitation of extraocular movements
Atopic dermatitis	Sensitivity to allergen with skin manifestation	Dry, raised plaque
Basal cell carcinoma	Neoplasm	Umbilicated elevated lesion with telangiectasia, with possible ulceration

(continued)

TABLE 30.2 Differential Diagnosis of Eyelid Swelling (*continued*)

Disease	Pathophysiology	Signs and Symptoms
Blepharitis	Inflammation of the eyelid margin and base of eyelashes	Erythema of eyelid margin with irritation, itching and dandrufflike scales
Capillary hemangioma	Hamartomatous proliferation of vascular endothelial cells	Superficial red raised lesion or deep dark blue lesion; size increases with crying
Cavernous sinus thrombosis	Thrombosed superior ophthalmic vein and cerebral veins	Ophthalmoplegia, fever, headache, and altered consciousness
Chalazion	Obstruction (blockage or inflammation) of a meibomian gland of the eyelid	Painless discrete mass within the eyelid
Conjunctivitis (allergic, bacterial, or viral)	Inflammation of the conjunctiva	Injection and/or chemosis of the conjunctiva, associated with tearing and itching
Contact dermatitis	Reaction to allergen or irritant	Erythema and edema associated with pruritus
Dacryoadenitis	Inflammation of the lacrimal gland	Superolateral orbital painful swelling
Dacryocystitis	Inflammation of the lacrimal sac and duct	Painful erythematous elevation of the medial aspect of the lower eyelid
Endophthalmitis	Intraocular inflammation, usually caused by infection	Painful vision loss with injection of the conjunctiva
Herpes zoster ophthalmicus	Reactivation of a varicella zoster virus infection affecting the first division of the trigeminal nerve (V_1)	Erythematous macules, papules, and vesicles; dermatomal distribution to the forehead and upper eyelid; respects midline
Hordeolum or stye	Hordeolum: infection of the meibomian (sebaceous) glands Stye: infection of the sweat gland (gland of Zeis) of the eyelid	Tender erythematous elevation at the eyelid margin
Impetigo and erysipelas	Bacterial infection	Impetigo—pustular lesions and round red patches with yellow crusts; can be painful or itchy Erysipelas—raised, tender, well-defined bright red skin lesion
Medication effects (eg, allopurinol, cephalosporins, corticosteroids, valproic acid)	Drug reaction	Periorbital cutaneous inflammation
Orbital neoplasm	Intraorbital neoplasm	Painless proptosis, usually unilateral
Periorbital ecchymosis	Disruption of blood vessels, common in trauma	Blue or purple discoloration of skin
Squamous cell carcinoma	Neoplasm	Erythematous scaly patches or ulcers

MANAGEMENT

Preseptal Cellulitis

Once preseptal cellulitis is confirmed, treatment with antibiotics targeted toward *S aureus*, *Streptococcus* species, and, possibly, anaerobes should be started. If the patient appears to have severe disease or is less than one year of age, admission to the hospital should be considered. Owing to the rise of methicillin-resistant staphylococcus aureus (MRSA), it is recommended to start patients on trimethoprim-sulfamethoxazole or clindamycin plus amoxicillin-clavulanic acid or cefpodoxime or cefdinir for a course of 5 to 7 days.[8] Treatment should produce a prompt and complete response; however, if outpatient treatment fails after 24 to 48 hours, hospitalization with IV broad-spectrum antibiotics is the next step. Further workup with a CT scan and surgical consultation should be considered.[8]

Orbital Cellulitis

Once the diagnosis of orbital cellulitis is confirmed, broad-spectrum IV antibiotic treatment including MRSA coverage is paramount. If there are concerns for intracranial extension, anaerobic coverage should be added with metronidazole. With normal renal function, IV vancomycin with ceftriaxone, cefotaxime, ampicillin-sulbactam, or piperacillin-tazobactam is a standard recommendation.

Clinical improvement is expected after 48 to 72 hours of IV antibiotics. In these instances, transition to oral antibiotics and outpatient treatment is feasible with regimens that include oral clindamycin, or trimethoprim-sulfamethoxazole plus amoxicillin, amoxicillin-clavulanate, cefpodoxime, or cefdinir for a total of 14 days. For complicated cases, treatment should cover 21 days.

In complicated cases where there is no clinical improvement with continued fever, swelling, proptosis, pain, or changes in visual function, after 48 to 72 hours of IV antibiotics, further workup should include investigating for large subperiosteal or orbital abscesses and intracranial extension. Abscesses larger than 10 mm and those that are in a nonmedial location should be evaluated for surgical drainage.[9]

Pediatric Issues

Preseptal cellulitis is a common childhood illness and can rapidly progress to orbital cellulitis and involve intracranial structures.[10] In a retrospective pediatric study, the most common predisposing factors for preseptal cellulitis were trauma or dental abscesses.[10] Even though the risk of orbital spread is low, clinicians typically have a lower threshold for admission and IV antibiotics in pediatric patients. Fever, headache, nausea, and vomiting should raise concern for orbital cellulitis and warrant further imaging and an ophthalmology consultation.[11] "Graves eye sign," particularly ophthalmoplegia, chemosis, proptosis, pain on movement of the eye, diplopia, and elevated C-reactive protein (CRP), should prompt concern for severe orbital cellulitis. Proptosis is a specific indicator for surgical management for periorbital or preseptal cellulitis.

Orbital cellulitis is most commonly associated with sinus infections. Because orbital cellulitis in children is usually caused by a single gram-positive organism, surgical intervention is less likely to be needed in children 9 years and younger. Failure of medical management of periorbital or preseptal cellulitis should prompt consideration for further workup, including imaging and surgical intervention to prevent life-threatening complications from orbital cellulitis.[12]

TIPS AND PEARLS

- If a patient with preseptal cellulitis fails to improve on oral antibiotic for 24 to 48 hours as an outpatient, they should begin treatment if 48 to 72 hours of IV antibiotics. All cases of orbital cellulitis should be admitted for IV antibiotic treatment.
- For concurrent sinusitis, add oxymetazoline nasal spray for 3 days and saline nasal irrigation to drain sinuses.
- Serious complications of orbital cellulitis include those that extend into the central nervous system (CNS), including cavernous sinus thrombosis, meningitis, and intracranial abscess. New sixth nerve palsy in the setting of acute orbital cellulitis that is not improving is worrisome for cavernous sinus thrombosis with the cranial nerve VI running along the wall of the cavernous sinus.

EVIDENCE

Are steroids useful in the treatment of orbital cellulitis?

Owing to the variation of clinical practice, there is insufficient evidence to support the use of steroids in the management of orbital cellulitis. Further high-quality randomized controlled studies need to be performed.[13]

Do blood cultures assist in the identification of the causative organism for orbital cellulitis?

In the workup of orbital cellulitis, blood cultures have a low yield, of less than 20%. Surgical aspiration of periosteal or orbital abscess is the definitive test to find the etiology.[9]

References

1. Stimes GT, Girotto JE. Applying pharmacodynamics and antimicrobial stewardship to pediatric preseptal and orbital cellulitis. *Paediatr Drugs*. 2019;21(6):427-438.
2. Carlisle RT, Digiovanni J. Differential diagnosis of the swollen red eyelid. *Am Fam Physician*. 2015;92(2):106-112.
3. Adamson J, Waterfield T. Fifteen-minute consultation: preseptal and orbital cellulitis. *Arch Dis Child Educ Pract Ed*. 2019;104(2):79-83. Erratum in: *Arch Dis Child Educ Pract Ed*. 2019;104(5):280.
4. Wong SJ, Levi J. Management of pediatric orbital cellulitis: a systematic review. *Int J Pediatr Otorhinolaryngol*. 2018;110:123-129.
5. Fay A, Dolman P. *Diseases and Disorders of the Orbit and Ocular Adnexa*. 1st ed. Elsevier; 2017.
6. Gordon AA, Phelps PO. Management of preseptal and orbital cellulitis for the primary care physician. *Dis Mon*. 2020;66:101044.
7. Santos JC, Pinto S, Ferreira S, et al. Pediatric preseptal and orbital cellulitis: a 10-year experience. *Int J Pediatr Otorhinolaryngol*. 2019;120:82-88.
8. Bae C, Bourget D. Periorbital cellulitis (November 19, 2020). In: *StatPearls* [Internet]. StatPearls Publishing; 2021.
9. Mejia E, Vohra V, Braiman M. Ocular cellulitis (Updated February 15, 2021). In: *StatPearls* [Internet]. StatPearls Publishing; 2021.
10. Cürebal B, Şahin A, Dalgıç N. Preseptal cellulitis in children: a single-center experience. *Sisli Etfal Hastan Tip Bul*. 2019;53(4):409-412.
11. Ibrahim LF, Babl FE, Hopper SM, Bryant PA. What is the risk of missing orbital cellulitis in children? *Arch Dis Child*. 2021;106(9):896-899.
12. Murphy DC, Meghji S, Alfiky M, Bath AP. Paediatric periorbital cellulitis: a 10-year retrospective case series review. *J Paediatr Child Health*. 2021;57(2):227-233.
13. Kornelsen E, Mahant S, Parkin P, et al. Corticosteroids for periorbital and orbital cellulitis. *Cochrane Database of Syst Rev*. 2021;4:CD013535.

CHAPTER 31

Eyelid Lacerations

Kyle J. Godfrey
Sirivalli Chamarti

THE CLINICAL CHALLENGE

Eyelid trauma is a common presentation to the emergency department (ED). Eyelid lacerations account for 7.7% of all complaints of eye trauma presenting to the ED.[1,2] The eyelids contain complicated and sensitive anatomy that is easily damaged in trauma. Care must be taken to ensure that the anatomic structures and functional relationships are preserved and repaired in a timely manner. The eyelids must maintain proper position relative to the ocular surface and visual axis, have adequate functional excursion with dynamic blink, and facilitate tear drainage through the nasolachrymal system. The lacrimal outflow system must remain patent, and the punctum must maintain proper apposition to the ocular surface and tear lake. Inadequate eyelid reconstruction can cause eyelid malposition, resulting in ptosis, secondary ocular surface problems, and chronic tearing (epiphora).

PATHOPHYSIOLOGY

As a concise review of the relevant anatomy, the upper and lower eyelids should rest in close apposition to the globe and tear film. At the eyelid margin, the eyelid can be conceptualized as containing four layers organized into two lamellae: the anterior lamella, composed of eyelid skin and the circumferential orbicularis oculi muscle, and the posterior lamella, composed of the tarsus and palpebral (eyelid) conjunctiva. In the upper eyelid, the tarsus is approximately 10 mm in height and in the lower eyelid, approximately 4 mm in height.[3,4]

Beyond the tarsus, the eyelid anatomy becomes somewhat more complex. In both the upper and the lower eyelids, beneath the eyelid skin is the orbicularis oculi muscle, the circumferential protractor muscle, innervated by the temporal and zygomatic branches of the facial nerve, which enables both voluntary and involuntary blinking. Deep to the orbicularis oculi muscle is the orbital septum. The orbital septum defines the anterior boundaries of the orbit, and fuses with the periosteum of the orbital bones at the arcus marginalis, which circles the anterior margin of the bony orbital rim.

Beneath the orbital septum is orbital fat, which is generally superficial to the eyelid retractors. The eyelid retractors in the upper eyelid include the more superficial levator palpebrae superioris, which inserts on the anterior aspect of the tarsus and the deeper, sympathetically innervated Mullers muscle, which inserts at the superior border of the tarsus. In the lower eyelids, the rudimentary lower eyelid retractors insert near to the inferior tarsal border.[5] Deep to the retractors is the conjunctival epithelium, which contacts the tear film and ocular surface.

The canalicular anatomy is highly relevant in eyelid trauma. In the upper and lower eyelids, the puncta are medial and lateral to the plica semilunaris, respectively, and have a diameter of approximately 0.3 mm at the mucocutaneous junction directed posteriorly into the tear lake. The puncta overlie the canaliculi, which travel approximately 2 mm vertically, turn medially at 90° angles, and travel 8 to 10 mm within the orbicularis oculi muscle before entering the lacrimal sac. In most individuals, the upper and lower canaliculi converge to form a common canaliculus before entering the posterolateral nasolachrymal sac deep and slightly superior to the anterior crus of the medial canthal tendon. Without support from the tarsus, which terminates near the punctum, the medial eyelid has only soft tissue support and is vulnerable to injury.[6]

Owing to their relative proximity, concurrent injury to both the canaliculi and the medial canthal tendon complex is common. A high index of suspicion for canalicular laceration or medial canthal tendon avulsion should be maintained in all cases of eyelid trauma, particularly when there is evidence of trauma medial to the punctum. Canthal avulsions and canalicular lacerations most commonly occur secondary to blunt trauma, animal bites, motor vehicle collisions, falls, and assault with lateral traction to the eyelid. They are often associated with avulsion of the medial canthal tendon. Lacerations of the inferior system are more common than the superior.[7]

APPROACH/THE FOCUSED EXAM

After life-threatening injuries are addressed and the patient is stabilized, the priority in assessing any ocular adnexal injury should be to evaluate the status of the globe. Once any globe injuries have been evaluated and appropriately addressed, a careful examination of the eyelids and lacrimal system should be performed. Collecting a focused history regarding the circumstances of the injury is critical in guiding the examination. In assessing the eyelids, several clinical features are important to recognize, including (1) laceration extent and depth, (2) status of the eyelid margins, (3) involvement of the canthal tendons, (4) involvement of the canalicular system. Additionally, in any ocular adnexal trauma, care should be taken to evaluate for an orbital compartment syndrome caused by a retrobulbar hemorrhage. In the presence of significantly elevated orbital compartment pressure, consideration may be given to lateral canthotomy and cantholysis to relieve orbital tension and/or delayed repair of eyelid lacerations to prevent containing an expanding hemorrhage.

Regarding depth, abrasions and superficial lacerations will involve the skin and possibly muscle layer only. Knowing that deep to the orbicularis oculi muscle and orbital septum is orbital fat, the presence of orbital fat in any eyelid wound signifies violation of the orbital septum and should raise suspicion for deeper injury to the globe, orbital structures, and the possibility of a retained orbital foreign body (**Figure 31.1**). Depending on the mechanism of injury, and when safe to do so, orbital imaging (typically computed tomography) should be performed in this context.

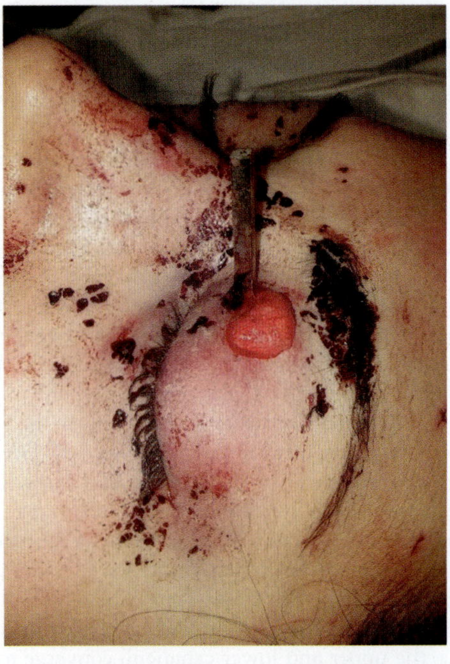

Figure 31.1: Orbital fat protruding through the site of a left upper eyelid penetrating injury, suggesting violation of the orbital septum and deeper orbital involvement.

After excluding orbital extension of the laceration, it is critical to evaluate the status of the eyelid margin. Any laceration involving the eyelid margin requires specialized repair to prevent notching, eyelid malposition, and ocular surface injury.

Next, the eyelid should be evaluated for any possible injury to the lacrimal canaliculi. Canalicular injury should be suspected with any laceration medial to the lacrimal puncta on the eyelid margin. In cases of suspected canalicular injury, punctal exploration should be performed (**Figure 31.2**). In most cases, canalicular exploration should be performed by an ophthalmologist to minimize risk of iatrogenic injury to the delicate canalicular system.

Finally, the eyelid should be evaluated for any injury to the medial or lateral tendon complexes. Medial canthal avulsion is suggested by laxity of the medial canthal complex with increased distractibility of the lower eyelid laterally and anteriorly (**Figure 31.3**). Similarly, lateral canthal

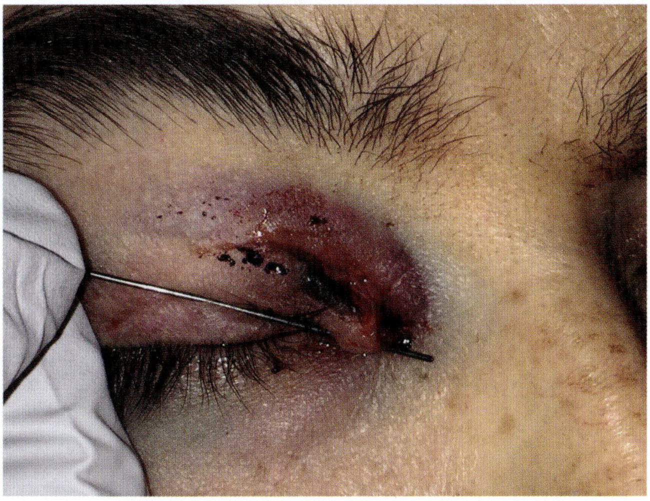

Figure 31.2: Canalicular exploration is demonstrated in a medial, right upper eyelid injury. After being passed through the dilated punctum, the Bowman probe is clearly visible externally, confirming laceration of the upper eyelid canaliculus proximal to the lacrimal sac.

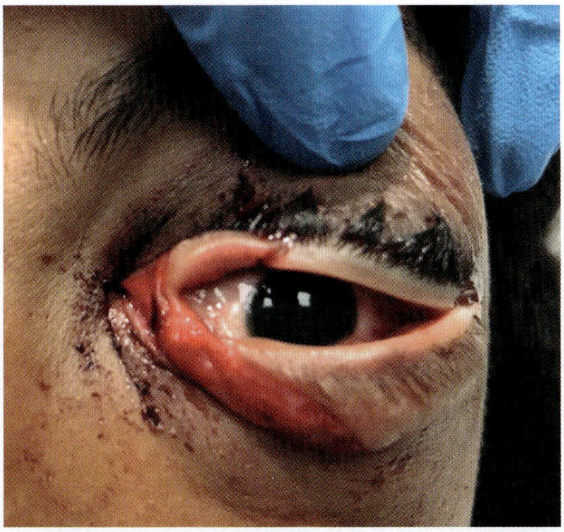

Figure 31.3: Medial canthal tendon avulsion in upper and lower eyelid laceration, demonstrated by lateralization of the medial canthal tendon complex and significantly decreased medial canthal tendon tone.

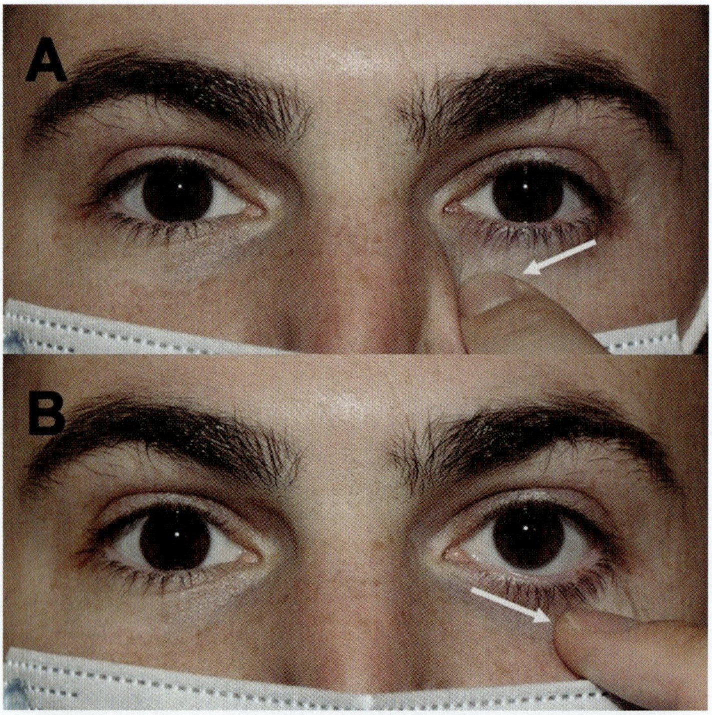

Figure 31.4: Normal lateral canthal and medial canthal tendon tone are demonstrated. A, Lateral canthal tendon tone is assessed by attempting to distract the lateral eyelid medially with a single finger. B, Medial canthal tendon tone is assessed by attempting to distract the medial eyelid laterally with a single finger.

tendon injury should be suspected with increased distractibility of the lower eyelid laterally and anteriorly. Comparison with the contralateral, unaffected eyelid may be useful for practitioners unfamiliar with normal horizontal eyelid tone (**Figure 31.4**). Additionally, a "snapback" test can be performed, where the lower eyelid is distracted inferiorly toward the cheek with a single finger. On release, a normal eyelid will "snap back" into its normal position touching the globe. A positive test is marked by slow or incomplete return of the lower eyelid to its normal position. Although age-related laxity may also produce a positive snapback test, any significant delay in return, particularly with asymmetry in comparison with the contralateral, unaffected side should raise suspicion for tendon injury.

DIFFERENTIAL DIAGNOSIS

- Simple, superficial eyelid lacerations involving the *skin and orbicularis oculi muscle*
- Lacerations with any concern for concomitant deeper injury of the globe or orbit
- Lacerations involving the eyelid margin
- Lacerations with associated eyelid tendon injury
- Lacerations involving the *canalicular* system

MANAGEMENT

Given the delicate anatomy of the eyelids, and the critical structure-function relationships therein, ophthalmology should, whenever possible and as resources allow, be consulted for eyelid laceration repairs, particularly in cases of (1) full thickness laceration, (2) marginal involvement, (3) canalicular involvement, or (4) canthal tendon involvement. Eyelid lacerations should be repaired as soon as it is safe to do so within the context of the patient's other injuries and necessary interventions. Ideally, eyelid lacerations should be repaired within 24 to 48 hours.

If the associated lacerations and adnexal trauma are substantial, or if there is contamination of the wound, copious irrigation and cleaning should be performed, with balanced salt solution if available, and oral or intravenous antibiotics should be considered. Tetanus vaccination status should be confirmed and updated if needed.

In cases where there is no involvement of the eyelid margin, canalicular systems, or tendons, repair can be considered at the bedside by ophthalmology or the emergency provider in appropriate cases. For complex lacerations, the operating room may afford increased patient comfort and provide a more controlled setting.

Preoperative surgical preparation and draping should be performed with betadine in the standard fashion for ophthalmic plastic surgery. Local anesthetic, such as lidocaine 2% with 1:100 000 epinephrine can be injected prior to exploration and repair. If possible, 5% betadine can be used in and around the eyes (or diluted to this strength with balanced salt solution). Copious irrigation, exploration, and gentle debridement of the laceration using moist cotton-tipped applicators is essential prior to repair. Tissue should not be excised primarily unless frankly necrotic. If there is no concomitant ocular injury, a rigid protective contact lens (or a Morgan-style lens) can be placed (with ophthalmic ointment) to protect the ocular surface from injury during repair.

As discussed, the critical structural elements of the eyelid are balanced vectors between the anterior and posterior lamella, the medial and lateral canthal tendons, and the structural integrity of the tarsus.[8] In repairing any eyelid laceration, care must be taken to recreate these naturally existing vectors of support.

Given the consequences of even small vectors of induced tension, an effort should be made to preserve and incorporate all native tissue. The laceration should be irrigated and thoroughly explored to rule out occult, deeper injury, including the tarsus, septum, or eyelid retractors. The tissue should generally be repaired by starting closest to the eyelid margin and working away, because the tension and alignment adjacent to the eyelid margin are most consequential to position and function. In repairing lacerations, small bites should be taken when possible and gentle eversion achieved. Simple interrupted sutures are best, but simple running sutures can be placed as appropriate for long, straight lacerations. Layered closure of the thin eyelids is not always necessary, although in cases where the laceration is perpendicular to the orbicular oculi fibers, closure of the orbicularis oculi can be considered with a small gauge buried interrupted absorbable type suture (eg, 7-0 or 8-0 polyglactin). Closure of deeper layers, including the orbital septum, fat, or deeper orbital contents, should never be performed because this can lead to eyelid retraction or lagophthalmos.[9]

Regarding suture selection, 6-0 or 7-0 suture should generally be used in the eyelids. Lacerations of the eyebrow or thicker skin adjacent to the lateral canthus may require 5-0 suture. Magnification, in the form of surgical loupes or a microscope, may enable increased precision in the repair of delicate eyelid tissues with small-gauge sutures. Absorbable sutures should be used if there is any concern regarding follow-up.[10] Absorbable suture options include plain gut or fast absorbing plain gut. Chromic gut can be considered but often lasts longer than necessary and induces undesirable scarring or will need to be manually removed. Removable suture options include polypropylene, nylon, and silk. Silk, used by some for the theoretical advantage of soft tails in the event of contact with the ocular surface, should be removed as early as possible owing to its inflammatory nature. Staples should not be used in the eyelid. Tissue adhesives should generally be avoided around the eyelids because multiple reports have described iatrogenic closure of the eyelids with cyanoacrylate glues.[11] Following laceration repair, particularly if absorbable sutures are used, antibiotic ophthalmic ointment should be liberally applied and prescribed for use on discharge. Oral antibiotics can also be considered.[12,13] For any canalicular involving laceration, it is practice to prescribe patients topical steroid-antibiotic drops.

PEDIATRIC ISSUES

Eyelid and eyebrow lacerations are common in the pediatric population. The most common causes of these injuries include dog bites, handlebar injuries, and traumatic collisions. Careful consideration should always be given for rabies prophylaxis in the appropriate setting. For isolated injuries, even in the pediatric setting, delayed closure for up to 24 hours may be considered because there would be less swelling. [14] If laceration repair is performed with an awake pediatric patient, with or without sedation, and there is additional concern for potential iatrogenic globe puncture, an additional safety measure of the application of tetracaine plus a Morgan Lens or corneal shield during the entire procedure can be considered. Absorbable sutures should be utilized preferentially.[15]

TIPS AND PEARLS

- Suture selection: use the smallest possible, but largest necessary, gauge of suture
  - 6-0 or 7-0 for eyelid skin closure
  - 5-0 or 6-0 suture for the eyebrows and lateral canthal area
- Staples should not be used in the eyelid. Tissue glues should be avoided in the eyelids.
- Start laceration repair at the edge of the laceration that is closest to the eyelid margin and work away from the eyelid margin.
- When in doubt, it is often better to delay repair than proceed with an inappropriate repair. If a delayed repair is necessary, the eye should be kept well lubricated with antibiotic ophthalmic ointment and be protected with an eye shield in the interim.[16]
- Canalicular laceration and medial canthal tendon avulsion should be suspected in any laceration medial to the upper or lower eyelid puncta and are common in injuries where the eyelids are pulled laterally.
- Tetanus booster should be initiated for those who have had more than 5 years since their last vaccination.

EVIDENCE

What is the optimal timeline for eyelid laceration repair?

Regarding timing of closure, one retrospective study showed that there was no statistical significance for poor outcomes following delayed eyelid laceration repair over 24 hours.[17] A proposed theory is that the extensive vascular supply of the eyelids contributes to a more amendable healing environment with increased oxygen perfusion and decreased risk of infection, even after delayed closure. In their series, operating room repair was indicated for those lacerations affecting children, those involving the canalicular system or deeper tissue planes, and complex lacerations requiring extensive reconstruction or exploration. Delayed repair can occur in the cases of medical conditions delaying anesthesia, delay of greater than 24 hours in seeking care, or a missed diagnosis by their providers. The authors of this review concluded that any complications after eyelid laceration were more likely caused by technical aspects of the repair rather than the timing of repair. In their study, none of the pediatric cases that had delayed closure had any complications.[17]

When should patients receive systemic antibiotics after eyelid laceration?

Following repair of an eyelid laceration, patients can be placed on a topical ophthalmic antibiotic ointment, such as erythromycin ophthalmic, twice daily. Consideration can also be given to oral antibiotics. One clear indication for oral antibiotics for eyelid lacerations is for animal bites.[18] Animal bites are often contaminated with polymicrobial pathogens from the animal's saliva, so it is of essence to give antibiotic prophylaxis and monitor the area closely for developing infection. Possible pathogens include *Pasteurella, Streptococcus,* and *Bacteroides* species and should be covered with oral antibiotics such as amoxicillin-clavulanic acid, ampicillin-sulbactam, or cefazolin. In patients who are status post splenectomy, gram negative *Capnocytophaga canimorsus* infection is a potentially life-threatening infection, which can be treated with clindamycin.[18] If a clinician has a high index of suspicion for underlying accompanying infection after eyelid trauma, further imaging such as a contrast computed tomography of the orbits should be obtained.

References

1. Iftikhar M, Latif A, Farid UZ, et al. Changes in the incidence of eye trauma hospitalizations in the United States from 2001 through 2014. *JAMA Ophthalmol*. 2019;137(1):48-56.
2. McGwin G Jr, Hall TA, Xie A, et al. Trends in eye injury in the United States, 1992–2001. *Invest Ophthalmol Vis Sci*. 2006;47(2):521-527. PMID: 16431945.
3. Gordon AA, Tran LT, Phelps PO. Eyelid and orbital trauma for the primary care physician. *Dis Mon*. 2020;66(10):101045.
4. Ko AC, Satterfield KR, Korn BS, et al. Eyelid and periorbital soft tissue trauma. *Facial Plast Surg Clin North Am*. 2017;25:605-616.
5. Lin B. Closing the gap, wound closure for the emergency practitioner. 2016. https://lacerationrepair.com/special-situations/ear-lacerations-part-ii/
6. Singer AJ, Gulla J, Hein M, et al. Single-layer versus double-layer closure of facial lacerations: a randomized controlled trial. *Plast Reconstr Surg*. 2005;116:363-368; discussion 9-70.
7. Murchison AP, Bilyk JR. Canalicular laceration repair: an analysis of variables affecting success. *Ophthalmic Plast Reconstr Surg*. 2014;30:410-414.
8. Chowdhury HR, Rose GE, Ezra DG. Long-term outcomes of monocanalicular repair of canalicular lacerations. *Ophthalmology*. 2014;121:1665-1666.e1.
9. Chu YC, Wu S-Y, Tsai Y-J, et al. Early versus late canalicular laceration repair outcomes. *Am J Ophthalmol*. 2017;182:155-159.
10. Nicks B, Ayello E, Woo K, et al. Acute wound management: revisiting the approach to assessment, irrigation, and closure considerations. *Int J Emerg Med*. 2010;3(4):399-407.
11. Coutts SJ, Sandhu R, Geh VS. Tissue glue and iatrogenic eyelid gluing in children. *Pediatr Emerg Care*. 2012;28(8):810-811. doi:10.1097/PEC.0b013e31826288fa
12. Roberts JR, Custalow CB. *Roberts and Hedges' Clinical Procedures in Emergency Medicine and Acute Care*. Elsevier; 2019.
13. Singh S, Ganguly A, Hardas A, et al. Canalicular lacerations: factors predicting outcome at a tertiary eye care centre. *Orbit*. 2017;36:13-18.
14. Tintinalli JE, Ma OJ, Yealy DM, et al. *Tintinalli's Emergency Medicine: A Comprehensive Study Guide*. McGraw-Hill Education; 2020.
15. Brophy M, Sinclair S, Hosteler SG, Xiang H. Pediatric eye injury-related hospitalizations in the United States. *Pediatrics*. 2006;117:e1263-e1271.
16. Walls, RM, Hockberger RS, Gausche-Hill M. *Rosen's Emergency Medicine: Concepts and Clinical Practice*. Elsevier; 2018.
17. Chiang E, Bee C, Harris GJ, Wells TS. Does delayed repair of eyelid lacerations compromise outcome? *Am J Emerg Med*. 2017;35(11):1766-1767.
18. Butler T. Capnocytophaga canimorsus: an emerging cause of sepsis, meningitis, and post-splenectomy infection after dog bites. *Eur J Clin Microbiol Infect Dis*. 2015;(7):1271-1280.

CHAPTER 32

Herpes Zoster Ophthalmicus

Alexandra Ortego
Paul Petrakos

THE CLINICAL CHALLENGE

Herpes zoster, commonly known as shingles, occurs when the human herpesvirus type 3, the virus responsible for varicella infection, is reactivated in the neurosensory ganglia, often years or decades after the primary infection. Herpes zoster classically results in a unilateral inflammatory reaction causing pain and a vesicular rash in the distribution of a neurosensory dermatome (**Figure 32.1**). According to the Centers for Disease Control and Prevention, there are an estimated 1 million annual cases of herpes zoster in the United States, and nearly one in three people will develop herpes zoster in their lifetime.[1] Herpes zoster ophthalmicus (HZO) is a commonly encountered disorder in emergency departments (EDs) and urgent care settings and accounts for 10% to 20% of herpes zoster cases.[2]

Herpes zoster and HZO primarily affect the elderly and immunocompromised. Decreased cellular immunity as a result of advanced age, immunosuppression, or physical stress allows the virus that had been dormant for years and suppressed by the immune system to reactivate. Early diagnosis, treatment with antivirals, and, when there is concern for eye involvement, ophthalmologic consultation is essential in decreasing the duration of symptoms and complications of herpes zoster and HZO such as permanent vision loss, prolonged or permanent pain, and scarring.

PATHOPHYSIOLOGY

HZO results from the reactivation of the varicella virus (human herpesvirus 3) in the ophthalmic branch of the trigeminal nerve (**Figure 32.2**). Primary varicella infection most commonly occurs in childhood and presents as a febrile illness and diffuse pustular rash. During the primary infection, viral particles are believed to spread from infected skin along sensory nerve endings to the nerve ganglia. An alternative hypothesis is that the virus gains access to the nerve ganglia via hematologic spread during primary illness. Viral particles then remain dormant for years in the spinal and cranial nerve ganglia, suppressed by the host's immune system.[1]

Reactivation of the varicella virus occurs when the host's cellular immunity fails to continue suppressing the virus. This may occur secondary to advanced age, immunocompromised states, physical stress, or malnutrition. When no longer suppressed, the viral particles replicate and migrate peripherally along sensory nerves, triggering an inflammatory response. During this period of viral replication, some patients may experience a prodromal phase with symptoms of fatigue and low-grade fever. Local inflammatory response to the virus as it reaches distal nerve endings leads to neuropathic pain in affected dermatome, the vesicular rash and, when affecting the ophthalmic nerve, ocular inflammation.

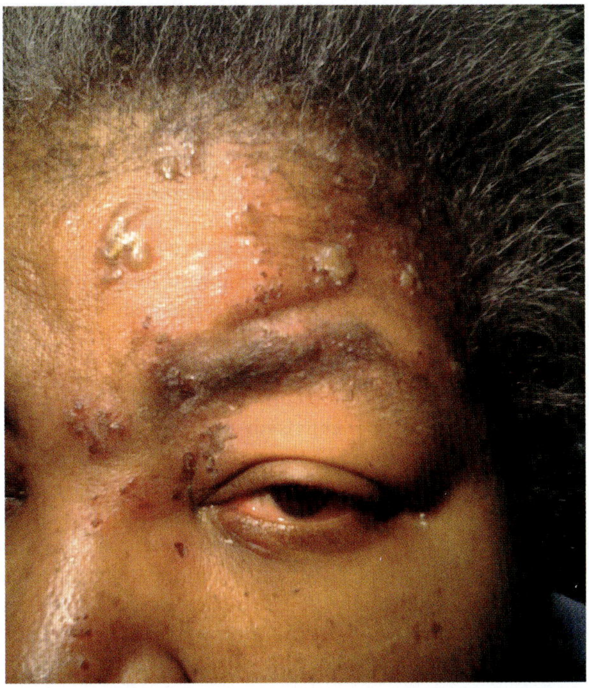

Figure 32.1: Herpes zoster affecting the ophthalmic branch of the trigeminal nerve. (From Rapuano CJ. *Wills Eye Institute: Cornea*. 3rd ed. Wolters Kluwer; 2019. Figure 7.9a.)

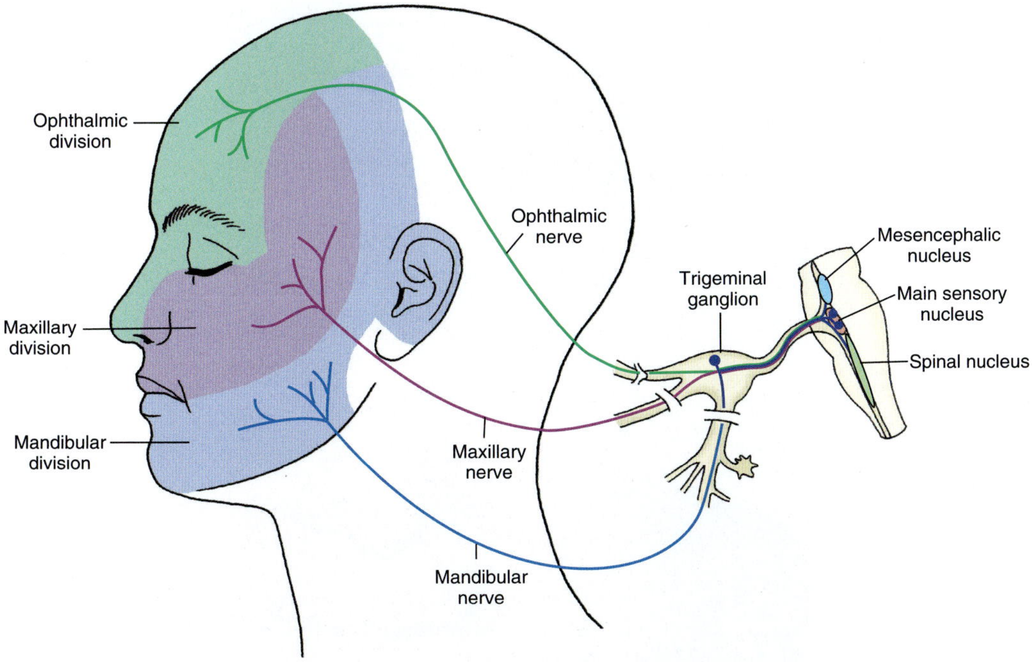

Figure 32.2: Dermatomes of the trigeminal nerve. (From Parent A. *Carpenter's Human Neuroanatomy*. 9th ed. Wolters Kluwer; 1996:505.)

When herpes zoster involves the ophthalmic nerve, patients typically develop pain over the affected V1 dermatome and a unilateral erythematous rash over the forehead with progression to vesicles that erupt and crust over. Rash over the tip of the nose, Hutchinson sign (**Figure 32.3**) indicates involvement of the nasociliary nerve (a branch of the ophthalmic nerve) and is highly correlated with ocular involvement.[3] Ocular involvement may manifest as a rash over the eyelid, conjunctivitis (35% to 70%), keratitis (13% to 75%) (punctate epithelial keratitis, pseudodendritic lesions, erosions, persistent defects), uveitis (18% to 47%), acute retinal necrosis, optic neuritis or rarely oculomotor palsies.[4] Ocular complications could progress to permanent visual loss, scarring, and pain.[2]

Keratitis typically develops within a month of dermatitis and may affect all layers of the cornea (epithelium, stroma, and endothelium). Early signs include punctate epithelial keratitis, presenting 2 days after vesicle formation, and pseudodendrites, about 4 to 6 days after presentation. These signs are seen in 5% to 51% of patients with ocular involvement. Other complications include blepharitis and secondary glaucoma.[4]

Necrotizing retinitis is an uncommon complication of HZO that can lead to retinal tears, retinal detachment, and subsequent permanent vision changes. These patients typically present in the acute setting with far worse visual acuity. There are two forms of necrotizing retinitis: acute retinal necrosis (ARN) and progressive outer retinal necrosis (PORN).

ARN (**Figure 32.4**) is typically seen in immunocompetent individuals. Patients typically report pain, decreased vision, and floaters at the time of presentation. ARN commonly causes retinal detachments (50% to 75%) with multiple holes and giant retinal tears, conferring poor visual prognosis. Only 30% of patients achieve final visual acuity better than 20/200.[5]

PORN (**Figure 32.5**) is typically found in immunocompromised patients. Although there is less inflammation owing to their immunocompromised state, and therefore lower incidence of floaters, it has a much faster progression and worse outcome when compared with ARN.[6]

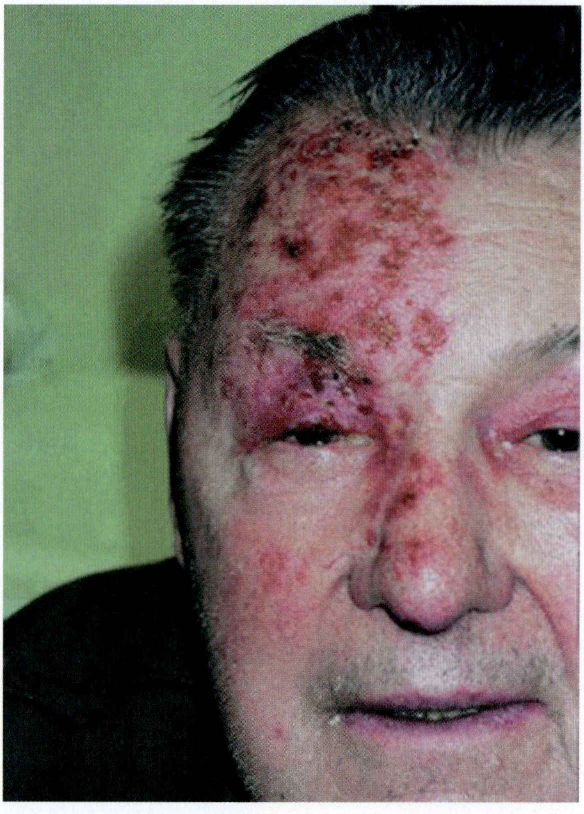

Figure 32.3: Hutchinson sign.

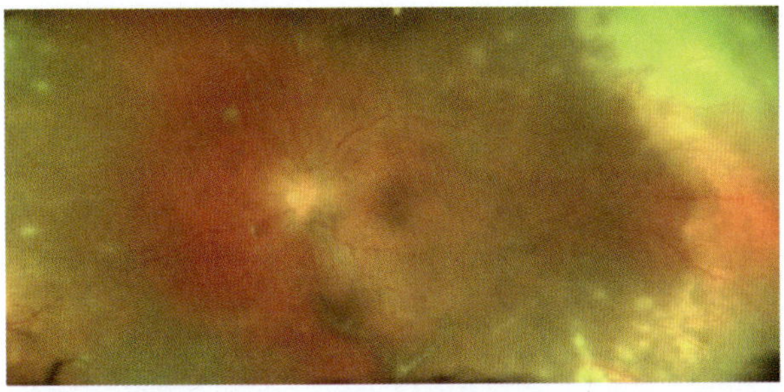

Figure 32.4: Acute retinal necrosis. (Courtesy of Dr. Thanos Papakostas, Weill Cornell Medical Center.)

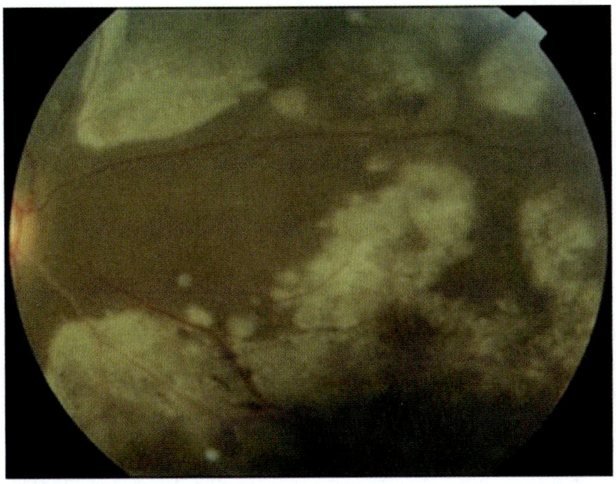

Figure 32.5: Progressive outer retinal necrosis.

Additionally, patients with HZO commonly develop postherpetic neuralgia (PHN). PHN is defined as pain in a dermatomal distribution that is sustained for at least 90 days after the rash and occurs in about 20% of patients with herpes zoster. It is caused by nerve damage secondary to an inflammatory response induced by viral replication within a nerve. Risk factors include older age, severe prodrome or rash, severe acute zoster, ophthalmic involvement, immunosuppression, or chronic conditions.[7]

APPROACH/THE FOCUSED EXAM

Patients with a painful, vesicular rash in the V1 distribution should be evaluated for HZO. Evaluation includes the following:

- Visual acuity
- External examination of eyelids, periocular skin, scalp, and nose
- Intraocular pressure
- Slit lamp examination of anterior segment
- Dilated fundus examination by ophthalmology

When evaluating the vesicular rash, care should be taken to identify any involvement of the tip of the nose (Hutchinson sign) as this is a strong predictor of ocular inflammation and corneal denervation in HZO.[3] Focused anterior segment slit lamp examination should be performed looking for conjunctivitis, keratitis, pseudodendrite on corneal staining (**Figure 32.6**), corneal epithelial defects, stromal opacities, and anterior chamber cell or flare. Elevated intraocular pressure can be seen from trabeculitis in patients with HZO.

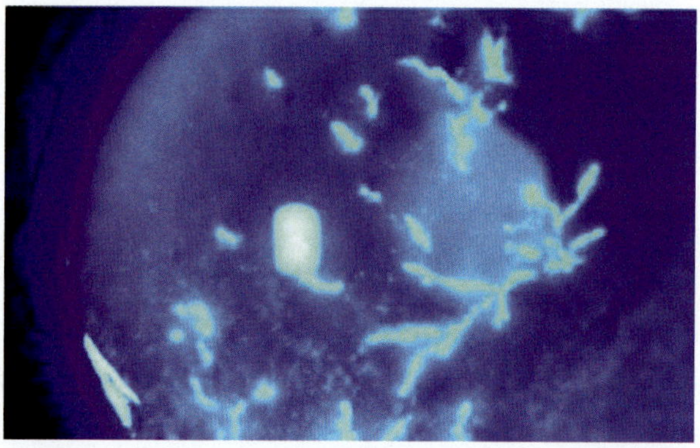

Figure 32.6: Pseudodendrites.

DIFFERENTIAL DIAGNOSIS

The differential diagnosis of decreased vision and a red eye is broad; however the presence of a dermatomal rash, pseudodendritic corneal epithelial defects, and Hutchinson sign help narrow the differential to HZO. The differential diagnosis of the corneal involvement includes herpes simplex epithelial disease, severe dry eye with filamentous disease, exposure keratopathy, corneal abrasion, Epstein-Barr virus, mumps, and syphilis. The retinal manifestations of HZO may be similar to those seen in sarcoidosis, cytomegalovirus retinitis, posterior uveitis, endophthalmitis, and lupus retinopathy.[1]

Herpes simplex epithelial disease shares some characteristics of HZO in that it may cause a vesicular rash; however, the rash of herpes simplex will not respect a dermatomal distribution. The dendritic lesions seen in herpes simplex may be mistaken for the pseudodendritic lesions seen in HZO. Dendritic lesions are formed by a true epithelial defect in the cornea in which epithelium is absent in the affected area, whereas the pseudodendritic lesions of HZO are heaped-up epithelial cells with "negative" fluorescein staining from stain collecting at edges of epithelium.[1]

MANAGEMENT

The treatment for HZO, like herpes zoster in other distributions, begins with systemic antiviral agents. Treatment within 72 hours of the rash results in decreased virus shedding, severity and duration of rash, acute pain, and incidence of ocular involvement.[4] Antiviral therapy should not be delayed while awaiting definitive diagnosis or ophthalmology evaluation. Typically, antiviral therapy is continued for 7 to 10 days. For immunocompetent adults, oral acyclovir (800 mg 5 times daily), valacyclovir (1000 mg 3 times daily), or famciclovir (500 mg 3 times daily) are typically used. Immunocompromised patients may require intravenous acyclovir 10 to 12 mg/kg/day every 8 hours. Intravenous foscarnet is an alternative for acyclovir-resistant disease.[6]

Supportive care for HZO includes artificial tears, cold compresses, and analgesics. Topical antibiotic ointments to the affected skin (erythromycin or bacitracin 2 to 3 times daily) are given to prevent secondary bacterial infections.

Keratitis, Uveitis, and Trabeculitis

On slit lamp evaluation, patients may have corneal edema, cells in the anterior or posterior chamber, and/or elevated intraocular pressure. Both topical and systemic corticosteroids may be used in disease management of HZO for keratitis, uveitis, and trabeculitis. Clinical trials, however, have shown variable results, and this should not be started without the involvement of ophthalmology. The clinician must weigh potential benefit and risk for adverse events, including cataract formation and elevated intraocular pressure. Topical corticosteroid utility is typically determined through an ophthalmic examination on a case-by-case basis.

Topical antivirals may also be considered for keratitis, but there is limited evidence regarding their utility in managing HZO.[8] Elevated intraocular pressure can occur from herpetic trabeculitis.

These patients require topical aqueous suppressants such as timolol, brimonidine, dorzolamide drops, or acetazolamide pills. Typically, these pressure lowering drops are given in combination with topical corticosteroids for the treatment of trabeculitis.

Retinal Necrosis

Treatment for both ARN and PORN requires evaluation by a retina or posterior uveitis specialist. Systemic and/or intravitreal antiviral therapy are the mainstays of treatment. Intravenous foscarnet or cidofovir may be effective in infections resistant to acyclovir. Intravitreal ganciclovir or oral valganciclovir may also be used. A 3-month course of oral acyclovir has been shown to reduce the incidence of involvement of the second eye.[4]

Postherpetic Neuralgia

Management of PHN may include tricyclic antidepressants, gabapentin, pregabalin, opioids, topical analgesics, or oral steroids. For postherpetic itching, diphenhydramine can also be useful. Rarely, it may require nerve block or botulinum map injections. Capsaicin cream applied to the rash may decrease pain as well.[7]

Vaccination

Prevention is key in herpes zoster. Zostavax is recommended for all patients over 60 years of age. It has been shown to reduce the risk to developing zoster by 51.3% and demonstrated a 66.5% efficacy for preventing PHN. It shortens the duration and decreases severity of disease. Shingrix is indicated for adults over 50 years of age. Efficacy of the recombinant zoster vaccine against the development of zoster and PHN is higher than that of live attenuated vaccine.[9]

TIPS AND PEARLS

- Early identification and initiation of antiviral treatment, within 72 hours of vesicular rash formation, remains the most crucial component of management.
- Complete eye exam for all HZO patients
  - Visual acuity
  - Pupils
  - Intraocular pressure
- Prompt referral to ophthalmology for further evaluation.[10]

EVIDENCE

What is the preferred antiviral treatment?

Acyclovir, valacyclovir, and famciclovir have all been shown in clinical trials to be effective in treating HZO. Valacyclovir or famciclovir are preferred to acyclovir for their simpler dosing regimen. They have also both been shown to reduce the incidence, duration, and severity of PHN. No significant difference has been shown when comparing valacyclovir to famciclovir for reducing pain associated with herpes zoster and PHN. Acyclovir being as effective as valacyclovir and famciclovir in treating HZO is debatable with various conflicting studies.[11,12]

Should you give topical antivirals over oral antivirals?

This question was raised by findings of differences in absorption of oral and topical acyclovir. Topical acyclovir achieves higher levels in the aqueous humor when compared to oral acyclovir. However, despite achieving higher levels, topical acyclovir is associated with worse outcome and increased complications. Neoh et al. treated 57 patients with HZO within 72 hours of rash with either topical acyclovir ointment or oral acyclovir (800 mg orally 5 times per day) for 7 days and followed them for 12 months. Patients who received topical acyclovir had a higher likelihood of ocular complications, and anterior uveitis was more frequent and more severe. Corneal hypoesthesia was significantly more frequent and severe at 1 month for the topical acyclovir group. From

2 weeks on, the patients receiving acyclovir ointment were more likely to have pain, and their pain was more severe, but it was not statistically significant. Topical acyclovir seems to have no prophylactic value despite better penetration.[7]

Is prolonged antiviral therapy helpful?

The Zoster Eye Disease Study (ZEDS), funded by the National Eye Institute and the National Institute of Health, was a randomized controlled clinical trial that sought to determine whether prolonged suppressive valacyclovir treatment 1000 mg daily for 1 year reduces complications of HZO, including eye disease and/or PHN compared to placebo. An internet-based survey was distributed to 170 investigators regarding their practice patterns in treating recent onset or chronic HZO. Valacyclovir was the preferred antiviral for both recent onset and chronic by responders. About 70% of them believed prolonged antiviral prophylaxis could prevent or reduce recurrent and/or chronic signs of HZO during the period of administration. Despite frequent use of prolonged suppressive antiviral treatment in HZO, it is currently not evidence based.[13] Previous prospective clinical trials showed no evidence regarding the efficacy of prolonged antiviral therapy to reduce chronic and/or recurrent disease.[9]

References

1. Vrcek I, Choudhury E, Durairaj V. Herpes zoster ophthalmicus: a review for the internist. *Am J Med.* 2017;130(1):21-26.
2. Johnson JL, Amzat R, Martin N. Herpes zoster ophthalmicus. *Prim Care.* 2015;42(3):285-303.
3. Zaal MJ, Voker-Dieben HJ, D'Amaro J. Prognostic value of Hutchinson's sign in acute herpes zoster ophthalmicus. *Graefes Arch Clin Exp Ophthalmol.* 2003;241(3):187-191.
4. Li JY. Herpes zoster ophthalmicus: acute keratitis. *Curr Opin Ophthalmol.* 2018;29:328-333.
5. Kaiser PK, Friedman NJ, Pineda R. *The Massachusetts Eye and Ear Infirmary Illustrated Manual of Ophthalmology*. 4th ed. Elsevier; 2014.
6. Riordan-Eva P, Cunningham ET Jr. *Vaughn & Asbury's General Ophthalmology*. 8th ed. The McGraw-Hill Companies; 2011.
7. Saguil A, Kane S, Mercado M. Herpes zoster and postherpetic neuralgia: prevention and management. *Am Fam Physician*. 2018;96(10):656-663.
8. Neoh C, Harding SP, Saunders D, et al. Comparison of topical and oral acyclovir in early herpes zoster ophthalmicus. *Eye (Lond)*. 1994;8:688-691.
9. Oxman MN, Levin MJ, Johnson GR, et al. A vaccine to prevent herpes zoster and postherpetic neuralgia in older adults. *N Engl J Med.* 2005;352:2271-2284.
10. Minor M, Payne E. Herpes zoster ophthalmicus. [Updated 2021 Jan 5]. In: *StatPearls* [Internet]. StatPearls Publishing; 2021.
11. Beutner KR, Griedman DJ, Forszpaniak C, et al. Valaciclovir compared with acyclovir for improved therapy for herpes zoster in immunocompetent adults. *Antimicrob Agents Chemother.* 1995;39:1546-1553.
12. Colin J, Prisant O, Cochener B, et al. Comparison of the efficacy and safety of valaciclovir and acyclovir for the treatment of herpes zoster ophthalmicus. *Ophthalmology*. 2000;107:1507-1511.
13. Lo DM, Jeng BH, Gillespie C, Wu Mengfei, Cohen EJ. Current practice patterns and opinions in the management of recent onset or chronic herpes zoster ophthalmicus of Zoster Eye Disease Study Investigators. *Cornea*. 2019;38(1): 13-17.

CHAPTER 33

Eyelid Lesions

Lora R. Dagi Glass
Juliana Wilson

THE CLINICAL CHALLENGE

Eyelid lesions commonly present in the emergency department (ED) or urgent care settings. There are an estimated two million visits a year to the ED for eye complaints, almost 50% of which are nontraumatic complaints. Eyelid lesions are the sixth most common cause of nontraumatic eye complaints. Most nontraumatic complaints can be discharged home.[1] Although eyelid lesions are typically not threatening to the vision, patients are often symptomatic and may be concerned about the cosmetic appearance.

Eyelid lesions should be approached by taking a detailed history of timing, pain or discomfort, discharge, attempted treatment, and any visual symptoms. Examination should include a detailed external review of the face and eyelid region, looking at the nature of the lesion from a dermatologic perspective. Where is it located? Is it macular or papular, inflamed or cool, draining or bleeding, ulcerated or otherwise causing local destruction (such as eyelash loss, or madarosis), tender, or itchy? Are there associated lesions elsewhere on the face?

Lesions of eyelids can be categorized by their anatomic location: epithelial layer, glandular, and mucosal layer. Here, we describe common lesions that plague each anatomic region and explore their differential diagnosis. As with any other epithelialized area, molluscum contagiosum lesions commonly present on the eyelid. Specialized sebaceous glands of the eyelid, or meibomian glands, cause chalazia or hordeola when inflamed. Pyogenic granuloma occurs when the nonkeratinized, or mucosal, inner epithelial lining suffers from inflammation just as the mouth or other mucosal regions of the body can.

MOLLUSCUM CONTAGIOSUM

Pathophysiology

Molluscum contagiosum is a pox virus infection of the skin that is commonly seen in children and immunocompromised persons but that may occur at any age and in any immune state. It spreads easily via contact with persons or infected surfaces. It can occur in any location but commonly occurs on the face and eyelids. It is painless, skin colored, and can be pruritic.

Approach/The Focused Exam

There may be single or multiple lesions (sometimes even conglomerated), and these lesions may be limited to the eyelid or periocular region or present in multiple regions. Molluscum lesions classically present as small umbilicated nodules that are skin colored or slightly lighter/pearly (**Figure 33.1**). They can also present as a giant lesion or as an erythematous lesion. They can be itchy and irritated and may cause surrounding dermatitis and/or conjunctivitis.

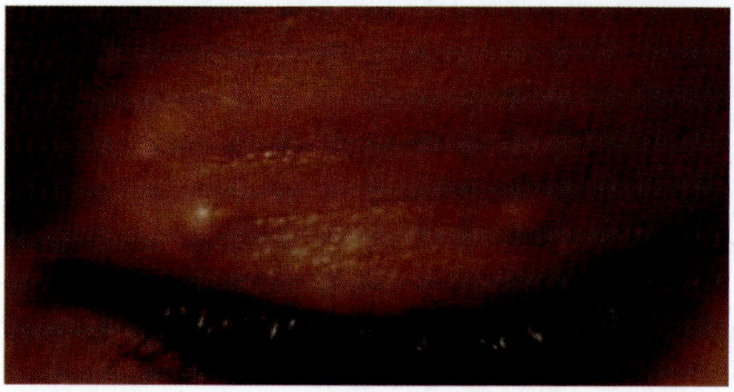

Figure 33.1: Molluscum contagiosum lesions on the upper eyelid.

Differential Diagnosis

Small growths that can be mistaken for molluscum include benign periocular lesions such as epidermal inclusion cysts (**Figure 33.2**), hidrocystomas (**Figure 33.3**), papillomas (**Figure 33.4**), syringomas (**Figure 33.5**), and chalazia (**Figure 33.6**). Also, although able to present across the age

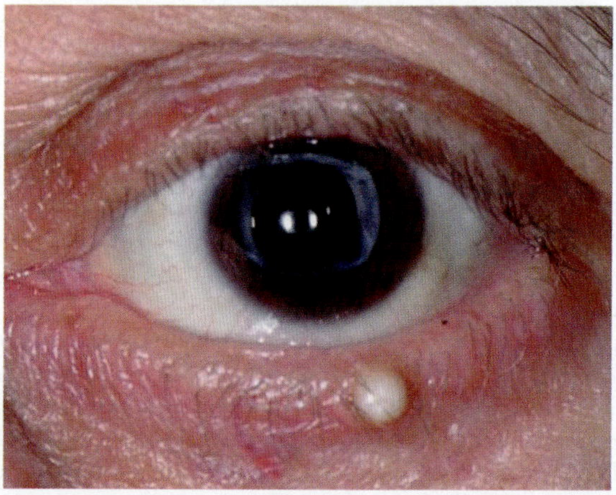

Figure 33.2: Small epidermal inclusion cyst on the central lower eyelid lashline. (From Eyelid cystic lesions simulating neoplasms. In: Shields JA, Shields CL. *Eyelid, Conjunctival, and Orbital Tumors: An Atlas and Textbook*. 3rd ed. Wolters Kluwer; 2016:195-206. Figure 11.20.)

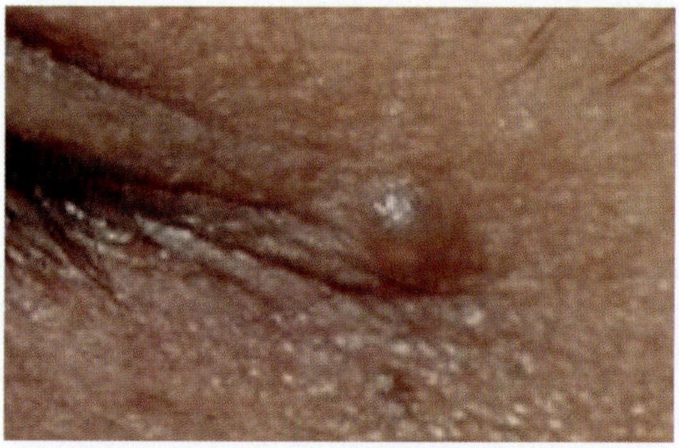

Figure 33.3: Hidrocystoma of the lateral canthus. Note the slightly blue hue, attributable to the cyst's transparency.

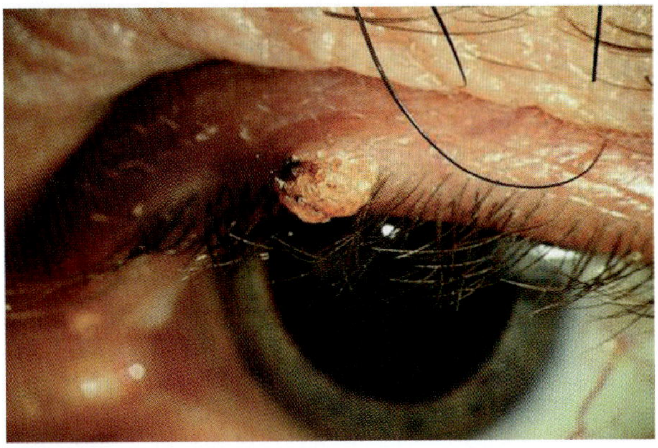

Figure 33.4: Papilloma of the upper eyelid. (From Benign tumors of the eyelid epidermis. In: Shields JA, Shields CL. *Eyelid, Conjunctival, and Orbital Tumors: An Atlas and Textbook*. 3rd ed. Wolters Kluwer; 2016:3-18. Figure 1.2.)

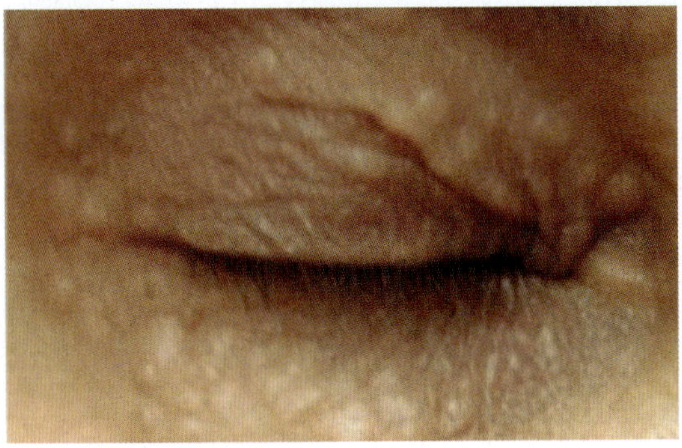

Figure 33.5: Periocular syringomas. These typically present with innumerable lesions.

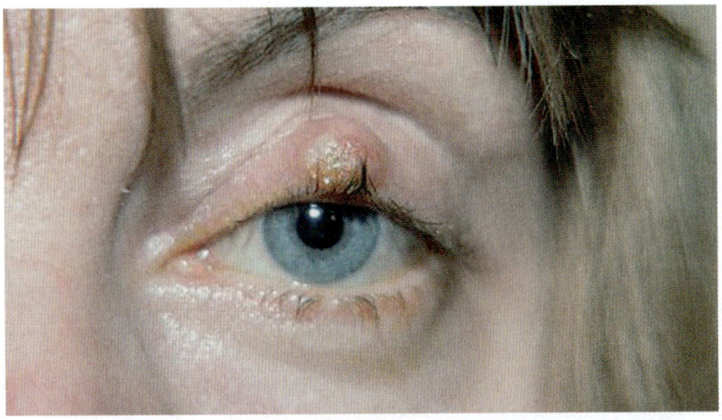

Figure 33.6: Chalazion of the upper eyelid. (From Eyelid inflammation. In: Penne R. *Wills Eye Hospital Color Atlas and Synopsis of Clinical Ophthalmology: Oculoplastics*. 3rd ed. Wolters Kluwer; 2019:24-29. Figure 2.1b.)

spectrum, most occur more commonly in adults. Hidrocystomas transilluminate, whereas molluscum does not. Cancerous periocular lesions such as basal cell carcinoma (**Figure 33.7**) and squamous cell carcinoma are more common in adults (**Figure 33.8**) and tend to present with a chronic, singular lesion. They may also have overlying telangiectasia, madarosis (eyelash loss), or other destruction of the surrounding architecture. Other causes of conjunctivitis, including infectious or allergic conjunctivitis, will not be associated with the typical molluscum lesion. Other causes of

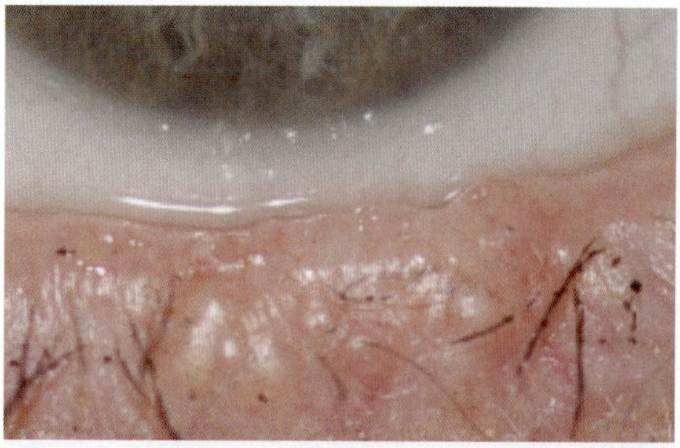

Figure 33.7: Basal cell carcinoma of the lower eyelid margin. Note the eyelash loss (madarosis).

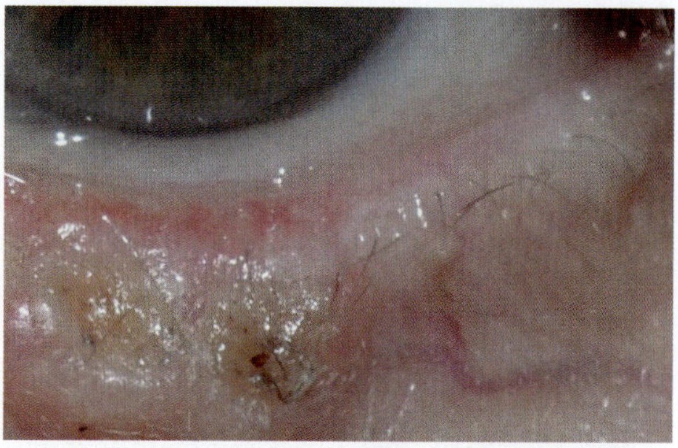

Figure 33.8: Ulcerating squamous cell carcinoma of the lower eyelid margin.

dermatitis, including infectious, allergic, or atopic dermatitis (**Figure 33.9**), will also not present with the typical molluscum lesion.

Management

Patients should avoid scratching the lesions to prevent spread and ocular irritation. Treatment of molluscum on the eyelid consists of surgical removal or waiting for natural resolution. Lesions typically self-resolve within 12 to 18 months. However, in the case of cosmetic disruption or other

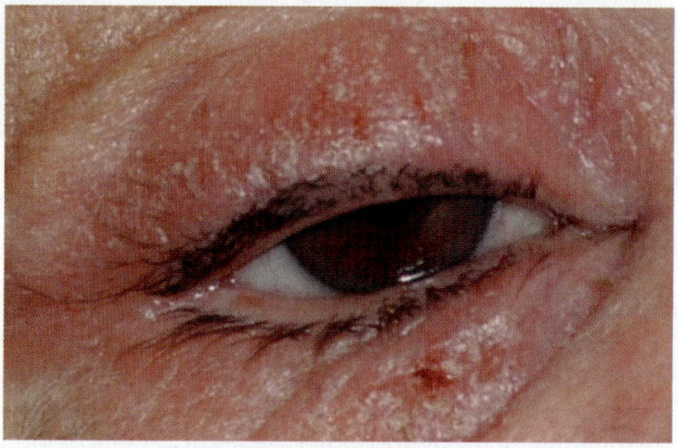

Figure 33.9: Severe periocular dermatitis with thickened, inflamed, crusting and bleeding skin.

symptoms (ie, conjunctivitis, dermatitis, irritation), curettage or excision is preferred. Topical options considered elsewhere on the body are typically unsafe for periocular use.

CHALAZION/HORDEOLUM

Pathophysiology

Chalazia (Figure 33.6) and hordeola (**Figure 33.10**) can occur in all age groups but are most common at ages 30 to 50. They often occur as a single lesion but can present as concurrent or asynchronous lesions involving one or both eyes. A chalazion is a benign granulomatous inflammatory process caused by obstructed specialized eyelid sebaceous glands (meibomian, Zeis, and Moll glands). Patients may report a small sensation of irritation with a quickly appearing painless bump, a chronic painless bump, or a chronic painless bump that may wax and wane. A hordeolum is similar in etiology but has developed a secondary infection; thus, hordeola are red, inflamed, and tender or painful. Chalazia are not always apparent in a hordeolum but may present after the hordeolum has cooled down. Clinically, chalazia and hordeola are on a spectrum. A resolving hordeolum may leave a residual chalazion, and a chalazion may become infected and thus become a hordeolum.

For further comparison between the two related entities, please see **Table 33.1**.

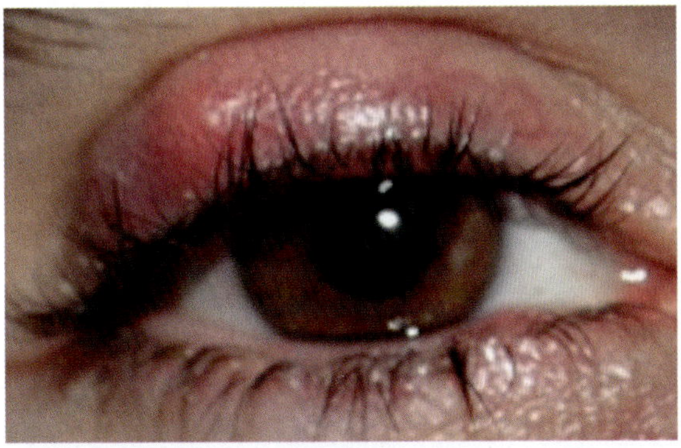

Figure 33.10: Hordeolum of the upper eyelid; in addition to a preseptal appearance with limited erythema and edema of the eyelid, one can see an underlying nidus of inflammation laterally. This nidus may persist as a chalazion after the infection is treated.

TABLE 33.1 Chalazion versus Hordeolum

	Chalazion	Hordeolum
Appearance	Sterile, typically firm, nontender nodules	Hot, erythematous, inflamed, infected, and tender
Emergency department (ED) treatment	Warm compresses; refer for outpatient eye care	Warm compresses, oral antibiotics such as doxycycline or azithromycin; refer for outpatient eye care
Definite treatment	Time, rarely need anti-inflammatory injections, oral anti-inflammatories, or excisions	Oral antibiotics, may need incision & drainage if abscess present
Time course	Acute-chronic	Acute

Approach/The Focused Exam

All chalazia and hordeola are centered on the eyelids themselves, because they involve the sebaceous glands of the eyelid. The clinician often sees evidence of underlying blepharitis—dandruff or crusting on eyelashes, or small domes of clogged oil (looks cream/white) on the eyelid margin (inspissated meibomian glands). The clinician may also see evidence of facial rosacea, which can cause the blepharitis typically underlying chalazia and hordeola.

A patient may have more than one chalazion or hordeolum at a time. Chalazia are sterile, typically firm, nontender nodules. Hordeola are hot, erythematous, inflamed, infected, and tender; typically, infection is with a gram-positive bacterium like *Staphylococcus aureus*.

Differential Diagnosis

Nodular growths of the eyelid include skin cancers (eg, basal cell, squamous cell, or sebaceous cell carcinoma). Skin cancers are typically slow growing. If a chalazion recurs repeatedly in the same location—especially if it never occurs elsewhere—one must have increased concern for a masquerading sebaceous cell carcinoma (**Figure 33.11**). Epidermal inclusion cysts and hidrocystoma cysts can also grow quite large; a deep epidermal inclusion cyst can mimic a chalazion. Hidrocystomas should transilluminate with light, unlike a chalazion. Hordeola may turn into a more severe preseptal cellulitis or present with an abscess. If blepharitis is identified on examination, this can be associated with demodicosis (demodex mites; invisible to the naked eye), more rarely vitamin A deficiency, smoking, some glaucoma medications (ie, prostaglandin analogues), some systemic medications (dupilumab, bortezomib), and likely comedogenic periocular products, including false eyelash glue.

Management

For both chalazia and hordeola, treating the commonly underlying blepharitis is the first-line treatment to calm the current inflammatory state, as well as to prevent future occurrences. Warm compresses and eyelid cleansers (often special preparations of dilute hypochlorous acid) can help keep lashes clean and eyelids less inflamed and are all that is needed for many cases of chalazia. Topical antibiotics (eg, erythromycin ointment) or combination antibiotic-steroid ointments (eg, tobramycin-dexamethasone) may augment conservative therapy by treating any associated infection or inflammation. In cases with developing cellulitis, oral antibiotics with anti-inflammatory properties, such as doxycycline or azithromycin, will be more effective.[2,3] Hordeola with a visible

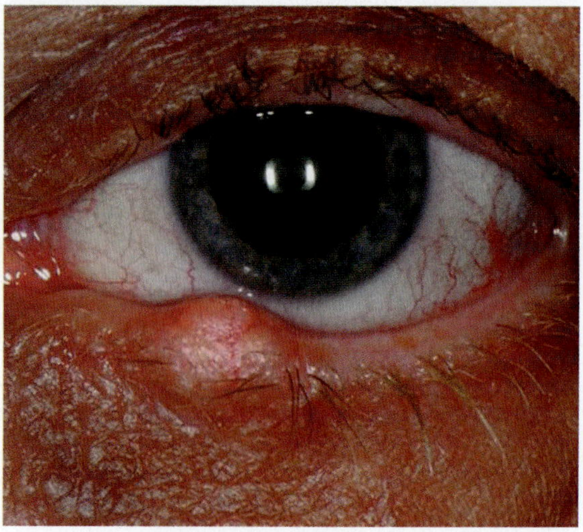

Figure 33.11: A sebaceous cell carcinoma of the lower eyelid.

abscess benefit from incision and drainage at the time of presentation and warrant immediate referral to an ophthalmologist.

Lesions that have been present for days to weeks or that have failed conservative treatment can be managed by an ophthalmologist on an outpatient basis. Even though many lesions will resolve with time, it may take weeks to months. Ophthalmologists may opt to treat with injections of steroid or more definitive management with incision and curettage.

PYOGENIC GRANULOMA

Pathophysiology

As sterile and nongranulomatous capillary-based lesions, pyogenic granulomas (**Figure 33.12**) are poorly named. The more accurate term is lobular capillary hemangioma. The exact pathophysiology is unknown, but pyogenic granulomas tend to occur in sites of previous inflammation, such as surgical sites, trauma sites, or even chalazion sites.

Approach/The Focused Exam

Patients will often notice a sudden large, red-colored lesion inside their eyelid that "pops" into view with certain eyelid manipulation. They may recall a recent history of chalazion or trauma (including iatrogenic trauma). The lesion itself is typically easily visualized with traction on the eyelid. They are similar or slightly darker in color compared with the surrounding conjunctiva and are most frequently pedunculated, although they can sometimes look sessile. Because of their vascularity, the provider must take care during examination because the lesions bleed easily, even with gentle manipulation.

Differential Diagnosis

A chalazion typically appears less pedunculated than a pyogenic granuloma, although pyogenic granulomas may grow over a chalazion. A conjunctival neoplasm typically shows less discrete pedunculation, has greater spread, and may appear more white, gray, or gelatinous (rather than red or dark red). However, if a patient has recurring pyogenic granulomas in the same region, a neoplasm should be suspected.

Management

Topical steroid drops or ointment may help shrink the lesion; topical timolol has more recently been described as a noninvasive treatment as well. Excision is a common and typically definitive treatment. Other less frequently used options include laser, cryotherapy, and cautery.

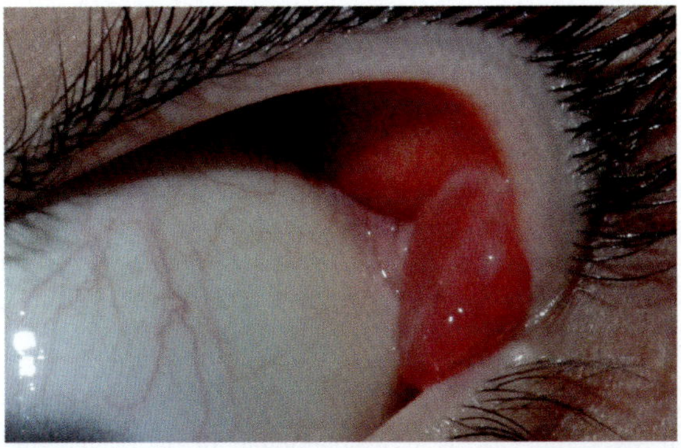

Figure 33.12: A pyogenic granuloma of the lateral upper eyelid is most visible when the eyelid is gently pulled. (From Eyelid. In: Gervasio K, Peck T. *The Wills Eye Manual*. 8th ed. Wolters Kluwer; 2021:136-153. Figure 6.11.2.)

TIPS AND PEARLS

- There is a wide spectrum of eyelid lesions, most of which are benign or can be referred to an ophthalmologist on a routine basis.
- Lesions that cause ulceration, eyelash loss, or recurrence in the exact same location are concerning for neoplasm.
- Both chalazia and hordeola benefit from warm compresses.
- Hordeola benefit from immediate antibiotic treatment, and anti-inflammatory antibiotics may also be helpful in resolving chalazia if there is no resolution with warm compresses owing to their impact on typically underlying blepharitis.

EVIDENCE

What is the role of topical or oral antibiotics with a chalazion?

Topical ophthalmic antibiotics or combination steroid-antibiotics, such as erythromycin or tobramycin-dexamethasone preparations, can help calm chalazia owing to their anti-inflammatory properties; these properties can theoretically help calm acute inflammation (although not studied in chalazia specifically) and are commonly used to treat underlying blepharitis. In addition, oral doxycycline and azithromycin can help calm down chalazia and underlying blepharitis for the same reasons.[2,3] Doxycycline (and others within the tetracycline family) inhibits a number of matrix metalloproteinases, protease-activated receptor 2, cytokine release, leucocyte chemotaxis, nitric oxide synthase, and IgE production, in addition to protecting against oxidative stress and, in vitro as well as anecdotally, granuloma formation.[4] Azithromycin, as part of the macrolide family, also inhibits cytokine production and release, neuotrophil migration and T-cell proliferation and chemotaxis, the production of reactive oxygen species, and the expression of costimulatory B-cell molecules; increases T-cell apoptosis; and modulates selective toll-like receptors.[5]

However, the mainstay of treatment is warm compresses and gentle cleansing, and a large retrospective review of nearly 3000 patients at the University of California, San Francisco, found that in the 320 patients prescribed oral antibiotics, these prevented chalazion recurrence but did not seem to impact initial chalazion treatment success overall; notably, chalazion duration was not studied.[6] If chalazia do not resolve with warm compresses, as well as potentially antibiotic therapy, patients can be referred for steroid or 5-fluorouracil injections or excision of the chalazia on a nonurgent basis.[7,8]

When is it appropriate to prescribe a topical steroid or topical beta-blocker for pyogenic granuloma?

A pyogenic granuloma is bothersome and even fearsome looking at times but it is not a life- or organ-threatening condition. One can consider topical steroids to see if the lesion decreases in size, but this would require monitoring of intraocular pressure (IOP) to avoid unrecognized asymptomatic IOP spikes. Thus, consideration of this treatment is best considered on nonurgent referral.[9,10] Because pyogenic granulomas are vascular and beta-blockers have been used to successfully treat infantile hemangiomas, there has been interest in their use in pyogenic granulomas. The mechanism of action is posited to be attributable to vasoconstriction. A case series of four pediatric patients demonstrated successful ocular surface pyogenic granuloma resolution with topical timolol drops.[11] Notably, topical timolol can have systemic beta-blocker effects (stronger in infants) and should be weighed accordingly.

References

1. Channa R, Zafar SN, Canner JK, et al. Epidemiology of eye-related emergency department visits. *JAMA Ophthalmol.* 2016;134(3):312-319. doi:10.1001/jamaophthalmol.2015.5778
2. Geerling G, Tauber J, Baudouin C, et al. The international workshop on meibomian gland dysfunction: report of the subcommittee on management and treatment of meibomian gland dysfunction. *Invest Ophthalmol Vis Sci.* 2011;52(4):2050-2064. doi:10.1167/iovs.10-6997g

3. Lam-Franco L, Perfecto-Avalos Y, Patiño-Ramírez BE, Rodríguez García A. IL-1α and MMP-9 tear levels of patients with active ocular rosacea before and after treatment with systemic azithromycin or doxycycline. *Ophthalmic Res*. 2018;60(2):109-114. doi:10.1159/000489092. Epub 2018 Jun 6. PMID: 29874670.
4. Henehan M, Montuno M, De Benedetto A. Doxycycline as an anti-inflammatory agent: updates in dermatology. *J Eur Acad Dermatol Venereol*. 2017;31(11):1800-1808. doi:10.1111/jdv.14345. Epub 2017 Jun 7. PMID: 28516469.
5. Steel HC, Theron AJ, Cockeran R, Anderson R, Feldman C. Pathogen- and host-directed anti-inflammatory activities of macrolide antibiotics. *Mediators Inflamm*. 2012;2012:584262. doi:10.1155/2012/584262. Epub 2012 Jun 21. PMID: 22778497; PMCID: PMC3388425.
6. Alsoudi AF, Ton L, Ashraf DC, et al. Efficacy of care and antibiotic use for chalazia and hordeola. *Eye Contact Lens*. 2021;48(4):162-168.
7. Aycinena AR, Achiron A, Paul M, Burgansky-Eliash Z. Incision and curettage versus steroid injection for the treatment of chalazia: a meta-analysis. *Ophthalmic Plast Reconstr Surg*. 2016;32(3):220-224.
8. Wladis EJ, Bradley EA, Bilyk JR, Yen MT, Mawn LA. Oral antibiotics for meibomian gland-related ocular surface disease: a report by the American Academy of Ophthalmology. *Ophthalmology*. 2016;123(3):492-496.
9. DeMaria LN, Silverman NK, Shinder R. Ophthalmic pyogenic granulomas treated with topical timolol-clinical features of 17 cases. *Ophthalmic Plast Reconstr Surg*. 2018;34(6):579-582. doi: 10.1097/IOP.0000000000001116. PMID: 29634609.
10. Herwig-Carl MC, Grossniklaus HE, Müller PL, Atzrodt L, Loeffler KU, Auw-Haedrich C. Pyogenic granuloma associated with conjunctival epithelial neoplasia: report of nine cases. *Br J Ophthalmol*. 2019;103(10):1469-1474. doi:10.1136/bjophthalmol-2018-312960. Epub 2019 Feb 1. PMID: 30709809.
11. Oke I, Alkharashi M, Petersen RA, Ashenberg A, Shah AS. Treatment of ocular pyogenic granuloma with topical timolol. *JAMA Ophthalmol*. 2017;135(4):383-385. doi:10.1001/jamaophthalmol.2017.0110. PMID: 28301661.

CHAPTER 34

Ptosis

Harsha S. Reddy
Di Coneybeare

THE CLINICAL CHALLENGE

Eyelid droop, called blepharoptosis, is often abbreviated to simply ptosis. Ptosis is defined as the inferior displacement of upper eyelid margin from its anatomic position, normally, about 1 to 2 mm inferior to the corneoscleral limbus. Approximately 5% to 13% of adult populations worldwide experience ptosis.[1] The underlying etiology for ptosis is broad with a wide range of acuity, making management of ptosis in the emergency setting challenging. In addition, the severity of ptosis does not always correlate with the degree of pathology or risk to vision and health. Furthermore, patients may not be aware of the time of onset of ptosis and may not present until their eyelid obstructs the visual axis or has significantly decreased their quality of life.

PATHOPHYSIOLOGY

Elevation of the upper eyelid requires coordination of the structural musculature and nervous components that innervate them. The tarsal plates (connective tissue) provide the general structural integrity of the eyelids. Elevation of the upper eyelids occurs by coordinated action of the levator palpebrae superioris and the superior tarsal muscle (Müeller muscle). The oculomotor nerve (cranial nerve III) provides innervation to the levator palpebrae muscle, whereas the superior tarsal muscle receives innervation from the sympathetic fibers of the superior cervical ganglion. The frontalis muscle innervated by the facial nerve (cranial nerve VII) raises the eyebrows.

Disruption to any of the components responsible for upper eyelid elevation can cause ptosis. The pathophysiology can be dichotomously divided into congenital and acquired. This chapter concentrates on the underlying pathophysiology of acquired ptosis that will present in the emergency setting. Pathophysiology of acquired ptosis can be categorized as mechanical, aponeurotic, myogenic, neuromuscular junction, and neurogenic disorders.

Any mass occupying lesions (eg, orbital tumors) or eyelid cellulitis can cause ptosis that can be categorized under mechanical disruption. Thinning of the aponeurosis, caused by aging or iatrogenic intervention, of the levator palpebrae muscle contributes to the aponeurotic causes of ptosis. Myogenic causes of ptosis can involve mitochondrial dysfunction or underlying genetic defects that often cause bilateral ptosis as a result of skeletal muscle dysfunction. Neuromuscular junction causes of ptosis most commonly involve antibodies attacking the acetylcholine receptor (AChR) at the neuromuscular junction of the levator palpebrae muscle. Lastly, neurogenic disorders involve oculomotor nerve palsy or the disruption of the cervical sympathetic chain.

APPROACH/THE FOCUSED EXAM

In evaluating patients with ptosis, emergency providers should inquire about any history of trauma, the course of the lid droop (onset, progression, variation), the presence and nature of eye pain, headache, and double vision. Patients should be asked about a history of eye surgery, eye drops, allergies, eye rubbing, and keratoconus, all of which can lead to eyelid retractor dehiscence.

A complete intraocular exam should be preceded by a cranial nerve exam, ocular motility exam, and evaluation of globe dystopia. Anterior displacement of the eye (proptosis or exophthalmos) should be noted, by either observation ("ant's eye view" or "worm's eye view") or measurement (with an exophthalmometer). Orbital tumors are discussed in Chapter 29.

Careful examination of an acutely ptotic eyelid may reveal a focal eyelid lesion (eg, hordeolum or chalazion) or another process limited to the eyelid. A diffusely edematous pink eyelid associated with tearing and red eye suggests viral conjunctivitis, whereas an edematous lid with surface scale associated with itching is more likely to be allergic dermatitis. For many patients, it is impossible for them to distinguish whether the lid is drooping (ptosis) or swollen, and they may simply describe either condition as a "heavy" lid. Comparison with old photographs (eg, on a driver's license or social media accounts) can be helpful to establish their baseline appearance. In some cases, a new presentation will be identified as a preexisting condition.

Specific measurements to precisely elucidate the ability of the upper eyelid to elevate include the margin reflex distance-1 (MRD1) and levator function (LF), also known as levator excursion. MRD1 measures the distance from the corneal light reflex (with a bright focal light source held at eye level) to the upper eyelid margin (**Figure 34.1**). LF, normally 15 to 20 mm, is measured by holding a ruler next to the patient's eyelid margin when they are looking down and then measuring the maximal superior position of the eyelid when they are asked to look up while the examiner fixates their frontalis by pressing firmly on the forehead (**Figure 34.2**).

The most important elements of the intraocular exam for a ptotic patient are the pupillary exam: evaluate for anisocoria, direct response, consensual response, relative afferent pupillary defect (rAPD), visual acuity, and intraocular pressure. Decreased vision is generally not caused by ptosis alone, so some other cause must be found either on the intraocular exam or, if there is an rAPD, on the optic nerve/visual pathways.

In many acute presentations, neuroimaging is appropriate. A thin-sliced orbital computed tomography (CT) is sufficient for most cases of orbital trauma where the pathology is limited to the orbit, but magnetic resonance imaging (MRI) is the diagnostic modality best suited for deep orbital and intracranial pathology. If an autoimmune etiology is suspected, laboratory workup may be indicated.

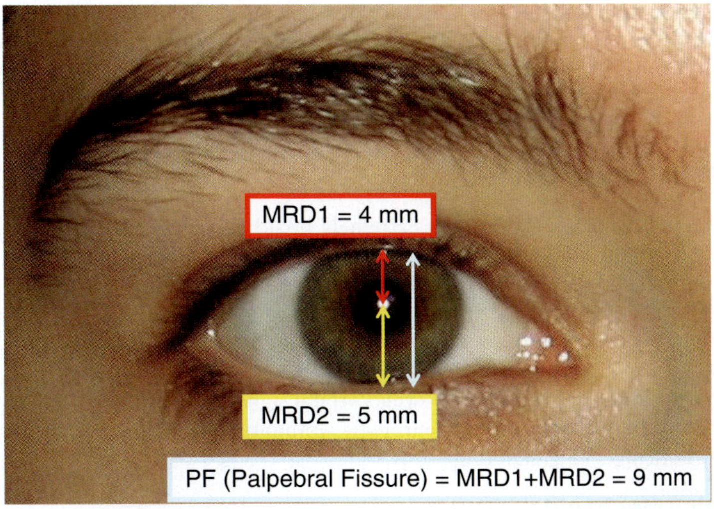

Figure 34.1: The upper eyelid (MRD1); this is the distance in mm from the corneal light reflex to the upper eyelid margin. MRD2 = distance from the corneal light reflex to the lower eyelid margin. Ptosis is defined as a low MRD1 value. MRD, margin to reflex distance. (Courtesy of Harsha S. Reddy, MD.)

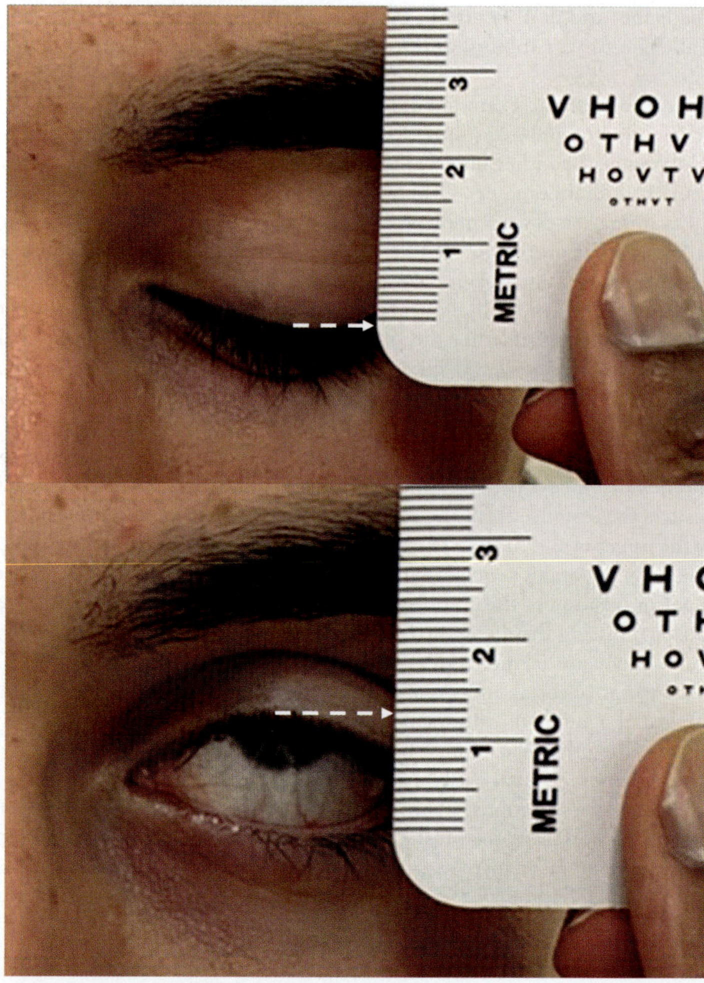

Figure 34.2: Levator function (levator excursion) is measured by aligning a ruler with the eyelid margin when the patient is looking down. The patient is then asked to look up (while the examiner looks up), and the maximal upper eyelid position is marked against the same ruler—in this case 13.5 mm. (Courtesy of Harsha S. Reddy, MD.)

DIFFERENTIAL DIAGNOSIS

The differential diagnosis for ptosis is extremely broad given the numerous possible underlying causes. Some common and possible dangerous presentations are highlighted here.

Aponeurotic Ptosis

Thinning and involution of the aponeurosis of the levator apparatus related to aging is by far the most common cause of acquired ptosis.[1] This often presents in the elderly with symmetric and bilateral ptosis. In the absence of focal eyelid/orbital signs, pupillary involvement, vision changes, extraocular motility defects, or other neurologic symptoms or findings, it is possible that the patient is suddenly noticing a long-standing ptosis.

Traumatic (Mechanical) Ptosis

Ptosis can result from edema/hemorrhage weighting down the eyelid (mechanical ptosis) or blunt trauma or transection of the levator aponeurosis/muscle or from a neurogenic cause (covered separately later). Mechanical ptosis is readily visible externally (**Figure 34.3**). Damage to the levator can be more subtle—suspicion should be high in any full thickness horizontal laceration above

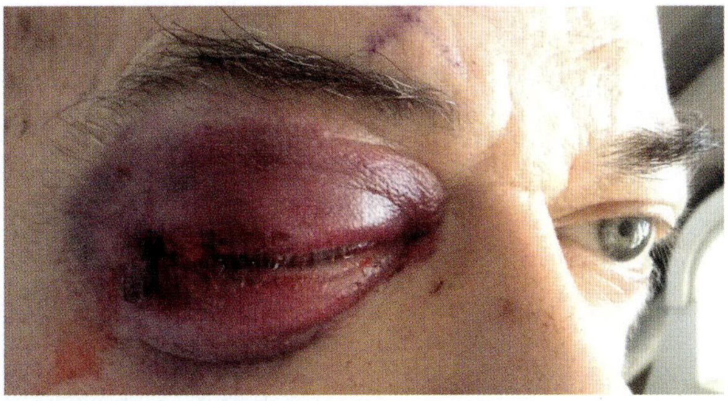

Figure 34.3: Eyelid hematoma causing mechanical ptosis of the upper eyelid. (Courtesy of Harsha S. Reddy, MD.)

the tarsus or any laceration in which orbital fat is visible in the upper eyelid. Blunt trauma to the levator is less well understood and can spontaneously resolve as late as 6 months post trauma. Measurement of LF and comparison with the unaffected side is helpful for diagnosis and monitoring for improvement. Occasionally, a process that causes enophthalmos such as an orbital floor fracture can give the appearance of ptosis (pseudoptosis) because the recessed position of the globe makes the palpebral fissure smaller.

Neurogenic Ptosis

Third Nerve Palsy

A complete third nerve palsy results in a fixed dilated pupil, severe eyelid ptosis with extremely low LF (<5 mm), and an eye that is "down and out" owing to the unopposed action of the lateral rectus and superior oblique. However, patients may present with an incomplete third nerve palsy with paresis of the extraocular muscles or only partial ptosis. Involvement of only the superior rectus and levator (the lid is ptotic and the eye cannot look up) suggests damage to only the superior division of the cranial nerve three (CNIII). A thorough cranial nerve exam should identify involvement of other nerves, which may suggest anatomic location or specific etiologies.

A vast array of pathologies can result in compression, stretching, or hemorrhage of the oculomotor nerve and result in CNIII palsy: vascular, traumatic, infectious/inflammatory, neoplastic, migraines, and neurodegenerative disorders.[1] Aneurysms of the superior cerebellar artery and posterior communicating artery in the cisternal space generally compress the parasympathetic pupillary fibers that run along the nerve, resulting in mydriasis. A ruptured aneurysm can cause direct hemorrhagic damage to the nerve or lead to uncal herniation, which can damage the oculomotor nerve directly or indirectly.[2] The CNIII can also be compressed in the cavernous sinus by space-occupying lesions, including carotid-cavernous fistulas (CCF). In that case, CN IV, V_1, and VI are also often affected, and the patient may present with proptosis and dilated "corkscrew" episcleral vessels and high intraocular pressure (**Figure 34.4**).

Horner Syndrome

Horner syndrome is a clinical constellation of ptosis, miosis, and (sometimes) anhidrosis that results from disruption along the three-neuron oculosympathetic pathway. The pathway originates from the hypothalamus, where the first-order neuron descends along the brainstem to the spinal cord. From here, the second-order neurons travel as the sympathetic chain to the superior cervical ganglion, with some fibers wrapping around the subclavian artery. Finally, some third-order sympathetic neurons travel along the internal carotid artery, connecting the superior cervical ganglion to the pupillary dilator muscle and Müeller muscle of the eyelid. Other third-order sympathetic neurons travel along the external carotid to the sweat glands of the face.

The classic triad of Horner syndrome is ptosis, miosis, and anhidrosis. Etiologies of Horner syndrome are divided into first-order neuron processes (ie, hypothalamic, brainstem, or cervical cord tumor/stroke/demyelination); second-order neuron processes (ie, apical lung tumor, subclavian artery aneurysm, cervical rib injury, thyroid cancer); and third-order neuron processes (ie, internal carotid artery dissection or aneurysm, cavernous sinus process, neck trauma).

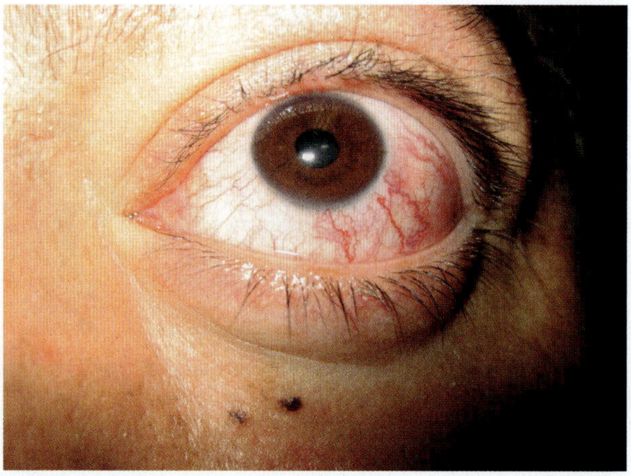

Figure 34.4: This patient presents 1 month after blunt trauma with proptosis, dilated episcleral vessels, and high intraocular pressure. An orbital computed tomography revealed an enlarged superior ophthalmic vein, and a magnetic resonance imaging/magnetic resonance angiogram showed a high-flow carotid-cavernous fistula. (Courtesy of Harsha S. Reddy, MD.)

Neuromuscular Junction Ptosis

Myasthenia Gravis

Myasthenia gravis is a rare neuromuscular disorder characterized by fatigable weakness in skeletal muscle. It can be systemic or limited to the eye (ocular myasthenia gravis). Systemic findings include facial muscle weakness (dysarthria, dysphagia) and proximal limb weakness. Eye findings in the absence of systemic findings occur in 50% of presenting patients.[3] The ptosis is typically described as dramatically worse at the end of the day or with prolonged use of the eyes and better immediately on waking. The pathophysiology of disease is an antibody-mediated immune attack on the nicotinic AChR.[4]

Suspicion of myasthenia gravis is based on clinical exam. Because extraocular muscles are also commonly affected, these patients may also have motility abnormalities (paresis) that cause diplopia but do not match cranial nerve patterns. To assess whether ptosis is caused by myasthenia, two tests are routinely performed. First, the patient is asked to maintain a sustained upward gaze for 1 minute. In myasthenic patients, the eyelids become significantly lower toward the end of the test as the levator muscle fatigues (**Figure 34.5**). Conversely, the patient can be asked to close the eyes to rest the levator muscle for 2 minutes. Approximately 50% of patients with myasthenia will show an improvement in their MRD1 of 2 mm immediately after this test.[5] Placing cold compress over the closed eyelids is an alternative version of the "rest test." Other etiologies of ptosis will not be dramatically affected by either the sustained upward gaze or rest tests. Once an eyelid is fatigued, the LF will also be abnormally low. Patients with myasthenia do not have pupillary abnormalities. A general neurologic exam for muscular weakness should be conducted, with particular attention paid to neck flexors that are relatively weak compared with the neck extensors in patients with systemic disease.

Lab testing for AchR antibodies is routinely performed in an outpatient setting, although 30% to 65% of patients with purely ocular myasthenia gravis will be seronegative.[6,7] Single fiber electromyography (EMG) testing can also be useful. The tensilon test (Edrophonium), previously a well-established test, is a less commonly used test today given concern for systemic side effects and potentially high false positives.[5] All patients with confirmed or suspected myasthenia gravis should also get a chest CT to check for thymoma, which is present in 10% to 15% of patients.[8] In many cases, the lab workup is negative, and the diagnosis of myasthenia remains a clinical one. Response to systemic steroids and acetylcholinesterase therapy can serve as an empiric trial in these patients.

Myogenic Ptosis

In contrast to myasthenia, which affects the neuromuscular junction, several other acquired ptosis disease entities affect the muscle fibers themselves. These include chronic progressive external

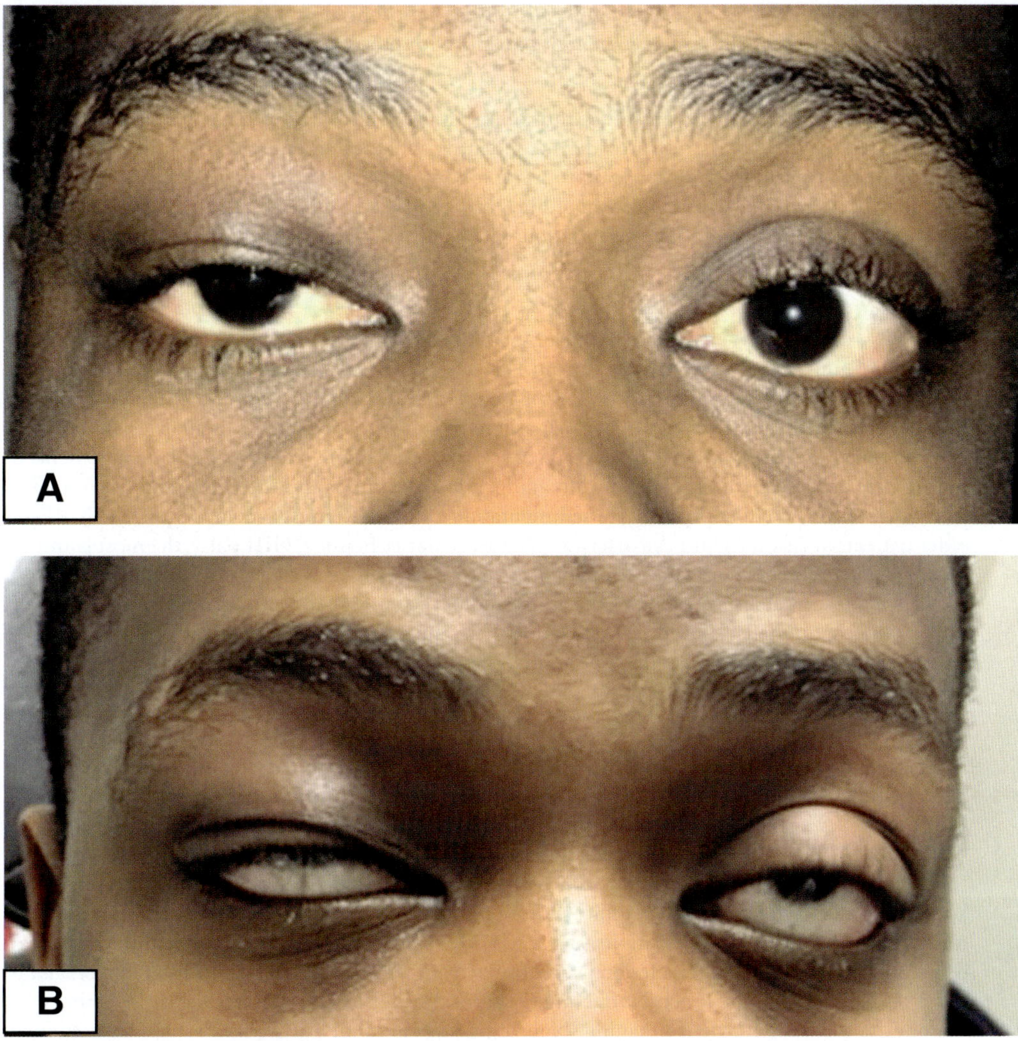

Figure 34.5: A, A young patient with variable ptosis of the right upper eyelid who had recurrent ptosis after an initially successful ptosis repair. B, Fatigue of the right upper eyelid and worse ptosis after sustained upgaze. Both eyes exhibit this feature, but the right eye is more obvious. (Courtesy of Harsha S. Reddy, MD.)

ophthalmoplegia (CPEO) and various types of muscular dystrophy, including oculopharyngeal dystrophy. All of these conditions are characterized by both ptosis and limited ocular motility (ie, both the levator and the extraocular muscles are affected), and pupillary function and visual acuity are normal. In addition, the orbicularis oculi muscle is commonly affected (ie, patients may have trouble both opening and closing their eyes normally). Because these conditions are bilateral and symmetric, most patients do not have symptomatic double vision. A full review of these conditions are beyond the scope of this chapter.

Hereditary myopathies, such as CPEO and oculopharyngeal muscular dystrophy (OPMD), are rare but significant causes of ptosis. They present in middle age (30-60 years). Progression is usually gradual, but they may become symptomatic suddenly, as with other forms of ptosis. Patients my tilt their chin up to overcome the ptosis. CPEO may be isolated or part of Kearns-Sayre syndrome, which includes night blindness, life-threatening cardiac conduction abnormalities, and cerebellar ataxia. In OPMD, patients experience bulbar symptoms such as dysphagia or dysphonia, and atrophy may progress to proximal muscles and even to distal muscles. Muscle biopsy and genetic testing can confirm the diagnosis. Even though there is no cure for these conditions, their ptosis can be managed. Therefore, family history and appropriate referral are important components of the evaluation and management of patients with ptosis.

Management

Management of patients with ptosis depends on the etiology and cause of ptosis. The most important first step for the emergency provider is to identify whether an emergent condition is present. For subacute or chronic conditions, appropriate follow-up with an ophthalmologist, oculoplastics specialist, or neuro-ophthalmologist should be arranged based on the suspected diagnosis. If there is any doubt about the diagnosis, consultation with ophthalmology, neuro-ophthalmology, or neurology may be necessary based on availability.

CNIII Palsy

A diagnosis of third nerve palsy (complete or incomplete) is an emergency. The initial management is neuroimaging. While a noncontrast head CT may detect obvious intracranial hemorrhage or skull base fracture, CT angiogram (CTA) or magnetic resonance angiogram (MRA) is generally indicated to detect vascular pathology such as aneurysms or fistulas. If a vascular lesion is found, interventional radiology and neurosurgery services are often involved for surgical management. In the absence of a focal etiology on neuroimaging, a lab workup is indicated for inflammatory and infectious causes, notably erythrocyte sedimentation rate (ESR) and C-reactive protein (CRP) in older patients at risk for giant cell arteritis. Microvascular ischemic CNIII palsy, the most common etiology of oculomotor nerve palsy in patients over 50 years old, is a diagnosis of exclusion.[9]

Once life-threatening etiologies are addressed in the emergency setting, a neuro-ophthalmologist or ophthalmologist should be involved early in the care of these patients. Clinical stability of symptoms (diplopia, ptosis) for 6 to 12 months should be observed prior to surgical consideration (eg, strabismus surgery, frontalis sling), which can partially improve patient symptoms.

Horner Syndrome

In a patient presenting with acute Horner syndrome, especially if it is associated with head or neck pain, emergent neuroimaging is recommended to visualize the entire oculosympathetic pathway. MRI and MRA of the head and neck are best to diagnose masses and infarcts causing Horner, but CT and CTA are reasonable in patients for whom MRI is contraindicated.

Response to certain medications can help determine the level of disruption. Applying 0.5% apraclonidine (or, less commonly, topical cocaine) to the miotic pupil will result in dilation of the miotic pupil owing to hypersensitivity of the iris dilator muscle. Hydroxyamphetamine drops can be used to determine whether a lesion is pre- or postganglionic (ie, pupillary dilation in response to the drop suggests that the lesion is affecting the second-order neuron). However, drop testing does not obviate the need for neuroimaging. Neuroimaging does not always find a localizing etiology for the Horner syndrome. In one study of 88 patients with clinically isolated Horner syndrome, MRI/MRA found a causative etiology in only 20%.[10] Management should occur in consultation with neuro-ophthalmology.

TIPS AND PEARLS

- In lieu of identification cards, social media photos can be used to detect acuity of ptosis presentation.
- Ptosis in the context of any other cranial nerve involvement highly suggests neurogenic causes, and neuroimaging should be pursued.

EVIDENCE

Can wearing contacts cause ptosis?

In a recent meta-analysis, Hwang et al. analyzed five retrospective studies comparing findings of ptosis in contact wearing and contact nonwearing populations. They found a significant increase in the presentation of ptosis in patients wearing hard contacts and even sometimes soft contacts.[11] The proposed mechanism involves injury and stretching of the levator muscle and its aponeurosis in the process of placing and removing the contacts.[11] This acquired ptosis can be corrected merely by cessation of contact wearing for several months; if ptosis does not spontaneously resolve despite avoidance of further injury, surgical correction is recommended. In cases of symmetric ptosis, a history of contact lens wear may be helpful to identify the underlying cause.

Can ocular surgery cause ptosis?

Although most ocular surgery does not directly intervene on the apparatus affecting eyelid function, the incidence of postoperative ptosis in patients undergoing ocular surgery can range from 4% to more than one-third of the time.[12] In a recent systematic review and meta-analysis, the combined incidence of nontransient postoperative ptosis mounted to 11%.[12] The type of surgery and the preexisting levator apparatus integrity of the patient may contribute to the heterogeneity of the initial data. They identified two risk factors associated with increased incidence: glaucoma surgery and the female gender.[12] The exact mechanism causing postoperative ptosis is not well established but thought to be multifactorial. However, given the high incidence of postoperative ptosis, a careful surgical history can potentially help elucidate the cause of ptosis presentation.

References

1. Bacharach J, Lee WW, Harrison AR, Freddo TF. A review of acquired blepharoptosis: prevalence, diagnosis, and current treatment options. *Eye*. 2021;35:2468-2481.
2. Palazzolo L, Wang, D, Elmalem VI. *Neuro-Opththalmic Trauma in Pediatric Ophthalmology in the Emergency Room*. Springer Nature Switzerland AG; 2021.
3. Gilbert ME, Savino PJ. Ocular myasthenia gravis. *Int Ophthalmol Clin*. 2007;47:93-103, ix.
4. McGrogan A, Sneddon S, de Vries CS. The incidence of myasthenia gravis: a systematic literature review. *Neuroepidemiology*. 2010;34:171-183.
5. Kubis KC, Danesh-Meyer HV, Savino PJ, Sergott RC. The ice test versus the rest test in myasthenia gravis. *Ophthalmology*. 2000;107:1995-1998.
6. Porter NC, Salter BC. Ocular myasthenia gravis. *Curr Treat Options Neurol*. 2005;7:79-88.
7. Monsul NT, Patwa HS, Knorr AM, Lesser RL, Goldstein JM. The effect of prednisone on the progression from ocular to generalized myasthenia gravis. *J Neurol Sci*. 2004;217:131-133.
8. Silvestri NJ, Wolfe GI. Treatment-refractory myasthenia gravis. *J Clin Neuromuscul Dis*. 2014;15:167-178.
9. Kung NH, Van Stavern GP. Isolated ocular motor nerve palsies. *Semin Neurol*. 2015;35:539-548.
10. Beebe JD, Kardon RH, Thurtell MJ. The yield of diagnostic imaging in patients with isolated Horner syndrome. *Neurol Clin*. 2017;35:145-151.
11. Hwang K, Kim JH. The risk of blepharoptosis in contact lens wearers. *J Craniofac Surg*. 2015;26:e373-e374.
12. Wang Y, Lou L, Liu Z, Ye J. Incidence and risk of ptosis following ocular surgery: a systematic review and meta-analysis. *Graefes Arch Clin Exp Ophthalmol*. 2019;257:397-404.

CHAPTER 35

Corneal Trauma: Abrasions, Lacerations, Foreign Bodies, Burns, and Contact Lenses

Leejee H. Suh
Daniel L. Overbeek

INTRODUCTION

The surface of the eye, comprised of the cornea and conjunctiva, is susceptible to injuries from exposure or trauma. Eyelids and eyelashes act as physical barriers to the outside environment and, along with the blink reflex, protect the globe from many oncoming threats. Tears bathe the ocular surface with nutrients and immune factors but also trap and sweep away small particles.

The cornea is the eye's main focusing layer as it bends or refracts light so that images are focused onto the retina. The hallmark transparency of the cornea is caused by the highly organized arrangement of collagen fibers contained in the stroma, which is bordered externally by the corneal epithelium and internally by the endothelium. Disruption of the corneal stroma caused by a laceration results in scar formation, opacification of the cornea, and potential loss of vision.

The endothelium is a single layer of cells on the inner surface of the cornea that maintains desiccation of the stroma. Damage or loss of corneal endothelial cells, which do not regenerate, causes loss of corneal clarity from ensuing corneal edema.

Finally, the cornea is one the most sensitive tissues of the body as it is densely innervated with sensory nerve fibers from the ophthalmic division of the trigeminal nerve, making corneal injuries notably painful.

ABRASIONS

Even minor trauma to the corneal surface can cause epithelial cells to separate from their underlying attachments. A corneal abrasion, also interchangeably called "corneal epithelial defect," is the loss of part or all of the corneal epithelium without injury to the underlying stroma.

APPROACH/THE FOCUSED EXAM

Common causes of corneal abrasion include injury from fingernails, paper, makeup applicators, tips of eye drop dispensers, dust or dirt particles, and other objects. In chronic contact lens wearers, malpositioned lenses can cause a corneal epithelial injury. If the patient is unable to identify a discrete injury, the physician should be concerned about serious spontaneous causes of an epithelial defect, which include severe dry eye and exposure keratopathy from incomplete blink or inadequate closure of the eyelids, such as in sedation or an altered mental status, seventh nerve palsy, eyelid deformity, proptosis, floppy eyelid syndrome, and Parkinson disease.

The patient will complain of intense pain, photophobia, and foreign body sensation and tearing and likely have difficulty voluntarily opening the affected eye. For this reason, instillation of a topical anesthetic drop such as proparacaine or tetracaine can temporarily relieve the discomfort and facilitate the rest of the exam.

On examination, the visual acuity of a patient with a corneal abrasion may be decreased if the abrasion disrupts the central cornea. Fluorescein stain and cobalt blue illumination will best highlight the presence and dimensions of a corneal epithelial defect (**Figure 35.1**). Ideally, the cornea is evaluated with slit lamp magnification, noting the extent of any abrasion and any underlying tissue disturbance. A cotton-tipped applicator soaked in topical anesthetic can be used to debride loose epithelium and aid in a careful evaluation. The de-epithelialized corneal stroma underneath should be smooth and transparent. If the denuded area is not smooth or is disrupted, there may be a laceration or perforation of the cornea. If the area is not transparent, a cellular infiltrate may have caused opacification of the underlying stroma, and infectious keratitis must be considered (**Figure 35.2**). In either case, immediate evaluation by an ophthalmologist is essential.

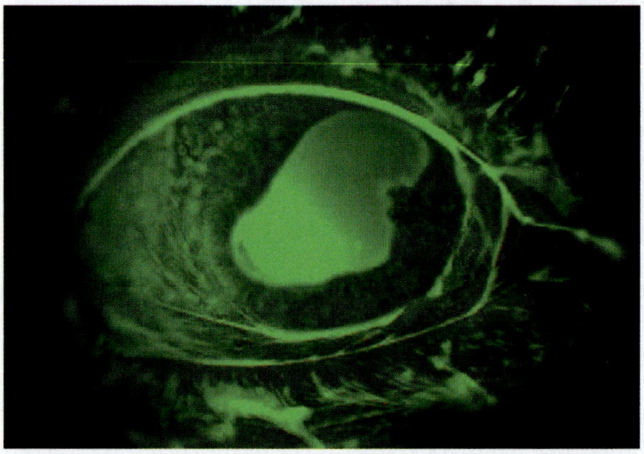

Figure 35.1: Corneal abrasion—fluorescein staining delineates the margins of the corneal abrasion. (From Casper DS, Cioffi CA, eds. *The Columbia Guide to Basic Elements of Eye Care: A Manual for Healthcare Professionals*. Springer; 2019. Reproduced with permission from Springer International Publishing.)

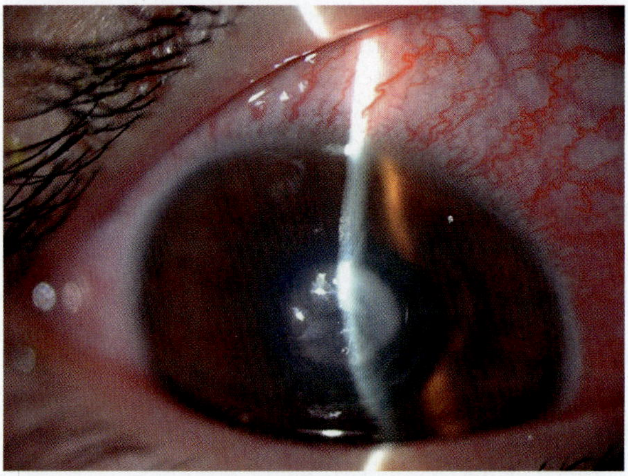

Figure 35.2: Corneal ulcer—also known as keratitis, the area under the corneal abrasion shows a whitish infiltrate in the corneal stroma. (From Casper DS, Cioffi CA, eds. *The Columbia Guide to Basic Elements of Eye Care: A Manual for Healthcare Professionals*. Springer; 2019. Reproduced with permission from Springer International Publishing.)

In evaluating the anterior chamber, the clinician should look for a normal chamber depth, a normal iris, and a round and reactive pupil. Any disruption of these structures may indicate a perforating injury, with an occult intraocular foreign body presumed to be present.

DIFFERENTIAL DIAGNOSIS

Corneal abrasions are usually easily diagnosed. Entities that present in a similar fashion include infectious keratitis (corneal ulcer from bacterial, fungal, or viral etiologies), recurrent erosion syndrome, ultraviolet keratitis (welder's "burn"), and severe dry eye syndrome. Recurrent erosion syndrome is a common condition of the epithelial and/or epithelial basement membrane characterized by recurrent corneal abrasions that typically occur on awakening when the eyelids are rubbed and opened. Common etiologies include a history of traumatic corneal abrasion and anterior corneal basement membrane dystrophy. Finally, one must entertain a very high degree of suspicion for infectious keratitis in any patient who has a history of injury from organic matter or one who wears contact lenses, particularly with overnight lens wear, poor contact lens hygiene, and a history of sleeping and/or swimming with contacts.

MANAGEMENT

The prognosis for corneal abrasion is excellent because the corneal epithelium will usually regenerate without scar formation within 1 week and restore normal visual acuity. The primary complication of concern, however, is secondary infectious keratitis, which can cause scarring and subsequent vision loss. For this reason, all patients with a corneal abrasion are started on prophylactic topical antibiotics. Proper topical antibiotic selection is important and may not be the same in all cases. For a noncontact lens wearer, topical ophthalmic erythromycin ointment, bacitracin or bacitracin/polymyxin ophthalmic ointment or polymyxin B/trimethoprim drops are all commonly used. If the patient is a contact lens wearer, or the injury was from a fingernail or organic matter (eg, tree branches), a broader spectrum antibiotic, such as a topical fourth generation fluoroquinolone such as moxifloxacin, is usually the antibiotic of choice.

Antibiotic treatment is typically continued for 5 to 7 days 4 times daily or until the epithelial defect has resolved. In the case of abrasions from organic matter, the patient must be followed by an ophthalmologist to monitor for delayed-onset fungal infection. For large abrasions, a cycloplegic agent (ie, cyclopentolate 1%) is often used to reduce photophobia caused by ciliary body spasm. Contact lens wearers should forgo any contact lens wear for at least 1 week beyond full recovery and the completion of a complete antibiotic course. The patient should then be referred to an ophthalmologist for continued care to ensure appropriate healing and resolution and to confirm that no secondary keratitis is present. Patching the eye can be considered for pain control but should not be done if the injury involves fingernails or organic matter or if the patient wears contact lenses, because in these cases patching may enhance bacterial growth.[1]

LACERATIONS

A corneal laceration is caused by a sharp object cutting through the epithelium and into the stroma. When a laceration is full thickness, it is termed a corneal perforation and results in an open globe. These wounds can often be self-sealing, especially when caused by a high-velocity projectile. The patient may report significant pain, photophobia, and reduced vision, as in a corneal abrasion, or may have more subtle symptoms.

Slit lamp examination should include examination of not only the cornea but also the adjoining conjunctiva and sclera to look for extension beyond the peripheral cornea. The anterior chamber depth of the affected eye should be compared with the contralateral eye as a shallower anterior chamber signifies a wound leak and likely full thickness laceration.

A Seidel test is very useful in identifying a wound leak from a corneal perforation. In this test, the eye is anesthetized with topical anesthetic, and then a moistened fluorescein strip is applied directly over the potential site of perforation while observing the area under the cobalt blue light in slit lamp examination. If there is a wound leak, the fluorescein dye will be diluted by the escaping aqueous humor and appear as a green stream (**Figure 35.3**). This is called a "positive Seidel test."

Once a corneal laceration and perforation are detected, immediate ophthalmology evaluation is required to decide whether treatment can be performed at the slit lamp or with surgical intervention. Full thickness corneal lacerations greater than 2 mm generally require surgical intervention in the operating room with primary closure (**Figure 35.4**). If the anterior chamber is flat, the repair should be done within 24 hours to avoid permanent damage to the lens and cornea and creation of peripheral scarring or synechiae between these two areas. If there is concomitant iris prolapse through the corneal laceration, repair should be done in the operating room to either reposition the iris into the anterior chamber or debride areas that appear necrotic or

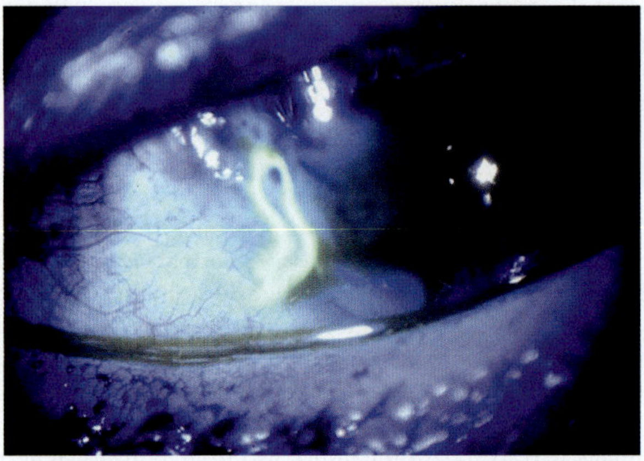

Figure 35.3: Positive Seidel test—under cobalt blue illumination, the area of perforation is highlighted by the "green" stream of fluid. (From Casper DS, Cioffi CA, eds. *The Columbia Guide to Basic Elements of Eye Care: A Manual for Healthcare Professionals*. Springer; 2019. Reproduced with permission from Springer International Publishing.)

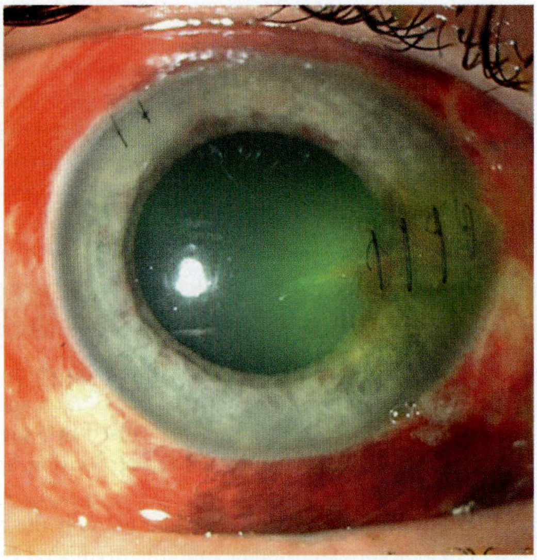

Figure 35.4: Corneal laceration repair—10-0 nylon sutures are used to primarily close the corneal laceration. (From Casper DS, Cioffi CA, eds. *The Columbia Guide to Basic Elements of Eye Care: A Manual for Healthcare Professionals*. Springer; 2019. Reproduced with permission from Springer International Publishing.)

infected. Extensive lacerations with avulsion and large amount of tissue loss may require corneal transplantation.

Smaller corneal lacerations that are 1 to 2 mm can be managed by ophthalmology at the slit lamp. Bandage soft contact lens may be sufficient for a small self-sealing, beveled, or edematous corneal laceration to protect the wound as it heals. Prophylactic topical antibiotics, such as moxifloxacin, are started in addition to topical aqueous suppressants such as topical timolol to reduce aqueous production. The United States Food and Drug Administration has not approved cyanoacrylate glue for use in the eye, but its usage for small corneal perforations is still commonplace by ophthalmologists.[2]

FOREIGN BODIES

Most superficial foreign bodies spontaneously dislodge from the cornea into the tear film. Reflex tearing rinses loose foreign bodies from the eye. Foreign bodies can embed into the cornea, and patients will often have symptoms similar to a corneal abrasion but can be slightly delayed after the initial trauma. Metallic foreign bodies are usually retained within the corneal epithelium or stroma (**Figure 35.5A**) and often exhibit "rust rings," consisting of oxidized ferrous materials, owing to reaction with the overlying tear film, which leach into the surrounding tissue (**Figure 35.5B**).

Vertical corneal abrasions suggest a retained foreign body under the upper or lower eyelid causing repeated trauma to the cornea. The upper and lower lids should be everted and examined for any foreign material. This exam can be facilitated by sweeping underneath the lid. With the eye anesthetized and the patient in opposite gaze, a cotton tip applicator can be used to gently sweep the upper and lower fornix to remove or rule out any foreign body.

A history of injury from high-speed projectiles; machines such as drills, saws, grinders, sanders, hammering metal-on-metal; or explosions warrants a full dilated exam to rule out intraocular penetration. The deeper corneal stroma, iris, lens, and anterior chamber should be intact, and if there is any concern for intraocular penetration, computed tomography (CT) of the orbits can be helpful in identifying radiopaque foreign bodies.

MANAGEMENT

If a corneal foreign body is present, and if it is safely determined that the cornea is not perforated, the foreign body should be removed under slit lamp magnification after instillation of topical anesthetic and an eyelid speculum. A superficially embedded foreign body can sometimes be removed with a cotton-tipped applicator alone. However, it is often necessary to use a 25-to-30-gauge needle to gently remove the corneal foreign body. Prevention of keratitis is then managed with topical antibiotic treatment and referral to ophthalmology, similarly to the management of corneal abrasions. If a metallic foreign body has been retained for 12 to 24 hours, a rust ring may form, which can be managed by ophthalmology with removal with a corneal burr at the slit lamp. It is sometimes safer

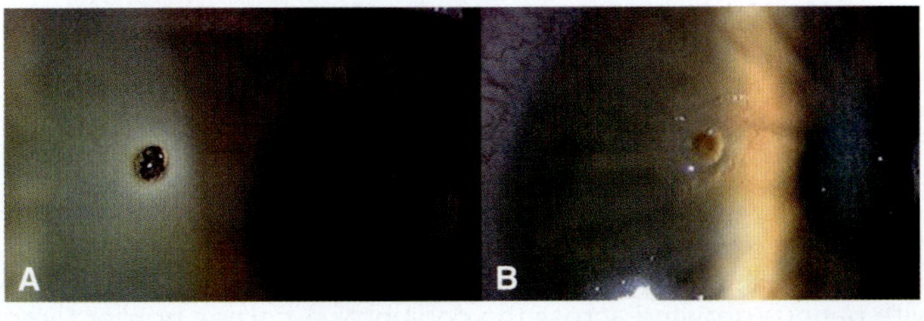

Figure 35.5: Metallic corneal foreign body (A) and associated rust ring (B). (From Casper DS, Cioffi CA, eds. *The Columbia Guide to Basic Elements of Eye Care: A Manual for Healthcare Professionals*. Springer; 2019. Reproduced with permission from Springer International Publishing.)

to leave a deeper, central rust ring to allow time for the rust to migrate anteriorly, at which removal will be more accessible. This is especially important in injuries involving organic matter, which carry higher risks of infection.

BURNS

Chemical burns make up a significant proportion of ocular injuries, and severe cases can have significant long-term morbidity. Chemical burns to the eye are frequently related to industrial exposures, including in the construction and chemical industries.

PATHOPHYSIOLOGY

The thin and fragile nature of the cornea makes it prone to caustic damage. Tear layers work to protect the cornea and maintain appropriate corneal pH. Chemical burns caused by alkali agents tend to be more severe because the lipophilic nature of the chemicals leads to deeper penetration into the cornea. Acid burns tend to be more superficial owing to buffering by corneal proteins. Severe injury can also be damaging to the limbal stem cells. Limbal stem cell deficiency (LSCD) is a long-term complication (**Figure 35.6**), with poor healing and chronic epithelial injuries. Additionally, ongoing inflammation after the initial injury can worsen chronic symptoms, including vision impairment.

EMERGENT EVALUATION AND MANAGEMENT

Initial evaluation and management after a suspected corneal burn focuses on halting any ongoing damage to the corneal surface. Copious irrigation of the eye is the most important step to attempt to normalize pH and should be started even before the patient arrives in the emergency department (ED). Early irrigation is critical to decrease complications, need for surgery, and improve visual acuity.[3] If available, balanced irrigation solutions such as specialized eyewash solutions, balanced saline solutions, lactate ringers, or diphoterine should be used. If unavailable, tap water or normal saline can also be utilized, because they are readily available, but can have longer times to pH normalization. Time to irrigation should be minimized, and initial aggressive irrigation should not be delayed to obtain specialized solutions.[4]

Some toxins, such as calcium oxide (cement/lime), will react with water to produce other caustic substances. However, these toxins will also react with the aqueous component of natural tears, so high-volume irrigation should still be performed as early as possible in these exposures, and water should be used if no other solution is available.

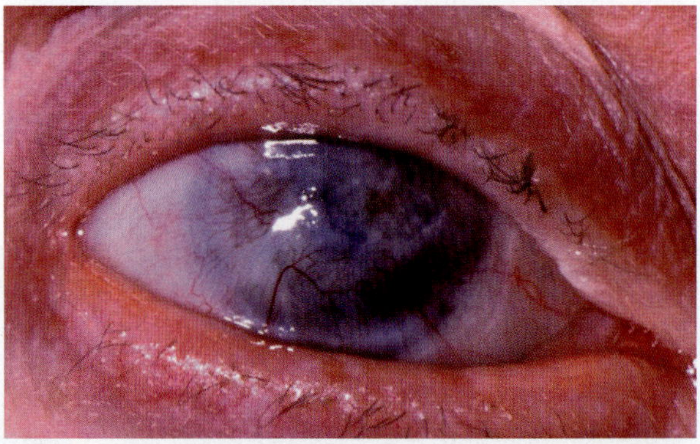

Figure 35.6: Limbal stem cell deficiency after chemical burn—there is "conjunctivalization" of the corneal surface with pannus growing across the conjunctiva-cornea border (limbus). (Courtesy of Daniel S. Casper, MD, PhD. In: Casper DS, Cioffi CA, eds. *The Columbia Guide to Basic Elements of Eye Care: A Manual for Healthcare Professionals*. Springer; 2019. Reproduced with permission from Springer International Publishing.)

To satisfactorily irrigate the eye, topical anesthesia will likely be required. The eye can be manually irrigated, with one individual retracting the eyelids and the other flushing the eye. Special care should be taken to ensure no foreign material remains under the lids in the cul-de-sac, and any particles need to be carefully extracted. pH testing should be performed if available, and the eye should be irrigated until the pH normalizes, or for at least 30 minutes if testing is not available.

In the short term following a significant corneal chemical injury, epithelial regeneration is critical, and treatments attempt to avoid further damage, encourage reepithelialization, and decrease corneal inflammation. Ensuring appropriate lubrication with artificial tears or ointments can protect from further epithelial damage. Topical corticosteroids are also used in the early phase to reduce the inflammatory response in both the cornea, conjunctiva, and anterior chamber. Topical antibiotics should also be utilized to prevent invasive infection while the protective epithelial layer is damaged. Ophthalmologic follow-up will be needed for any patient with a corneal burn requiring irrigation.

CONTACT LENS CONSIDERATIONS

Contact lens wearers can have myriad reasons for urgent evaluation, including retained lenses, corneal abrasions, and corneal infections (keratitis). Contact lenses disrupt the three-layer tear film and enhance tear evaporation, leading to the lack of corneal oxygenation and the symptoms of dry eye.

Contact lens wearers can present to the ED or urgent care setting for a retained or displaced contact lens in their eye. The normal position of the contact lens is over the cornea, but it may occasionally relocate over the sclera or in various parts of the eye, including under the upper eyelid. The patient will report discomfort and foreign body sensation with a history of difficulty removing the contact lens. Although the contact lens usually falls out of the eye, the eye must be examined to rule out retention. Fluorescein and topical anesthetic are placed into the eye. The fluorescein stains the contact lens, making identification easier (**Figure 35.7**). Retained lenses are usually found in the superior fornix and may require eversion of the upper eyelid for removal.

Contact lens wearers are at increased risk for developing infectious keratitis because extended and continual use of contacts can cause corneal hypoxia that allows more susceptibility to infections. The risk increases with extended contact lens use, such as overnight wear, and activities such as swimming with contact lenses or poor contact lens hygiene. Micro-corneal abrasions from contact lens use may allow organisms from the ocular surface to enter the corneal stroma. Bacterial infections are the most common etiology for contact lens-related keratitis.

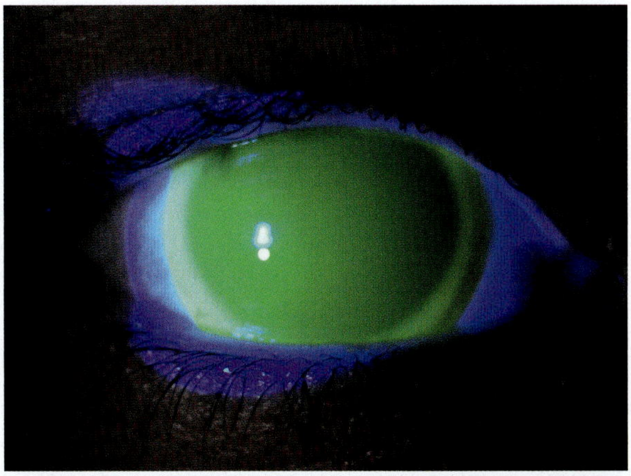

Figure 35.7: Fluorescein-stained contact lens. (Courtesy of Suzanne Sherman, OD.)

A history of swimming with contacts or washing them with tap water makes the patient more susceptible to infections from the parasite *Acanthamoeba*. On presentation, the patient will have symptoms similar to those of a corneal abrasion. If the patient still has the contact lens in the eye, the lens should be removed and can be cultured. On examination, the conjunctiva will be injected, and the cornea will have an infiltrate in the stroma with possible coexisting iritis in the anterior chamber (Figure 35.2). Urgent referral to the ophthalmologist is required for culture of the corneal infiltrate.[5] Topical antimicrobial therapy should be initiated in the ED or urgent care setting, such as a fourth-generation fluoroquinolone. Larger, sight threatening corneal ulcers must be treated with fortified topical antibiotics such as vancomycin and tobramycin and should be seen urgently by ophthalmology.

TIPS AND PEARLS

- Consider the visual acuity as the vital sign of the eye—any patient with significantly impaired visual acuity should trigger ophthalmologic consultation.
- Contact lens wearers are at increased risk for complications, should receive broad spectrum antimicrobial therapy for corneal injuries, and should discontinue contact lens use during any acute injury until ophthalmologic follow-up.
- Fluorescein staining can be utilized to identify a displaced and retained contact lens.
- Immediate copious irrigation should be utilized for corneal chemical exposures, utilizing balanced solutions if available.

EVIDENCE

Can repeated topical anesthetic use cause toxicity?

Topical ophthalmic anesthetics are used for initial assessment of eye trauma, removal of foreign bodies, and measurement of intraocular pressure. Repeated application of topical anesthetics should be avoided, however, owing to evidence that has shown complications of the cornea such as persistent epithelial defects, stroma edema, sterile infiltrates, corneal thinning, and even perforation.[6,7] Most providers do not prescribe topical anesthetic for corneal abrasions, owing to concern for masking of possible keratitis pain, and delayed wound healing increasing risk of ulceration. Repeated use can mask symptoms and may discourage follow-up. However, because the benefit would only be to manage foreign body sensation, we recommend against prescribing anesthetics.[8,9] Topical corticosteroids or antibiotic-steroid combinations should also be avoided, owing to an associated increased risk of infection and delayed healing.

Does the use of specialized irrigation matter?

For patients with corneal burns from caustic agents, normalization of the pH is critical to decreasing corneal damage and to improving long-term outcomes. Multiple studies have investigated the use of a variety of irrigation solutions. Animal studies, such as from Rihawi et al., have shown faster normalization of pH with specialized irrigation solutions such as Cederroth or Diphoterine solutions.[10] Observational studies have also supported specialized solutions.[11] However, these are often unavailable in the ED or urgent care setting. Immediate irrigation with tap water has also been shown to reduce severity and shorten healing time.[12] As such, we recommend immediate irrigation as the priority, with the choice of solution often dependent on what is immediately available in the ED or urgent care setting.

References

1. Lim CH, Turner A, Lim BX. Patching for corneal abrasion. *Cochrane Database Syst Rev*. 2016;7(7):CD004764.
2. Mascai MS. The management of corneal trauma: advances in the past twenty-five years. *Cornea*. 2000;19(5):617-624.

3. Kuckelkoran R, Schrage N, Keller G, Redbrake C. Emergency treatment of chemical and thermal eye burns. *Acta Ophthalmol Scand*. 2002;80(1):4-10.
4. Kompa S, Redbrake C, Hilgers C, Wustemeyer H, Schrage N, Remky A. Effect of different irrigating solutions on aqueous humour pH changes, intraocular pressure and histological findings after induced alkali burns. *Acta Ophthalmol Scand*. 2005;83(4):467-470.
5. Lin A, Rhee MK, Akpek EK, et al. Bacterial keratitis preferred practice pattern. *Ophthalmology*. 2019;126(1):P1-P55.
6. McGee HT, Fraunfelder FW. Toxicities of topical ophthalmic anesthetics. *Expert Opin Drug Saf*. 2007;6(6):637-740.
7. Katsimpris JM Sarantoulakou M, Kordelou A, Petkou D, Petropoulos IK. Clinical findings in patients with topical anaesthetic abuse keratitis: a report of five cases. *Klin Monbl Augenheilkd*. 2007;224(4):303-308.
8. Yu CW, Kirubarajan A, Yau M, Armstrong D, Johnson DE. Topical pain control for corneal abrasions: a systematic review and meta-analysis. *Acad Emerg Med*. 2021;28(8)890-908.
9. Waldman N, Winrow B, Densie I, et al. An observational study to determine whether routinely sending patients home with a 24-hour supply of topical tetracaine from the emergency department for simple corneal abrasion pain is potentially safe. *Ann Emerg Med*. 2018;71(6):767-778.
10. Rihawi S, Frentz M, Schrage NF. Emergency treatment of eye burns: which rinsing solution should we choose? *Graefes Arch Clin Exp Ophthalmol*. 2006;244(5):845-854.
11. Merle H, Donnio A, Ayeboua L, et al. Alkali ocular burns in Martinique (French West Indies): evaluation of the use of an amphoteric solution as the rinsing product. *Burns*. 2005;31(2):205-211.
12. Ikeda N, Hayasaka S, Hayasaka Y, Watanabe K. Alkali burns of the eye: effect of immediate copious irrigation with tap water on their severity. *Ophthalmologica*. 2006;220(4):225-228.

CHAPTER 36

The Red Eye: Keratitis, Conjunctivitis, Episcleritis, Scleritis, Pterygium/Pinguecula

David Peak
Neha Shaik

THE CLINICAL CHALLENGE

The etiology of the red eye includes the spectrum from nonemergent conditions to potentially sight-threatening true emergencies. The terminology can be challenging because some terms such as conjunctivitis and keratitis merely refer to pathology of a particular part of the eye, but the clinician must infer the cause of the pathology in order to effectively treat the patient. Inciting pathology can also affect multiple parts of the eye simultaneously and be related to infection, toxins, trauma, or inflammatory conditions. An understanding of the various conditions will help inform the urgency of ophthalmology consultation or follow-up.

PATHOPHYSIOLOGY

The conjunctiva covers the anterior portion of the eye (except the cornea) and provides eye protection, lubrication, and a degree of immune defense. The conjunctiva can be subdivided into three parts: the palpebral/tarsal conjunctiva, which lines the eyelids; the bulbar conjunctiva, lining the globe to the limbus; and the fornices, which form the junction between the bulbar and the palpebral conjunctiva. The palpebral conjunctiva is somewhat loose and flexible, allowing for movement, unlike the bulbar conjunctiva. The conjunctiva consists of a superficial epithelial layer, the substantia propria, and a deep fibrous layer. The epithelial layer is composed of nonkeratinized stratified squamous and columnar epithelial cells, goblet cells (more numerous close to the fornix), blood vessels, fibrous tissue, lymphatics, melanocytes, T- and B-cell lymphocytes, Langerhans cells, and accessory lacrimal glands. The middle substantia propria contains numerous lymphocytes, mast cells, plasm cells, and neutrophils. The deepest fibrous layer contains nerves and blood vessels.

Bulbar conjunctival vessels are normally invisible to barely visible to the naked eye. They dilate and cause redness owing to multiple stimuli, including allergens, irritants, fever, infections, and even some emotional states. The bulbar conjunctiva may also reveal other pathology such as icterus in the case of significant elevations in serum bilirubin concentrations.

The palpebral conjunctiva is normally pink and smooth. It may become pale with significant anemia or injected and swollen with inflammatory and infectious conditions. In patients with severe allergic vernal keratoconjunctivitis, there may be a cobblestoning-type pattern with giant papillae (>1 mm diameter).

The cornea is a dome-shaped transparent ocular tissue extending from the sclera at the limbus. The cornea is made up of multiple avascular layers, normally transparent and highly innervated with unmyelinated nerve endings. The cornea is considered to have the highest density of pain receptors in the entire body (roughly 300-600 times greater than skin), making it highly sensitive to touch, which results in reflexive closing.

Nutrients and oxygen diffuse through the cornea from tears on the outside and the aqueous humor on the inside surface. Because transparency is so important, the cornea is thought to have what is referred to as immunologic immunity, meaning that it will generally tolerate introduction of minor antigens with little or no inflammatory response.

The episclera is a fibrous, elastic structure consisting of two layers that both contain vessels originating from the anterior ciliary arteries that stem from the ophthalmic artery. The episclera lies between Tenon capsule and the sclera. Compared to the scleral stroma, the collagen bundles of the episclera are less dense, thinner, and more irregularly arranged.

The sclera is mostly collagenous and avascular and provides strength and some degree of flexibility to the globe, covering the posterior five-sixths of its surface with an anterior opening for the cornea and a posterior opening for the optic nerve. The sclera is continuous with the stromal layer of the cornea at the junction between them, which is called the limbus and, posteriorly, with the optic nerve's dura and arachnoid sheaths. The sclera is composed of fibrils of Type I collagen that are arranged in irregular and interlacing bundles (which account for the opaque quality as well as strength and flexibility), elastic fibers, fibroblasts, and proteoglycans and glycoproteins. The tendons of the rectus muscles inset into the superficial scleral collagen. If one were to make a model of the eye using a tennis ball, the sclera would be akin to the rubber core of the ball, functioning to protect and maintain the shape of the eye.

A small portion of the anterior sclera (the "white of the eye") is visible. The sclera may appear more brownish in individuals with more melanin, which deposits in the conjunctiva and sclera, and this is normal. In osteogenesis imperfecta type 1, the sclera is much thinner, revealing the blue choroid. The sclera is almost avascular but is surrounded by both the vascular episclera externally and the richly vascular choroid internally. At the limbus, however, there is an intrascleral venous plexus, which is contiguous with the episcleral veins and ciliary venous plexus. The sclera does contain sensory nerves, which cause pain with inflammation.

Conjunctivitis ("pink eye") refers to inflammation of the bulbar conjunctiva. Common etiologies include inflammatory conditions, irritants/allergens, and infections (viral and bacterial). Viral conjunctivitis is the most common etiology in both pediatric and adult populations. *Adenovirus* is common and is usually associated with other viral symptoms such as fever, pharyngitis, and cough, although isolated ocular symptoms may also occur. Viral conjunctivitis is highly contagious and spread by direct contact of ocular secretions.

Keratitis refers to inflammation of the cornea. Ultraviolet keratitis occurs from exposure in the absence of eye protection (eg, welders, skiers/snowboarders). Keratitis can also be caused by autoimmune diseases (eg, rheumatoid arthritis, lupus, Wegener granulomatosis), dry eye syndrome (keratoconjunctivitis sicca), vitamin A deficiency, and infection. Most infectious keratitis is bacterial. However, viral, fungal, and protozoal infections can also occur (outbreaks of *Acanthamoeba* have been reported). A delay in diagnosis and treatment may result in ocular complications, including corneal perforation, cornea scar, persistent infiltrates and/or vascularization of the cornea, and even blindness.

Episcleritis usually presents with mild episcleral inflammation that is usually diffuse (>80%) but can be nodular and is considered generally benign. The inflammation is confined to the superficial episcleral tissue with hyperemia, dilated and congested vessels, and nongranulomatous infiltrates consisting of lymphocytes and plasma cells. Patients may present with a bright red or salmon pink eye from vascular dilation, epiphora, mild pain, photophobia, foreign body sensation, and decreased vision, which usually resolve within a few days to weeks. Uncommon complications include decreased vision, anterior uveitis, and ocular hypertension. Episcleritis is not thought to progress to scleritis.

Scleritis, inflammation and edema of the sclera, is an uncommon, severe inflammatory disorder often associated with ocular complications. Scleritis can often be the first manifestation of an underlying systemic disease, such as rheumatoid arthritis. The inflammation can involve a nongranulomatous or granulomatous process with or without necrosis. Scleritis may be delineated as anterior, posterior, or diffuse, which is most common (approximately 75%). Anterior scleritis can be subdivided as diffuse, nodular, necrotizing with or without inflammation, and scleromalacia perforans (especially with rheumatoid arthritis).

In the anterior group, diffuse is most common and least severe. Necrotizing anterior scleritis is the least common type but most dangerous with ocular complications. It is more often associated with systemic inflammatory diseases and more likely to lead to ocular complications. Purely posterior scleritis (posterior to the insertion of the medial and lateral rectus muscles) is uncommon (10%-20%) but potentially dangerous given that it may lack anterior signs that suggest the diagnosis, may affect the retina and optic nerve, and usually requires intensive immunosuppressive therapy.[1] Complications of scleritis are common and include permanent decreased visual acuity, anterior uveitis, peripheral keratitis, choroiditis, and glaucoma. These complications may also require additional therapy.

Differentiating episcleritis from scleritis is important mainly because of the differences in ocular complications. The two conditions have many similarities, including rare frequency, mostly monocular, female predominance, middle-aged patient distribution, and association with systemic connective tissue or vasculitis disease. The most common etiology for both processes is idiopathic.[2]

Other benign conditions that can cause a red eye are pinguecula and pterygium. These are both acquired, raised lesions of the submucosal conjunctiva. There is controversy about the etiology. Exposure to UV radiation is thought to be one of the most common risk factors. Both conditions occur more commonly in populations closer to the equator and rural populations. There may be genetic predispositions, and both are more common with advancing age and in men. Pinguecula lesions represent collagen, elastic tissue, and other connective tissue degeneration associated with lipid and lipofuscin deposition,[3] calcium deposits, fibrosis, and scar tissue.[4,5] Pterygia additionally exhibit significant squamous metaplasia and angiogenesis that invades the cornea and may cause astigmatism as well as obstruction of vision if invasion crosses the visual axis. Both conditions occur near the limbus and are usually at the 3-o'clock and 9-o'clock positions, with the nasal side being more common for both.

APPROACH/THE FOCUSED EXAM

The approach to the history and exam for the red eye is somewhat straightforward given that, except for isolated posterior scleritis, all the associated conditions will have abnormalities on physical examination. Important features of the history include timing, associated features, and exacerbating features. In addition to the ocular examination, inspection of the head, face, and neck for abnormalities, including swelling, erythema, rash, trauma, or infection, should be performed. A neurologic exam including visual acuity, extraocular muscle function, and visual field testing is helpful to exclude other causes. The slit-lamp examination allows an examination of the eye with magnification. Whenever pain or visual impairment is present, measuring intraocular pressure is essential. The use of fluorescein staining is helpful to identify corneal abrasions and other epithelial changes, such as dendritic lesions or punctate epithelial erosions.

Conjunctivitis

In most of the red eye conditions, there will be some degree of conjunctival injection, making the history and exam critical to rule out other etiologies. In isolated conjunctivitis, patients may describe watery, serous, or purulent discharge with crusting around the eyelids in the morning. Usually, there are minimal vision complaints. The patient may report a history of recent exposure to sick contacts or recent travel history. If both eyes are involved, usually one eye developed symptoms first. Upper respiratory symptoms may indicate a viral etiology.

Allergic conjunctivitis is usually bilateral, symmetric, and characterized by itching and tearing. The exam will demonstrate a diffusely injected red eye or eyes (including both the bulbar and palpebral conjunctiva). The eyelids may be swollen, and discharge may be apparent (**Figure 36.1**).

Purulent discharge may indicate a bacterial etiology or epidemic keratoconjunctivitis (EKC), a severe and highly contagious adenoviral infection. In cases of copious discharge, gonococcal or

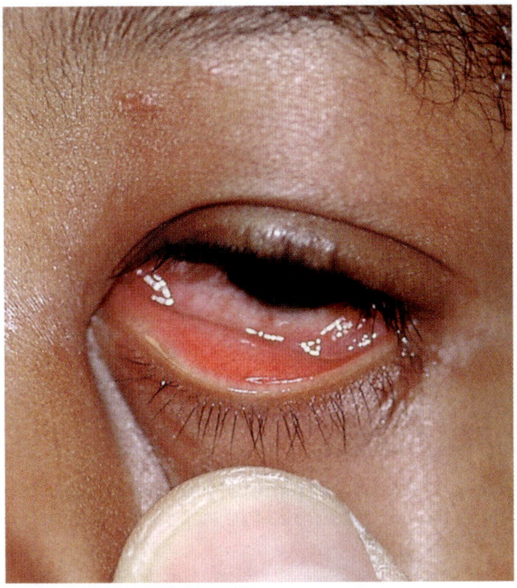

Figure 36.1: Allergic conjunctivitis demonstrating lid edema and conjunctival injection without discharge. (From Fleisher GR, Ludwig W, Baskin MN, *Atlas of Pediatric Emergency Medicine*. Lippincott Williams & Wilkins; 2004. Figure 15.10.)

chlamydial conjunctivitis should also be considered. In addition to examination of the eyes, palpable preauricular lymph nodes may also support the diagnosis of EKC.

Keratitis

While evaluating keratitis, the history is important to differentiate between self-limited and severe causes. First, infectious keratitis must be ruled out. Contact lens wear is a common cause of keratitis, corneal abrasions, and ulcerations (Chapter 35).[6] Previous herpetic infection may indicate reactivation of herpetic keratoconjunctivitis, although this should be considered in all cases. Bacterial and fungal keratitis may be preceded by trauma or foreign body sensation. Acanthamoeba is more likely in patients who use well water.

The slit-lamp examination of the cornea is imperative. This is best done with a slit beam directed at an angle to the corneal surface. Pan across the cornea while focusing on the layers of the cornea and then into the anterior chamber. First look for irregularities in the corneal epithelium, which may include sloughed epithelium, corneal opacity, or scarring. An early corneal ulcer may appear like a round white dot, whereas large ulcers will appear as an opaque, possibly purulent infiltration of the cornea. Looking deeper may reveal white infiltrate in the superficial and middle layers of the cornea. Looking past the cornea may reveal cell and flare in the anterior chamber, a sign of intraocular inflammation described in Chapter 38. Fluorescein staining may reveal corneal abrasions, ulcerations, dendritic lesions, or punctate epithelial erosions (**Figure 36.2**). A Wood lamp may be used in children, uncooperative patients, or when a slit lamp is not available.

Episcleritis

Episcleritis can present with unilateral or bilateral (bright) red eye redness, which is usually sectorial/localized (**Figure 36.3**) but can be more diffuse. It usually presents with minimal discomfort, tearing, and sometimes a foreign body sensation and occasionally with blurred vision. In contrast to the deep episcleral vascular injection notable in scleritis, the vascular congestion with episcleritis will usually blanch with application of topical phenylephrine (2.5% or 10%), which may help discriminate between the two diagnoses. Given that episcleritis can be complicated by decreased visual acuity, increased intraocular pressure, and anterior uveitis, examination should include these possibilities.

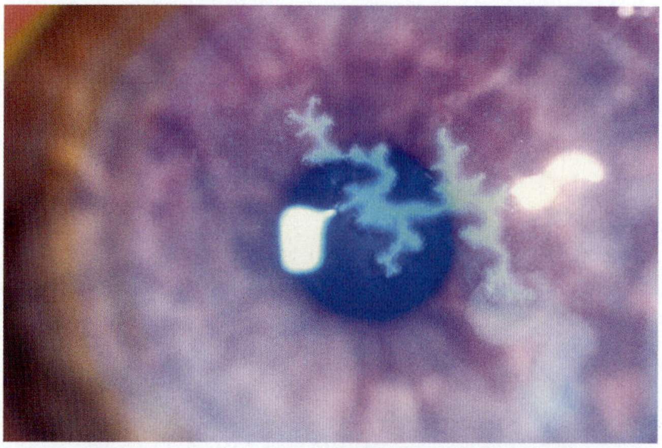

Figure 36.2: Herpes simplex keratitis demonstrating dendrites on the corneal epithelium visualized with a cobalt blue light. (From Rapuano CJ. *Wills Eye Institute - Cornea*. 3rd ed. Wolters Kluwer; 2019. Figure 7.5a.)

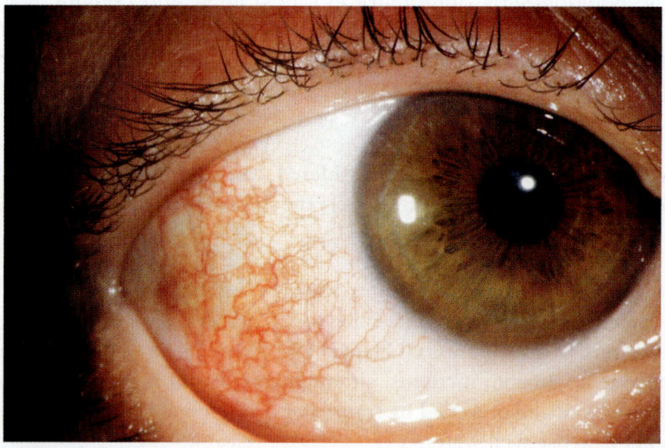

Figure 36.3: Localized injection of the episcleral vessels in episcleritis. (From Rapuano CJ. *Wills Eye Institute - Cornea*. 3rd ed. Wolters Kluwer; 2019. Figure 9.1a.)

Scleritis

In contrast to episcleritis, the sclera has rich sensory innervation, and patients will usually present with deep, throbbing, ocular pain. Extraocular movements may exacerbate the pain, which can radiate to the jaw or face. The history may also reveal photophobia, epiphora, decreased vision, and insomnia caused by pain. Examination with the slit lamp will reveal a violaceous injected eye (or eyes) described as a diffuse, deep red/blue/purple hue (**Figure 36.4**). The violaceous hue will usually not blanch with topical phenylephrine. Scleral edema and congestion of the deeper episcleral vessels observed during slit-lamp exam are considered a sine qua non sign. Given that scleritis can be complicated by decreased visual acuity, increased intraocular pressure, anterior uveitis, and peripheral keratitis, examination should assess for these possibilities. For advanced evaluation, B-scan ultrasound may show scleral thickening, resulting in a T-sign at the insertion of the sclera and optic nerve.

Pinguecula and Pterygium

Direct visualization of the eye without the need for magnification is often sufficient to make these diagnoses, although slit lamp will improve the exam. Pinguecula appear as small, yellow, "fleshy,"

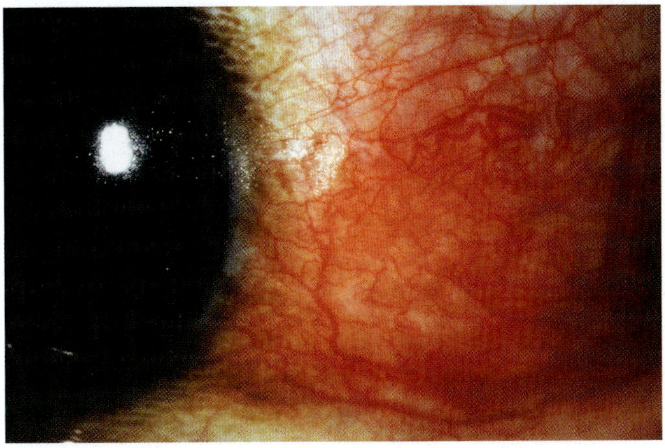

Figure 36.4: Diffuse inflammation of the conjunctiva and sclera is present in this eye with diffuse scleritis. (From Rapuano CJ. *Wills Eye Institute - Cornea*. 3rd ed. Wolters Kluwer; 2019. Figure 9.2a.)

"fatty," submucosal interpalpebral lesions that do not encroach the cornea (**Figure 36.5**). A pterygium, on the other hand, will be noted at the same positions at the limbus but will encroach over/onto the cornea. Pterygium (also known as "surfer's eye") is usually a triangularly shaped structure resembling an "insect wing" that encroaches onto the cornea and includes distinctive lines of neovascularization (**Figure 36.6**).

DIFFERENTIAL DIAGNOSIS

The differential diagnosis for the red eye includes traumatic injuries (eg, corneal abrasions), acute angle closure glaucoma, subconjunctival hemorrhage, endophthalmitis, blepharitis, iritis, and dry eye syndrome in addition to conjunctivitis, keratitis, episcleritis, scleritis, pinguecula, and pterygium. Uveal and conjunctival cancers may present with a complaint of a red eye. Other infections and/or thrombosis (eg, cavernous vein thrombosis) may present with eye complaints or abnormalities. The lack of significant pain, photophobia, and visual changes in conjunctivitis is helpful in ruling out more serious conditions. Keratitis is usually quite painful and often associated with visual changes neither of which is common with episcleritis. Uveitis typically presents

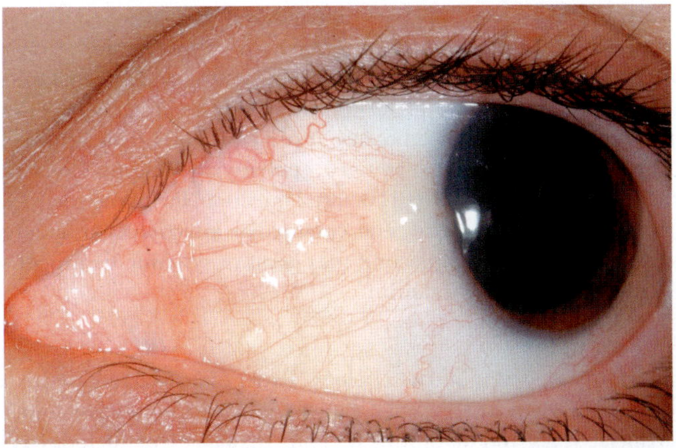

Figure 36.5: Nasally located pinguecula. (From Shields JA, Shields CL. *Eyelid, Conjunctival, and Orbital Tumors: An Atlas and Textbook*. 3rd ed. Wolters Kluwer; 2016. Figure 24.69.)

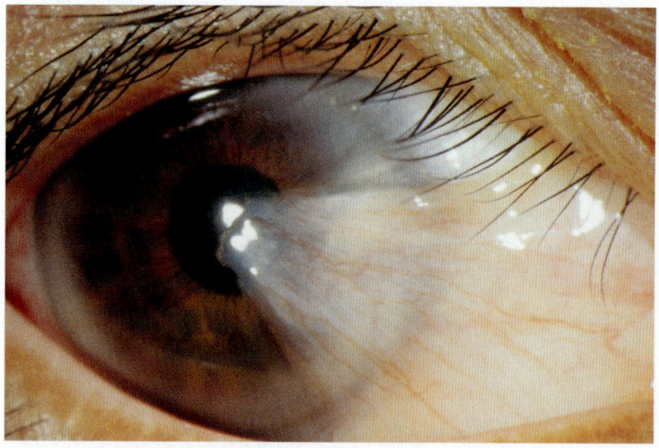

Figure 36.6: A nasal wing-shaped fibrovascular growth is apparent in this patient's right eye with a classic nasal pterygium. This pterygium is reaching into the visual axis. (From Rapuano CJ. *Wills Eye Institute - Cornea*. 3rd ed. Wolters Kluwer; 2019. Figure 2.1c.)

with significant pain and perilimbal redness and may be associated with a poorly reactive pupil. When evaluating pinguecula and pterygium, the differential includes intraepithelial neoplasm and squamous cell conjunctival carcinoma, localized conjunctivitis or episcleritis, symblepharon and pseudo-pterygium.

MANAGEMENT

Conjunctivitis

Conjunctivitis is usually a benign, self-limited disease that can often be treated without ophthalmology consultation. In cases of viral conjunctivitis, no testing or treatment is necessary, and it usually self-resolves in 7 to 10 days. Viral conjunctivitis can start in one eye and spread to the fellow eye within 2 to 3 days. It is important to discuss hand hygiene given the highly transmissible nature of the illness. Patients may benefit from topical antihistamines or decongestants, warm compresses and/or topical lubricants. Patients may request antibiotics given that there are some protocols for schools/workplaces that require 24 hours of topical antibiotic therapy in order to return.

Patients with ocular herpes virus infections may also present with some degree of conjunctivitis but will usually also have symptoms/signs of keratitis. Ocular herpes infection is best managed by an ophthalmologist and usually involves oral and/or topical antiviral therapy.

Unlike viral conjunctivitis, bacterial conjunctivitis is mostly unilateral and is not as contagious in nature (**Figure 36.7**). Bacterial conjunctivitis is also usually self-limited, although topical antibiotics may shorten the clinical course. Ointment may be preferred over eye drops in children and in patients with poor compliance because it persists longer than drops. Common choices include erythromycin ointment and trimethoprim-polymyxin B drops. Conjunctivitis with copious purulent discharge may indicate a severe bacterial infection, including methicillin-resistant Staphylococcus aureus (MRSA), gonococcal, and chlamydial infections. An emergent ophthalmology referral is warranted, because the infection may require systemic treatment. Cultures should be obtained to identify the causative organism.

Keratitis

Treatment for keratitis depends on the etiology. Patients that have keratitis related to UV radiation (welders, skiers/snowboarders, etc.), can be managed with reassurance and topical lubrication with artificial tears and/or ointment. Pain management includes systemic nonsteroidal anti-inflammatory drugs (NSAIDs) and cycloplegic eyedrops (eg, atropine, homatropine) to reduce photophobia from ciliary spasm. Symptoms usually resolve in 1 to 2 days as cornea reepithelializes.

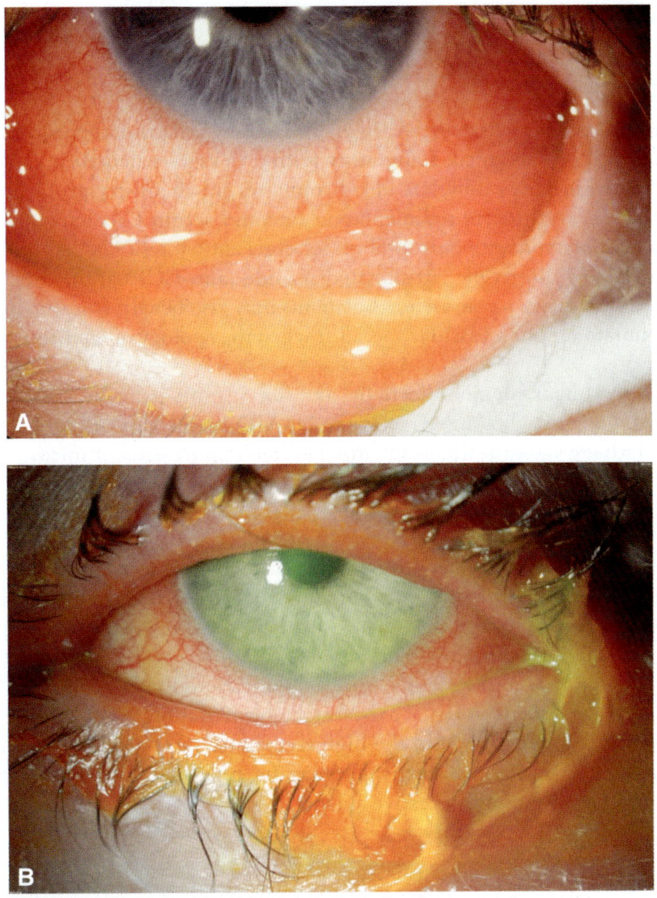

Figure 36.7: A, Diffuse conjunctival injection and a purulent discharge are present in this eye with bacterial conjunctivitis. B, A severe purulent discharge with crusting can be seen in this patient who has bacterial conjunctivitis. There is also moderate conjunctival injection. (From Rapuano CJ. *Wills Eye Institute - Cornea*. 3rd ed. Wolters Kluwer; 2019. Figure 1.3ab.)

Obtaining corneal cultures should be considered with severe infection (central or large >2 mm infiltrates, multifocal lesions, or evidence of stromal melting), history of recent corneal surgery or when a nonbacterial etiology is presumed. For contact wearers, antibiotic coverage must include coverage for *Pseudomonas* species. Empiric treatment should be initiated with broad-spectrum antibiotic drops given hourly for the first 24 to 48 hours. Typical monotherapy includes a fourth-generation fluoroquinolone. Drops are preferred because ointments tend to have poor corneal bioavailability. Patients need ophthalmologic evaluation and are usually reevaluated daily for the first few days of treatment.

Episcleritis

For minimally symptomatic, first episode episcleritis without visual changes or systemic symptoms, treatment with topical lubricants and/or topical NSAID therapy (eg, ketorolac or diclofenac drops 2-4 times daily) with referral to an ophthalmologist is appropriate because most patients will not have serious ocular complications and do not have an underlying systemic inflammatory disease. Referral to primary care, rheumatologist or vascular specialist for further evaluation and laboratory testing should be routine when a systemic disorder is suspected as the etiology for episcleritis. Routine referral to ophthalmology is prudent for refractory symptoms because patients may benefit from topical steroids (eg, fluorometholone acetate 0.1% or prednisolone acetate 1% 4 times daily) or other therapy. Urgent or even emergent ophthalmology consultation may be indicated when there is visual impairment or significant increase in intraocular pressure or when the diagnosis is in question.

Scleritis

Given that scleritis is a rare, destructive, sight-threatening inflammatory condition, emergent ophthalmology referral is warranted. Laboratory testing in cases when an underlying inflammatory disease is suspected includes complete blood count, serum chemistry profile, urinalysis and acute phase reactants (eg, erythrocyte sedimentation rate and serum C-reactive protein) but also may include rheumatoid factor, antineutrophil cytoplasmic antibodies (ANCA) testing, antinuclear antibody (ANA) testing, anticyclic citrullinated peptide (anti-CCP) antibodies, rheumatoid factor. Chest X-ray is also usually recommended. Patients may also benefit from evaluation from internal medicine, rheumatology, or a vascular specialist when the etiology of scleritis is related to a systemic disease.

Common treatment for noninfectious, anterior scleritis includes topical steroids as well as NSAID agents. Patients who are refractory to NSAID agents may be started on oral prednisone. In cases of underlying systemic illness, treatment often requires oral or intravenous systemic glucocorticoids or immunosuppressive therapy.

Pinguecula and Pterygium

For symptomatic pinguecula or pterygium (or for cosmetic concerns), patients can be educated and treated symptomatically with artificial tears and outpatient referral to ophthalmology for consideration of further treatment. Given the other diseases on the differential, it is important for an ophthalmologist to evaluate the patient. Ophthalmologists also may use nonsteroidal anti-inflammatory agents or steroids for symptomatic relief. Surgical indications for pterygium include induced astigmatism, encroachment over the visual axis, intractable irritation, restricted eye movement, or significant cosmetic concerns. Owing to the high recurrence rate, surgery is usually combined with adjunctive therapy, including conjunctival autografts, topical or subconjunctival medications (eg, cyclosporine or other immunosuppressive agents).[7,8]

TIPS AND PEARLS

- Most red eye conditions have at least some degree of conjunctivitis
- Adenovirus, a common cause of "pink eye," is not adequately killed with alcohol. If this diagnosis is suspected, use bleach or peroxide wipes to disinfect all surfaces between patients.
- EKC is a severe, highly contagious form of adenoviral conjunctivitis.
- Conjunctivitis, keratitis, episcleritis, and scleritis can all be a complication of autoimmune disease.
- Always consider herpetic disease when you see uptake on fluorescein staining.
- Ask about contact lens wear.
- Episcleritis blanches with phenylephrine, but scleritis typically does not.

EVIDENCE

Are antibiotics necessary for conjunctivitis?

In 2019, the American Academy of Ophthalmology, in "Conjunctivitis Preferred Practice Pattern," recommended against universally prescribing topical antibiotic drops for mild conjunctivitis.[9] Most cases of acute, infectious, conjunctivitis are viral, whereas indiscriminate use of antibiotics increases health care costs and may contribute to antibiotic resistance. Furthermore, predicting the etiology of mild conjunctivitis based on signs and symptoms is generally inaccurate.[10]

There may be instances in which antibiotics are beneficial. When given early, antibiotics resulted in faster remission of bacterial conjunctivitis.[11] The greatest benefit over placebo occurred when drops were started within the first 2 days of symptom onset. No antibiotic has shown a superior effect, so treatment choice is empirical.[9] If used, topical antibiotics should be administered for 5 to 7 days. A preparation with steroids should not be given empirically in eyes with a suspected infection. Patients started on steroids need close follow-up with an ophthalmologist.

References

1. Sainz de la Maza M, Molina N, Gonzalez-Gonzalez LA, et al. Clinical characteristics of a large cohort of patients with scleritis and episcleritis. *Ophthalmology*. 2012;119(1):43-50.
2. Honik G, Wong IG, Gritz DC. Incidence and prevalence of episcleritis and scleritis in Northern California. *Cornea*. 2013;32(12):1562-1566.
3. Utine CA, Tatlipinar S, Altunsoy M, et al. Autofluorescence imaging of pingueculae. *Br J Ophthalmol*. 2009;93(3):396-399.
4. Kim KW, Kim JC. Current approaches and future directions in the management of pterygium. *Int J Ophthalmol*. 2018;11(5):709-711.
5. Shahraki T, Arabi A, Feizi S. Pterygium: an update on pathophysiology, clinical features, and management. *Ther Adv Ophthalmol*. 2021;13:25158414211020152.
6. Cope JR, Collier SA, Nethercut H, et al. Risk behaviors for contact lens-related eye infections among adults and adolescents – United States, 2016. *MMWR Morb Mortal Wkly Rep*. 2017;66(32):841-845.
7. Fonseca EC, Rocha EM, Arruda GV. Comparison among adjuvant treatments for primary pterygium: a network meta-analysis. *Br J Ophthalmol*. 2018;102(6):748-756.
8. Kaufman SC, Jacobs DS, Lee WB, et al. Options and adjuvants in surgery for pterygium: a report by the American Academy of Ophthalmology. *Ophthalmology*. 2013;120(1):201-208.
9. Varu DM, Rhee MK, Akpek EK, et al. Conjunctivitis preferred practice pattern. *Ophthalmology*. 2019;126(1):P94-P169.
10. Azari AA, Arabi A. Conjunctivitis: a systematic review. *J Ophthalmic Vis Res*. 2020;15(3):372-395.
11. Sheikh A, Hurwitz B, van Schayck CP, McLean S, Nurmatov U. Antibiotics versus placebo for acute bacterial conjunctivitis. *Cochrane Database Syst Rev*. 2012;2012(9):CD001211.

CHAPTER 37

The Pediatric Red Eye: Ophthalmia Neonatorum, Conjunctivitis, and Uveitis

Ashley A. Foster
Tamiesha A. Frempong

INTRODUCTION

A red eye is one of the most common pediatric eye conditions evaluated in the emergency department (ED). Careful diagnosis is critical because the causes vary by age and presentation. Neonatal conjunctivitis carries some of the most significant potential for morbidity and mortality because it may progress to sepsis and death. Conjunctivitis beyond the neonatal period, commonly referred to as pink eye, is broadly defined as inflammation of the conjunctiva and has many distinct causes.

THE CLINICAL CHALLENGE

Ophthalmia Neonatorum

Neonatal conjunctivitis, or ophthalmia neonatorum, is defined as conjunctivitis that occurs in a *newborn less than 1 month of age*. Causes include chemical, bacterial, or viral agents.[1] The risk of morbidity from the infection is severe, because the infection can rapidly destroy the eyes and cause corneal ulceration, endophthalmitis, and subsequent blindness.[2] It can also disseminate and lead to sepsis, meningitis, arthritis, or other severe manifestations of invasive disease. Fortunately, rates of ophthalmia neonatorum have been declining since initiation of preventative measures, including neonatal prophylaxis and identification and treatment of maternal infections during pregnancy (**Table 37.1**). Nevertheless, this diagnosis should not be missed.

Conjunctivitis

Conjunctivitis beyond the neonatal period is a relatively benign condition. The etiologic causes fall into two categories: infectious (bacterial/viral) and noninfectious (allergic/toxic). Although infectious conjunctivitis is highly contagious and inconvenient owing to discomfort and missed days from school or work, it is self-limiting or manageable with medications. However, notable exceptions with high morbidity cannot be overlooked. *Neisseria gonorrhoeae* (NG) conjunctivitis that can occur in adolescents and adults carries the risk of corneal ulceration, endophthalmitis, or subsequent blindness. Chemical conjunctivitis caused by acid or alkali burns to the eye are true ocular emergencies. Because alkali agents penetrate ocular tissue deeper than acidic chemicals, they are potentially more devastating to the eye and vision.

TABLE 37.1 Etiology of Ophthalmia Neonatorum and Time Frame of Onset of Symptoms

Etiology of Symptoms	Time Frame of Onset of Symptoms
Chemical conjunctivitis	Within 24 hours of birth
Neisseria gonorrhoeae	Within 1 week of birth
Chlamydia trachomatis	Within days to weeks of birth
Herpes simplex virus	Within 1-3 weeks of birth

Uveitis

Uveitis is often accompanied by conjunctivitis, causing a red eye. It can be extremely challenging to diagnose because children may have a range of symptoms, including severe pain or vision loss, or they may be completely asymptomatic. Uveitis can occur as anterior (iris and ciliary body), intermediate (vitreous and pars plana), posterior (choroid or retina), or pan uveitis (all structures). Uveitis can be infectious or noninfectious or represent a masquerade syndrome (eg, leukemia).[3] Pediatric uveitis denotes an important disease to detect because of the risk of poor visual outcomes if there is a delay to diagnosis or treatment. Noninfectious anterior uveitis is the most common type in the United States, representing a majority of cases (61.9%).[4] Although most cases of anterior uveitis are idiopathic, more than ¼ of patients have underlying systemic disease.[2] Early diagnosis and aggressive treatment improve morbidity associated with this disease. Uveitis can also develop after nonpenetrating or penetrating trauma to the eye, especially in males.

PATHOPHYSIOLOGY

Conjunctivitis

The underlying cause of conjunctivitis in the pediatric population is influenced by the age of the child (**Figure 37.1**). Clinical signs and symptoms can help in distinguishing among the various causes of conjunctivitis (**Table 37.2**).

Viral and allergic causes are more common in school-aged children, whereas bacterial causes of acute conjunctivitis are twice as likely in infants and toddlers. The exception is in adolescents with copious, mucopurulent discharge associated with conjunctivitis concerning for NG or *Chlamydia trachomatis* (CT) infection.

The most implicated bacteria in the younger cohorts are *Haemophilus influenza, Streptococcus pneumonia, Staphylococcus aureus,* and *Moraxella catarrhalis*. Notably, otitis media occurs in 25% of patients with conjunctivitis even in the absence of ear pain.[1] Therefore, every child with conjunctivitis also requires an ear exam owing to the risk of concurrent infection, most commonly caused by *H influenza*.

Adenovirus is the most common viral cause of infectious conjunctivitis, accounting for 20% of all cases, particularly in the fall and winter months.[1] Primary herpes virus conjunctivitis occurs between the ages of 1 and 5 years.[1] Eighty percent of cases are unilateral. Fifty percent of patients have corneal involvement evidenced by corneal dendrite.[1] Contact with another person with an active lesion may also be elicited in the history of present illness.

Uveitis

Uveitis can be divided into isolated uveitis or a manifestation of systemic disease. Juvenile idiopathic arthritis represents the most common systemic disease to cause anterior uveitis.[5] Additional systemic diseases associated with uveitis are listed in **Table 37.3**.

Uveitis can present with eye pain, redness, or light sensitivity and is more likely to have bilateral eye involvement. Patients may have conjunctival injection with photophobia or vision changes. Slit lamp examination is recommended and will often reveal white blood cells in the anterior chamber, described as "cell and flare" (**Figure 37.2**).[2] Cells may settle in the front of the eye, forming a hypopyon.[2]

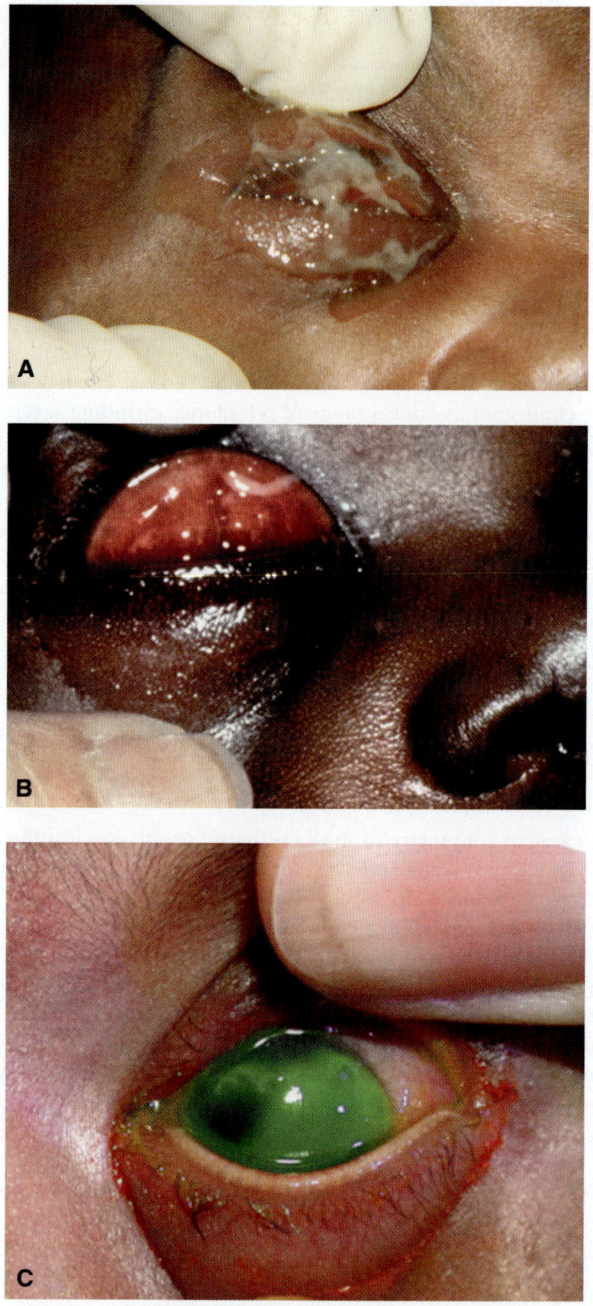

Figure 37.1: A, Neonatal gonorrheal conjunctivitis with associated lid swelling and significant purulent discharge. (From Bachur RG, Shaw KN, Chamberlain J, Lavelle J, Nagler J, Shook JE, eds. *Fleisher & Ludwig's Textbook of Pediatric Emergency Medicine*. 8th ed. Wolters Kluwer; 2021. Figure 123.6.) B, Neonatal conjunctivitis caused by Chlamydia trachomatis with pseudomembrane formation. (From Nelson LB, Olitsky SE. *Harley's Pediatric Ophthalmology*. 6th ed. Wolters Kluwer; 2014. Figure 9.12.) C, Neonatal conjunctivitis and keratitis caused by HSV in a neonate. A corneal dendrite is seen with associated epithelial defect. (From *Taylor and Hoyt's Pediatric Ophthalmology and Strabismus*. 5th ed. Elsevier; 2017:109-112. Figure 13.1.C.)

TABLE 37.2 Signs, Symptoms, and Patient Characteristic in Postneonatal Conjunctivitis

Etiology	Discharge	Eyelid Edema	Corneal Involvement	Itchiness	Preauricular Adenopathy	Patient Age Group
Bacterial	Mucopurulent	+	Gonococcal ulceration	–	+	Infants/toddlers
Viral	Clear, serous	++	EKC/ Subepithelial infiltrates	–	+++	School age, late childhood, early adulthood
HSV	Clear	++ (vesicles)	Dendrites	–	++	Ages 1-5 years
Allergic	Clear, ropy	+++ (allergic shiners)	Shield ulcer in severe allergy	+++	–	School age, late childhood, early adulthood

HSV, herpes simplex virus; EKC, epidemic keratoconjunctivitis.

TABLE 37.3 Systemic Disease Associated With Uveitis

Causes of Pediatric Uveitis		
Rheumatologic		
Juvenile idiopathic arthritis	Systemic lupus erythematosus	Fuchs heterochromic iridocyclitis
Sarcoidosis	Inflammatory bowel disease	Kawasaki disease
HLA-B27-associated disease	Juvenile xanthogranuloma	Tubulointerstitial nephritis and uveitis
CINCA/NOMID	Behcet disease	
Infectious		
Herpetic disease	Syphilis	Leprosy
Lyme disease	Tuberculosis	Viral syndromes
Fungal disease	HIV	
Other		
Postbacterial infection	Multiple sclerosis	Sympathetic ophthalmia
Trauma	Leukemia	Drug induced

CINCA, chronic infantile neurologic, cutaneous, and articular syndrome; NOMID, neonatal-onset multisystem inflammatory disease.

Additionally, the pupil may have abnormalities, including small size, poor dilation, or irregular shape.[2] For patients with known systemic illness that carry increased risk of uveitis (**Table 37.3**), the emergency provider should have high suspicion of the potential diagnosis of uveitis with any ocular complaint.

APPROACH/THE FOCUSED EXAM

The examination starts the minute the provider enters the examination room, and critical components to the examination are noncontact. Is the child guarding or refusing to open the eyes? Are the eyelids involved? Is the problem unilateral or bilateral? Is there visible discharge? Are there visible lesions such as vesicles around the eye or on the face? Visual acuity assessment can be made

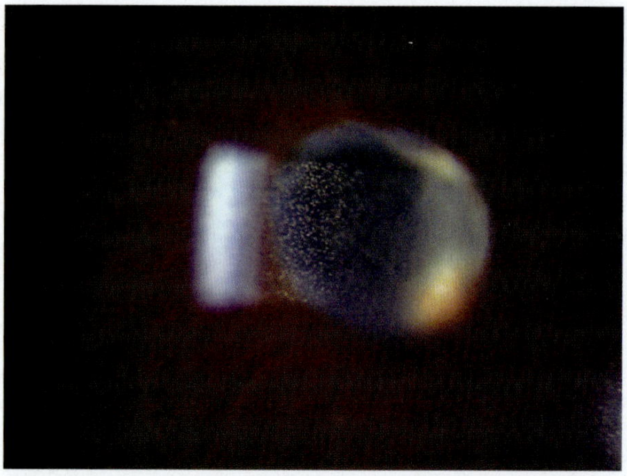

Figure 37.2: Slit-lamp view of cell and flare. (From Allingham RR, Damji KF, Freedman SF, Moroi SE, Rhee DJ, Shields MB. *Shields Textbook of Glaucoma*. 6th ed. Wolters Kluwer; 2011. Figure 22.1b.)

crudely by shining a bright light on the eye and eliciting a wince to the light. This should be done one eye at a time and can be achieved through closed eyelids. Also asking the child to count fingers is another crude assessment of vision.

If the child is refusing to open the eye owing to eye pain, a topical anesthetic may reduce guarding, as is seen in corneal pathology. Turning down the room lights may also be helpful in examining a child with photophobia. Fluorescein testing may aid in visualizing corneal pathology, highlighting the lesions in green.

If a slit lamp examination is indicated, make sure to set up the slit lamp first before inviting the child to engage with the instrument. When evaluating the anterior chamber, make sure to turn the light beam to the smallest diameter, with the highest brilliance on the highest magnification to ensure optimal viewing of the anatomy.

DIFFERENTIAL DIAGNOSIS

The differential diagnosis for pediatric patients who present with a red eye with or without pain can be best described in age categories. For the neonate, potential diagnoses include chemical conjunctivitis, bacterial conjunctivitis, viral conjunctivitis, congenital glaucoma, birth trauma (particularly if forceps delivery was performed), corneal abrasion, or foreign body.

The differential diagnosis for red eye in pediatric patients beyond the neonatal period includes chemical, viral, bacterial, or allergic conjunctivitis, corneal abrasion, foreign body, globe rupture, uveitis, orbital cellulitis, infectious keratitis, blepharitis, Sturge-Weber Syndrome, or Kawasaki disease.

Vernal conjunctivitis is a rare severe allergic conjunctivitis. It is typically bilateral and presents with severe photophobia, large "shield" ulcers on the cornea, and cobblestone-like papillae on the everted upper lids (**Figure 37.3**). Its presentation is often notable, and these patents should be referred to ophthalmology immediately.[6]

There are several clinical signs and symptoms useful in distinguishing "pink eye" from these other, more serious "red eye" conditions. For instance, conjunctival injection of the tissue bordering the cornea, the limbus, is spared in conjunctivitis. Limbal involvement occurs in keratitis and uveitis.

With the exception of adenoviral keratoconjunctivitis, pain and photophobia are not typical features of conjunctivitis and may therefore point in the direction of a corneal abrasion, keratitis, uveitis, or glaucoma (congenital or acute). Significantly decreased vision is also a sign/symptom of a more serious eye condition. Extraocular motility limitation, proptosis, or sinus disease are more consistent with an orbital process such as orbital cellulitis. Fever, red eyes, characteristic rash on the hands, feet and body, as well as red lips and tongue ("strawberry tongue") are all signs and symptoms of Kawasaki disease.

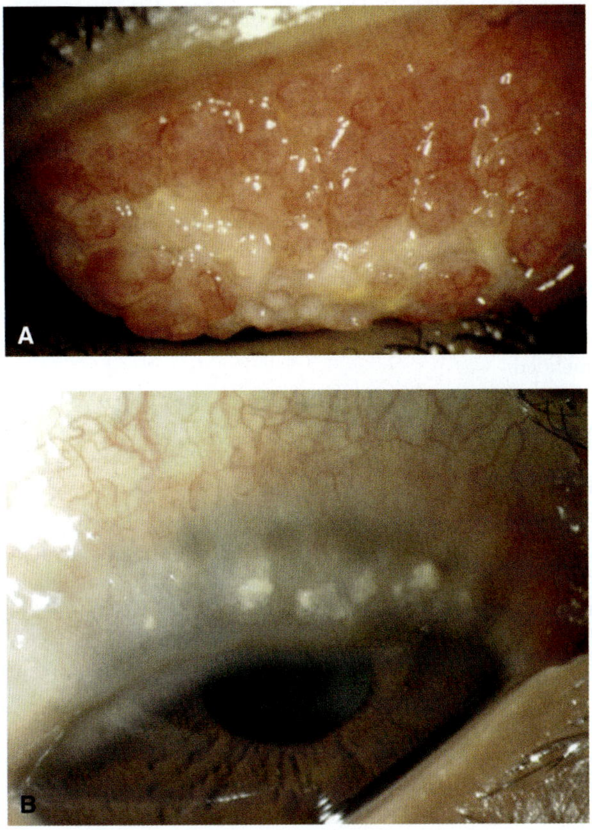

Figure 37.3: Vernal Conjunctivitis. A, Horner-Trantas dots, a collection of degenerated epithelial cells and eosinophils. B, Giant papillae at superior tarsus. (From *Taylor and Hoyt's Pediatric Ophthalmology and Strabismus*. 5th ed. Elsevier; 2017:130-155. Figures 16.21, 16.22.)

MANAGEMENT

Ophthalmia Neonatorum

All neonates who present with concern for conjunctivitis require a careful prenatal history with special attention paid to sexually transmitted infection screening and whether ocular prophylaxis was administered at birth. If chemical conjunctivitis is suspected, provide reassurance and consider follow-up to a pediatric ophthalmologist within 24 hours. The condition is self-limited and requires no treatment.[1]

Neonates with suspected NG conjunctivitis require culture and gram stain of eye drainage and full sepsis evaluation: blood culture, labs, urinalysis and urine culture, cerebrospinal fluid (CSF) studies, NG and CT polymerase chain reaction (PCR).[2] Additionally, hospitalization is recommended with initiation of IV ceftriaxone 25 mg/kg maximum dose 125 mg (alternatively IV cefotaxime).[1] Copious eye irrigation is necessary both immediately on presentation and at frequent intervals until eye discharge is eliminated.[1] Additionally, consultation with ophthalmology and infectious disease is recommended. Patients should be tested for other potential concomitant sexually transmitted infections, including CT, syphilis, and HIV. Furthermore, prompt treatment of the mother and sexual partners is indicated.[1]

For patients with suspected CT, culture of eye discharge should be obtained. For treatment, oral erythromycin for 14 days and close pediatrician follow-up within several days from ED visit is recommended. There is an association with erythromycin and pyloric stenosis, and therefore infants started on this therapy should be monitored closely in the outpatient setting. Similar to NG conjunctivitis, the patient should be tested for concomitant infections and, additionally, eye drainage should be tested for NG conjunctivitis but not treated unless diagnostic assessment is positive. Follow-up with ophthalmology is recommended within 1 to 2 months after infection.

In the setting of suspected herpes simplex virus (HSV) conjunctivitis, viral culture of the multiple areas, including the mouth, nasopharynx, rectum, and conjunctivae, should be obtained. Full sepsis evaluation including blood culture, serum HSV PCR, labs, urinalysis and urine culture, CSF studies, and CSF HSV PCR should be obtained, and the child should be hospitalized. Obtaining liver function test (LFT) studies can help to determine whether the neonate has disseminated HSV, as elevations in LFTs are often found in neonates with disseminated infection.[7] IV acyclovir (60 mg/kg/day divided into 3 doses) for 14 to 21 days and topical antiviral therapy are the recommended treatments of choice.[7] Additionally, consultation with ophthalmology and infectious disease is recommended.

MANAGEMENT

Conjunctivitis

Typically, the diagnosis of pediatric conjunctivitis is clinically based on signs and symptoms. Culture is not indicated except in the case of neonatal conjunctivitis or in adolescents suspected to have NG or CT conjunctivitis. Although bacterial conjunctivitis is self-limited, topical antibiotics have been shown to eradicate bacteria from the conjunctiva and improve clinical symptoms sooner. Topical antibiotics that are well tolerated, inexpensive and have broad-spectrum coverage include bacitracin-polymyxin (Polysporin) and trimethoprim-polymyxin (Polytrim). If a child has concurrent otitis media, then oral antibiotics are indicated, making topical antibiotics unnecessary. The child can often safely return to school or daycare 24 hours after starting antibiotics.

Contact lens wearers with conjunctivitis are a special group. Conditions as simple as contact lens overwear can present with a red eye, but early signs of vision threatening infection may first present as conjunctivitis as well. These patients should be started on a topical fluoroquinolone antibiotic with *Pseudomonas* coverage such as moxifloxacin or ciprofloxacin, and they require a slit lamp examination by an ophthalmologist, who should see the patient the next day at the latest.

For viral conjunctivitis, studies show no difference in the effectiveness of artificial tears compared to antiviral and anti-inflammatory medications. Treatment for most cases of viral conjunctivitis is therefore supportive: cold compress, artificial tears, and decongestants if necessary. Steroids should be avoided because they may prolong the infection or cause bacterial superinfection, glaucoma, or cataracts. Resolution of a viral conjunctivitis may take 1 to 2 weeks. The child does not need to stay out of school for the full duration of the conjunctivitis but certainly during the period with active upper respiratory symptoms.

HSV eye infection is treated with topical antiviral medication or oral acyclovir. In patients with frequent return of HSV eye infection, chronic low dose oral therapy is helpful in keeping recurrences at bay. If HSV is suspected, fluorescein staining of the cornea should be performed to look for dendrites. The absence of a dendrite does not eliminate herpes as the cause of the conjunctivitis. The use of steroids is absolutely contraindicated in herpes keratitis because it may worsen infection. Suspected herpes eye infection always requires immediate referral to and management by an ophthalmologist.

Uveitis

If uveitis is suspected, urgent ophthalmology evaluation within 24 hours is recommended for diagnosis confirmation with a dilated fundus exam and potential initiation of systemic therapy.[2] Initial treatment in the ED should be discussed with ophthalmology and may include topical corticosteroids and/or cycloplegics.[2] Additionally, if systemic disease is associated, treatment of underlying disease may aid in the improvement of uveitis.[2] Once diagnosis is confirmed by an ophthalmologist, treatment may range from topical corticosteroids to immunomodulatory therapy.[3] Patients with uveitis require close follow-up with ophthalmology at regular intervals to ensure no development of ocular complications or vision loss occurs.

TIPS AND PEARLS

- Approaching an eye exam in a child requires planning, patience, and creativity.
- Toys or videos on a phone can draw the child's attention to gaze in different directions.
- Caregiver involvement can be incredibly helpful—consider having the child sit in the caregiver's lap, or demonstrate the exam on the caregiver or a stuffed animal first to gain rapport with the child.
- If there is a concern for serious injury such as globe rupture and the child will not tolerate an eye exam, consider anxiolysis such as intranasal midazolam with a papoose to ensure safe examination of the eye.
- When trying to examine the eye of a neonate, consider dimming the ambient lights, or hold the neonate upright to encourage spontaneous eye opening.
- For children with concern for infectious conjunctivitis, wear gloves and thoroughly clean any equipment used for examination.

EVIDENCE

Are antibiotics really necessary for bacterial conjunctivitis?

A literature review evaluated the effects of empirical treatment in adults and children with suspected bacterial conjunctivitis and treatment in those with culture-proven bacterial infection.[8] The findings revealed that in those with culture-positive nongonococcal bacterial conjunctivitis, antibiotics significantly increased clinical and microbiologic cure rates over 2 to 10 days compared to placebo. In those treated empirically, there was only marginal benefit from antibiotics. This finding may highlight the clinical uncertainties of the diagnosis and therefore management. Consequently, if prescribing topical antibiotics empirically, consider recommending that caregivers wait 1 to 2 days before starting treatment and only if symptoms have not resolved at that time.

Can you send a child home with topical anesthetic?

Topical anesthetics such as tetracaine or proparacaine provide significant pain relief in the setting of a corneal abrasion. A recently published double-blind, randomized clinical trial included 118 adults, aged 18 to 80 years with uncomplicated corneal abrasions: 50% received tetracaine and the other half placebo.[9] Subjects were asked to use the drops every 30 minutes as needed for 24 hours. All study participants were given a prescription for hydrocodone/acetaminophen 7.5/325 mg and were instructed to use 1 or 2 tablets as needed every 6 hours for breakthrough pain. The researchers reported that pain was significantly lower in the tetracaine group and that those patients used less hydrocodone. However, the study was not powered for safety. There are no similar studies in the literature including subjects younger than 18 years. Therefore, topical anesthetic for home use is not yet recommended for the pediatric population because there is no evidence in the literature to support this as a safe practice.

References

1. Teoh DL, Reynolds S. Diagnosis and management of pediatric conjunctivitis. *Pediatr Emerg Care*. 2003;19(1):48-55.
2. Iqbal A, Langhan ML, Rotruck J, et al. An evidence-based approach to nontraumatic ocular complaints in children. *Pediatr Emerg Med Practice [Internet]*. 2021;18(2):1-28. www.ebmedicine.net
3. Wentworth BA, Freitas-Neto CA, Foster CS. *Management of Pediatric Uveitis*. F1000Prime Reports; 2014:6.
4. Ferrara M, Eggenschwiler L, Stephenson A, et al. The challenge of pediatric uveitis: tertiary referral center experience in the United States. *Ocular Immunol Inflamm*. 2019;27(3):410-417.
5. Mehta PJ, Alexander JL, Sen HN. Pediatric uveitis: new and future treatments. *Curr Opin Ophthalmol*. 2013;24(5):453-462.

6. Richards A, Guzman-Cottrill JA. Conjunctivitis. *Pediatr Review [Internet]*. 2010;31(6):196-207. http://pedsinreview.aappublications.org/
7. Sanders JE, Garcia SE. Pediatric herpes simplex virus infections: an evidence-based approach to treatment. *Pediatr Emerg Med Pract*. 2014. 11(1):1-19. www.ebmedicine.net
8. Epling J. Bacterial conjunctivitis. *BMJ Clin Evid [Internet]*. 2012;2012:0704. www.clinicalevidence.com
9. Shipman S, Painter K, Keuchel M, Bogie C. Short-term topical tetracaine is highly efficacious for the treatment of pain caused by corneal abrasions: a double-blind, randomized clinical trial. *Ann Emerg Med*. 2021; 77(3):338-344.

CHAPTER 38

Anterior Uveitis, Hypopyon, and Hyphema

Adria Simon
Anjum F. Koreishi

THE CLINICAL CHALLENGE

Anterior uveitis, hypopyon, and hyphema represent a spectrum of pathologies affecting the anterior segment of the eye. The anterior segment is the space between the iris and the cornea. Uveitis is a general term for inflammation within the eye. The uveal tract consists of the iris and ciliary body anteriorly and the choroid posteriorly. Anterior uveitis involves inflammation of the iris and/or ciliary body, encompassing terms like iritis and iridocyclitis,[1] which are clinically essentially interchangeable. Hypopyon refers to a collection of white blood cells in the anterior chamber and is a clinical presentation of anterior uveitis. Hyphema is a collection of red blood cells in the anterior chamber. Whereas anterior uveitis can affect any age group or gender, hyphema most commonly results from blunt or penetrating trauma and is seen more often in children and young males.[2]

The etiology of anterior uveitis can be challenging to parse out in the emergency setting. This umbrella term represents a group of heterogeneous disorders unified by the presence of inflammation in the anterior uveal tract (iris and/or ciliary body). Anterior uveitis can be acute, subacute, or chronic, although it is typically acute in the emergency setting. It is typically immune mediated, but notable infectious etiologies must be ruled out.[3] Trauma can also cause uveitis. Anterior uveitis shares many presenting symptoms with other common forms of ocular pathology, including redness, photophobia, tearing, pain, and blurry vision. Distinguishing between these conditions necessitates a comprehensive history and ocular examination. This variability in presentation and etiology causes a clinical challenge as workup, management, and prognosis vary in each case.

Most appreciable hyphemas can be easily diagnosed on visual inspection. Hyphema most often occurs in conjunction with ocular trauma, and severe pathology such as open globe must be excluded. Secondary hemorrhage can be difficult to predict in a patient without clear clinical risk factors and is associated with complications like corneal blood staining, elevated intraocular pressure, and formation of synechiae.[2] Careful documentation and communication of the initial degree of hyphema between emergency providers and ophthalmologists at follow-up is necessary to determine appropriate treatment if secondary hemorrhage occurs.

PATHOPHYSIOLOGY

Anterior Uveitis and Hypopyon

Whether infectious, traumatic, or secondary to systemic infection, anterior uveitis results from an underlying inflammatory process with subsequent transudation of proteins and leukocytes from inflamed vessels. The hallmark clinical finding of anterior uveitis is cells, visible leukocytes in the anterior chamber, and flare, when the aqueous fluid is visible owing to protein leakage (**Figure 38.1**).

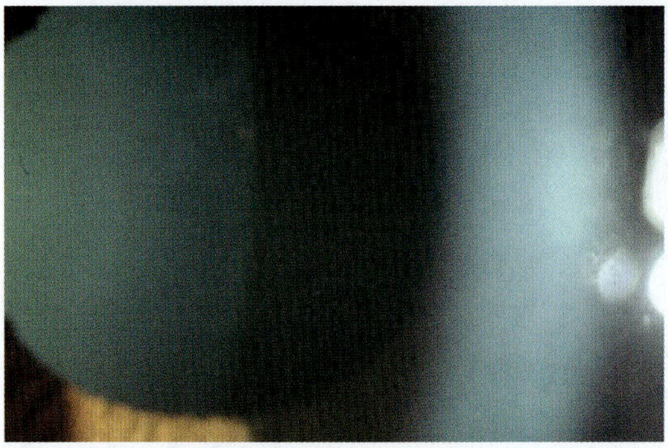

Figure 38.1: Slit lamp photo showing cells (small white specks between the light beam). These are not visible without a slit lamp. (Courtesy of Dr. Debra Goldstein.)

Inflammation of the iris ciliary muscles causes ciliary spasm and pain. Inflammation of the ciliary body may cause low intraocular pressure, such as in HLA-B27 related uveitis. Inflammation of the trabecular meshwork, which drains aqueous fluid from the eye, can cause elevated intraocular pressure, as in Herpesviridae-related uveitis.[4]

Hypopyon can often be visualized with the naked eye (**Figure 38.2**). This finding does not occur in isolation; rather, hypopyon is a sequela of other underlying conditions such as severe uveitis, bacterial keratitis, or, most concerningly, endophthalmitis.[5]

Hyphema

Hyphema is most commonly the result of blunt or penetrating trauma to the eye. Rupture of vessels supplying the ciliary body and iris results in accumulation of blood in the anterior chamber (**Figure 38.3**). Pathophysiology of spontaneous hyphema is particular to the etiology, including retinal ischemia, typically because of retinal vein occlusion or diabetic retinopathy, ocular ischemia from carotid occlusion, or intraocular tumors. Rebleeding, which is recurrence of hyphema usually after 3 to 7 days, occurs in about 5% of cases owing to clot retraction.[6] Elevated intraocular pressure can develop owing to trabecular meshwork obstruction in the setting of rebleeding or clot. Particular caution is warranted in patients with underlying sickle cell disease or trait. The relative hypoxia and acidic pH of the anterior chamber induces sickling of red blood cells in the trabecular meshwork, reducing outflow of aqueous and causing significant elevations in intraocular pressure.[7]

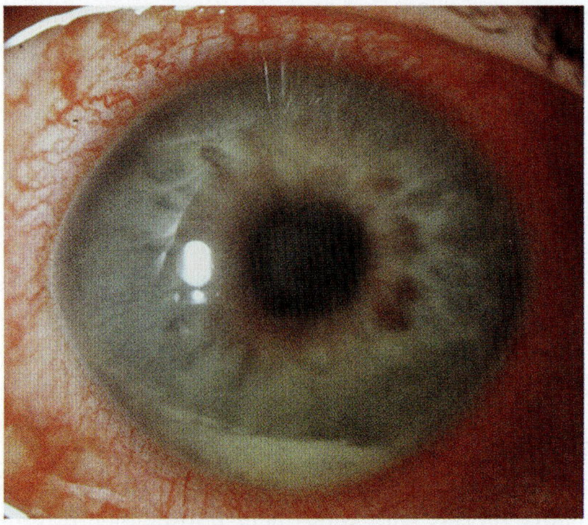

Figure 38.2: Hypopyon in a patient with acute HLA-B27 uveitis. (Courtesy of Dr. Debra Goldstein.)

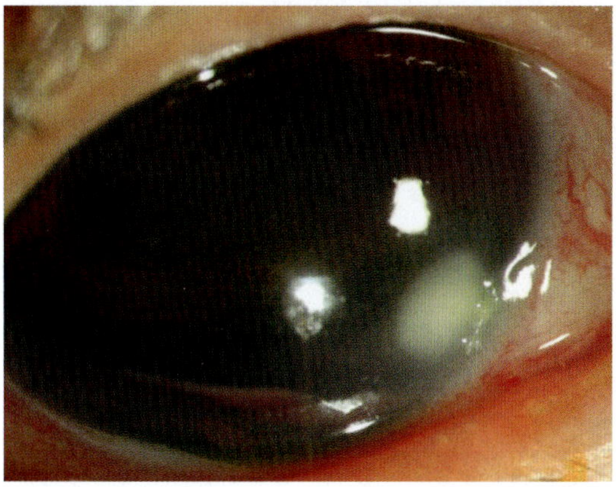

Figure 38.3: Layered hyphema (dark red layer in inferior anterior chamber) in a patient with a corneal ulcer (white lesion on right of photo) and iris neovascularization.

APPROACH/THE FOCUSED EXAM

Anterior Uveitis and Hypopyon

Anterior uveitis should be considered in patients presenting with pain, conjunctival injection, blurred vision, and photophobia. A careful history should include recent trauma/foreign body or ocular surgery, full review of systems relating to inflammatory or infectious conditions such as axial stiffness from ankylosing spondylitis and oral ulcers/skin lesions from Herpesviridae (specific concerns listed in **Table 38.1**). Examination should always include visual acuity and intraocular pressure. Ocular discharge should not be present and helps distinguish anterior uveitis from other etiologies of the painful red eye. Inspection of the eye may reveal perilimbal injection known as ciliary flush,[8] although diffuse conjunctival injection may be present. A red eye that is significantly tender to palpation should raise concern for scleritis. Examination of the pupil can reveal a poorly reactive pupil secondary to ciliary spasm[8] or an irregular pupil caused by posterior synechiae, scarring of the iris to the lens (**Figure 38.4**). Consensual photophobia, the presence of pain when illuminating the unaffected pupil, is suggestive of anterior uveitis.[3] Fluorescein staining of the cornea can assess other causes of the acutely painful red eye such as keratitis or corneal abrasion. Hypopyon may be seen without the slit lamp as a white deposit in the inferior anterior chamber (Figure 38.2). Slit lamp examination, notably the presence of cells and flare (Figure 38.1), is the key to evaluation of anterior uveitis. Inflammatory deposits on the corneal endothelium, known as keratic precipitates, may be noted on slit lamp exam. Dilated examination is necessary to rule out posterior uveitis and to evaluate for optic disc or macular edema, which can be manifestations of anterior uveitis and are vision threatening. **Table 38.2** highlights key ocular findings.

Hyphema

Patients most often present with blurred vision after trauma. Hyphema can occur with relatively insignificant mechanisms; any ocular trauma warrants evaluation for hyphema.[2] The emergency provider should first evaluate for more significant traumatic injury such as globe rupture and retrobulbar hematoma. Fluorescein staining allows for evaluation of concurrent corneal abrasion or penetrating injury to the globe. Visual acuity, pupillary response, and intraocular pressure should be measured (unless there is concern for open globe). Layered hyphema can be visible without the slit lamp (Figure 38.3). Small hyphema, microhyphema (red blood cells in anterior chamber without layering), and corneal blood staining (blood deposited in the cornea) are evaluated with the slit lamp.

TABLE 38.1 Select Etiologies of Uveitis With Anterior Involvement and Descriptions

	Etiology	Anatomy	Age	Suggestive Signs	Ocular Involvement	Diagnosis	Treatment
Immune-mediated etiologies	*HLA-B27 related*	Unilateral	Younger	Low IOP, +/− hypopyon, aggressive	Anterior	HLA-B27	Steroid, cycloplegia
	Sarcoidosis	Any		Possible high IOP	Any	CXR, ACE lysozyme	Steroids
	TINU	Bilateral	Younger	Younger, recent malaise	Anterior +/− other	Urine b2-microglobulin	Steroids
	IBD	Any		Blood/mucus in stool	Any	HLA-B27, colonoscopy	Steroids
	Behcet disease	Any	Younger	+/− Hypopyon, oral aphthous ulcers	Anterior, posterior	Clinical	Steroids, IMT
	VKH	Bilateral	Younger	Younger, recent headache/ meningismus	Disc edema, serous RD	Clinical	Steroids, IMT
Trauma/ mechanical etiologies	Traumatic iritis	Any	Younger	Younger, pigment in anterior chamber	Anterior	Clinical	+/− Steroids, cycloplegia
	UGH	Unilateral		Possible high IOP, malpositioned IOL	+/− Hyphema	Clinical	Steroids, +/− surgical
Infectious etiologies	*HSV/VZV*	Unilateral		High IOP, +/− corneal edema	Evaluate for retinitis	Aqueous PCR	PO valacyclovir, steroid
	CMV	Unilateral		High IOP, central keratic precipitates	Evaluate for retinitis	Aqueous PCR	PO valgancyclovir, steroid
	Toxoplasmosis	Unilateral		Possible high IOP	Must have retinitis	Clinical	Antibiotics, steroids
	Endophthalmitis	Unilateral		+/− Hypopyon, recent surgery/trauma	Vitritis	Culture	Injection/surgery
	Syphilis	Any	Any	Any	Any	Syphilis IgG/ reflex RPR	Intravenous penicillin
Malignancies	Lymphoma	Any	Older	Older, larger cells, less flare	Vitreous, retina	Cytology	Variable
	Leukemia	Any	Younger	Younger, +/− hypopyon/ blood	Any, +/− masses	Cytology	Variable

ACE, angiotensin converting enzyme; CMV, cytomegalovirus; CXR, chest X-ray; HSV, herpes simplex virus; IBD, inflammatory bowel disease; IgG, immunoglobulin G; IMT, systemic immunomodulatory therapy; IOL, intraocular lens; IOP, intraocular pressure; PCR, polymerase chain reaction; RD, retinal detachment; RPR, rapid plasma reagin; TINU, tubulointerstitial nephritis and uveitis; UGH, uveitis-glaucoma-hyphema syndrome; VKH, Vogt-Koyanagi-Harada syndrome; VZV, varicella-zoster virus.

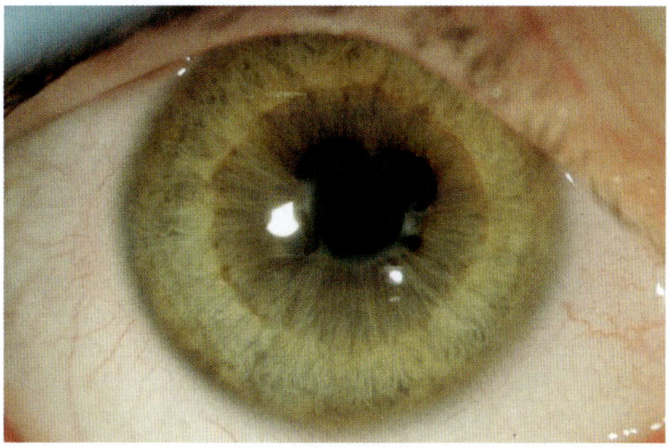

Figure 38.4: Posterior synechiae, scarring of the iris to the lens, causing irregular pupil. Occurs in most etiologies of anterior uveitis. Occurs in chronic or severe acute disease.

TABLE 38.2 Possible Clinical Findings in Anterior Uveitis

Sclera/conjunctiva	Injection
Cornea	Edema, keratic precipitates
Anterior chamber	Cells, flare, hypopyon
Iris	Posterior synechiae, nodules

DIFFERENTIAL DIAGNOSIS

Anterior Uveitis and Hypopyon

The first step is to diagnose uveitis by seeing cells in the anterior chamber of the eye. Other conditions that can mimic symptoms of uveitis should be ruled out, including corneal abrasion, corneal ulcer, and scleritis. Traumatic anterior uveitis, known as traumatic iritis, presents after blunt trauma, is highly symptomatic, and has a mix of white blood cells (may be minimal) and pigment.

There are myriad etiologies of anterior uveitis, which can be immune-mediated, infectious, traumatic, or malignant. A selection that may present acutely is shown in Table 38.1, with select points discussed in the text. Immune-mediated uveitis is commonly "idiopathic," but sarcoidosis and HLA-B27 are commonly known etiologies. HLA-B27 causes highly symptomatic unilateral anterior uveitis with or without hypopyon. It may be associated with ankylosing spondylitis, psoriatic arthritis, reactive arthritis, and arthritis of inflammatory bowel disease. Behcet disease can cause hypopyon, especially when bilateral. However, occlusive retinal vasculitis is the most pressing issue.

Infectious etiologies are important to consider. Anterior uveitis secondary to viral infections such as herpes simplex virus (HSV) or varicella zoster virus (VZV) is relatively common and typically present unilaterally with elevated intraocular pressures. Hypopyon with blood should raise concern for Herpesviridae infection. It is imperative to evaluate for necrotizing herpetic retinitis (acute retinal necrosis) with dilated examination when concerned for Herpesviridae infection.

Endophthalmitis is the most severe and urgent diagnosis in the differential. It presents after surgery or penetrating trauma and can cause hypopyon but also significant vitreous and retinal inflammation. Patients with significant systemic illness may present with endogenous endophthalmitis without history of trauma or surgery.

Tuberculosis is a less common cause, but can cause granulomatous anterior inflammation, usually in the setting of chorioretinal involvement and without active pulmonary disease. Last, syphilis can cause any type of uveitis and ought to be considered in all cases.

The diagnostic workup depends on the clinical presentation and history. In the absence of a clear history of ocular trauma or predisposing condition, patients with uveitis should undergo laboratory testing, including complete blood count, complete metabolic panel, and evaluation for sarcoidosis and syphilis. HLA-B27 should be obtained in cases of unilateral disease. Tuberculosis testing (interferon gamma release assay) is obtained in most cases because it can impact treatment even if it is not the cause of uveitis. Further testing is based on the clinical scenario (Table 38.1).

Hyphema

Traumatic hyphema does not have a significant associated differential diagnosis. Hyphema may occur concurrently with traumatic iritis, corneal abrasion, open globe, or penetrating foreign body.

Spontaneous hyphema requires more search for a possible underlying cause. In adults, spontaneous hyphema can be caused by iris neovascularization (typically secondary to retinal vein occlusion or diabetic retinopathy), clotting abnormalities, anticoagulation, Herpesviridae infection, malignancy, or intraocular lens problems (uveitis-glaucoma-hyphema syndrome). Spontaneous hyphema in children can be caused by juvenile xanthogranuloma, retinoblastoma, or leukemia. Testing for sickle cell disease should be considered in patients presenting with spontaneous hyphema owing to a higher rate of complications.

MANAGEMENT

Anterior Uveitis and Hypopyon

The goal of treatment in anterior uveitis is to reduce inflammation. Corticosteroids are the mainstay of treatment and should be initiated in consultation with an ophthalmologist. Close ophthalmology follow-up is warranted to ensure treatment response and to evaluate for adverse effects of medication and specific findings that can help direct management. If a dilated exam cannot be done in the emergency setting, expeditious ophthalmology follow-up is necessary because posterior involvement can cause long-term visual complications.[1]

For anterior uveitis and noninfectious hypopyon, topical corticosteroid therapy with prednisolone acetate 1% every 1 to 2 hours or difluprednate 0.05% 4 times daily should be initiated and then tapered based on clinical response. Difluprednate has a higher rate of intraocular pressure elevation and should hence be used with caution. More severe cases may require systemic or locally injected corticosteroids, but this should be deferred to ophthalmology.

Traumatic iritis is generally self-limited. However, severe inflammation or symptoms are treated with topical steroids and cycloplegia.

If hypopyon is caused by endophthalmitis, treatment is surgical or procedural and should be referred to ophthalmology emergently. Topical steroids can still be used, but antibiotic therapy is necessary.

Herpetic anterior uveitis, caused by HSV or VZV, may also present with hypopyon and should be treated with valacyclovir 1 g orally 3 times per day in conjunction with topical steroids.[9] Empiric antiviral therapy is commonly employed without definitive diagnosis, with suggestive signs like unilateral disease, elevated intraocular pressure, or corneal edema. Such patients should be urgently evaluated by ophthalmology. Viral infection in the retina requires emergent ophthalmology evaluation and more intensive therapy.[10]

Cycloplegic agents can help pain by reducing ciliary spasm and also prevent formation of posterior synechiae, thus reducing the risk of angle-closure glaucoma that can happen with 360° of posterior synechiae.[4] Typically, cyclopentolate 1% is used nightly or twice per day. Topical atropine is very long lasting and may cause synechiae in the dilated position, and tropicamide is generally not strong enough.

Hyphema

The goal of treatment is to control pain and inflammation, treat/prevent elevated intraocular pressure, and prevent rebleeding. Topical steroids such as prednisolone acetate 1% and cycloplegia using cyclopentolate 1% are used to treat pain and inflammation. Steroids are thought to inhibit fibrinolysis, leading to decreased risk for rebleeding.[7] Cycloplegia reduces ciliary spasm and prevents posterior synechiae formation. With a small hyphema (<1/3 of the anterior chamber), and no clinical risk factors, observation and close follow-up may be appropriate.

Behavioral modifications to reduce risk of rebleeding are generally recommended but do not have strong supporting evidence.[7] These include relative bed rest, an eye shield to prevent secondary injury, elevation of the head of the bed, and avoidance of aspirin or nonsteroidal anti-inflammatory drugs (NSAIDs). Patients can photograph their eye to document the clinical course and ensure appropriate clearing.

If the intraocular pressure is elevated, this must be treated with ocular hypotensive agents. Carbonic anhydrase inhibitors should be avoided in the setting of possible sickle cell trait or disease owing to pH changes. Elevated intraocular pressure can cause glaucoma or corneal blood staining.

Hyphema that does not resolve or causes persistent elevated intraocular pressure may require surgical washout of the anterior chamber to prevent associated secondary glaucoma, corneal blood staining, and synechiae.[7]

Hyphema of any size in the presence of sickle cell disease/trait, large hyphema, or elevated intraocular pressure warrants urgent ophthalmologic evaluation.

Close follow-up is necessary to monitor for rebleeding and commonly causes elevated intraocular pressure.[6]

TIPS AND PEARLS

- Photophobia, injection, and lack of discharge are suggestive of anterior uveitis.
- Intraocular pressure can vary with etiology and should be checked in all patients.
- Anterior uveitis can only be diagnosed after dilated exam ruling out posterior pathology.
- Topical corticosteroids are the mainstay of treatment for both uveitis and hyphema.
- Patients with uveitis should have close follow-up with ophthalmology to ensure appropriate resolution and facilitate evaluation for precipitating etiologies if undetermined at the time of diagnosis.
- Evaluate for the presence of concurrent traumatic ocular injury in patients with hyphema.
- All African American patients with hyphema should be tested for sickle cell disease/trait.
- Patients presenting with large hyphema, hyphema concurrent with sickle cell disease/trait, or high intraocular pressure require urgent evaluation by ophthalmology.

EVIDENCE

What is the evidence for steroid formulations in the treatment of uveitis?

Multiple formulations exist for corticosteroid therapy. Difluprednate 0.05% and prednisolone acetate 1% are the most commonly used topical agents for uveitis. The literature shows that difluprednate 4 times daily is noninferior to prednisolone acetate 8 times daily, suggesting that it may be more effective for anterior uveitis.[7] Larger randomized trials to compare the two medications are ongoing. There are no clear data on frequency of topical steroid use in relation to uveitis severity, so this is based on clinical judgment. There are no studies comparing systemic, periocular, or intraocular steroids in anterior uveitis, so their use is based on clinical judgment.

What evidence supports the use of aminocaproic acid or TXA in traumatic hyphema?

Evidence for the treatment of traumatic hyphema is variable without demonstrable benefit in the prevention of secondary complications like elevated intraocular pressure. Some physicians advocate for the use of tranexamic acid or aminocaproic acid in traumatic hyphema with the goal of stabilizing clot formation and ultimately reducing the risk of secondary hemorrhage. A recent Cochrane review found that administration of antifibrinolytic medications conferred some small benefit in visual acuity but with prolonged time to clearance of hyphema and with associated systemic side effects; as such, routine administration is not recommended.[7]

References

1. Harthan JS, Opitz DL, Fromstein SR, Morettin CE. Diagnosis and treatment of anterior uveitis: optometric management. *Clin Optom*. 2016;8:23-35.
2. SooHoo JR, Davies BW, Braverman RS, Enzenauer RW, McCourt EA. Pediatric traumatic hyphema: a review of 138 consecutive cases. *J AAPOS*. 2013;17(6):565-567.
3. Deibel JP, Cowling K. Ocular inflammation and infection. *Emerg Med Clin North Am*. 2013;31(2):387-397.
4. Hom J, Sarwar S, Kaleem MA, Messina CR, Sepah YJ, Nguyen QD. Topical mydriatics as adjunctive therapy for traumatic iridocyclitis and iritis. *Cochrane Database Syst Rev*. 2020;2020(8):CD013260.
5. Kim CH, Chen MF, Coleman AL. Adjunctive steroid therapy versus antibiotics alone for acute endophthalmitis after intraocular procedure. *Cochrane Database Syst Rev*. 2017;2017(2):CD012131.
6. Bansal S, Gunasekeran DV, Ang B, et al. Controversies in the pathophysiology and management of hyphema. *Surv Ophthalmol*. 2015;61(3):297-308.
7. Gharaibeh A, Savage HI, Scherer RW, Goldberg MF, Lindsley K. Medical interventions for traumatic hyphema. *Cochrane Database Syst Rev*. 2019;2019(1):CD005431.
8. Heng LZ, Hamilton RD. Ocular emergencies. *Medicine*. 2018;46(12):754-749.
9. Chan NS, Chee SP. Demystifying viral anterior uveitis: a review. *Clin Exp Ophthalmol*. 2019;47(3):320-333.
10. Sheppard JD, Toyos MM, Kempen JH, Kaur P, Foster CS. Difludpredate versus prednisolone acetate for endogenous anterior uveitis. *Invest Ophthalmol Vis Sci*. 2014; 55(5):2993-3002.

CHAPTER 39

Lens Dislocation

Elizabeth Yetter
Khurram Chaudhary

THE CLINICAL CHALLENGE

There are a number of challenges with ectopia lentis, more commonly known as lens dislocation. The symptoms of dislocation of a patient's natural lens or an implanted lens may vary. Patients may report immediate or gradual vision loss and may have associated large floaters or diplopia—either monocular or binocular. Depending on the etiology, the vision loss may or may not be accompanied by pain.

As such, lens dislocation becomes a part of the differential in a patient that presents with sudden loss of vision. When the lens is not in place, there is a major loss of refraction, and the eye becomes severely hyperopic, causing difficulty with distance vision. When the lens becomes partially dislocated, this is referred to as lens subluxation. A subluxated lens can also impair vision by causing irregular refractive surfaces when the lens is tilted. The lens can split the visual axis and lead to an optical defect where two or more blurred images are formed, leading to monocular diplopia.

Pathophysiology

The lens is located posterior to the iris and supported in 360° by zonules, tiny threadlike fibers, which attach the lens to the ciliary body. The tightening and relaxing of the zonules adjust the lens for near or far vision. Disruption of the zonules can lead to subluxation (partial dislocation), where the lens either hangs from the ciliary body, or dislocation, where the lens lies in the posterior segment of the eye.

Traumatic injury of the eye is the most common cause of lens dislocation. The lens usually dislocates posteriorly because the iris limits the lens's movement anteriorly. It may float in the vitreous humor if it is tethered to intact zonules or settle onto the retina.[1] However, other rare causes of anterior lens dislocation have been reported, such as a 51-year-old male with no history of eye or systemic disease who presented with painless vision loss in his right eye after vomiting for 4 hours. It was theorized that the increased neck and chest pressure from vomiting with subsequent increased intraocular pressure from the back to the front of the eye caused disruption of the zonules and led to anterior dislocation.[2] The severity and location of the zonular disruption will dictate the degree of dislocation the lens will undergo anatomically. It is also worth noting that patients with connective tissue disorders, such as Ehlers-Danlos or Marfan syndrome, are at risk for lens dislocation even from minor trauma. Some conditions usually diagnosed in the pediatric years, such as homocystinuria or microspherakia (a congenitally spherical, smaller lens), also increase the risk of lens dislocation. In cases such as chronic uveitis or syphilitic uveitis, it has been theorized that the zonules become weakened by humoral and cellular effects of the disease.[3]

Rarely, iatrogenic trauma can cause lens dislocation (eg, after cataract surgery in 0.2% to 3% of cases).[4] Intraocular lens (IOL) dislocation may be caused by asymmetric fixation, intraoperative complications, zonular weakness, inadequate capsular complex, pseudoexfoliation syndrome, myopia/increased axial length of the globe, retinitis pigmentosa, uveitis and Marfan syndrome, and other connective tissue disorders.

APPROACH/THE FOCUSED EXAM

A thorough medical history can be useful in ascertaining the underlying etiology of the vision loss along with a full ophthalmic exam. As lens dislocations seen in the emergency department (ED) are often caused by trauma, providers should perform complete primary and secondary surveys. During the secondary survey, the identification of any visual disturbance warrants further investigation.

When assessing past medical history, inquire whether the patient wears glasses or contacts and whether they were wearing them at the time of the injury in order to assess for other complicating factors such as corneal abrasions, foreign bodies, or globe rupture. Ask about history of connective tissue disorders, glaucoma, infections of eye, or any medical intervention to the eye preceding the injury. In assessing past surgical history, ask whether the patient has had any prior eye surgeries such as cataract removal, lens insertion, retinal surgery, and/or glaucoma surgery.

Note any facial swelling, ecchymosis, lacerations to the eyelid or surrounding structures. If there is significant eyelid edema, a second person may be required to help hold the eyelids open for a full examination of the eye. Note pupillary responses and extraocular movements, and complete a visual acuity test with a Snellen chart. Perform a fluorescein exam to assess for Seidel sign in globe rupture and presence of corneal abrasions. Intraocular pressures should be obtained provided there is no concern for globe rupture. These assessments may help lead to the cause of vision loss but are inadequate alone to diagnose lens dislocation. All of this is predicated on patient cooperation, because one prospective study was unable to perform visual acuity evaluation in 60% of over 300 ED patients, and is a possible issue in trauma patients presenting with pain.[5]

If available in the ED and if the patient can cooperate, a slit-lamp examination can aid in the diagnosis of lens dislocation. The patient's chin should be placed on the chin rest, with the forehead touching the top band and the eyes aligned with the black markings on the side of the stabilization frame. Adjust the width of the beam and angle the slit lamp to 45° to get an adequate view of the anterior chamber. The lens can dislocate within the lens plane, posteriorly into the vitreous cavity, or, less commonly, anteriorly into the anterior segment. When examining a patient with a subluxated lens via slit-lamp biomicroscopy, the observer can usually appreciate a deep anterior chamber and phacodensis (tremulousness of the lens during eye movement), signaling instability of the zonular fibers. A subluxated lens will often, but not inevitably, dislocate.

Phakia/phakic refers to the presence of the natural lens. Pseudophakia/pseudophakic refers to the presence of an artificial lens in place of the natural lens, such as those seen after cataract surgery. The following figures show patients with a normal phakic lens (**Figure 39.1A**), an intraocular/implant lens (Figure 39.1B), **a** partially dislocated phakic (Figure 39.1C) and pseudophakic lens (Figure 39.1D).

Computed tomography (CT) remains the most widely used imaging platform for diagnosis of lens dislocation. CT scan of the facial bones or a dedicated orbital CT scan can not only diagnose lens dislocation but can also evaluate concomitant pathology such as retrobulbar hematomas, entrapped inferior rectus muscle, or globe rupture.

Although CT scan is often the means of evaluating ocular trauma in the ED (including lens dislocation) owing to its high osseous and soft tissue resolution,[1] point-of-care ultrasound (POCUS) is another rapid alternative (**Figure 39.2**). It can be performed as part of a complete trauma survey if globe rupture is not suspected. (POCUS is discussed in depth in Chapter 26.) Remember to scan in both transverse and sagittal planes, and ask the patient to look horizontally and vertically to assess for pathology. In the case of lens dislocation, the lens may be partially attached (**Figure 39.3**) or completely detached (**Figures 39.4** and **39.5**), resting at the most dependent region of the posterior segment.

DIFFERENTIAL DIAGNOSIS

The differential diagnoses relate to the underlying cause of the lens dislocation. Although there are many possible causes of lens dislocation, the most common cause for those presenting to the ED is trauma. However, in cases of minor trauma, other causes of lens dislocation should be considered and communicated during referral to ophthalmology. Additional eye trauma may be present, such as vitreous hemorrhage or globe rupture.[6]

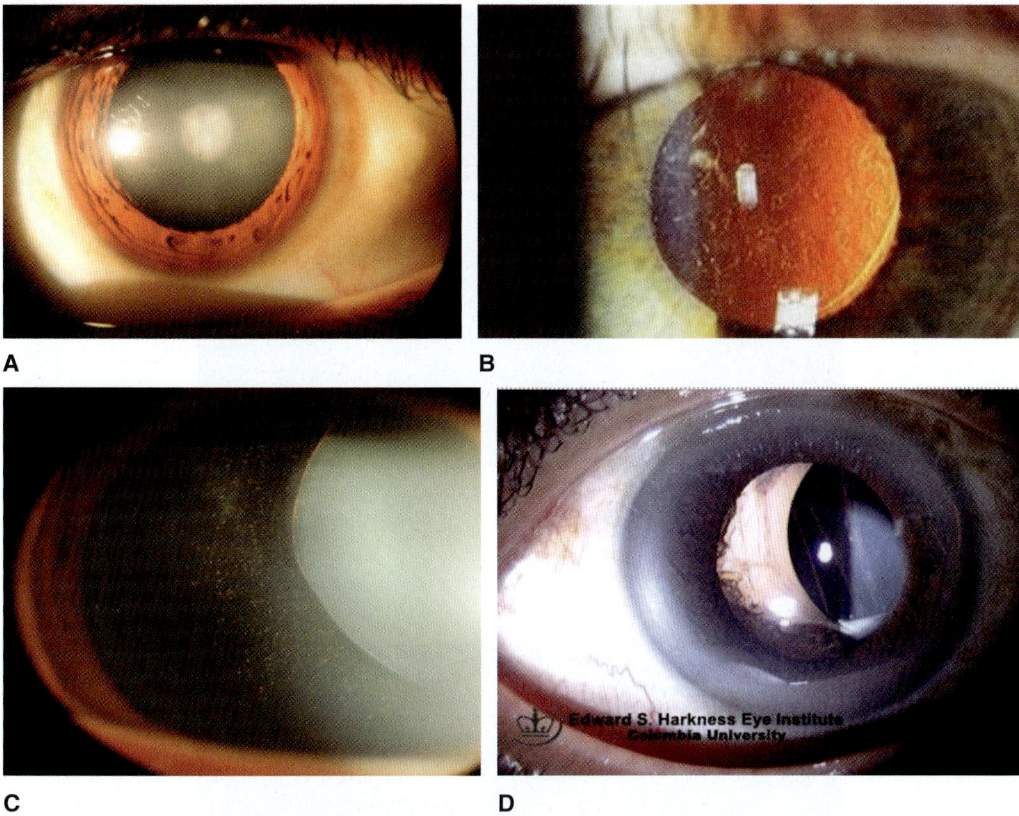

Figure 39.1: A, Normal phakic lens. The central white dot is a congenital posterior polar cataract, which is an uncommon, but nonpathologic finding. B, Implant/intraocular lens. The lens is not perfectly clear owing to a posterior capsule opacity, which occurs commonly after cataract surgery. When it affects vision, it can be removed electively with a laser procedure in clinic. C, Partially dislocated phakic lens and D, partially dislocated pseudophakic lens. (Courtesy of Khurram Chaudhary, MD, Edward S. Harkness Eye Institute, Columbia University.)

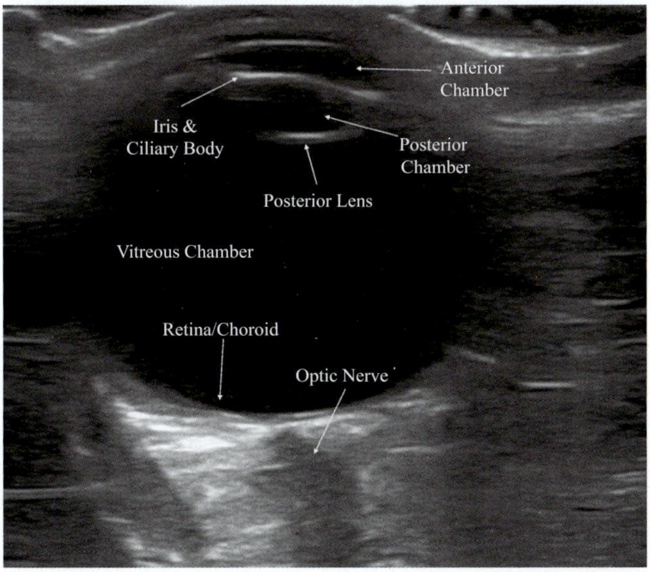

Figure 39.2: Point-of-care ultrasound demonstrating normal eye in transverse plane using a linear probe. Note that the anterior eye is at the top of the image and the posterior eye at the bottom of the image.

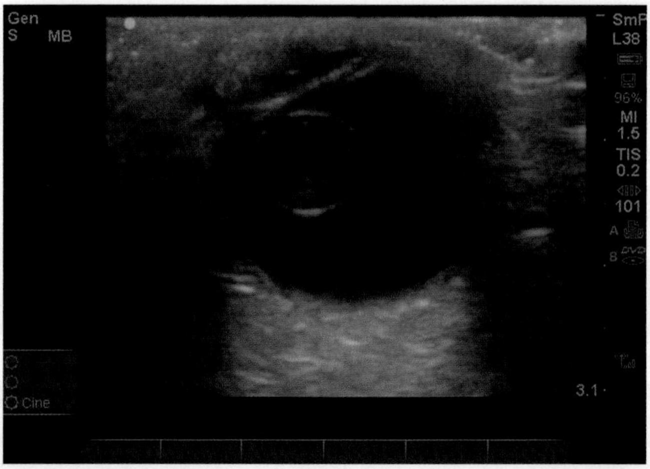

Figure 39.3: Point-of-care ultrasound in the emergency department demonstrating lens dislocation, tethered on one end. (Courtesy of Turandot Saul, MD RDMS FACEP, Mount Sinai Morningside & West.)

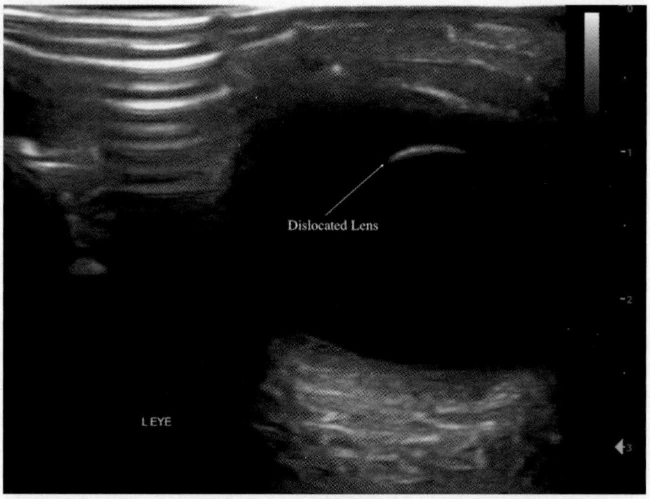

Figure 39.4: Point-of-care ultrasound demonstrating a dislocated artificial lens floating in vitreous chamber in transverse plane using a linear probe. Note how the lens orientation appears flipped compared with the normal lens. (Courtesy of Zilin Zhou, MD and Nicholas Buffin, MD, Mount Sinai Morningside & West.)

Ocular contusion may cause subluxation of the lens, particularly in patients with concomitant latent syphilis, or previous ocular surgery. Self-injurious behavior may be considered. Deliberate dislocation of the lens has been performed in certain parts of the world for the treatment of cataracts, called "couching," where the lens is pushed into the vitreous cavity with surgical instruments.

Atraumatic causes of lens dislocation require further investigation. As mentioned previously, ectopia lentis can also be caused by genetic diseases such as Marfan syndrome, homocystinuria, and microspherophakia. In the case of Marfan syndrome or homocystinuria, subluxation may occur in utero or within the first decade of life. Rarely, autosomal recessive disorders can cause ectopia lentis without other phenotypic changes. Other diseases that can lead to lens dislocation include intraocular tumors, uveitis, severe myopia, and buphthalmos (enlarged eye).

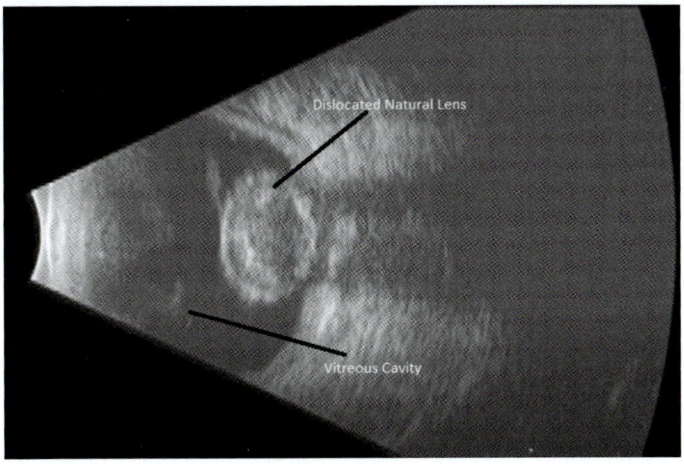

Figure 39.5: Ophthalmology ultrasound of a complete dislocation of the natural crystalline lens. Note that the anterior eye is to the left of the image and the posterior eye to the right of the image.

MANAGEMENT

The diagnosis of dislocation of either a natural or implanted lens requires ophthalmology consultation. The decision whether to have an emergent versus an urgent consultation depends on the clinical scenario. If the patient presents with pain, high intraocular pressure, flashes of light or a curtain coming over the vision, emergent consult is indicated. Significant vitreous traction can lead to a retinal tear and a subsequent retinal detachment. The edge of an artificial IOL in the posterior segment can also potentially embed itself within the retina and cause a retinal tear with subsequent detachment. Conversely, the natural lens has a smooth capsule and can safely remain in the posterior chamber. If the lens dislocates anteriorly, it may cause pupillary block and severely increased intraocular pressure.[7] These scenarios can lead to irreversible vision loss and in turn would need to be addressed with topical medication, laser surgery, or other surgical intervention immediately to prevent permanent vision loss.

Patients with chronic vision loss and normal intraocular pressure with no other concomitant pathology besides phacodonesis or pseudophacodonesis can be seen the next day in clinic for outpatient management because the risk of permanent vision loss is minimal if not addressed emergently.

Whether or not surgical intervention is necessary varies. When visual acuity is significantly affected such as seeing the IOL within the pupillary axis in the absence of dilation, the IOL dislocation must be surgically treated.[4] However, IOL dislocation sometimes does not affect visual acuity, and in those cases most clinicians would proceed with conservative treatment.

TIPS AND PEARLS

- POCUS is a valuable tool to identify ocular pathology such as lens dislocation in cases that exclude obvious globe rupture.
- Complete lens dislocation into the posterior segment or anterior chamber associated with elevated intraocular pressures warrants emergent ophthalmology consultation and intervention.
- Consider further investigation in patients with atraumatic lens dislocation or subluxation.

EVIDENCE

What is the sensitivity and specificity of POCUS in diagnosing lens dislocation?

One prospective cohort study evaluating 351 eyes in patients with suspected traumatic eye injuries used CT scanning reviewed by a radiologist compared with a bedside ocular examination by an ophthalmologist as the gold standards to determine sensitivity and specificity of POCUS for six types of eye injuries, including lens dislocation. Sensitivity and specificity of POCUS for lens dislocation was 96.8% (95% CI 83.3%-99.9%) and 99.4% (95% CI 97.8%-99.9%) respectively, when compared with orbital CT. Positive likelihood ratios were high and negative likelihood ratios were low, suggesting that a positive POCUS result was highly associated with presence of dislocation and that a negative ultrasound was associated with absence of dislocation. Like many POCUS studies, the amount of training in ocular ultrasound and operator experience may limit its generalizability.[5] This study demonstrates similar sensitivity and specificity seen in previous studies[8]; sensitivity and specificity improved after providing 16 hours of focused POCUS ocular education and 48 hours of hands-on ocular POCUS training.

References

1. Thelen J, Bhatt AA, Bhatt AA. Acute ocular traumatic imaging: what the radiologist should know. *Emerg Radiol.* 2017;24:585-592. doi:10.1007/s10140-017-1528-0
2. Wang M, Gao Y, Li R, Wang S. Monocular lens dislocation due to vomiting: a case report. *BMC Ophthalmol.* 2018;18(3):3. doi:10.1186/s12886-017-0651-8
3. Rapkin JS, Bogorad DD. Bilateral dislocation of the crystalline lens in a patient with presumed syphilitic uveitis. *Henry Ford Hosp Med J.* 1986;34(3):207-210.
4. Yang S, Nie K, Jiang H, Feng L, Fan W. Surgical management of intraocular lens dislocation: a meta-analysis. *PLoS One.* 2019;14(2):e0211489. doi:10.1371/journal.pone.0211489. eCollection 2019.
5. Ojaghi Haghighi S, Lombardi KM, Davis S, Vahdati SS, Sorkhabi R, Pourmand A. Diagnosis of traumatic eye injuries with point-of-care ocular ultrasonography in the emergency department. *Ann Emerg Med.* 2019;74(3):365-371 doi:10.1016/j.annemergmed.2019.02.001
6. Frasure SE, Saul T, Lewiss RE. Bedside ultrasound diagnosis of vitreous hemorrhage and traumatic lens dislocation. *Am J Emerg Med.* 2013;31(6):1002.e1-1002.e2. doi:10.1016/j.ajem.2013.02.013. Epub 2013 Apr 18. PMID: 23602749.
7. Pyle M, Gallerani C, Weston C, Frasure SE, Pourmand A. Point of care ultrasound and ocular injuries: a case of lens dislocation and a comprehensive review of the literature. *J Clin Ultrasound.* 2021;49:282-285. doi:10.1002/jcu.22904
8. Ojaghi Haghighi SH, Morteza Begi HR, Sorkhabi R, et al. Diagnostic accuracy of ultrasound in detection of traumatic lens dislocation. *Emergency (Tehran).* 2014;2(3):121-124. PMID: 26495362; PMCID: PMC4614573.

CHAPTER 40

Leukocoria

Kei U. Wong
Matthew S. Pihlblad

THE CLINICAL CHALLENGE

Leukocoria, or "white pupil," is an abnormal clinical finding of a white pupillary reflex (**Figure 40.1**). It is often the initial manifestation of a wide range of serious intraocular disorders involving the retina (eg, retinoblastoma), lens (eg, cataract), or vitreous (eg, hemorrhage).[1] The mean age of children at presentation with the chief complaint of "abnormal red reflex" or "leukocoria" is 22.0 + 32.5 months.[2] In a study by Lin et al., almost 40% of children referred to pediatric ophthalmology for leukocoria had a visually significant diagnosis (retinoblastoma; refractive error requiring glasses; amblyopia; cataracts; strabismus; or a cornea, retina, or iris condition).[2]

Despite recommended routine pediatric screening with the red reflex test, most children with retinoblastomas initially present with leukocoria detected by a family member.[3] Abramson et al.[4] reported 80% of children with retinoblastoma had their presenting sign of leukocoria initially detected by a parent or a friend, compared with 8% by a pediatrician. As most conditions of leukocoria are vision threatening, the discovery of leukocoria necessitates rigorous etiologic workup and urgent ophthalmology evaluation to assess for life-threatening conditions, in particular retinoblastoma, to avoid serious morbidity and mortality.

PATHOPHYSIOLOGY

The human eye's red reflex is caused by the retro-illumination of normal choroidal vasculature reflecting through the various ocular structures, including the cornea, pupil, lens, vitreous, and retina. The abnormal white pupillary reflex of leukocoria is caused by interference in any of these structures.[5] As the etiologies of leukocoria are expansive, their pathogenesis, clinical features, and treatment will differ depending on the underlying cause.

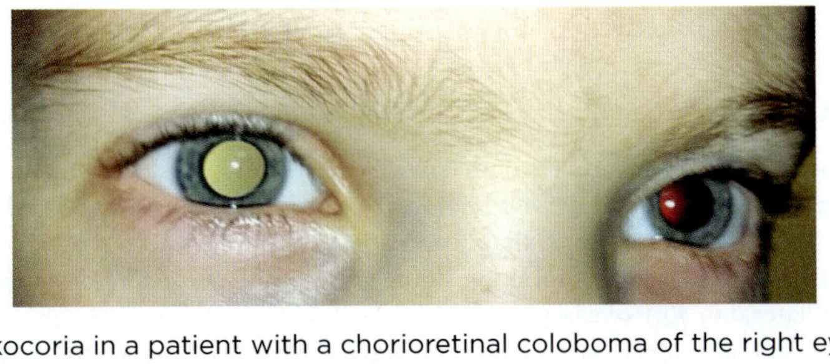

Figure 40.1: Leukocoria in a patient with a chorioretinal coloboma of the right eye.

APPROACH/THE FOCUSED EXAM

Although the differential diagnosis of leukocoria is broad, it can be further narrowed down based on patient history (including history of present illness, birth history with prematurity or trauma), full family history, additional clinical examination findings, and a good ophthalmic examination (including indirect ophthalmoscopy and fundus photography). Whereas older children are often incidentally diagnosed with leukocoria from photographs, infants are mostly diagnosed by fundoscopic examination with finding of asymmetry of the red reflex.[1]

Whereas a detailed history is paramount to provide diagnostic clues, a thorough clinical examination is pivotal to the diagnosis of leukocoria. The method of detection of leukocoria depends on the age of onset, certain positions or conditions (eg, dark environment, dilated pupil) to allow for better visualization.[1,3] In addition, the more peripheral a lesion is within the retina, the more important positioning and lighting become.[2]

The evaluation begins with age-appropriate vision assessment and external examination for the presence or absence of proptosis, orbital mass, signs of ocular trauma, infection, or inflammation (including regional lymphadenopathy).[1] Any child presenting with leukocoria should be evaluated for visual acuity, pupillary reflexes, indirect ophthalmoscopy, and slit lamp examination of both anterior segment and fundus.[5]

The pupils are examined for reactivity and relative afferent defect. A markedly diminished pupillary reflex, a white reflex, dark spots in the reflex, or asymmetry (ie, Brückner reflex) are all considered to be abnormal findings.[5,6] The color of the pupillary reflex also gives a hint of the diagnosis. As an example, white pupillary reflex is typical for retinoblastoma, whereas a yellow reflex (or xanthocoria) could be indicative of Coats disease, and a blue-gray pupil is commonly seen in congenital cataracts.[7]

Extraocular muscle abnormalities can be evaluated by observing gross eye movements, assessing for alignment by observing the corneal light reflex of a single point light source (eg, from a pen light or an otoscope), and the cover/uncover test. Signs of misalignment can be a common finding seen in retinoblastoma. The slit lamp examination can be used to detect cataract, cornea opacity, or anterior chamber inflammation. Lastly, a dilated funduscopic examination can assess the status of the retina (eg, retinal detachment), detect retinal vascular abnormalities or exudates, or the presence of mass lesions.[1,3] Ophthalmology follow-up or urgent consultation is appropriate for this examination.

Ocular point-of-care ultrasound (POCUS) can give accurate and clinically relevant information on intraocular disease in a leukocoria patient. Ultrasound is readily available in the emergency department (ED) without the use of potentially harmful ionizing radiation.[8] Guidelines no longer recommend computed tomography (CT) imaging for leukocoria owing to the concern for possible retinoblastoma.[9]

DIFFERENTIAL DIAGNOSIS

The differential diagnosis of leukocoria is extensive. Primary diagnostic considerations and clinical findings associated with the commonly diagnosed conditions of leukocoria are summarized as follows.

RETINOBLASTOMA

Retinoblastoma (**Figure 40.2**) affects both sexes equally without significant racial or ethnic predilection.[5,7] Nearly all cases are diagnosed before 5 years of age; median age at diagnosis is younger for the bilateral form (<12 months) than for the unilateral unifocal form (24 months).[7,10] Approximately 90% of diagnosed cases of retinoblastoma are sporadic. Overall, retinoblastoma is unilateral in 70% and bilateral in 30% of cases.[7]

Retinoblastoma results from malignant transformation of the primitive retinal cells, caused by a mutation in the RB1 tumor suppressor gene. Heritable retinoblastoma is associated with germline mutations in the RB1 gene. Patients present at an early age and have bilateral and/or multifocal disease, and approximately 10% have a positive family history.[7] In contrast, children presenting

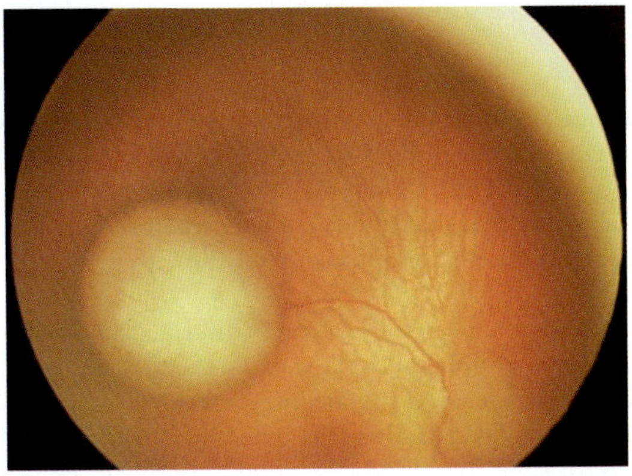

Figure 40.2: Right eye showing multifocal retinoblastoma lesions. One along the superior vessel arcade and one nasal to the optic nerve.

with nonheritable retinoblastoma typically have unilateral and unifocal disease, have a negative family history, and usually present at a later age. The nonheritable form results from somatic RB1 mutations in the tumor only.[1]

Any child presenting with unequivocal leukocoria should prompt urgent referral to an ophthalmologist within 1 week of detection, and sooner when practical, because patient survival in retinoblastoma is highly dependent on early detection and the degree of tumor extension at the time of initial diagnosis.[1,4]

PEDIATRIC CATARACT

Cataract (**Figure 40.3**) is opacification of the lens, which can cause partial or total blindness if not diagnosed and treated promptly. The most common etiology is idiopathic, but an autosomal-dominant inheritance is also possible.[11] Infants and children with cataracts may present with an asymmetric red reflex, leukocoria, strabismus, nystagmus in one or both eyes.[2,11] Cataract in children may be congenital or acquired, unilateral or bilateral.

Cataracts may also be associated with congenital infections such as rubella, toxoplasmosis, herpes simplex virus, and cytomegalovirus (CMV).[11] Unilateral cataracts are usually sporadic, whereas bilateral cataracts are associated with other systemic diseases like intrauterine infections (eg, TORCH infection), metabolic disorders (eg, galactosemia), and chromosomal anomalies.[5] Acquired cataracts may be caused by ocular trauma, uveitis, associated with long-term systemic corticosteroid therapy, and ionizing radiation.[1,11]

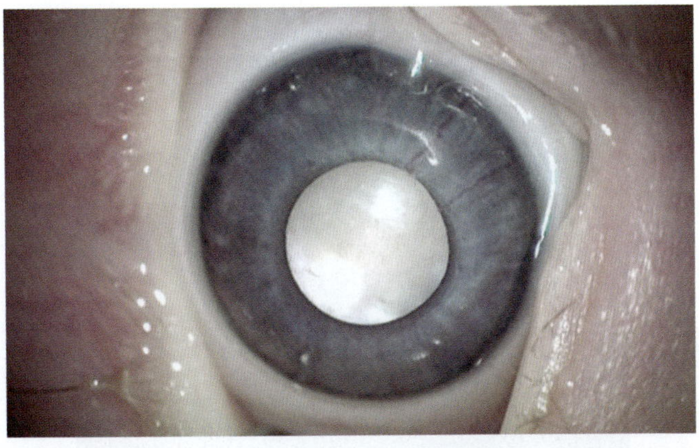

Figure 40.3: Congenital cataract in an infant during exam under anesthesia and cataract surgery with white reflex.

COATS DISEASE

Coats disease (**Figure 40.4**) is a nonheritable, sporadic disorder with an incidence of 0.09 per 100 000 population. Coats disease has a bimodal age distribution (under 18 years of age and middle-aged), primarily affecting males, representing 80% to 90% of cases.[1,7] In contrast to younger age of diagnosis in retinoblastoma patients (18 months), the average age presenting with Coats disease is 5 years.[11] Shields et al.[12] reported that of 604 patients who presented with pseudo-retinoblastoma conditions, Coats disease accounts for approximately 30% to 40% of those referred for suspected retinoblastoma.

Coats disease is an exudative retinal vascular disorder characterized by retinal telangiectasias (most prominent in the peripheral), yellow exudates, and retinal detachment.[1,7] Findings are mostly unilateral (nearly 90% of cases) and include strabismus, gradual decrease in visual acuity, or leukocoria.[11] The leukocoria in Coats disease is generally more yellow (also known as xanthocoria) owing to the presence of subretinal lipid exudation.[5,7] In advanced cases, ocular ultrasound will show intraretinal exudation that can cause complete retinal detachment but absence of calcium.[7,11] It is critical to recognize that calcification (on exam or ultrasound) is almost never seen with Coats disease, whereas it is common in advanced retinoblastoma.[7]

PERSISTENT FETAL VASCULATURE

Persistent fetal vasculature (PFV), formerly known as persistent hyperplastic primary vitreous (PHPV), is the second most common cause of infantile leukocoria in the presence of a microphthalmic eye.[7,12] PFV is nonheritable and commonly presents unilaterally.[5] It results from failure of regression of the embryonic primary vitreous and hyaloid vascular system during gestation.[1,13] The most common ocular finding is the presence of fibrovascular tissue on the posterior surface of the lens, with or without an associated cataract.[7]

Children with PFV may go on to develop early cataract and closed-angle glaucoma, and the visual prognosis is generally poor.[13] Ocular ultrasound evaluation may demonstrate the posterior segment findings of a stalk extending from the optic nerve to the posterior lens and can measure the axial lengths for comparison between the eyes.[7]

VITREOUS HEMORRHAGE

Vitreous hemorrhage can result from many conditions, including trauma, uveitis, vascular abnormalities (eg, advanced ROP, PFV), leukemia, or other blood dyscrasias. Trauma, including abusive head trauma, is the most common cause of vitreous hemorrhage in young children.[1,11] Vitreous hemorrhage causes leukocoria when there is extensive reorganization followed by transformation

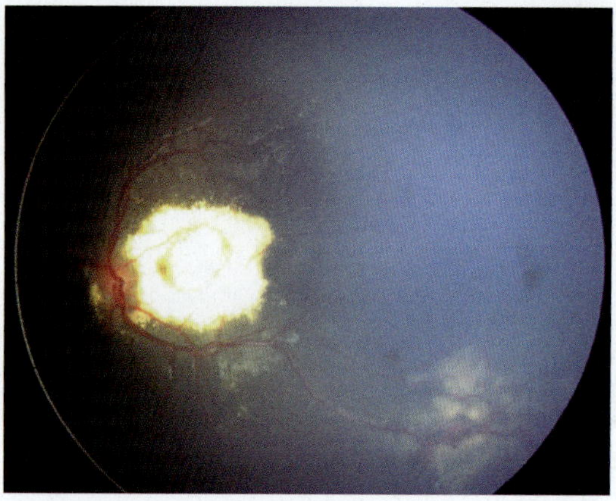

Figure 40.4: Fundus photo of the left eye of a patient with Coats disease with extensive exudates in the macula and peripheral telangiectatic vessels.

of the blood into white or yellow debris prior to its degradation.[1] Ocular ultrasonography is helpful in distinguishing vitreous hemorrhage from retinoblastoma; the absence of a retinal-based mass and/or calcifications exclude retinoblastoma.[1]

OCULAR TOXOCARIASIS (OCULAR LARVA MIGRANS)

Ocular toxocariasis is an infection caused by ascarid *Toxocara canis* or *T catis*. It occurs most commonly in children and adolescents (2-14 years), acquired through the ingestion of larvae (often with a history of the young child playing in infested areas).[7,11] Ocular toxocariasis is mostly unilateral and presents with strabismus, blurred vision, and leukocoria.[5]

Ocular toxocariasis clinically presents as retinal granuloma (localized at the posterior pole or periphery), endophthalmitis, vitreous abscess, and tractional retinal detachment.[5] Anterior segment findings may include iritis. Dilated exam or ultrasonography may show vitritis, similar to endophthalmitis. The ocular lesions may be confused with retinoblastoma, particularly if there is associated calcification.[1,11] One distinguishing feature from retinoblastoma is the presence of retinal and/or vitreous traction, which is almost always present with toxocariasis.[7]

Serology tests can also help to confirm previous exposure and support the suspected diagnosis of toxocariasis, as well as elevated serum IgE.[7] In difficult cases, an anterior chamber tap can be performed to show eosinophils or vitreous for *Toxocara* antibodies but could lead to tumor dissemination in retinoblastoma.

RETINOPATHY OF PREMATURITY

Retinopathy of prematurity (ROP) (**Figure 40.5**) results from abnormal vascular proliferation of incompletely vascularized retina in premature (under 32 weeks of gestation) or low-birth-weight (less than 1500 grams) infants and can lead to permanent blindness.[5,11] It presents as leukocoria when ROP is severe and results in extensive fibrovascular proliferation and/or tractional retinal detachment (stages 4-5).[1,7]

ROP commonly have bilateral and symmetric presentation. The retinal findings are not typically present at birth but develop in infants (7-9 weeks of age).[7] Infants present with signs of ROP typically between 35 and 45 weeks of postconceptional age and have usually received oxygen therapy.[1,5] Diagnosis of ROP can be made with a history of prematurity, bilateral and symmetric presentation, and presence of tractional retinal detachment on ocular examination.[1] Bilateral retinal avascularity and nonperfusion affecting the temporal peripheral retina are characteristic findings on fundoscopy, but more advanced cases present with fibrovascular proliferation.[7]

RETINAL DYSPLASIA

Retinal dysplasia refers to aberrant differentiation of retinal tissues, consists of oval or circular groupings of dysplastic retinal cells in variable shapes and sizes (unlike those seen in retinoblastoma,

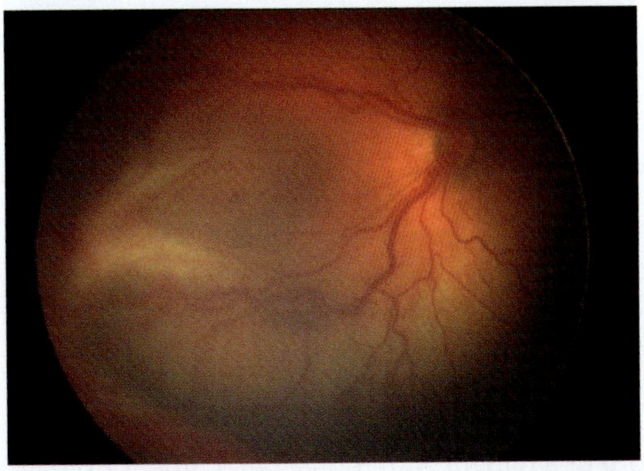

Figure 40.5: Retcam fundus photo of the right eye showing retinopathy of prematurity (Zone II, Stage 4a, with plus disease): Moderate abnormal blood vessel growth with venous dilatations and arteriolar tortuosity within the posterior retinal vessels.

which are uniform in size).[1] Retinal dysplasia may be hereditary (eg, trisomy 13, trisomy 18, Norrie disease) or caused by intrauterine infections (eg, TORCH infections, Zika virus); both forms are commonly associated with retinal detachment.[11] Affected children with inherited retinal dysplasia may present with bilateral leukocoria with retinal detachments. In contrast, retinal dysplasia caused by congenital infections are rarely associated with leukocoria if there is diffuse retinal involvement or retinal detachment.[1]

FAMILIAL EXUDATIVE VITREORETINOPATHY (FEVR)

FEVR (**Figure 40.6**) is a hereditary retinal vascular disorder characterized by avascularity of the temporal retina, with associated peripheral fibrovascular proliferation, and subretinal exudates, leading to tractional retinal detachment in advanced cases.[5,7] Patients with onset of symptoms before 3 years of age are at increased risk for poor visual outcome.[11]

FEVR is caused by genetic abnormality (aberrant Wnt signaling) that affects the growth and development of retinal blood vessels.[5] The mode of inheritance is autosomal dominance with 100% penetrance.[1,5,7] Unlike ROP, the fundus findings of FEVR are often highly asymmetric (with severe findings in one eye and minimal findings in the other eye) and not associated with a history of prematurity or low birth weight.[7] Furthermore, owing to the hereditary component of FEVR, family members will exhibit similar exam findings such as peripherally avascular retina.[1,5]

OTHER

Refractive error (high refractive error, anisometropia), strabismus, normal reflex (~15° off axis when capturing normal optic nerve in pupil on photography), tumors, congenital malformations, infectious, ocular trauma, cornea opacity.

MANAGEMENT

Leukocoria is a sign of an underlying ocular or systemic disease. The management of each ocular condition varies depending on the underlying etiology. Immediate evaluation by an ophthalmologist with a comprehensive examination of the fundus is essential in all cases of leukocoria, even in the emergency setting.

Early detection of retinoblastoma is strongly correlated with increased patient survival, and this must be ruled out in every case. Because of the significant morbidity and mortality associated with undiagnosed retinoblastoma, it is imperative that prompt follow-up be arranged for a child presenting with unequivocal leukocoria before discharge from the ED. If prompt follow-up cannot be arranged or there is concern with compliance of follow-up, it is necessary to transfer the patient to a tertiary care center or ophthalmologist evaluation.[12]

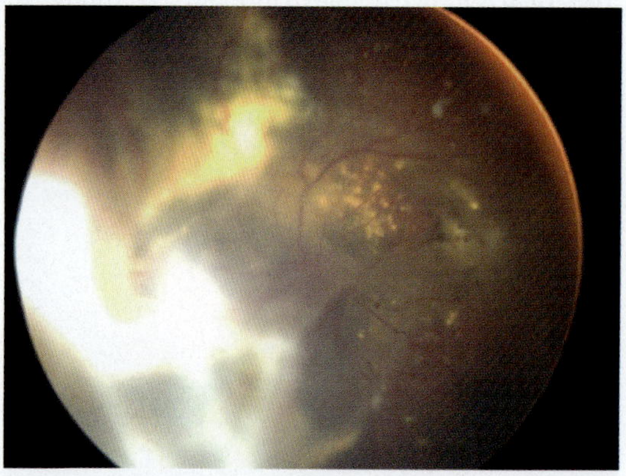

Figure 40.6: Fundus photo of a patient with retinal detachment from FEVR with tractional retina elevation with fibrosis and exudates.

It is important to emphasize that retinoblastoma is diagnosed clinically under dilated fundus examination with support from other imaging, including B-scan ultrasound and magnetic resonance imaging (MRI); intraocular biopsy is always contraindicated. Calcification within the ocular mass may be demonstrated on CT scans; however, clinicians should recognize possible RB1 mutation in children secondary to radiation exposure. MRI is helpful to assess extraocular extension and optic nerve involvement and allows confirmation of the diagnosis in most cases (ie, advanced Coats disease or intracranial spread of retinoblastoma).[7,9] If the cause of leukocoria is uncertain, laboratory investigations (including serologic test for TORCH infections, genetic testing) may be useful for congenital infections, infections for cataracts, or metabolic studies (ie, galactosemia).[5,10]

TIPS AND PEARLS

- The red reflex test (**Figure 40.7**) described by Swiss ophthalmology Brückner is performed with a direct ophthalmoscope set to 0 about 2 to 3 feet from the patient, with the largest aperture light turned to the brightest setting with the room lights off. The red reflexes from both pupils illuminated simultaneously are compared as well as the position of the cornea light reflections. The "red" reflex should be light orange/yellow in less pigmented eyes and deep red in more darkly pigmented eyes. The reflexes should be identical in color, brightness, and size. The examiner can then move closer to each eye to examine in more detail. The red reflex test is an easy test even in uncooperative patients that can screen for vision and life-threatening conditions.
- Ultrasound can be very helpful and is readily available in most EDs (which can differentiate cataract, retinoblastoma, and retinal detachment).
- Urgent referral within 1 week or less to an ophthalmologist is required.

EVIDENCE

What is the sensitivity of the Red Reflex test (Brückner Test)?

When performed by pediatric ophthalmologists as a screening exam, one study showed a sensitivity of 82.6% and a specificity of 98.7% of the Brukner test to identify posterior pathology.[14] A meta-analysis of the red reflex testing in neonates showed a sensitivity of 23% and a specificity of 98%.[15] Most (61.8%) patients presenting to a pediatric ophthalmologist with the chief complaint of an abnormal red reflex had a normal eye exam. Even with varying sensitivities and specificities, the red reflex test is an easy, low-cost exam that can be easily performed by ED and primary care providers. Therefore, it is recommended as part of routine screening exams[3,4] because it can detect significant diagnoses.[2]

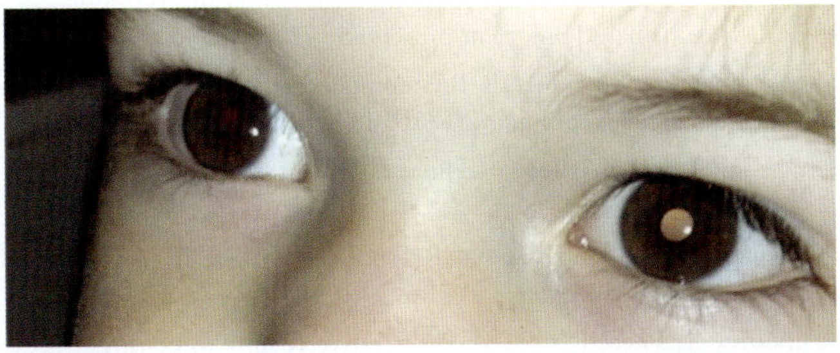

Figure 40.7: External photos of a child with a normal eye exam. The picture was taken ~15° off axis, which caputured the normal optic nerve in the reflex of the left eye.

What should the emergency provider do if they detect an abnormal red reflex?

- Need to rule out retinoblastoma: Early detection of retinoblastoma saves vision/eyes/life.[4]
- Recommend ophthalmology consultation if available or consider referral to facility with ophthalmology coverage.
- Recommend Ocular POCUS: Noninvasive test that can be easily performed at the bedside in most EDs, which can provide critical diagnostic information.[8,16]
    - If detects mass, or calcium would warrant MRI brain (to check for trilateral retinoblastoma) and orbits with pre- and postcontrast enhancement, CT not recommended.[9]
    - If shows cataract without mass (ciliary body or posteriorly) or other abnormalities (eg, foreign body, vitreous hemorrhage), would warrant urgent outpatient ophthalmology evaluation (within a week).
        - Congenital cataract requires timely removal to improve visual outcomes caused by critical period for visual development: cataract surgery should be performed by 4 to 6 weeks of age in unilateral cases and 6 to 8 weeks in bilateral cases for the best visual outcomes and can prevent additional problems of severe deprivation amblyopia, sensory strabismus, and nystagmus.[17]

References

1. Kaufman PL, Saunders R. Approach to the child with leukocoria. UpToDate. Waltham, MA: UpToDate. 2012. Accessed December 15, 2020. https://www.uptodate.com/contents/approach-to-the-child-with-leukocoria.
2. Lin SY, Yen KG, Zhu H, et al. Abnormal red reflex: etiologies in a pediatric ophthalmology population. *Clin Pediatr*. 2020;59(8):760-765.
3. Loh AR, Chiang MF. Pediatric vision screening. *Pediatr Rev*. 2018;39(5):225.
4. Abramson DH, Beaverson K, Sangani P, et al. Screening for retinoblastoma: presenting signs as prognosticators of patient and ocular survival. *Pediatrics*. 2003;112(6):1248-1255.
5. Kanukollu VM, Tripathy K. Leukocoria. StatPearls [Internet]. Treasure Island (FL): StatPearls Publishing. 2022. Accessed December 12, 2020. https://www.ncbi.nlm.nih.gov/books/NBK560794.
6. Roe LD, Guyton DL. The light that leaks: Brückner and the red reflex. *Surv Ophthalmol*. 1984;28(6): 665-670.
7. Kim JW, Singh AD. Differential diagnosis of leukocoria. In: Berry JL, Kim JW, Damato BE, et al., eds. *Clinical Ophthalmic Oncology: Retinoblastoma*. Springer International Publishing; 2019:11-26.
8. Giacalone M, Mastrangelo G, Parri N. Point-of-care ultrasound diagnosis of retinoblastoma in the emergency department. *Pediatr Emerg Care*. 2018;34(8):599-601.
9. de Graaf P, Göricke S, Rodjan F, et al. Guidelines for imaging retinoblastoma: imaging principles and MRI standardization. *Pediatr Radiol*. 2012;42(1):2-14.
10. Cassoux N, Lumbroso L, Levy-Gabriel C, et al. Retinoblastoma: update on current management. *Asia Pac J Ophthalmol*. 2017;6(3):290-295.
11. Damasco CVC, Dire DJ. A child with leukocoria. *Pediatr Emerg Care*. 2011;27(12):1170-1174.
12. Shields CL, Schoenberg E, Kocher K, et al. Lesions simulating retinoblastoma (pseudoretinoblastoma) in 604 cases: results based on age at presentation. *Ophthalmology*. 2013;120(2):311-316.
13. Payabvash S, Anderson JS, Nascene DR. Bilateral persistent fetal vasculature due to a mutation in the Norrie disease protein gene. *Neuroradiol J*. 2015;28(6):623-627.
14. Saiju R, Yun S, Yoon P, et al. Bruckner red light reflex test in a hospital setting. *Kathmandu Univ Med J*. 2012;10(2):23-26.
15. Taksande A, Jameel PZ, Taksande B, et al. Red reflex test screening for neonates: a systematic review and meta analysis. *Indian J Ophthalmol*. 2021;69(8):1994.
16. Skidmore C, Saurey T, Ferre RM, et al. A narrative review of common uses of ophthalmic ultrasound in emergency medicine. *J Emerg Med*. 2021;60(1):80-89.
17. Medsinge A, Nischal KK. Pediatric cataract: challenges and future directions. *Clin Ophthalmol (Auckland, NZ)*. 2015;9:77.

CHAPTER 41

Vascular Retinopathies

Avnish Deobhakta
Daniel J. Egan

THE CLINICAL CHALLENGE

Vascular retinopathies can represent a sentinel event for serious systemic illness. As such, once the diagnosis of a vascular retinopathy is made or suspected, careful examination and testing for the underlying cause is critical. For patients with ischemic retinopathy, secondary prevention of further vascular insults like stroke can prevent significant morbidity. Identification of these processes can be challenging for the emergency provider given the heterogeneity of the descriptions of symptoms by patients. The experience of visual changes described by patients overlaps between diagnoses. Therefore, maintaining a broad differential diagnosis with a systematic approach to the complaints is important to prevent future events or progression of vision loss.

PATHOPHYSIOLOGY

A general understanding of anatomy is helpful to get a clear grasp of the vascular processes that affect the retina. The ophthalmic artery is the first intracranial branch of the internal carotid artery and enters the orbit accompanied by the optic nerve. The retinal artery branches off to enter the cerebrospinal space supplying the retina. The central retinal artery provides blood flow to the center of the retina, including the macula and fovea, and its branches perfuse the rest of the retina. Notably, up to 50% of the population has a cilioretinal artery that arises from either the choroid or the posterior ciliary arteries and provides most of the macular circulation.[1] In these individuals, cases of retinal artery occlusion (RAO) may have preservation of the middle field of vision owing to this variant. Acute retinal ischemia is usually embolic from an ipsilateral carotid artery, the aortic arch, or the heart (valvular disease or thrombus from atrial fibrillation). Patients with sickle cell disease also carry an increased risk of retinal ischemia in vaso-occlusive crises.

Transient Monocular Vision Loss (TMVL)

TMVL, also known as amaurosis fugax, is the most common form of retinal ischemia and the retinal equivalent of a TIA. Approximately 14 to 15 per 10 000 individuals experience this annually.[2,3] TMVL typically presents with sudden, episodic, unprovoked, painless monocular blindness lasting seconds to minutes. The causes of TMVL vary, but all eventually result in dysfunction of the neural visual system itself (retina, optic nerve) or the vascular supply to it (choroid). The pathology is usually thromboembolic, causing occlusion of flow through the retinal artery or one of its branches, the primary source of the occlusion being the ipsilateral carotid artery or an inflamed ipsilateral temporal artery.[4] As a nonvascular cause, demyelinating disease can present as TMVL secondary to optic neuritis. When chronic severe ipsilateral carotid artery stenosis is the cause of TMVL, it may be attributable to *ocular ischemic syndrome*.

Retinal Artery Occlusion (RAO)

Pathophysiologically, the occlusion lies within the retinal arterial circulation (either the central retinal artery itself or a distal branch of the central retinal artery) with the type of vision loss dependent on the location of the clot. Central retinal artery occlusion (CRAO) is associated with profound loss, whereas a branch retinal artery occlusion (BRAO) has a partial scotoma corresponding to the location of the pathology. The cause of RAO is thromboembolic, and, like TMVL, often arises from similar sources. In ocular ischemic syndrome, critical stenosis of the carotid artery reduces central retinal artery perfusion pressure by up to 50%, placing these individuals at high risk for subsequent RAO. Additionally, giant cell arteritis (GCA), carotid artery dissection, vasculitis, sickle cell disease, and various hypercoagulable states can potentially be causative, though less likely.

Retinal Vein Occlusion (RVO)

In general, the major risk factor for RVO is systemic hypertension, along with advanced age (>65), smoking, and diabetes mellitus. Less common causes include hypercoagulable states (eg, multiple myeloma, polycythemia vera, and sickle cell disease), inflammatory diseases (eg, sarcoidosis), infectious diseases (eg, syphilis and tuberculosis), and pharmacologic causes (eg, oral contraceptive). RVO is the second most common retinal vasculopathy after diabetic retinopathy.[5]

Much like its arterial counterpart, RVO is broadly split into two types: central RVO (CRVO) and branch RVO (BRVO). In CRVO, the occlusion is thought to be caused by either a thrombus posterior to the lamina cribrosa of the optic nerve or turbulence initiated by central retinal arterial hypertension that compresses the nearby central retinal vein, the latter of which shares a sheath with its arterial counterpart. In BRVO, a similar thrombotic or inflammatory blockage can occur within one of the tributaries of the central retinal vein.

Hypertensive Retinopathy

In the context of long-standing and poorly controlled hypertension, the retina experiences progressive microvascular changes. Physiologically, retinal vessels have unique features that distinguish them from a generic vasculature, including the absence of a sympathetic nerve supply and the presence of a blood-retinal (brain) barrier. Long-standing elevated blood pressure damages retinal vessels, causing decreased neurosensory retinal function.[6] Damage to the endothelial cells leads to angiogenesis and neovascularization, which may further impair vision. Risk factors for this condition include any that are related to hypertension, including genetic factors and smoking.

APPROACH/THE FOCUSED EXAM

The American Heart and National Stroke Associations have amended the definition of stroke to include brain, spinal cord, or retinal cell death attributable to ischemia. As such, patients with acute vascular retinopathies are evaluated similarly to patients experiencing other stroke syndromes, including an assessment of risk factors. For all patients with a complaint of visual disturbances, the emergency provider should obtain a thorough medical history, including past ophthalmologic history, medications, and history of similar problems in the past. Focusing on the present illness, it is important to clarify certain key elements: onset of symptoms, monocular or binocular symptoms, duration of symptoms, associated symptoms (eg, headache or neck pain), and neurologic deficits. Furthermore, because GCA is associated with vascular retinopathies, a review of systems for this disease is critical. These patients are over age 50 and may report a history of jaw claudication, headache (particularly in the region of the temporal artery), tenderness of the scalp, constitutional symptoms, arthralgias, and fever (see Chapter 49). The physical examination will focus primarily on the eye, including a thorough examination of the retina, usually performed by an ophthalmologist after pupillary dilation. When GCA is suspected, measurement of inflammatory markers is recommended (erythrocyte sedimentation rate [ESR], C-reactive protein [CRP], and platelets).

Visual acuity and an assessment of the visual fields may uncover deficits. A comprehensive neurologic examination including cranial nerves is warranted. Given the association with underlying vascular disease, evaluation of the carotid arteries for bruits or evidence of other vascular disease on examination is important. Auscultation of the heart and assessment with electrocardiogram may identify a causative dysrhythmia like atrial fibrillation.

Transient Monocular Vision Loss

Patients will occasionally endorse a "vertically dropping black curtain" when describing their visual disturbance, although others may simply describe a "graying or darkening" of vision instead.

Symptoms are typically "negative" symptoms with loss of vision and do not characteristically include colors or flashes of light. It is important to keep in mind the inconsistency of symptomatic descriptions by patients. Most patients will report these episodes lasting anywhere from 2 to 30 minutes. Patients typically present for evaluation after symptoms have resolved. As a result, examination of the retina is expected to be normal.

Retinal Artery Occlusion

Like TMVL, this condition presents with sudden, painless, often profound, monocular vision loss that does not resolve. RAO is considered a stroke of the retina, and assessment of these patients should mirror a general stroke evaluation. Medical history will often reveal some combination of cerebrovascular risk factors like hypertension, hyperlipidemia, diabetes mellitus, or tobacco use. Examination includes a complete neurologic examination. Visual acuity often demonstrates profound vision loss when the occlusion is central. Some preservation of vision is possible with a BRAO or in patients with a cilioretinal artery. On assessment of the pupils, the affected eye will usually have an afferent pupillary defect. On fundoscopic examination, the retina demonstrates a white appearance because of retinal edema. The most obvious clinical finding for a CRAO is a cherry red spot noted in the central fundus, which is seen in 90% of patients (**Figure 41.1**) and related to preserved choroidal blood flow to the fovea.[7] In other cases, a frank embolus (termed a "Hollenhorst plaque") can be seen within the lumen of a vessel (**Figure 41.2**). In BRAO, segmental white discoloration of the retina is seen. The optic nerve should appear normal in both CRAO and BRAO.

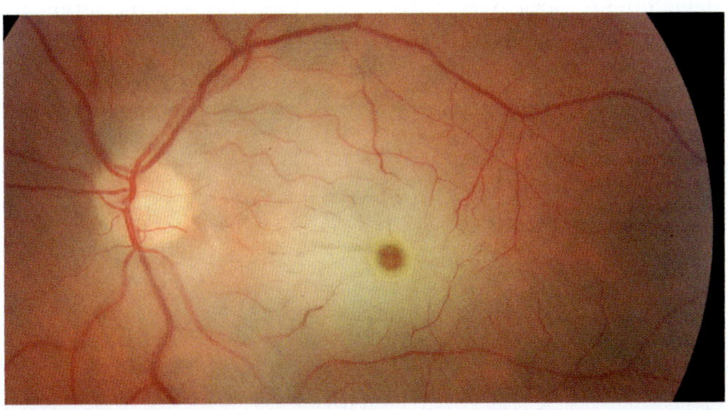

Figure 41.1: Central retinal artery occlusion, left eye. Note the whitening of the entire macula with a central sparing island akin to a cherry red spot. (Courtesy of Avnish Deobhakta, MD.)

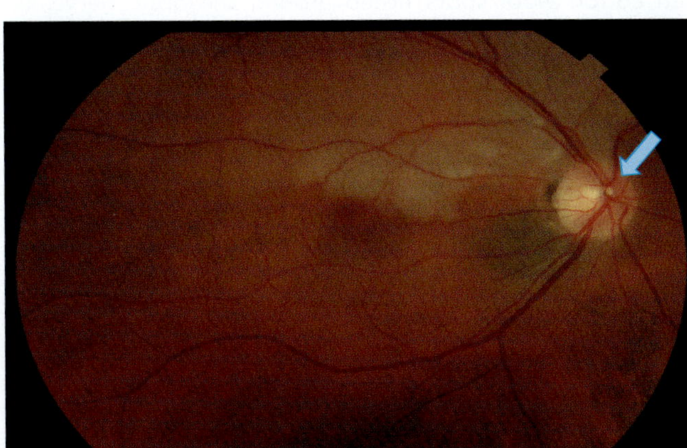

Figure 41.2: Branch retinal artery occlusion, right eye. Note the superior whitening of the retina. Close examination notes a Hollenhorst plaque in the superior retinal arterial arcade just after it branches from the central retinal artery within the optic nerve head (Arrow). (Courtesy of Avnish Deobhakta, MD.)

Retinal Vein Occlusion

Patients with RVO will often similarly complain of sudden, painless, and unilateral decreased central vision, typically less severe than that seen in RAO or TVML. Typically, a fundoscopic examination of a patient with a central RVO will reveal retinal hemorrhages in all four quadrants of the retina, along with optic nerve head swelling and possibly cotton wool spots (**Figure 41.3**). Although these findings are more limited and sectoral in those with a branch RVO, it is noteworthy that in *both* the central and branch varieties, the presenting feature can be vitreous hemorrhage, which itself often manifests with more profound vision loss (as blood is within the vitreous body, thus obscuring the entire retina).

Hypertensive Retinopathy

As compared with the foregoing, hypertensive retinopathy is often less symptomatically severe and bilateral. Patients will describe a much more progressive change in vision and not the acute change noted in the other conditions described in this chapter. Patients will have a history of poorly controlled hypertension. Approach to these patients should include an investigation for other signs of end organ damage from long-standing hypertensive disease.

The funduscopic examination of the patient will reveal a spectrum of blood vessel disruption. At its mildest, retinal arterioles will demonstrate narrowing, or retinal venules will be dilated or tortuous with few visual symptoms. However, prolonged elevated blood pressure can result in disruptions in the blood retinal barrier itself, causing focal areas of ischemia (cotton wool spots), retinal hemorrhages, and exudates. Moreover, in the most severe, malignant hypertensive situations, frank retinal detachments, optic nerve edema, and infarctions of the retina and choroid can occur with associated profound vision loss (**Figure 41.4**).[8]

Figure 41.3: Central retinal vein occlusion, right eye. Scattered hemorrhages can be seen throughout the fundus, with cotton wool spots noted around the optic nerve. (Courtesy of Avnish Deobhakta, MD.)

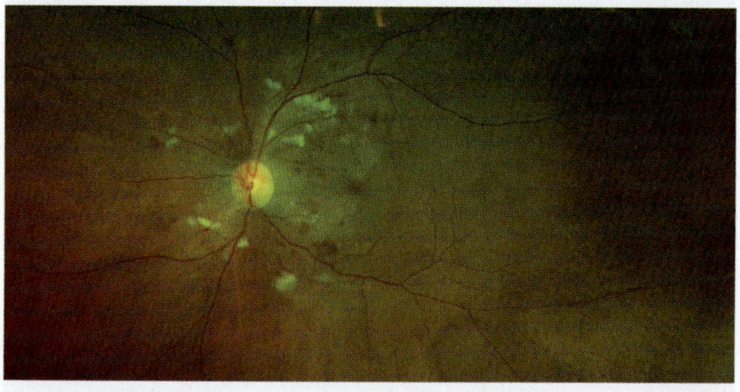

Figure 41.4: Malignant hypertension. Note the predominance of cotton wool spots clustered around the posterior pole. Also note the relative paucity of retinal hemorrhages in distinction to other retinal vasculopathies. (Courtesy of Avnish Deobhakta, MD.)

DIFFERENTIAL DIAGNOSIS

The four major forms of retinal vasculopathies are identified in **Table 41.1**. All of these are important to consider in the evaluation of patient with vision changes. In younger patients without typical stroke risk factors, consider the possibility of carotid artery dissection, which can occur spontaneously or secondary to trauma, neck manipulation, or in the setting of fibromuscular dysplasia. Primary thrombosis may occur in patients with an underlying hypercoagulable condition. Significantly elevated intraocular pressure may lead to compression of the central retinal artery, leading to ischemia.

Acute vision loss must prompt an assessment for a cerebral infarct. However, strokes associated with the visual cortex more typically cause a homonymous hemianopsia. The central vision often remains intact owing to preservation of the central retinal artery. Isolated ischemia of the optic nerve is also possible (see Chapter 50). Retinal vasospasm may lead to intermittent transient vision loss occurring over years and is a diagnosis of exclusion. Demyelinating diseases may present with TMVL, but, as a differentiating factor, typically have pain associated with optic neuritis. Inclusion of giant cell arteritis on the differential as a causative factor of TMVL and RAO is critical.

MANAGEMENT

Transient Monocular Vision Loss

Given that symptoms have resolved, the primary management of these patients involves investigation for underlying pathology and assessment for stroke. Up to 25% of these patients will have a stroke within 3 years of an episode of TMVL and may be at highest risk in the first 2 weeks after presentation.[3,9] The approach to the patient includes the evaluation and exclusion of associated causes and diseases (eg, giant cell arteritis). In cases where the clinical history is suggestive of giant cell arteritis and inflammatory markers are elevated, the emergency provider should initiate treatment with steroids pending biopsy diagnosis. The primary management of TMVL in the emergency setting is a search for the underlying cause including imaging of the brain as well as the vasculature of the neck, preferably with computed tomography (CT) or magnetic resonance (MR) angiogram. Engagement of ophthalmology and neurology consultants will assist in the workup and treatment plan for patients with TMVL.

Retinal Artery Occlusion

Given the often profound vision loss associated with this condition, the emergency provider should request an urgent ophthalmology consultation if RAO is suspected. If an RAO is indeed diagnosed, then a complete cardiovascular and stroke workup is needed, as there is a notable correlation with additional stroke or myocardial infarction in the immediate period post diagnosis.[10] In patients presenting with an acute RAO, ocular massage may be applied to the globe, where pressure is applied intermittently to the eye. With massage, the aqueous outflow increases and on release of the pressure perfusion to the retina may increase. The massage may also dislodge the embolus. Other treatment modalities like medications to decrease intraocular pressure have not demonstrated significant benefit. Patients presenting with symptoms less than 12 hours may benefit from intra-arterial (IA) tissue plasminogen activator within the ophthalmic artery.[11] Intravenous and IA

TABLE 41.1 Key features of Vascular Retinopathies

Retinal Vasculopathies	Laterality	Onset	Severity
Transient monocular vision loss (TMVL)	Monocular	Episodic	Temporary
Retinal artery occlusion (RAO)	Monocular	Sudden	Profound
Central branch	Monocular	Sudden	Partial scotoma
Retinal vein occlusion (RVO)	Monocular	Sudden	Moderate to Severe
Hypertensive retinopathy	Binocular	Gradual	Mild to Severe

thrombolysis have recently been supported as potential therapies in a scientific statement from the American Heart Association.[12] Nonetheless, historically, the visual outcomes for RAO—particularly those for CRAO—tend to be poor because there are very few ophthalmologic treatments that exist for it, so managing its attendant systemic risks is particularly poignant.[13]

Retinal Vein Occlusion

Although less severe in both the visual outcomes and systemic risks than the previous two conditions, RVO is still a vision threatening disease that often has an emergent presentation. Any patient under 50 years of age or with accompanying respiratory symptoms should receive particular attention for more esoteric etiologies (tuberculosis, sarcoidosis, thrombotic disease) and receive a broader workup (eg, chest X-ray) when appropriate.[13] In addition, a unique distinction between RAO and RVO is the potential presence of macular edema in the latter, which manifests as less severe central vision loss. Ophthalmology will treat this with intravitreal injections in the outpatient setting. In general, management in the ED involves blood pressure control and referral to ophthalmology.

Hypertensive Retinopathy

The prognosis of chronic hypertensive retinopathy rarely causes significant vision loss, and the retinal changes themselves can be halted or even reversed with treatment of the underlying hypertension. Although management of acute hypertensive emergencies is not within the scope of this book, it is important to note that visual changes may be a relevant symptom resulting from malignant or poorly controlled hypertension.

TIPS AND PEARLS

- In patients over the age of 50, consider GCA as a cause of RAO or TMVL.
- RAO should be considered as a stroke of the retina and evaluated in a similar fashion.
- Patients with acute retinal ischemia may have silent cortical infarcts present at the time of their retinal ischemia.
- Patients with hypertensive retinopathy have progressive, and usually bilateral, visual changes.

EVIDENCE

What is the effectiveness of IA thrombolysis for RAO?

There are many trials that suggest that there may be some benefit to vision recovery with the administration of IA thrombolysis. A systematic review in 2008 evaluated 8 studies for patients with IA thrombolysis and found visual improvement in 93% of patients.[14] Approximately 4.5% of patients experienced complications. The systematic review included mostly retrospective studies. One prospective study of 84 patients with RAO randomized to conservative treatment of IA thrombolytics found no difference in outcomes, calling its efficacy into question.[15] A recent case series of 15 patients with CRAO with a mean time to treatment of 8.83 hours did demonstrate a statistically significant improvement in visual outcome without adverse events.[11] The literature lacks many prospective, randomized controlled trials, limiting the adoption of this intervention for this condition.

References

1. Schneider M, Molnar A, Angeli O, et al. Prevalence of cilioretinal arteries: a systematic review and a prospective cross-sectional observational study. *Acta Ophthalmol*. 2021;99(3):e310-e318.
2. Dattilo M, Newman NJ, Biousse V. Acute retinal arterial ischemia. *Ann Eye Sci*. 2018;3.
3. Jeeva-Patel T, Kabanovski A, Margolin E. Transient monocular visual loss: when is it an emergency? *J Emerg Med*. 2021;60(2):192-196.

4. Frohman L, Wong AB, Matheos K, Leon-Alvarado LG, Danesh-Meyer HV. New developments in giant cell arteritis. *Surv Ophthalmol*. 2016;61(4):400-421.
5. Vortmann M, Schneider JI. Acute monocular visual loss. *Emerg Med Clin North Am*. 2008;26(1):73-96, vi.
6. Erden S, Bicakci E. Hypertensive retinopathy: incidence, risk factors, and comorbidities. *Clin Exp Hypertens*. 2012;34(6):397-401.
7. Hayreh SS. Ocular vascular occlusive disorders: natural history of visual outcome. *Prog Retin Eye Res*. 2014;41:1-25.
8. Henderson AD, Bruce BB, Newman NJ, Biousse V. Hypertension-related eye abnormalities and the risk of stroke. *Rev Neurol Dis*. 2011;8(1-2):1-9.
9. Biousse V, Nahab F, Newman NJ. Management of acute retinal ischemia: follow the guidelines! *Ophthalmology*. 2018;125(10):1597-1607.
10. Park SJ, Choi NK, Yang BR, et al. Risk and risk periods for stroke and acute myocardial infarction in patients with central retinal artery occlusion. *Ophthalmology*. 2015;122(11):2336-2343.e2.
11. Sobol EK, Sakai Y, Wheelwright D, et al. Intra-arterial tissue plasminogen activator for central retinal artery occlusion. *Clin Ophthalmol*. 2021;15:601-608.
12. Mac Grory B, Schrag M, Biousse V, et al. AHA Scientific Statement. Management of central retinal artery occlusion. A scientific statement from the American Heart Association. *Stroke*. 2021;52:e282-e294.
13. Hayreh SS, Zimmerman MB. Fundus changes in central retinal artery occlusion. *Retina*. 2007;27(3):276-289.
14. Noble J, Weizblit N, Baerlocher MO, Eng KT. Intra-arterial thrombolysis for central retinal artery occlusion: a systematic review. *Br J Ophthalmol*. 2008;92(5):588-593.
15. Schumacher M, Schmidt D, Jurklies B, et al. Central retinal artery occlusion: local intra-arterial fibrinolysis versus conservative treatment, a multicenter randomized trial. *Ophthalmology*. 2010;117(7):1367-1375.e1.

CHAPTER 42

Vitreous Detachment, Retinal Tear, and Retinal Detachment

Peter W. Clark

Christopher P. Hogrefe

THE CLINICAL CHALLENGE

The annual incidence of retinal detachment (RD) in the general population is reported to be between 0.8 and 1.8 per 10 000 persons per year for a lifetime prevalence of 1 in 300.[1,2] As such, RD is one of the most common ocular emergencies to present to an emergency department (ED). Prompt recognition and referral can significantly improve a patient's chances of meaningful visual recovery. However, the signs and symptoms of RD often share similarities with posterior vitreous detachment (PVD), which is more common and generally does not cause vision loss. The role of the emergency provider in this setting should be to identify those patients at high risk for current or impending RD in order to determine the urgency of ophthalmology referral.

RDs can be categorized into three distinct categories. Rhegmatogenous retinal detachment (RRD, from the Greek *rhegma,* meaning "break")[3] is the most common type and most likely to present acutely. Other categories include those produced by scar tissue pulling on the retina, known as tractional retinal detachments (TRD), and those produced by breakdown of the blood retina barrier (BRB) and fluid leakage under the retina, known as exudative retinal detachments (ERD). Accurate diagnosis is important because the risk factors, management, and prognosis between these types of RD are distinct.

Pathophysiology

RRDs are caused by tractional forces produced by the vitreous, an encapsulated gel made up of greater than 95% water incorporated into a matrix of collagen and hyaluronic acid.[4] Vitreous degeneration is a consequence of normal aging and results in gradual liquefaction (syneresis) and weakening of its attachments to the retina. Pockets of liquid vitreous form and dissect the adherent vitreous off the retina, producing a PVD (**Figure 42.1**). Optical aberrations caused by these pockets of fluid and separated fibrous adhesions to the retina and optic nerve cause small shadows, commonly described as "floaters."

Retinal breaks and tears (horseshoe tears) result from vitreous traction during the PVD (**Figure 42.2**) and are a required condition for RRD. Liquefied vitreous accesses the subretinal space through the tear, where it accumulates to produce an RD (**Figure 42.3**). It is of no surprise, then, that the age distribution of RRD closely tracks that of PVD, and factors that predispose to PVD also increase the rate of RRD. However, whereas PVD will occur in approximately 86% of the population, retinal tears are present in a very small fraction (7%), and the lifetime risk of RD is only around 0.33%.[1]

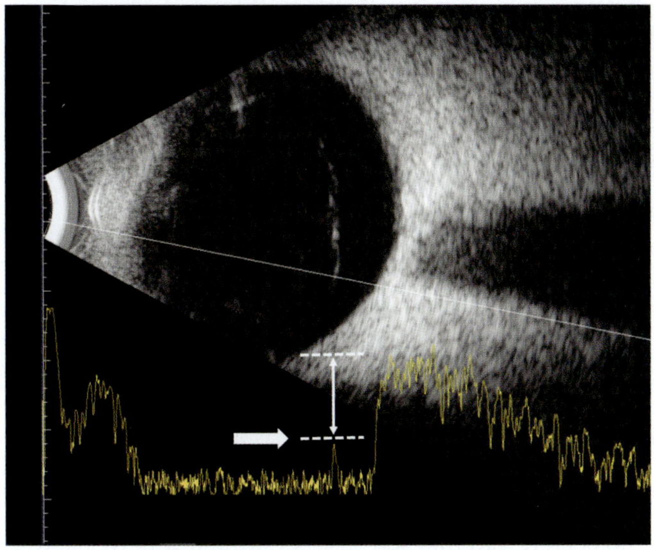

Figure 42.1: Ocular ultrasound (B-scan mode) demonstrating a posterior vitreous detachment. Accurate differentiation of the posterior vitreous (hyaloid) face from the retina is critical. Note the lower spike intensity of posterior vitreous demonstrated with superimposed amplitude scan (A-scan, white arrow). Posterior vitreous typically has a spike ratio of less than 80%, compared with higher density retinal tissue, which is typically 90% to 100% maximal spike height. It is also useful to perform "dynamic ultrasound" and observe the free swirling movements of the vitreous during eye movements as opposed to the "tethered" appearance of a retinal detachment. (Courtesy of Peter W. Clark, MD.)

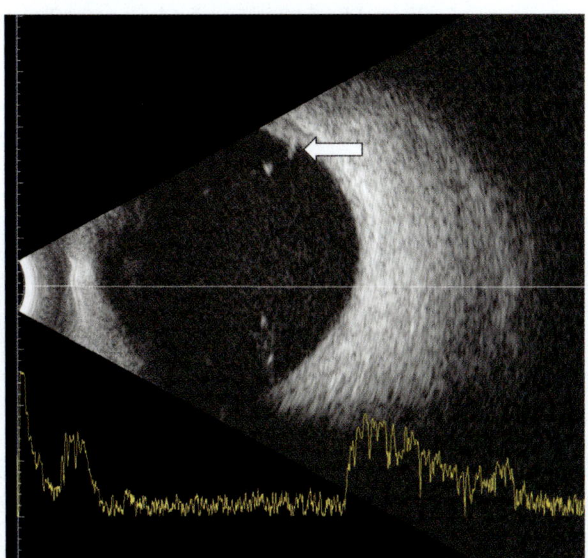

Figure 42.2: Ocular ultrasound image (9 o'clock transverse) demonstrating the presence of a retinal tear without associated detachment (white arrow). There is a small vitreous fiber with traction on the posterior lip of the tear, keeping it open. (Courtesy of Peter W. Clark, MD.)

Known risk factors for the development of RRD include nearsightedness (myopia), a history of prior ocular trauma, a history of cataract or other ocular surgery, previous RD in the contralateral eye, and a positive family history of RD. Myopic patients tend to have a higher rate of peripheral retinal degeneration, including areas of relative weakness that are predisposed to tears. Prior RD in one eye is a strong indicator that abnormal vitreoretinal adhesion and/or peripheral retinal

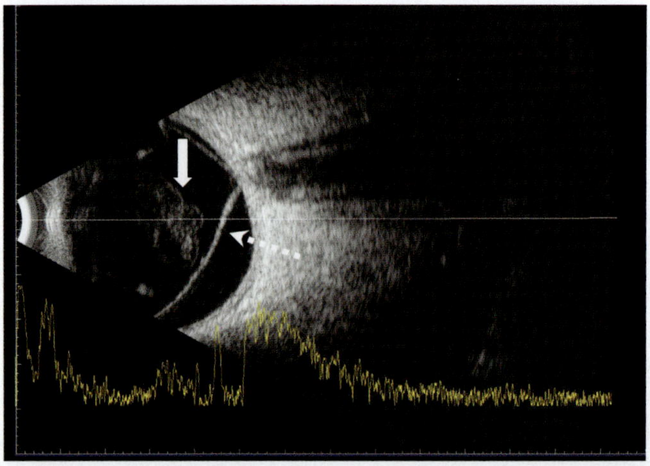

Figure 42.3: Ocular ultrasound image demonstrating a funnel retinal detachment emanating from the optic nerve. Note the central presence of a posterior vitreous detachment with low echogenicity (solid arrow), compared with the high spike associated with retinal tissue (dotted arrow). (Courtesy of Peter W. Clark, MD.)

degeneration is present and substantially increases the risk of RD in the contralateral eye. The rate of contralateral RRD during 5-year follow-up is as high as 23%.[5] Blunt trauma directly to the eye may result in compression and rebound expansion of the globe, causing immense vitreous traction, precipitating large retinal tears, particularly in younger patients with formed and adherent vitreous gel. Routine cataract surgery increases the risk of RRD by 6 to 8 times in the 6 years following surgery.[2] Cataract surgery complicated by posterior capsular rupture and vitreous loss carries a substantially higher rate of subsequent RRD.

In contrast to RRD, a TRD involves the proliferation of contractile membranes along the surface of the retina. They are generally secondary to chronic conditions such as proliferative diabetic retinopathy, recurrent RD, and posterior uveitis. These detachments are typically shallow and immobile (**Figure 42.4**) and are often characterized by gradual vision loss.

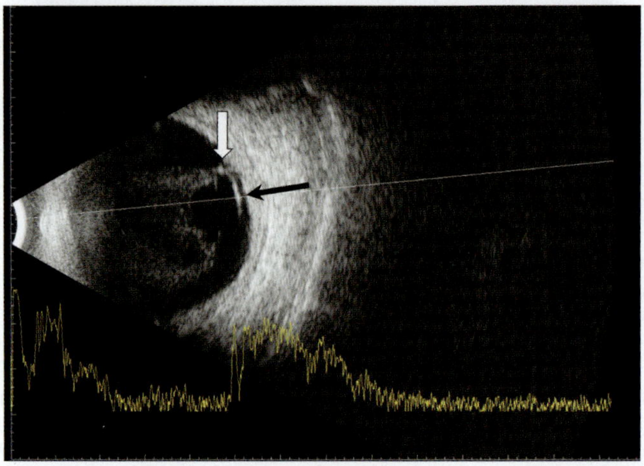

Figure 42.4: Ocular ultrasound image (3 o'clock transverse) demonstrating a small focal tractional retinal detachment in the setting of vitreous hemorrhage and proliferative diabetic retinopathy. Note the strong adherence of the vitreous to the retina (white arrow), creating a shallow elevation of the retina in the form of a tractional retinal detachment (black arrow). The hyperechoic medium in the center is diffuse blood mixed with vitreous. Also note the high spike associated with the retinal tissue. (Courtesy of Peter W. Clark, MD.)

ERDs occur from accumulation of subretinal fluid owing to breakdown of the BRB secondary to a variety of underlying causes, including malignant hypertension, preeclampsia/eclampsia, and a number of other vascular, inflammatory, infectious, and neoplastic conditions. A systemic workup is critical in these cases because visual symptoms often completely resolve with treatment of the underlying condition.

APPROACH/THE FOCUSED EXAM

The presentation of acute-onset new floaters (eg, black spots, strings, or cobwebs) or flashes (photopsias) in a single eye in the appropriate age group (ie, 50 or older) is highly likely to be secondary to acute PVD. Most (86%) of these patients will not have concomitant retinal tears or detachment.[1] However, the presence of symptomatic PVD accompanied by loss of central or peripheral vision (eg, a dark shadow or curtain) is highly correlated with the presence of RD.

The patient's best corrected vision should be assessed using their standard spectacle correction with and without pinhole occlusion to neutralize any residual refractive error. The intraocular pressure should be measured in both eyes. Asymmetrically low intraocular pressure readings in the single digits may be suggestive of RD because the aqueous outflow can be increased in the setting of RD. The visual fields should be mapped using confrontation. The location of the RD will be opposite of the visual field defect owing to the optical inversion of visual information entering the eye. A substantial RD may produce a positive afferent pupillary defect (APD) on swinging flashlight test.

A comparison of the pupillary red reflexes using the direct ophthalmoscope may alert the examiner to the presence of retinal pathology such as vitreous hemorrhage (VH), RD, or an opacity such as a cataract. An RD may show a lighter reflex owing to hydration of the retina. A media opacity may show a darker, less radiant reflex. Hemorrhage may give a rust or yellow reflex, whereas a cataract may cause a green-yellow or brown reflex.

Slit-lamp examination can reveal other signs of RD. "Shafer sign" is the clinical sign most highly correlated with the probability of a retinal tear or detachment and is defined as the presence of reddish pigment or red blood cells suspended in the anterior vitreous (so-called tobacco dust). This finding on slit-lamp examination (**Figure 42.5**) increases the probability of a retinal tear or detachment from a baseline rate of 14% up to 88%.[1] Although often difficult to visualize through an undilated pupil, it is extremely useful to document the absence or presence of Shafer sign when assessing a patient for possible retinal pathology on slit-lamp examination.

Imaging can be invaluable for evaluating an RD. Point-of-care ultrasound (POCUS) of the eye can identify and distinguish between a PVD (Figure 42.1), VH (Figure 42.4), and an RD (Figure 42.3). In some cases, retinal tears can also be identified (Figure 42.2). Chapter 26 discusses

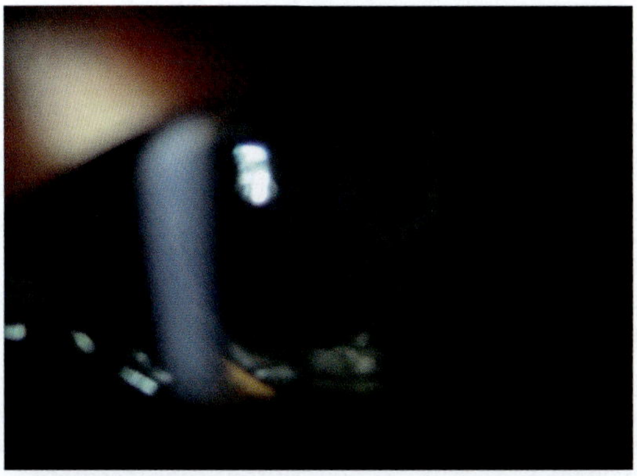

Figure 42.5: Slit-lamp photographs demonstrating "Shafer sign," the accumulation of reddish-brown pigmented cells in the anterior vitreous (behind the lens) also known as "tobacco dust." The presence of this sign significantly increases the probability of retinal tear or detachment. (Courtesy of Peter W. Clark, MD.)

the specifics of ocular POCUS. Fundus photography may become an alternative to dilated examination as the presence of nonmydriatic cameras becomes more common in EDs.

DIFFERENTIAL DIAGNOSIS

The differential diagnosis of PVD and RD includes other causes of flashes and floaters. The most common cause of visual flashes aside from acute PVD is the visual aura associated with migraines. These visual phenomena are produced by spreading depolarization of the visual cortex and are characterized by a colorful zigzagging pattern of light and visual distortion affecting one or both eyes simultaneously and lasting between 5 and 30 minutes, often terminating with a headache. Visual aura may also be present *without* a headache, the so-called *acephalgic* ocular migraine. The duration of symptoms helps distinguish an aura from a retinal tear. Whereas an aura lasts several minutes, flashes from vitreous traction are very quick, like electric sparks or shooting stars.

In rare cases, occipital lobe ischemia/infarction, transient ischemic attack (TIA), amaurosis fugax, or postural hypotension may present with limited episodes of visual photopsias or a curtain-like scotoma. These photopsias are of longer duration than typical flashes but shorter compared with migraine. Vision loss from an RD is not transient, distinguishing it from a vascular episode. If a cerebral or retinal infarction is suspected, a thorough neurologic examination should be performed to assess for a stroke.

An abrupt-onset burst of floaters, strings, or cobwebs in a patient with a history of uncontrolled diabetes is highly suspicious for VH secondary to proliferative diabetic retinopathy (PDR). The evaluation of these patients is often limited owing to the presence of fundus-obscuring VH and requires POCUS. In patients with advanced PDR, ocular ultrasound may demonstrate an underlying TRD (Figure 42.4).

MANAGEMENT

A suggested approach for patients with RRD proposed by Hollands et al. is a referral based on the presence of specific risk factors (**Table 42.1**). Any patient with acute progressive peripheral and/or central vision loss, a visual field defect by confrontation, or Shafer sign on slit-lamp examination

TABLE 42.1 Management of Patients With Presumed Posterior Vitreous Detachment (PVD)

Clinical Presentation	Referral Recommendation
Floaters/flashes with monocular visual field loss and/or "dark shadow"	Emergent referral to a retinal surgeon (owing to the high risk of retinal detachment)
New-onset floaters/flashes with subjective/objective visual reduction or vitreous hemorrhage/vitreous pigment on slit-lamp examination	Emergent referral to an ophthalmologist for a dilated eye examination
New-onset floaters/flashes without other symptoms	Dilated eye examination by an ophthalmologist within 2 weeks; counseling regarding high-risk features warranting urgent reassessment
Uncomplicated posterior vitreous detachment with new floaters/flashes and/or new subjective visual reduction	Ophthalmology referral to rule out a new retinal tear or detachment
Stable symptoms of floaters/flashes for weeks to months; minimally symptomatic without other features (eg, visual loss)	Outpatient referral to ophthalmology; counseling regarding high-risk features warranting urgent reassessment

Adapted from Hollands H, Johnson D, Brox AC, et al. Acute-onset floaters and flashes: is this patient at risk for retinal detachment? *JAMA*. 2009;302(20):2243-2249.

warrants same-day referral to an ophthalmologist. In many cases, direct referral to a retina specialist who can perform the repair may prevent progressive vision loss.

In patients with new-onset flashes or floaters *without* significant visual decrease, visual field defects, or Shafer sign, referral to ophthalmology may be made on a nonurgent basis within 1 to 2 weeks for a dilated examination. However, these patients must be counseled to see an ophthalmologist or ED physician immediately if they develop red flag signs, including an abrupt increase in flashes of light, burst of new floaters, acute visual loss, or development of a new dark shadow. Should a patient return to the ED with new symptoms following a previous diagnosis of uncomplicated PVD, an ophthalmologist should be consulted emergently. In patients with a history of floaters and flashes for several weeks and the absence of high-risk features, a nonurgent referral (within 1 week) to ophthalmology is appropriate. Stable floaters are very common in the elderly population owing to the presence of a preexisting PVD and are often monitored annually.

In terms of surgical management, the goal of the RD repair is reapposition of the sensory retina onto the underlying retinal pigment epithelium (RPE), followed by barricade of the causative retinal breaks to prevent redetachment either with thermal laser or freezing therapy (cryotherapy). These techniques create adhesive scars between the retina and the choroid of sufficient strength to block the continued passage of fluid from the intravitreal space into the subretinal space.

TIPS AND PEARLS

- RD is often associated with acute PVD and shares many symptoms, including new-onset flashes and floaters.
- High-risk signs and symptoms that require emergent referral to ophthalmology include significant vision loss, the subjective experience of a "dark shadow," a unilateral visual field defect, unexplained VH in a patient without risk factors, and the presence of Shafer sign on slit-lamp evaluation.
- Confrontation visual field testing is a quick and easy method to map out the area of detachment and assist in differentiating a bilateral defect consistent with a central nervous system process from a unilateral defect more suggestive of an ocular cause.
- POCUS provides a reliable method to accurately differentiate PVD, VH, and RD.

EVIDENCE

What is the sensitivity/specificity of POCUS for detecting PVD, RD, RT in the ED?

The development of POCUS has greatly enhanced the sensitivity of diagnosing PVD, retinal tear, and detachment in the ED. Multiple studies have validated the ability of emergency medicine physicians to accurately detect RDs using POCUS. In one large-scale multicenter study, emergency medicine physicians of varying experience with ocular ultrasound were able to diagnose retinal pathology with a sensitivity of 96.9% for RD, 81.9% for VH, and 42.5% for vitreous detachment and specificities of 88.1%, 82.3%, and 96.0%, respectively.[6] The use of ocular ultrasound is contraindicated in cases of trauma in which open globe injury is suspected, as any pressure applied to the globe may worsen injury.

What is the recommended timeline for treatment of RD?

The primary factor dictating the urgency of repair is the status of the macula. Cases presenting with the macula attached (macula-on) typically present with good central vision and are considered higher urgency. Macula-on detachments should be addressed as soon as possible and repaired in 1 to 2 days. If the patient cannot be sent directly to an outpatient clinic, then evaluation by an ophthalmologist in the ED is appropriate. Until the patient can be seen by a retina surgeon, minimizing ocular movement prevents progression of the detachment (eg, bilateral eye patching, although this may not be tolerated for extended periods of time).

Once the detachment progresses into the macula, the probability of visual recovery may decrease significantly. The percentage of patients with macula-on detachment achieving postoperative visual acuity (VA) of 20/40 or better was 80%, compared with 30% of those presenting with macula-off detachment.[7,8]

Even for macula-off RDs, recent large-scale observational analyses have suggested improved visual outcomes when repaired within 1 to 3 days of symptom onset, compared with 4 to 6 days.[9,10] However, these findings are not universally accepted. Thus, the consensus recommendation remains to repair macula-off detachments within 7 days from the time of central vision loss.[7,11] Therefore, any patient with a suspected or confirmed detachment should be evaluated by a retina specialist within 24 hours so that appropriate surgical management can be arranged.

References

1. Hollands H, Johnson D, Brox AC, et al. Acute-onset floaters and flashes: is this patient at risk for retinal detachment? *JAMA*. 2009;302(20):2243-2249.
2. Mitry D, Charteris DG, Fleck BW, et al. The epidemiology of rhegmatogenous retinal detachment: geographical variation and clinical associations. *Br J Ophthalmol*. 2010;94(6):678-684.
3. Blindbaek S, Grauslund J. Reply: Prophylactic treatment of retinal breaks—a systematic review. *Acta Ophthalmol*. 2016;94(1):e77-e78.
4. de Smet M, Elkareem A, Zwinderman, A. The vitreous, the retinal interface in ocular health and disease. *Ophthalmologica*. 2013;230(4):165-178.
5. Gonzales CR, Gupta A, Schwartz SD, et al. The fellow eye of patients with rhegmatogenous retinal detachment. *Ophthalmology*. 2004;111(3):518-521.
6. Lahham S, Shniter I, Thompson M, et al. Point-of-Care ultrasonography in the diagnosis of retinal detachment, vitreous hemorrhage, and vitreous detachment in the emergency department. *JAMA Netw Open*. 2019;2(4):e192162.
7. Wykoff CC, Flynn HW, Scott IU. What is the optimal timing for rhegmatogenous retinal detachment repair. *JAMA Ophthalmol*. 2013;131(11):1399-1400.
8. Salicone A, Smiddy WE, Venkatraman A, et al. Visual recovery after scleral buckling procedure for retinal detachment. *Ophthalmology*. 2006;113(10):1734-1742.
9. Yorston D, Donachie PHJ, Laidlaw DA, et al. Factors affecting visual recovery after successful repair of macula-off retinal detachments: findings from a large prospective UK cohort study. *Eye (Lond)*. 2021;35(5):1431-1439.
10. van Bussel EM, van der Valk R, Bijlsma WR, et al. Impact of duration of macula-off retinal detachment on visual outcome: a systematic review and meta-analysis of literature. *Retina*. 2014;34(10):1917-1925.
11. Hassan TS, Sarrafizadeh R, Ruby AJ, et al. The effect of duration of macular detachment on results after the scleral buckle repair of primary, macula-off retinal detachments. *Ophthalmology*. 2002;109(1):146-152.

CHAPTER 43

Infectious and Inflammatory Retinal Diseases

Brittany E. Powell
Victoria M. Hammond

THE CLINICAL CHALLENGE

Infectious and inflammatory retinal diseases are typically progressive and have significant ocular morbidity. Early and accurate diagnosis is critical to initiating immediate therapy and hinges on a high index of suspicion. The clinical challenge for the retinal pathology described in what follows is that the described disease entities are rare and might be encountered only occasionally during the career of any physician. However, a high index of suspicion with initiation of treatment and engagement with an ophthalmologist will result in dramatically improved outcomes.

PATHOPHYSIOLOGY

Infectious Retinal Inflammatory Syndromes

Exogenous Endophthalmitis

Endophthalmitis is an infection inside the eye. It most commonly occurs following surgery. Cataract surgery is the most frequent etiology, but it can also occur following glaucoma surgery, intravitreal injections, or rarely retina surgery. The incidence of endophthalmitis following cataract surgery has been reported to be from 0.012% to 1.3%.[1] By definition, it occurs within 6 weeks of anterior segment surgery, but usually it presents within the first week after surgery. The most common organisms are coagulase-negative *Staphylococcus* species, *Streptococcus* species, and gram-negative organisms, specifically *Pseudomonas* species.[1]

Posttraumatic endophthalmitis is associated with an open globe injury and has been reported to have an incidence as high as 15% to 30%.[2,3] The clinical presentation is variable and can be both rapidly progressive, as in posttraumatic *Bacillus* endophthalmitis, or more indolent, as in posttraumatic fungal endophthalmitis. In contrast to endophthalmitis following surgery, *Streptococcus pneumoniae* and gram-negative bacilli are much more prominent in these cases, although *Staphylococcal* infections also occur.[3] *Bacillus cereus* needs to be assumed in those cases with a soil-contaminated intraocular foreign body. The prognosis of posttraumatic endophthalmitis is much worse and can result in loss of the eye within hours after the injury.

Endogenous Endophthalmitis

Endogenous endophthalmitis via hematogenous spread of infectious organisms is rare, with an incidence of 0.04% to 0.4% but requires an extensive systemic workup and rapid treatment.[4] Endogenous endophthalmitis has been associated with intravenous drug use, endocarditis, diabetes mellitus, immune compromise, malignancy, prolonged hospital admission, and intravenous antibiotic administration.[5] Worldwide, common causes included liver abscesses, closely followed by pneumonia, endocarditis, sustained intravenous catheters, and meningitis. In cases of suspected endophthalmitis, while actively addressing the infection of the eye, it is important to simultaneously investigate for the underlying source of hematogenous spread.

Other Infectious Retinal Inflammatory Syndromes

Patients with retinal inflammatory syndromes from infection are typically immunocompromised and present with gradually decreasing vision and floaters. These infectious triggers lead to a severe immune-mediated inflammatory cascade on the retina and an obliterative vasculitis. Infections are most commonly caused by members of the herpes virus family (varicella zoster, herpes simplex viruses, cytomegalovirus, and Epstein-Barr virus). Other pathogens can result in retinal inflammation and should be considered in patients with known disease and eye symptoms, including syphilis, tuberculosis, toxoplasmosis, toxocariasis, Lyme disease, and West Nile virus. Viral meningoencephalitis has also been reported in association with viral necrotizing retinitis.

Noninfectious Retinal Inflammatory Syndromes

There are a variety of systemic inflammatory disorders that can affect the retina, including systemic lupus erythematosus-associated vasculitis, multiple sclerosis with pars planitis, sarcoidosis, and Bechet disease. The presence of a hypopyon in a patient who has not had intraocular surgery and no evidence infectious etiologies such a corneal ulcer has been reported in patients with Bechet disease and HLA-B27-associated acute anterior uveitis. Referral to an ophthalmologist should be considered if patients with known inflammatory disease are experiencing visual symptoms.

APPROACH/THE FOCUSED EXAM

The most important part of the exam is the medical history and timeline of symptoms in order to develop an adequate differential diagnosis. Endophthalmitis is rare but must be suspected in patients experiencing vision loss, pain, and photophobia following intraocular surgery or trauma. Endogenous endophthalmitis must be considered in those who are systemically ill or immunocompromised with gradual deterioration of vision or worsening of visual symptoms. Inflammatory retinal diseases typically present with gradually worsening photophobia, photopsias, floaters, and decreased vision. In contrast to iritis, vision loss is usually severe. Consideration for an undiagnosed systemic inflammatory condition in these patients is critical.

The history should include recent trauma, recent intraocular surgery, current medications, and the potential for immune suppression caused by underlying diseases or medication use. Is the patient experiencing vision loss, pain, eye discharge, redness, flashes, or floaters? When did the symptoms start? Have the symptoms progressed over hours, days, or weeks? Patients who have had glaucoma surgery are at risk for endophthalmitis even months or years after surgery, owing to the presence of a drainage bleb or implant. After cataract surgery or intraocular injection, the risk of endophthalmitis is significant only in the acute postoperative period.

The examination should consist of vital signs, visual acuity, intraocular pressure, and an external exam of the eyelids to assess for swelling, redness, and discharge. A slit lamp exam can assess for a red reflex, conjunctival injection, evidence of an open globe such as a corneal laceration, or a hypopyon (**Figures 43.1** and **43.2**). An ophthalmic ultrasound can also be helpful in showing vitritis but is not mandatory.

Any patient who presents with a hypopyon and concerning risk factors should be evaluated by ophthalmology for definitive diagnosis the same day. Endophthalmitis is the most likely diagnosis in a patient presenting within 6 weeks postoperative from ocular surgery or with any history of penetrating eye injury or prior glaucoma drainage surgery. However, other conditions that may present with the most common clinical findings of endophthalmitis can be considered and discussed with ophthalmology consultation. Hypopyon is present in up to 85% of patients with endophthalmitis but may also be present in conjunction with corneal ulcer or ulcerative keratitis.[6] Fluorescein testing of the cornea can be performed to evaluate for possible corneal ulcer, which would also require evaluation and treatment by ophthalmology. Other conditions that may present similarly to endophthalmitis include postoperative inflammation, vitreous hemorrhage, and iritis or uveitis, but these should be considered after evaluation for endophthalmitis is complete.

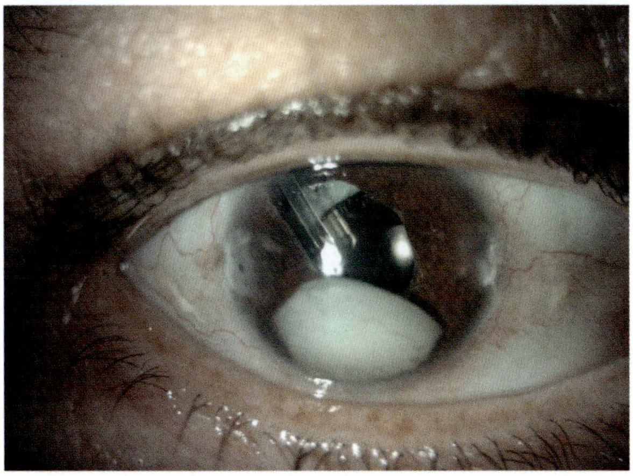

Figure 43.1: Photograph of right eye demonstrating hypopyon in a patient with a glaucoma drainage device.

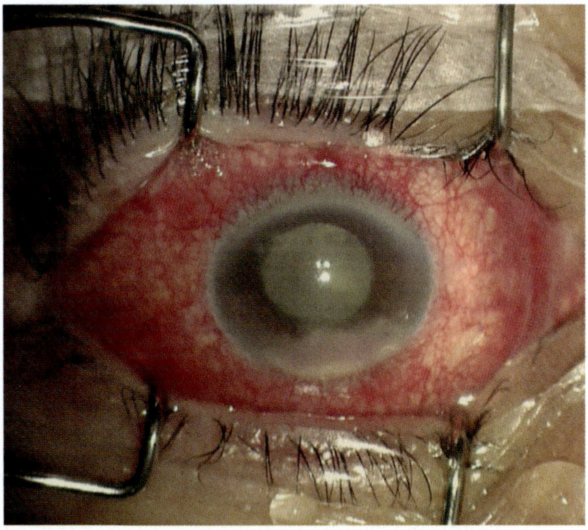

Figure 43.2: Photograph of right eye demonstrating hypopyon in a patient with endophthalmitis after cataract surgery.

MANAGEMENT

Management of endophthalmitis includes initiation of intravenous antibiotics (fluoroquinolones have better vitreous penetration and are recommended) and emergent ophthalmology evaluation for vitreous sampling, intravitreal antibiotics, and evaluation for surgical intervention (**Figure 43.3**). Although the standard of care is to treat with intravitreal and intravenous antibiotics, oftentimes topical and subconjunctival antibiotics are used to increase antibiotic concentration in the eye. In cases of posttraumatic endophthalmitis, orbital imaging with a computed tomography (CT) scan, initiation of intravenous antibiotics, and emergent referral to an ophthalmologist for vitreous sampling, intravitreal antibiotics, and evaluation for surgical intervention are indicated.

For patients with infectious retinal inflammatory syndromes and viral-associated retinal necrosis, early administration of antiviral medication is the cornerstone of the treatment. Given that this condition is seen primarily in immunocompromised patients, if this is not already documented, providers should evaluate for etiologies such as HIV.

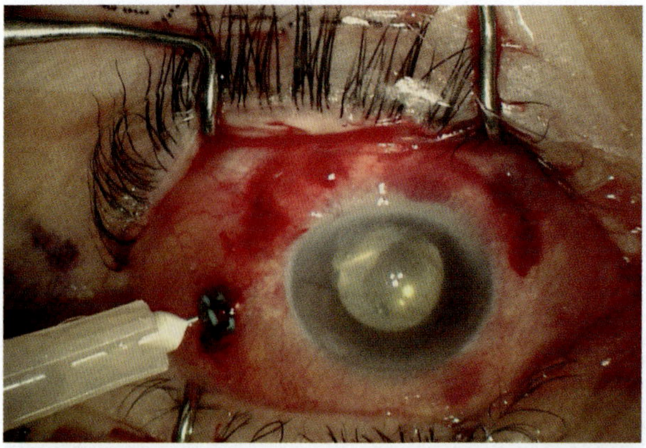

Figure 43.3: Photograph of right eye demonstrating intraocular injection of antibiotic in treatment of endophthalmitis.

DIFFERENTIAL DIAGNOSIS

	History	Presentation
Traumatic Endophthalmitis Endogenous Endophthalmitis Postsurgical Endophthalmitis	Does the patient have a history of immunosuppression, recent trauma, recent intraocular surgery, history of intravenous drug use?	Decreased vision, anterior chamber cell, hypopyon, pain, conjunctival injection, evidence of trauma/open globe, vitritis.
Infectious Uveitis	Does the patient have a history of immunosuppression, systemic evidence of infectious disease?	Decreased vision, anterior chamber cell, photophobia, conjunctival injection, vitritis.
Noninfectious/Inflammatory Uveitis	How long has the patient had symptoms; flashes, floaters, photophobia?	Decreased vision, anterior chamber cell, photophobia, conjunctival injection, vitritis.
Sympathetic Ophthalmia	Does the patient have a history of remote penetrating or perforating trauma in the fellow eye?	Decreased vision, bilateral eye pain, photophobia, evidence of anterior and/or posterior inflammation in uninvolved eye after ocular trauma.

PEDIATRIC ISSUES

Neonatal endogenous endophthalmitis is extremely rare (4.42 cases per 100 000 live births in the United States) but can occur in newborns as a complication of sepsis. Risk factors for neonatal endogenous endophthalmitis include candidemia, bacteremia, retinopathy of prematurity and low birth weight.[7] In case reports of neonatal endophthalmitis, the condition occurred as a result of sepsis and was not the presenting condition. This is different than adult patients in which endophthalmitis may be the presenting sign of underlying bacteremia. Therefore, it is unlikely to see a neonate present to the emergency department (ED) with endogenous endophthalmitis as the presenting complaint; however, this condition stresses the importance of ocular exams in clinical care of a septic neonate.[8]

Special consideration must also be mentioned for patients with a known diagnosis of juvenile idiopathic arthritis (JIA) because they are most likely to develop uveitis as an extra-articular manifestation of their condition. Although anterior uveitis is most common, panuveitis and posterior uveitis have been documented in up to 8% of patients with JIA. The symptoms of arthritis have been found to precede the development of uveitis in up to 90% of patients. Because of the high association of uveitis with JIA and the associated complications of ocular disease, regular screening eye exams have been suggested for patients diagnosed with JIA. It is important to consider retinitis in any patient who meets criteria for, or has a known diagnosis of, JIA.[9]

TIPS AND PEARLS

- The diagnosis of endophthalmitis is typically made clinically, and treatment is initiated empirically. An ophthalmologist will subsequently confirm the diagnosis with vitrectomy or vitreous aspiration.[10]
- Postcataract surgery is the most common cause of endophthalmitis and typically occurs within 6 weeks, with up to 75% occurring within the first 7 days.[11]
- Up to 85% of patients with endophthalmitis present with clinical hypopyon of the affected eye; thus, this clinical finding should increase suspicion and prompt consultation by ophthalmology.[6]
- The highest predictor of overall prognosis and visual recovery is the visual acuity at presentation. Visual acuity is necessary to determine the treatment plan and should be performed prior to consultation with ophthalmology.[6]
- Studies have shown only 10% of penetrating ocular injuries are complicated by endophthalmitis, but the risk is increased if there is a retained foreign body in the eye.[2]
- Studies have shown that only 50% of patients with endogenous endophthalmitis have systemic symptoms on presentation, with most common influential risk factors including diabetes, intravenous drug use, and HIV/AIDS.[5]
- 14 to 25% of endogenous endophthalmitis cases are bilateral, whereas only the affected injured/postoperative eye is involved in exogenous causes.[12]

EVIDENCE

Is it necessary to administer both intravitreal and systemic antibiotics for treatment of exogenous endophthalmitis?

Most of the data used to guide therapy in postoperative endophthalmitis are obtained from the Endophthalmitis Vitrectomy Study (EVS).[6] This study found that the addition of intravenous drug therapy to intravitreal drug therapy was not beneficial to treatment outcomes in postoperative endophthalmitis. However, these data cannot be extrapolated to posttraumatic endophthalmitis because the makeup of infectious etiology is vastly different in traumatic endophthalmitis, where it is standard of care to treat with both systemic and intravitreal antibiotics in order to provide coverage for both gram-positive and gram-negative organisms. Additional studies have proven benefit with the combination of therapy, and the standard of care in posttraumatic endophthalmitis is to administer broad spectrum antibiotics, specifically, vancomycin and ceftazidime, both systemically and intraocularly.[8]

Are systemic antibiotics or antifungals alone, without intravitreal therapy, sufficient to treat endogenous endophthalmitis?

Systemic antibiotics/antifungals are used to treat the underlying source of bacteremia/fungemia that embolized to ocular infection. If the ocular lesion has extended to involve the vitreous, then intravitreal antibiotic or antifungal therapy should be added to systemic therapy so as to allow rapid delivery of high drug concentrations because the intravitreal route bypasses the blood-retinal barrier. Often, the underlying source of infection is suspected during culture sampling of the vitreous and aqueous humor, and, therefore, empiric drug therapy is administered simultaneously during diagnostic vitrectomy or aspiration.[13]

References

1. Cao H, Zhang L, Li L, Lo S. Risk factors for acute endophthalmitis following cataract surgery: a systematic review and meta-analysis. *PloS One.* 2013;8:e7173.
2. Banker, TP, McClellan AJ, Wilson BD, et al. Culture-positive endophthalmitis after open globe injuries with and without retained intraocular foreign bodies. *Ophthalmic Surg. Lasers Imaging Retina.* 2017;48:632-637.
3. Gokce, G, Sobaci, G, Ozgonul, C. Post-traumatic endophthalmitis: a mini-review. *Semin Ophthalmol.* 2015;30:470-474.
4. Relhan N, Forster RK, Flynn HW. Endophthalmitis: then and now. *Am J Ophthalmol.* 2018;187:xx-xxvii.
5. Jackson TL, Paraskevopoulos T, Georgalas I. Systematic review of 342 cases of endogenous bacterial endophthalmitis. *Surv Ophthalmol.* 2014;59:627-635.
6. Results of the endophthalmitis vitrectomy study: a randomized trial of immediate vitrectomy and of intravenous antibiotics for the treatment of postoperative bacterial endophthalmitis. *Arch Ophthalmol.* 1995;113:1479-1496.
7. Moshfeghi AA, Charalel RA, Hernandez-Boussard T, Morton JM, Moshfeghi DM. Declining incidence of neonatal endophthalmitis in the United States. *Am J Ophthalmol.* 2011;151:59-65.e1.
8. Basu S, Kumar A, Kapoor K, Bagri NK, Chandra, A. Neonatal endogenous endophthalmitis: a report of six cases. *Pediatrics.* 2013;131:e1292-e1297.
9. Hawkins MJ, Dick AD, Lee RJW, et al. Managing juvenile idiopathic arthritis–associated uveitis. *Surv Ophthalmol.* 2016;61:197-210.
10. Bhagat N, Nagori S, Zarbin M. Post-traumatic infectious endophthalmitis. *Surv Ophthalmol.* 2011;56:214-251.
11. Lundström, M, Friling, E, Montan P. Risk factors for endophthalmitis after cataract surgery: predictors for causative organisms and visual outcomes. *J Cataract Refract Surg.* 2015;41:2410-2416.
12. Jackson TL, Eykyn SJ, Graham EM, Stanford MR. Endogenous bacterial endophthalmitis: a 17-year prospective series and review of 267 reported cases. *Surv Ophthalmol.* 2003;48:403-423.
13. Durand ML. Bacterial and fungal endophthalmitis. *Clin Microbiol Rev.* 2017;30:597-613.

CHAPTER 44

Nonaccidental Trauma

Kirsten Bechtel
Robin N. Ginsburg

THE CLINICAL CHALLENGE

Child abuse is a pervasive problem in the United States of America (USA), with rates of maltreatment up to 8.9/1000 children. Children under 12 months old have the highest rates of victimization (25.7/1000) and are most vulnerable to dying from maltreatment (22.9/100 000).[1] Abusive head trauma (AHT) is a catastrophic form of child abuse that includes cranial, ocular, and spinal injuries from shaking, blunt trauma, or both. Rates of AHT in the USA are thought to be 38.8 cases per 100 000 infants younger than 12 months old.[2]

Epidemiology and Pathogenesis

The histories provided by caregivers of infants with AHT are usually false. One should suspect AHT when there are inconsistencies between the history of the injury mechanism and the injury severity.[3] Additionally, children with persistent neurologic abnormalities, with a history of either no or low-impact trauma, are also more likely to have AHT. Clinical factors differentiating AHT from nonabusive head trauma include a seizure at or within 24 hours of presentation and apnea at presentation.

Infant crying is the most commonly reported trigger for a caregiver to shake an infant.[4] The developmental peak of crying in healthy infants occurs around 2 months of age. The characteristics of crying that may lead a frustrated caregiver to hurt an infant include the infant's unpredictable and inconsolable nature, the perception that it is painful, and prolonged duration.

Subdural hematoma (SDH) is the primary intracranial injury in AHT. The specificity of SDH for AHT is increased when associated with retinal hemorrhages (RHs) and underlying diffuse parenchymal injury.[5]

Ocular and Orbital Injuries Associated With Abuse

Physical child abuse can present with protean manifestations involving any part of the eye caused by either direct or indirect trauma. Ocular injury associated with unexplained neurologic findings or seizures should also prompt concern for abuse. Injuries presenting also include traumatic hyphema or new-onset strabismus from elevated intracranial pressure. RHs noted on routine examination in infants and children should be carefully documented and should raise suspicion of abuse if appropriate. RHs, a cardinal feature of AHT, are seen in over 50% of cases of AHT,5 of which most are bilateral. RHs are seldom seen without apparent ocular injury or evidence of significant head trauma. When assessing infants who are believed to be physically abused but present without neurologic symptoms of AHT, brain imaging should be strongly considered, and ophthalmic consultation is needed only to provide supportive evidence if AHT is suspected.

APPROACH/THE FOCUSED EXAM

It can be quite challenging to distinguish which ocular injury in children may be abusive. Blunt trauma can result in injury to any aspect of the eye or periocular structures. Many of these injuries are nonspecific and can be seen in both nonabusive and abusive head trauma and other systemic diseases. Owing to the transient presence of RHs, ocular evaluation, including indirect ophthalmoscopy, is ideally performed in the first 24 to 72 hours.[3]

The anterior segment can be evaluated with a penlight or slit lamp if necessary. Optic nerve injury can be assessed by examination for an afferent pupillary defect before pharmacologic dilation. Fractures to the orbital or frontal bones can occur but are less common in young children and infants, especially in cases of abuse.

Bilateral periorbital ecchymosis in children can be caused by direct forehead trauma or secondary to basilar skull fracture, blunt thoracic trauma, leukemia, and neuroblastoma. Corneal abrasions, lacerations, and iris damage can occur. Penetrating or blunt trauma can result in globe rupture; the globe should be protected with a shield as soon as its integrity is called into question.[6]

Subconjunctival hemorrhages are quite common in cases of abuse with ocular trauma and can be caused by direct or indirect etiologies (**Figure 44.1**). The extensive list of etiologies presenting with subconjunctival hemorrhages in childhood is well reported.[6] Causes are not specific for abuse and include infectious, hematologic, and neoplastic disease; Valsalva maneuver; increased intrathoracic pressure; vomiting, birth; and nonabusive trauma. In the absence of these etiologies, abusive injury must be considered.

Traumatic hyphema, defined as blood in the anterior chamber, can occur after high-velocity blunt or penetrating trauma .The complications of hyphema can lead to visual impairment and blindness caused by corneal blood staining, elevated intraocular pressure (IOP), optic atrophy, and glaucoma, making diagnosis and treatment essential for preserving vision. Nontraumatic hyphemas have been reported in retinoblastoma (masquerade syndrome), juvenile xanthogranuloma, and inflammatory conditions, including keratouveitis, leukemia, and hemophilia. Traumatic cataracts may be noted at the time of presentation or may occur later, necessitating a careful history of trauma if noted on routine examination.

Vitreoretinal Findings in AHT

Other than birth trauma, AHT is the leading cause of RH in infancy. Concomitant findings help distinguish RHs associated with AHT from other causes and should be well documented by detailed descriptions, drawings, and photo documentation when possible. Despite several attempts to provide a grading tool for RHs associated with AHT, no standard nomenclature has been accepted, highlighting the need for detailed documentation.[7] It is imperative to note that documentation should include the level of concern for suspected AHT, differential diagnosis, and suggestions for additional medical and ophthalmologic evaluation.

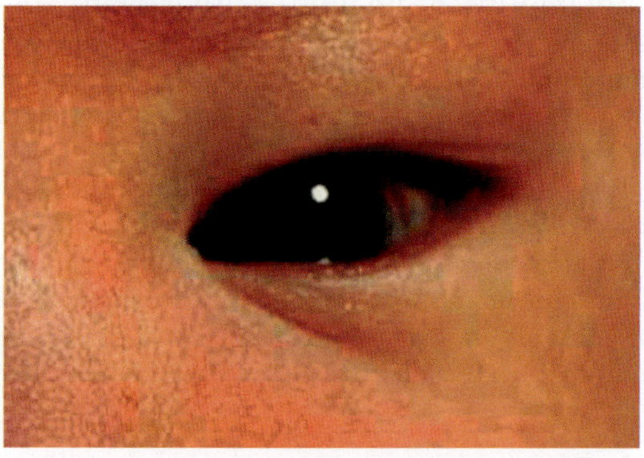

Figure 44.1: Subconjunctival hemorrhage in an infant. (Courtesy of Edna Asumang: Sub-conjunctival Haemorrhage Guidelines in Newborn Infants; Sheffield Children's NHS.)

It is essential that the ophthalmologist document the variability of RHs because this can be of significance in determining their etiology. RHs can vary in terms of size, shape, location, and number and be unilateral or bilateral.[5] The distribution of the hemorrhages in the posterior pole, periphery, or peripapillary area is vital, and the location or layer of the hemorrhages as subretinal, intraretinal, or preretinal or extending into the vitreous must also be documented, because such locations can help distinguish abusive from nonabusive injury. Particular attention should be paid to RHs too numerous to count because bilateral, multilayered hemorrhages extending to the periphery are highly specific for AHT[8] (**Figure 44.2**).

Other retinal ocular findings associated with, but not universally specific for, trauma include retinal detachment, retinoschisis (splitting of retinal layers), and retinal folds.[5] Retinal detachment has many etiologies and is not a common finding in AHT. Macular retinoschisis and folds are more specific for AHT but can also result from severe nonabusive trauma and childhood diseases such as sickle cell anemia and leukemia.[8] Distinguishing features between these entities might be better delineated with the help of history, concomitant findings, and optical coherence tomography (OCT).[9] The presence of extensive, multilayered RHs to the ora serrata, macular retinoschisis, and retinal folds are each highly suggestive of AHT but are not diagnostic, requiring careful history, testing, and examination to corroborate the etiology.

The direct ophthalmoscope allows for a limited view of the posterior pole of the retina and can be challenging with a small pupil and uncooperative child. This examination can sometimes suffice to confirm or refute the presence of RHs, particularly in cases of severe AHT with hemorrhagic retinopathy.

If neurologic status needs to be monitored by the pupillary response, short-acting mydriatics (eg, phenylephrine 2.5%), lenses that assist in small pupil exam, and performing indirect ophthalmoscopy on one dilated eye at a time can allow for pupillary response to remain intact. Indirect ophthalmoscopy through a dilated pupil by a trained ophthalmologist allows for a wide-angle stereoscopic view of the entire retina and a detailed documentation of all ocular findings to the ora serrata (anterior edge of the retina). In addition to RHs, retinoschisis, premacular folds, chorioretinal scars, and papilledema may be seen in instances of abuse.

Pathogenesis and Significance of RH

An effort to better elucidate the specificity of severe RH in diagnosing AHT in young children has led to a better understanding of their pathogenesis.[9] Two major theories on the cause of RHs attribute them to raised retinal venous pressure from sudden increases in the chest or head pressure. The second postulates that vitreoretinal traction from repeated acceleration-deceleration creates a direct mechanical effect of the shaking or impact itself. OCT has been helpful in demonstrating that vitreoretinal traction and shearing forces caused by shaking have been attributed to the formation of maculoschisis and RHs.[9] The appearance and extent of RH may be influenced by associated trauma, hypoxia, electrolyte imbalances, vascular shifts, coagulopathy, and intraocular pressure changes.

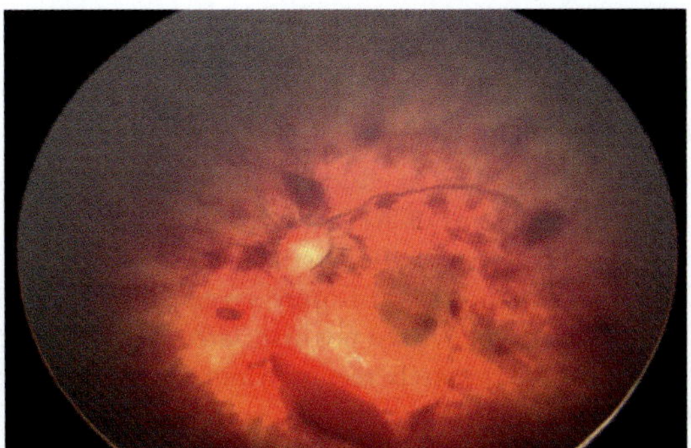

Figure 44.2: Left eye preretinal and intraretinal hemorrhages to the ora serrata in a 4-month-old infant with altered mental status and seizures due to AHT. (Courtesy of Kathleen Stoessel, MD.)

Visual Outcomes

Amblyopia can occur reasonably rapidly in young children if vision is not maximized in both eyes as quickly as possible. RHs usually resolve spontaneously and are not a source of visual morbidity. Approximately 45% of abused children will have abnormal vision in at least one eye, mainly owing to optic nerve or cortical injury. Retinal findings include macular scarring, retinal detachment, and nonclearing vitreous hemorrhage. Late ocular findings include strabismus, amblyopia, optic disk pallor, and cortical visual impairment.[10] Continued ophthalmic care after the ocular injury is essential to minimize permanent visual loss in this young population.

Postmortem Findings

Postmortem examination is essential to corroborate RH and retinoschisis viewed by indirect ophthalmoscopy and is critical in cases of unexplained death in infants and young children. Autopsy findings can reveal additional sites of hemorrhage to periorbital structures such as muscles, cranial nerve sheaths, fat, and the optic nerve sheath, findings that are more common in cases of abusive trauma.

TIPS AND PEARLS

- The retinal examination is an essential part of all encounters involving previously healthy children under the age of 5 who present with altered levels of consciousness, drowsiness with irritability, coma, convulsions, intracranial hemorrhage, injury, or unexplained death.
- In neurologically asymptomatic victims, brain imaging is essential and eye examinations are necessary if brain imaging demonstrates concern for AHT.
- Because RHs are transient, retinal evaluation should be done as early as possible, preferably within the first 24 hours but definitely within the first 72 hours of presentation.
- The ophthalmic examination should not be delayed even if pupillary dilation is of concern owing to the need to monitor pupillary response in severe intracranial injury. The presence of RHs can still be assessed through either direct or indirect ophthalmoscopy through a small pupil, fast-acting mydriatics, or consecutive pupillary dilation. A complete evaluation can be delayed until clinically appropriate.
- If AHT is suspected, an ophthalmologist should be consulted for a dilated retinal examination. Numerous bilateral, multilayered RH extending to the periphery should prompt a thorough evaluation of other injuries that would support a diagnosis of abuse. Detailed documentation of an afferent pupillary defect; anterior segment pathology; and the pattern, location, number, and type of RH is imperative to support the diagnosis of AHT.
- It should be remembered that all health care providers are mandated reporters of suspected child abuse and neglect. A reasonable suspicion of abuse or neglect is mandated to be reported to Child Protective Services.

EVIDENCE

Is it possible to differentiate nonabusive from abusive head trauma by ocular examination?

RH has been widely described in cases of child abuse, although it is not pathognomonic. Mild to moderate RHs is seen in most victims of AHT but has also been linked to many other pediatric conditions of differing severity.[6,7] Severe hemorrhagic retinopathy has been strongly associated with AHT, particularly with the presence of more severe intracranial injury.[8] It is important to note that cases of minor falls and blows are not associated with RHs unless there is also a severe life-threatening brain injury and are rarely seen in trauma without neurologic injury on imaging. In this setting, the hemorrhages are intraretinal or preretinal, confined to the posterior pole, and fewer in number.

The number, location with respect to the retina, and distribution of RHs can help substantiate the presumptive etiology as AHT in infants and young victims of abuse. Many investigators have demonstrated the high specificity and sensitivity of specific patterns of RH for AHT instead of nonabusive head trauma. In particular, extensive, multilayered hemorrhages extending to the ora serrata should raise serious concern for abuse.[7,8] Extensive intraretinal hemorrhages not associated with abuse have been described after crush injuries and ruptured aneurysms, presumably because of a rapid elevation in intracranial pressure. RHs confined to the posterior pole have been associated with epidural hemorrhages and occipital trauma in children.[11] Accurate description of RH is critical for appropriate differential diagnosis and requires a three-dimensional view of the entire retina with the indirect ophthalmoscope by ophthalmologists, through dilated pupils when possible.

How does birth trauma differ from AHT?

Hemorrhages from AHT and birth trauma may be indistinguishable in an infant aged 1 month or under. When diagnosing RHs in an infant, one must consider birth trauma as an etiology, occurring in 20% to 70% of deliveries.[12] It is important to note that RHs cannot be accurately dated. Birth-related RHs resorb in 2 to 6 weeks, depending on the type of hemorrhage, with flame-shaped hemorrhages resolving sooner than deeper dot-blot hemorrhages.[13] Weeks or months may be necessary to see the resolution of preretinal, foveal, or subretinal hemorrhages. This might help distinguish isolated preretinal hemorrhages with injuries of at least several days to a week old. Worsening of the degree of RH after admission and other associated retinal findings such as retinoschisis or retinal folds would help distinguish possible abuse from birth trauma.

An enormous number of ocular and systemic entities are associated with RH (**Table 44.1**), reinforcing the fact that RH alone should rarely, if ever, be used to diagnose child abuse without other supportive historic, physical, radiologic, and laboratory evidence. Except for birth trauma, severe coagulopathy, leukemia, or crushing head injury, most are not noted to occur with severe hemorrhagic retinopathy.[11]

Can CPR cause RH?

RHs have not been identified in cases of sudden infant death syndrome, severe coughing, seizures, apnea, or after vaccination.[5] A history of chest compressions during cardiopulmonary resuscitation in possible victims of abuse can complicate the interpretation of the finding of RHs in this population. RHs in this setting are rare and, if noted, are usually mild, confined to the posterior pole, and associated with coexisting risk factors for hemorrhage such as abnormal coagulation profile and platelet count.[14]

TABLE 44.1 Some Conditions of Childhood That Can Be Associated With Retinal Hemorrhage

Abusive head injury	Increased ICP
Nonabusive head trauma	Intraocular surgery
Anemia	Intracranial vascular malformations
Bacterial endocarditis	Leukemia*
Birth*	Maternal ingestion of cocaine
Blunt ocular trauma	Meningitis
Carbon monoxide poisoning	Osteogenesis imperfecta (with head trauma)
Cerebral aneurysm	Papillitis
Coagulopathy	Optic disc drusen
Convulsions	Retinal hemangioma
Cytomegalovirus retinitis	Retinopathy of prematurity
Extracorporeal membrane oxygenation	Sickle cell retinopathy
Galactosemia	Thrombocytopenia
Glutaric aciduria	Tuberous sclerosis
Henoch-Schonlein purpura	Vasculitis
Hemorrhagic disease of the newborn	X-linked retinoschisis
Hereditary bleeding disorders, eg, hemophilia, von Willebrand disease	
Hypernatremia/hyponatremia	
Hypertension (associated with exudates)	

References

1. https://www.acf.hhs.gov/cb/report/child-maltreatment-2019.
2. Shanahan ME, Zolotor AJ, Parrish JW, Barr RG, Runyan DK. National, regional, and state abusive head trauma: application of the CDC algorithm. *Pediatrics*. 2013;132(6):e1546-e1553.
3. Binenbaum G, Chen W, Huang J, Ying GS, Forbes BJ. The natural history of retinal hemorrhage in pediatric head trauma. *J AAPOS*. 2016;20(2):131-135.
4. Barr RG. Crying as a trigger for abusive head trauma: a key to prevention. *Pediatr Radiol*. 2014;44 (Suppl 4):S559-S564.
5. Christian CW, Levin AV, AAP Council on Child Abuse and Neglect, et al. The eye examination in the evaluation of child abuse. *Pediatrics*. 2018;142(2):e20181411.
6. Betts T, Ahmed S, Maguire S, Watts P. Characteristics of non-vitreoretinal ocular injury in child maltreatment: a systematic review. *Eye*. 2017;31:1146-1154.
7. Levin AV. Ocular manifestations of child abuse. *Ophthalmol Clin North Am*. 1990;3:249-264.
8. Bhardwaj G, Chowdhury V, Jacobs MB, Moran KT, Martin FJ, Coroneo MT. A systematic review of the diagnostic accuracy of ocular signs in pediatric abusive head trauma. *Ophthalmology*. 2010; 117(5):983-992.
9. Sturm V, Landau K, Menke MN. Optical coherence tomography findings in shaken baby syndrome. *Am J Ophthalmol*. 2008;146(3):363-368.
10. Weldy E, Shimoda A, Patnaik J, Jung J, Singh J. Long-term visual outcomes following abusive head trauma with retinal hemorrhage. *J AAPOS*. 2019;23(6):329.e1-329.e4.
11. Adams GG, Agrawal S, Sekhri R, Peters MJ, Pierce CM. Appearance and location of retinal haemorrhages in critically ill children. *Br J Ophthalmol*. 2013;97(9):1138-1142.
12. Zhao Q, Zhang Y, Yang Y, et al. Birth-related retinal hemorrhages in healthy full-term newborns and their relationship to maternal, obstetric, and neonatal risk factors. *Graefe's Arch Clin Exp Ophthalmol*. 2015;253(7):1021-1025. doi:10.1007/s00417-015-3052-9
13. Emerson MV, Pieramici DJ, Stoessel KM, Berreen JP, Gariano RF. Incidence and rate of disappearance of retinal hemorrhage in newborns. *Ophthalmology*. 2001;108(1):36-39.
14. Pham H, Enzenauer RW, Elder JE, Levin AV. Retinal hemorrhage after cardiopulmonary resuscitation with chest compressions. *Am J Forensic Med Pathol*. 2013;34(2):122-124.

CHAPTER 45

Blunt Trauma and Open Globes

Albert Lin
Nicholas Hoda

THE CLINICAL CHALLENGE

Severe blunt trauma to the eye can be a diagnostic dilemma owing to the wide variety of possible injuries. What makes this subject especially difficult is that examining the eye may be difficult or even contraindicated in certain instances, and the degree of posterior exam findings from trauma (which requires a dilated fundus exam) may not be deduced from the anterior segment appearance. When dealing with any severe trauma to the eye, perhaps the most important clinical and diagnostic question to answer is whether an open globe injury is present. In the United States, the estimated incidence of open globe injuries is 4.49 per 100 000 annually, and whereas open globes consist of 2.0% of ocular trauma cases, they are responsible for 8.3% of expenses related to ocular trauma.[1] Young men appear to be at most risk for open globe injuries, through either occupational or environmental hazards or from assault.

Blunt injuries involving the eye and orbit may make ophthalmologic evaluation difficult and risky, and other injuries may simulate open globe injury. Examination itself may be difficult or even impossible without advanced support owing to presentation, such as an uncooperative pediatric patient or a patient with altered mental status from medications or illicit substances. However, suspicion and rapid triage of open globe injuries is key to maximizing visual recovery and globe loss.

PATHOPHYSIOLOGY

The effects of blunt trauma to the eye vary depending on the amount and trajectory of force. Anterior segment injuries are from direct contusions to the eye itself or from force transmitted through the orbit or eyelid. Posterior segment injuries are typically from shockwave effects secondary to the anterior-posterior compression of the globe from blunt force trauma. The shockwave effects cause direct tissue damage and abnormal vitreous traction to the eye and subsequent injuries such as retinal dialysis, vitreous hemorrhage, and commotio retinae. In cases of severe compression, an open globe may even occur.

An open globe is defined as a full thickness wound of the sclera or cornea typically either after an injury that penetrates the eye or from an occult rupture after blunt injury. The largest proportion of volume of the internal contents of the eye is incompressible liquid (aqueous and vitreous humor). A blunt injury of significant force may cause the intraocular pressure (IOP) to rise to a point where the eyewall cannot contain the pressure and thus rupture at its weakest areas (limbus, posterior to the rectus muscles, and old wounds from intraocular surgery). Eyewall rupture results in expulsion of vital portions of the eye, including the lens, iris, retina, and choroid. Even if the globe is not ruptured, the force and the subsequently increased IOP and shockwave effects of the injury may cause other vision-decreasing pathology.

In contrast, the pathophysiology of open globe injuries from lacerating or penetrating injuries, usually from sharp objects or intraocular foreign body (IOFB) entry, is straightforward. These injuries typically enter through the anterior portions of the eye (cornea, limbus, anterior sclera) and typically do not cause damage to the surrounding orbital structures. The proper terminology to describe open globe injures is listed in **Table 45.1**.[2]

APPROACH/THE FOCUSED EXAM

History and Presentation

After any life-threatening injuries are addressed, a detailed history and exam of the eye should be obtained if possible. The timing of the injury and mechanism should be noted, especially if there is concern for an open globe injury. Although the mechanism is important, the severity or force of the mechanism is much more important in determining whether an open globe is present. Severe blunt trauma from bungee cords, assaults/fights, paintball injuries, falls, all-terrain and motor vehicular collisions, and sports injuries without protection are of particular risk in causing open globes.

The relative cleanliness of any penetrating injuries and the potential for a retained IOFB should also be investigated. Do not overlook the potential for retained foreign bodies from a wide variety of mechanisms such as hammering metal on metal, sharpening metal, or an explosion. Dirty or contaminated objects, especially if organic (like wood), may increase the risk of concurrent development of endophthalmitis with the open globe injury. In addition to the timing and mechanism of the injury, other important information includes whether the patient is experiencing pain or a decrease in vision and, if so, the timing of the pain or acuity change relative to the time of the injury.

Even with grievous injuries to the eye, a past medical and surgical history is important to obtain. Blunt injuries to the eye can sometimes precipitate or worsen existing systemic eye conditions that can cause vision loss. For example, in a diabetic patient with proliferative diabetic retinopathy, an accidental blow or fall can precipitate a diabetic vitreous hemorrhage, causing sudden vision loss. As noted earlier, a history of previous eye surgeries is important because surgical wounds may be a potential path for extraocular expulsion or wound dehiscence. It is important to know the patient's level of vision prior to the injury, including whether they wear corrective lenses or contacts. If the patient wears contacts, it is important to know if the patient had them on during the injury. Knowing the overall visual potential of the eye prior to the injury is helpful in setting expectations for the visual prognosis.

Physical Examination

Careful exam for a possible open globe injury is crucial, and, notably, this may include limiting the exam. On external exam, close visual inspection of the eyelids, orbit, and surrounding facial structures should first be performed, paying specific attention to any bruising pattern or lacerations on the eyelids and any injury to the lid margins and adnexa.

TABLE 45.1 Terminology for Open Globe Injuries

Term	Definition
Eyewall	Sclera and Cornea
Closed globe injury	No full thickness eyewall injury
Open globe injury	Full thickness eyewall wound present
Closed subgroups	
Contusion	No full thickness wound present
Lamellar laceration	Partial thickness eyewall wound present
Open subgroups	
Rupture	Full thickness wound present from blunt trauma
Laceration	Full thickness wound present from sharp object
Laceration subgroups	
Penetrating injury	Entrance wound without exit wound
Perforating injury	Entrance and exit wound present from same agent
Intraocular foreign body	Entrance wound with retained foreign object in eye (no exit wound)

It is not uncommon for the eyelids to be swollen shut owing to periorbital edema after blunt trauma. An attempt to open the eye may be performed, but extreme care must be taken to avoid applying pressure to the globe during examination, especially in an agitated, frightened, or uncooperative patient. Cavalier handling of the eye during examination in an open globe may result in expulsion of intraocular contents and potentially worsen the injury and prognosis. Measurement of visual acuity, confrontational visual fields, and evaluation of pupillary response and extraocular movements should be performed if possible. Evaluation for a relative afferent pupillary defect (RAPD) is crucial because the presence of an RAPD influences the overall prognosis. A "reverse RAPD" exam can be performed if the pupil is unrecognizable by looking for constriction of the contralateral pupil while light is shone into the injured eye. In a suspected open globe, measurement of IOP via tonometry is not recommended.

Ideally, a standard stationary or portable slit lamp should be used to examine the eye. On anterior segment examination, a full thickness laceration of the cornea or sclera may be readily apparent, with possible wound gaping. Other exam findings that are concerning for an open globe include the following:

Circumferential hemorrhagic conjunctival chemosis (**Figure 45.1**)
Hyphema, especially if 100% "eight ball" hyphema (indicating dark, clotted blood) (Figure 45.1)
Iris defects (transillumination defects), which may be caused by an intraocular foreign body (**Figure 45.2**, see black arrow)
Expulsed lens or dislocated intraocular lens and external vitreous humor (sticky, gelatinous texture) (**Figures 45.3** and **45.4**)
Black, stringy debris (uvea) subconjunctivally or overlying the conjunctiva (Figure 45.4)
Intraocular foreign body (**Figure 45.5**)

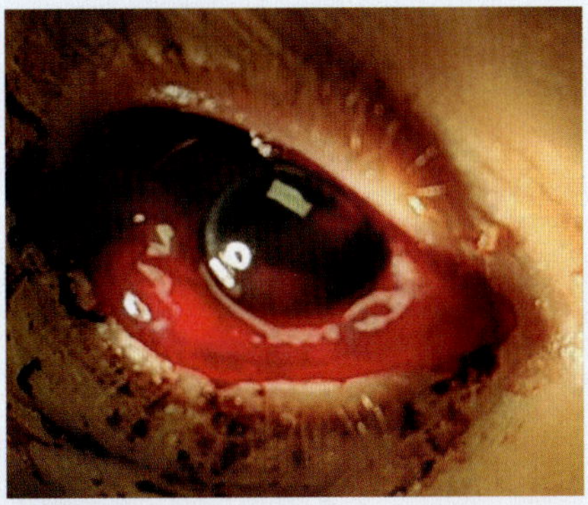

Figure 45.1: Open globe with circumferential hemorrhagic conjunctival chemosis and 8-ball hyphema. A peaked, irregular pupil indicative of early iris expulsion into the globe defect is noted. Additionally, a deflated globe with a flat anterior chamber is present.

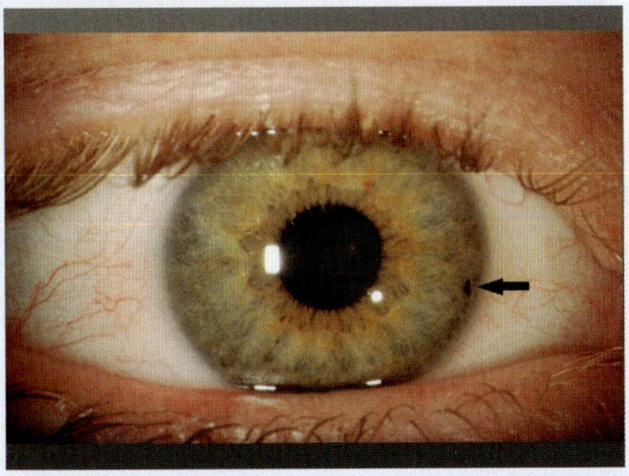

Figure 45.2: Iris transillumination defect (black arrow) from intraocular foreign body.

(continued)

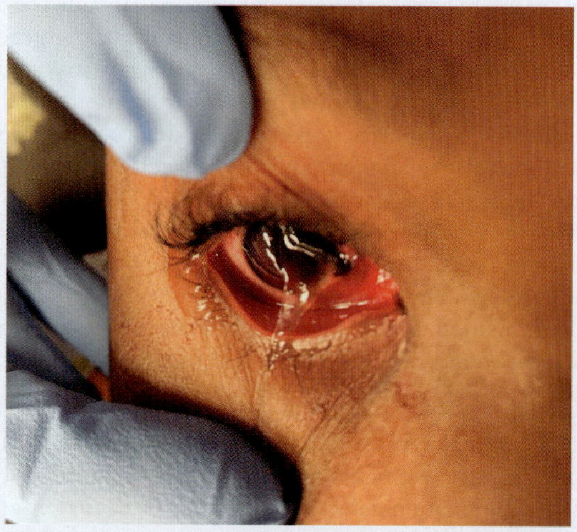

Figure 45.3: Vitreous humor prolapse noted by the sticky, gelatinous texture.

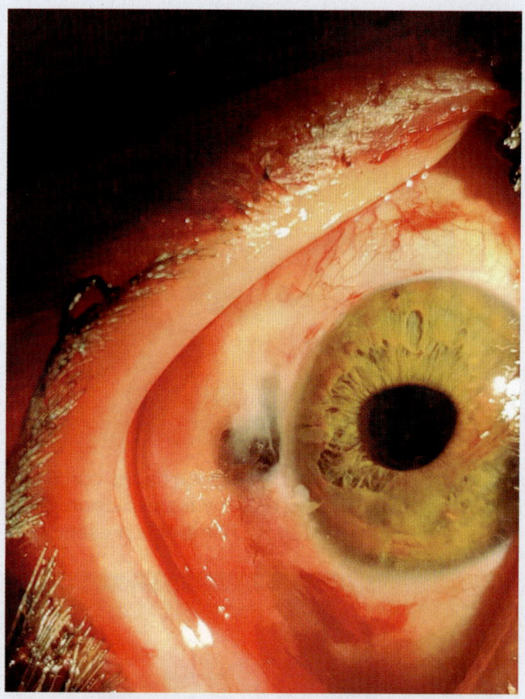

Figure 45.4: Uveal prolapse noted by black, stringy debris subconjunctivally or overlying the conjunctiva.

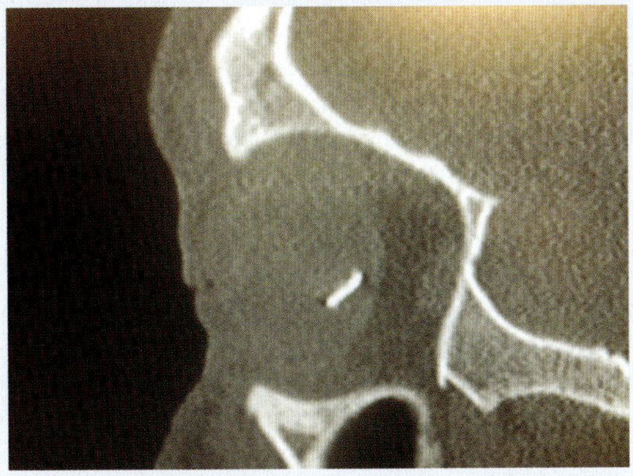

Figure 45.5: Computed tomography scan of metallic intraocular foreign body.

If the probability of an open globe is low or has been ruled out, a more assertive examination can be performed, although with any traumatic injury, overaggressive examination can sometimes worsen injuries to the eye. Owing to the specific skill sets and equipment required to perform a dilated fundus exam, examination techniques for posterior segment traumatic findings are outside the scope of this chapter.

Ancillary Imaging

If the presence of an open globe is uncertain, computed tomography (CT) scan may identify an occult open globe injury. CT is also helpful in determining both whether an IOFB is present and whether it is metallic. CT imaging clues that an occult open globe may be present include abnormal globe contour, volume loss, intraocular air, an absent or dislocated lens, vitreous hemorrhage, and retinal detachment. A CT orbit protocol is recommended to obtain as much detail of the globe as possible. Alternatively, in the trauma workup a CT face protocol is acceptable. A CT head may miss globe details that would suggest an open globe and is not recommended to evaluate ocular or orbital trauma.

Magnetic resonance imaging (MRI) provides much better detail of soft tissue injuries. It is a superior tool compared to CT for detecting organic foreign bodies in the eye and orbit. However, it is contraindicated in the setting of a possible metallic IOFB and is not recommended until metallic IOFBs have been ruled out.

Ultrasonography, or B-scan ultrasound, allows for the visualization of the globe, which can be very useful when the view is not clear or if the eyelids cannot be opened. Globe ruptures, vitreous hemorrhage, retinal detachments, lens dislocations, and intraocular foreign bodies can be detected via ultrasound.[3] However, in the setting of a potential open globe, it carries risk owing to the potential worsening of the injury. If an anterior wound (in the cornea or anterior sclera) is suspected or confirmed, further ultrasound is not necessary and not recommended by ophthalmologists; the risk of prolapse from an anterior wound is much higher than a posterior rupture during ultrasonography. For an open globe, any ultrasound attempts should be performed very lightly. Limitations to this include the provider's familiarity and experience with examining the eye, because it requires a very light touch. Image quality and reliability are also highly user dependent, which is crucial to keep in mind in the presence of an occult posterior rupture. Last, if the trauma has introduced air underneath the eyelids or into the globe, the air will obscure the image, limiting the exam. If the evaluating physician's comfort level performing an ultrasound for a suspected open globe is in doubt, it is better to defer to the ophthalmologist. Although the risk of prolapse with modern ultrasounds is low, a potentially salvageable open globe can lead to a devastating outcome if intraocular content extrusion occurs.

DIFFERENTIAL DIAGNOSIS

The differential diagnosis of an open globe is expansive owing to many traumatic eye findings that can cause decreased vision and pain and can accompany an open globe as well. In the setting of a sharp object or potential IOFB based on history, diagnosis may be straightforward, but blunt injuries may make it more difficult to determine whether an open globe is truly present. A table (**Table 45.2**) of potential differential diagnoses other than open globe rupture in the setting of blunt trauma is listed.

MANAGEMENT

Once an open globe is diagnosed or strongly suspected, further examination of the eye by any other care providers should be halted until a trained ophthalmologist can confirm the diagnosis. While awaiting that ophthalmologic consultation, it is best to protect the eye with a hard convex shield or covering such that inadvertent pressure to the eye is avoided. The use of an eye pad or gauze can apply pressure to the eye, so it is critical to avoid using these types of coverings. If a shield is not available, a paper cup can be fashioned for such use. Keep the edges of the shield over bony structures to avoid compression on the globe itself. A dedicated noncontrasted CT of the orbit should be obtained if there is suspicion of an IOFB. The head of the bed should be elevated to 30°, the patient's dietary status made NPO, and the patient's physical activity status made bed rest with bathroom privileges. The patient should be instructed to avoid Valsalva maneuvering, bending, straining, and strenuous activities.

Medical treatment consists of supportive and preventative measures intravenously. Antiemetics are recommended to prevent retching and emesis, and analgesics should be provided for pain relief to prevent excessive movement and agitation from pain. Intravenous antibiotics are recommended to prevent subsequent endophthalmitis, which may result in a catastrophic prognosis if it occurs after open globe injury.[4,5] Recommended empiric coverage for organisms that are commonly associated with posttraumatic endophthalmitis include the following:

TABLE 45.2 Differential Diagnosis of Blunt Trauma to the Eye

Diagnosis	Additional Signs/Symptoms
Corneal abrasion	Vision loss, photophobia, severe sharp pain, foreign body sensation
Traumatic iritis	Vision loss, photophobia (with light shined in either eye), sluggish pupil movements
Traumatic hyphema	Significant vision loss, photophobia
Orbital wall fracture	Periorbital edema/ecchymosis, +/− vision loss, decreased range of extraocular movements (EOM), pain with EOM, enophthalmos
Traumatic retrobulbar hemorrhage	Severe pain, proptosis with resistance to retropulsion, difficulty opening eyelids, eyelids tense to palpation, vision loss, RAPD, loss of color vision, increased IOP
Retinal tear or detachment	Flashing lights, floaters, painless sectoral or total vision loss, often seen as a curtain or seeing "underwater"
Subluxed or dislocated lens	Vision loss, with or without pain
Commotio retinae	Variable Vision loss, no pain
Choroidal rupture	Vision loss, no pain
Traumatic macular hole	Central vision loss, no pain
Optic nerve avulsion	Severe vision loss, RAPD present
Traumatic optic neuropathy	Severe vision loss, RAPD present

IOP, intraocular pressure; RAPD, relative afferent pupillary defect.

Adults: ceftazidime 50 mg/kg up to 2 g (TID dosing) + vancomycin 15 mg/kg up to 1.5 g (daily dosing). If there is no concern for IOFB, antibiotics may be narrowed to a fluoroquinolone such as moxifloxacin 400 mg. For the penicillin anaphylactic patient, a fluoroquinolone can be used in place of the cephalosporin.

Children less than 12 years: cefazolin 15 mg/kg (TID dosing), gentamicin 2 mg/kg (daily dosing).

Antifungals are not recommended unless there is very high suspicion of fungal introduction into the eye. Appropriate tetanus prophylaxis is recommended.

Repair of the open globe is recommended within 24 hours. Thus, if an ophthalmology service is not available or cannot provide surgical treatment, immediate transfer to a tertiary care center is warranted.

PEDIATRIC ISSUES

Pediatric patients with suspected open globes may be more difficult to examine compared to their adult counterparts. In addition to a reluctance to being examined, information about the mechanism of injury may be lacking, especially if no adults were present. The examination of a child who is struggling or actively fighting back may lead to increased IOP and further worsening of the injury. Ideally, physical restraint of the child to perform an examination should be avoided. Additional analgesia and even sedation may be necessary to allow for a proper examination of the patient, but this should be done only if the evaluating physician is comfortable evaluating eye trauma. However, this may also make subjective portions of the examination unreliable. An exam under anesthesia or procedural sedation should be deferred until an ophthalmologist is available to participate in the examination. One of the most important things the emergency physician can do is to keep the child calm to prevent any potential further harm to the eye.

TIPS AND PEARLS

- Periorbital edema and ecchymosis may suggest an open globe, but the appearance may be worse than it seems; the orbital structures help protect the eye and absorb impact from blunt trauma, thus keeping the eye from rupturing (**Figure 45.6**). If available, Desmarres retractors can be helpful in opening the eyes carefully, but, as always, avoid pressure on the globe. Alternatively, a paper clip can be opened and easily bent into a similar position with any device that can hold the paper clip tightly like a hemostat, needle holder, or sturdy forceps. Take care to ensure that there are no sharp edges after bending the paper clip before using this improvised tool.
- As before, if a severe injury is known to have occurred to the eye but the surrounding eyelid and orbital adnexa appear to be undamaged or undisturbed, this should raise more concern for an open globe, owing to the force of the injury likely being transmitted directly to the eye.
- If evidence of intraocular contents is noted immediately on the eyelids or cheek (usually a natural lens or intraocular lens implant), further examination is not recommended owing to the risk of further extrusion of contents.
- If in doubt and ophthalmologic consultation is not available, arrange for transfer for management quickly.

EVIDENCE

What is the evidence for presenting physical examination correlating with prognosis of open globe?

The ocular trauma score (OTS) is a method of determining the visual prognosis of an open globe injury.[6] The score was created by an analysis of 2500 open globe and eye injuries and has been

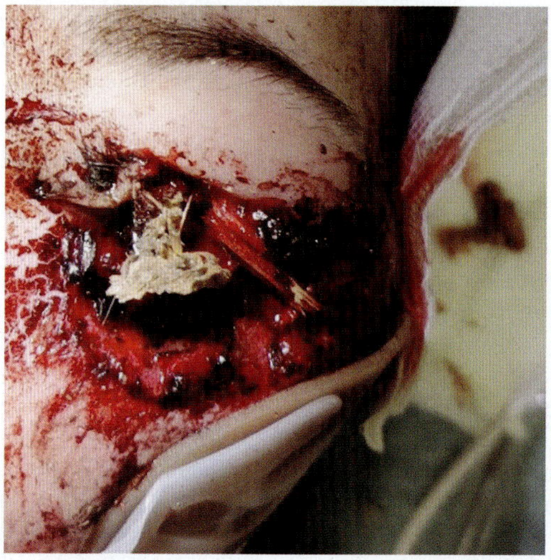

Figure 45.6: Severe periorbital trauma with periorbital edema without an open globe present.

supported in the literature over the past decades as a validating method to estimate visual prognosis. The score is calculated by setting a base score from presenting vision and subtracting from the base score if certain risk factors are present. The results are summarized in **Tables 45.3** and **45.4**.

What is the evidence for using CT scans for imaging open globes?

The sensitivity of a CT scan to detect an open globe injury ranges from 56% to 68%, depending on the interpreter, with a specificity range from 79% to 100%. In a study of 48 eyes, statistically significant findings for occult open-globe injury included change in globe contour, obvious volume loss,

TABLE 45.3 Calculating Ocular Trauma Score (OTS)

Risk Factor	Raw Points
Initial vision	
No light perception	60
Light perception/hand motion	70
1/200-19/200	80
20/200-20/50	90
>20/40	100
Rupture	−23
Endophthalmitis	−17
Perforating injury	−14
Retinal detachment	−11
Afferent pupillary defect	−10

TABLE 45.4 Visual Prognosis per Ocular Trauma Score (OTS)

Sum of Raw Points	OTS Score	No Light Perception (%)	Light Perception/ Hand Motion (%)	1/200-19/ 200 (%)	20/200-20/ 50 (%)	>20/40 (%)
0-44	1	74	15	7	3	1
45-65	2	27	26	18	15	15
66-80	3	2	11	15	31	41
81-91	4	1	2	3	22	73
92-100	5	0	1	1	5	94

an absent or dislocated lens, vitreous hemorrhage, and retinal detachment.[7] Although not considered statistically significant in the study, intraocular air has been suggested as a pathognomonic sign for globe rupture.

What is the evidence for intravenous antibiotics for open globes to prevent posttraumatic endophthalmitis?

A large study performed at Massachusetts Eye and Ear Infirmary on 675 patients demonstrated that the rate of posttraumatic endophthalmitis was less than 1% when patients were placed on intravenous antibiotics for 48 hours and were taken to surgery within 24 hours of presentation.[8] Antibiotics used in the study include vancomycin 1 g Q12 hours, ceftazidime 1 g Q8 hours, and fluoroquinolones. Oral antibiotics may theoretically be used instead of intravenous antibiotics, but owing to the high likelihood of these patients requiring surgery, it is not recommended, in order to keep the patient NPO.

References

1. Mir TA, Canner JK, Zafar S, Srikumaran D, Friedman DS, Woreta FA. Characteristics of open globe injuries in the United States from 2006 to 2014. *JAMA Ophthalmol*. 2020;138(3):268-275. doi:10.1001/jamaophthalmol.2019.5823
2. Kuhn F, Morris R, Witherspoon CD, Heimann K, Jeffers JB, Treister G. A standardized classification of ocular trauma. *Graefes Arch Clin Exp Ophthalmol*. 1996;234(6):399-403. doi:10.1007/BF00190717
3. Lahham S, Shniter I, Thompson M, et al. Point-of-care ultrasonography in the diagnosis of retinal detachment, vitreous hemorrhage, and vitreous detachment in the emergency department. *JAMA Netw Open*. 2019;2(4):e192162. doi:10.1001/jamanetworkopen.2019.2162
4. Huang JM, Pansick AD, Blomquist PH. Use of intravenous vancomycin and cefepime in preventing endophthalmitis after open globe injury. *J Ocul Pharmacol Ther*. 2016;32(7):437-441. doi:10.1089/jop.2016.0051
5. Tabatabaei SA, Soleimani M, Behrooz MJ, Sheibani K. Systemic oral antibiotics as a prophylactic measure to prevent endophthalmitis in patients with open globe injuries in comparison with intravenous antibiotics. *Retina*. 2016;36(2):360-365. doi:10.1097/IAE.0000000000000727
6. Kuhn F, Maisiak R, Mann L, Mester V, Morris R, Witherspoon CD. The Ocular Trauma Score (OTS). *Ophthalmol Clin North Am*. 2002;15(2):163-165, vi. doi:10.1016/s0896-1549(02)00007-x
7. Arey ML, Mootha VV, Whittemore AR, Chason DP, Blomquist PH. Computed tomography in the diagnosis of occult open-globe injuries. *Ophthalmology*. 2007;114(8):1448-1452. doi:10.1016/j.ophtha.2006.10.051
8. Andreoli CM, Andreoli MT, Kloek CE, Ahuero AE, Vavvas D, Durand ML. Low rate of endophthalmitis in a large series of open globe injuries. *Am J Ophthalmol*. 2009;147(4):601-608.e2. doi:10.1016/j.ajo.2008.10.023

CHAPTER 46

Open Angle and Traumatic Glaucoma

Soshian Sarrafpour
Magdalena Robak

THE CLINICAL CHALLENGE

Although often thought of as a disease of increased intraocular pressure (IOP), the term glaucoma refers to a group of diseases characterized by degeneration of retinal ganglion cells and is thus best understood as an optic neuropathy that is often, but not always, associated with elevated IOP. Glaucomatous damage occurs at the level of the ganglion cells, and thus thinning of the retinal nerve fiber layer (axons of the ganglion cells) and ganglion cell layer is seen in glaucoma. A variety of etiologies can present as open angle glaucomas, including traumatic glaucomas. Evaluation for other concerning ophthalmic conditions such as tumor or retinal detachment is essential in anticipation of treatment.

Glaucoma can lead to irreversible vision loss. The vision loss is classically peripheral vision (**Figure 46.1**); however, patients often describe blurry vision and require increased lighting to see well owing to a loss of contrast sensitivity.[1] More importantly, vision loss from glaucoma is oftentimes devastating to patients and can be associated with loss of independence, depression, falls, and motor vehicle collisions.[2,3] As such, whereas acute angle closure glaucoma is more readily recognized by emergency providers, the vision loss of open angle glaucomas may indirectly lead to a broader array of chief complaints, particularly in an aging population. Given the rapid irreversible vision loss that can happen, swift diagnosis and treatment are often essential to optimizing outcomes.

The most important and only known modifiable risk factor is elevated IOP. Other historical risk factors include increasing age, family history, race, and thinner central corneal thickness.[4] Other risk factors may include myopia, diabetes, systemic hypoperfusion, and trauma.[5]

Elevated IOP in open angle glaucomas presents a serious and urgent threat of damage to the optic nerve and thus the peripheral (and eventually central) vision of a patient. If left uncontrolled, persistently elevated IOPs can lead to irreversible blindness ("time is vision"). Patients usually present in the emergency setting because of pain and nausea associated with markedly high IOP, which may reduce penetrance and efficacy of traditional topical medications. Trauma-associated glaucoma can be challenging to evaluate owing to associated eyelid swelling, hyphema, vitreous hemorrhage, or corneal edema that limit ocular exam and visualization of the optic nerve. IOP measurement and other parts of the exam may also have to be deferred in the setting of trauma until a ruptured globe is ruled out. Additionally, patients presenting with trauma may have other life-threatening injuries that require immediate attention, leading to prolonged untreated elevations of IOPs and potential vision loss.

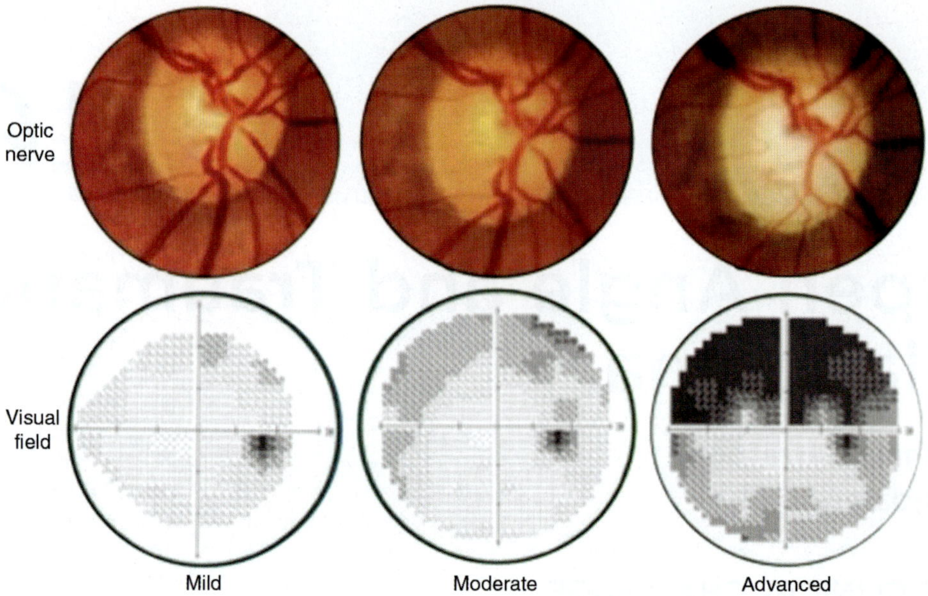

Figure 46.1: Optic Nerve and visual field findings of mild, moderate, and advanced glaucoma.

Open angle Glaucoma

Glaucoma is a leading cause of irreversible blindness in both the United States and abroad.[6] Globally, the prevalence of glaucoma in patients 40 to 80 years old is 3.54% as of 2014 and is predicted to impact almost twice as many people (111.8 million) by 2040.[7] In the United States, racial differences have been observed, although it is unclear due to methodological flaws whether this is due to genealogical differences or social injustices tracing back to slavery and continued structural racism. The most notable of these studies, "Racial Variations in the Prevalence of Primary Open-angle Glaucoma," identified at least a fourfold increase in age-adjusted prevalence of primary open angle glaucoma (POAG) in Black compared with white patients in East Baltimore. In the study, "race" was defined by self-reported census terms without respect to ancestry and all designations other than "Black" or "white" were included in the white cohort.[8]

Pathophysiology

The etiology of open angle glaucoma varies, and multiple mechanisms and etiologies are described. In general, outflow is typically obstructed past the visible trabecular meshwork (hence "open angle") or episcleral vascular pressures can be elevated (as in carotid-cavernous fistula, Sturge-Weber syndrome, etc.). Please refer to the differential diagnosis section for some potential etiologies of open angle glaucomas. POAG is a diagnosis of exclusion when no other cause is found.

Traumatic Glaucoma

Traumatic glaucoma is multifactorial and can occur following penetrating, blunt, chemical, and surgical trauma. Glaucoma occurs most commonly after blunt trauma, with an incidence of about 3.39% at 6 months after the inciting incident.[9] Risk factors include poor presenting visual acuity, older age, injury involving the lens, angle recession, presence of hyphema, and elevated IOP at presentation.[9] As a consequence of this, after emergency evaluation and treatment for acute conditions, referral to ophthalmology for follow-up and surveillance is appropriate.

Pathophysiology

Blunt trauma causes a sudden compression of the eye posteriorly, forcing the globe to expand at the equator and stretching tissues within the eye. This causes trauma to the pupil sphincter, the iris base, the ciliary body, the trabecular meshwork, the zonules holding the lens, and the peripheral retina.[10] Damage to the angle and trabecular meshwork can lead to lifelong glaucoma. Additionally, elevations in ocular pressure can occur from hyphema, vitreous hemorrhage, pigmentary debris, or inflammation after trauma.

Inflammation and dispersion of pigment and debris in the eye obstruct the trabecular meshwork and leads to IOP spikes. This is usually self-limited and clears spontaneously, although IOP control with medication may be required while waiting for resolution.

Traumatic hyphema can exacerbate posttraumatic IOP elevations by clogging the trabecular meshwork with red blood cells. Elevation of IOP can occur and should be managed appropriately, although these elevations tend to be self-limited. These patients should be followed closely for rebleeding, usually within the first 5 days of trauma.

Alkaline agents penetrate through tissue and cause glaucoma (uncommon in acid injuries). The IOP initially goes up to 40 to 50 mm Hg within 10 minutes, then returns to normal before gradually rising to high levels again over the next 1 to 2 hours. The initial IOP spike may be from distortion of the trabecular meshwork from contraction of the outer collagen layers of the eye, whereas the second elevation of IOP is thought to be from prostaglandin release. Long-term damage from inflammation can induce peripheral synechiae of the angle, which can lead to angle closure glaucoma.

Late manifestations of glaucoma from trauma can occur from a variety of etiologies as well. These include ciliary body muscle tears (angle recession), lens-induced glaucomas, ghost cell glaucoma (long-standing heme in the vitreous or anterior chamber can lead to khaki colored "ghost cells" which can obstruct outflow), choroidal hemorrhages, and retinal detachment. Lens-induced glaucomas are worth additional mention. Traumatic lens dislocation can lead to pupillary block or lens swelling that mechanically closes the angle (phacomorphic glaucoma). Additionally, if mature cataracts develop (phacolytic glaucoma) or if the lens capsule is violated (phacoantigenic or lens particle glaucoma), lens debris and inflammatory material can obstruct the outflow pathways.

APPROACH/THE FOCUSED EXAM

The initial evaluation should be systematic in the assessment of all eye emergencies; please refer to Chapter 25 for a detailed explanation of the general approach.

In the case of elevated IOP, a slit lamp examination can be helpful to understand the etiology. Corneal edema could suggest elevated IOP, and subtle pigment or inflammatory deposits on the posterior aspect of the cornea could suggest pigment dispersion syndrome or uveitis-related glaucomas. The anterior chamber depth can be evaluated to help distinguish between open angle and closed angle glaucomas. Ultimately, the gold standard is gonioscopy, but this is beyond the scope of emergency practice. Van Herick evaluation of the anterior chamber can be done without gonioscopy and can be a reasonably accurate way to assess for angle closure. This is done by creating a thin vertical slit beam and shining it onto the peripheral cornea at about a 60° angle. The anterior chamber depth to corneal thickness ratio is then estimated. A ratio of about 1 to 4 or less is concerning for risk of angle closure (**Figure 46.2**).

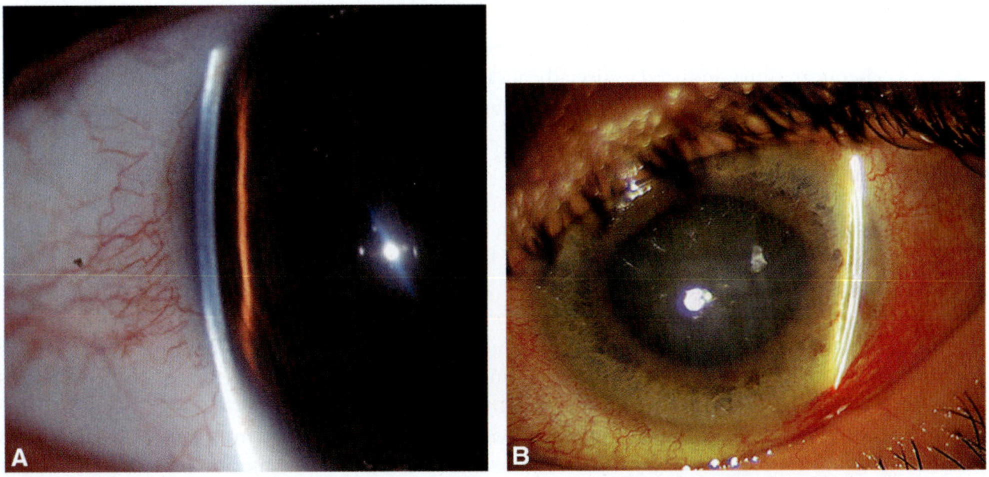

Figure 46.2: A, Van Herick on an eye with open angles. B, Van Herick on an eye in acute angle closure.

The anterior chamber is evaluated for hyphemas, cell, and flare. Careful evaluation of the iris can be done looking for transilluminating defects suggestive of pigmentary or pseudoexfoliation-related glaucoma. Checking for pseudoexfoliation deposits on the lens and lens status (mature cataracts or lens violation) is helpful to evaluate for lens-induced glaucomas and pseudoexfoliation glaucomas. Finally, a thorough dilated examination should be done to assess for other etiologies of elevated IOP like vitreous hemorrhage, tumors, or retinal detachment.

DIFFERENTIAL DIAGNOSIS

The differential diagnosis of open angle and traumatic glaucoma is large, and readers can refer to the chapter on closed angle glaucomas (Chapter 47) because those can be included in the differential diagnosis of glaucoma. Here is a list of common presentations in the differential for open angle glaucoma:

1. **Inflammatory Glaucomas**—Can be distinguished by the presence of cell and flare in anterior chamber examination or keratic precipitates (inflammatory collections on the endothelial layer of the cornea or in the angle). The etiologies include chronic uveitis, sarcoidosis, Posner Schlossman syndrome, Fuchs heterochromic iritis, and so on.
2. **Infectious Glaucomas**—Certain intraocular infections, including herpetic diseases (varicella zoster virus [VZV], herpes simplex virus [HSV]), syphilis, tuberculosis, and toxoplasmosis, can cause elevated IOPs. History and a full ocular and systemic exam can be helpful in distinguishing these.
3. **Tumors**—Ciliary body and other intraocular tumors can induce glaucoma by mechanical force (inducing angle closure), neovascularization, direct occlusion of the angle by malignant cells, and so on.
4. **Traumatic Hyphema**—Red blood cells in the anterior chamber can clog the trabecular meshwork and lead to elevations of IOP. Most clear spontaneously, although rebleeding can happen, most commonly 2 to 5 days after injury, so close follow-up is needed.
5. **Ghost Cell Glaucoma**—Occurs when injury to the globe disrupts the anterior hyaloid face and is associated with vitreous hemorrhage. IOP elevation can occur as soon as 1 to 3 weeks after injury from obstruction of the trabecular meshwork by rigid, khaki-colored remnants of red blood cells (ghost cells).
6. **Lens-Induced Glaucoma**—Lens-induced glaucoma includes angle closure induced by large cataracts (phacomorphic glaucoma) and obstruction of the trabecular meshwork by released lens particles or inflammatory debris. This can happen in mature white cataracts (phacolytic glaucoma), traumatic cataracts (phacoantigenic glaucoma), and postsurgery (lens particle glaucoma).
7. Other etiologies of glaucoma include elevated episcleral vasculature pressure from a carotid cavernous fistula or congenital abnormality (Sturge-Weber syndrome), pseudoexfoliation, pigment dispersion, retinal detachment (5%-10% present with elevated IOP), amyloidosis, chemical injury-induced (especially alkaline injury), and certain medications like steroids or certain sulfa drugs, including topiramate, hydrochlorothiazide, and acetazolamide.

MANAGEMENT

The most important treatment for any form of glaucoma, including open angle glaucoma and traumatic glaucoma, involves lowering the IOP. First-line agents are topical medications and oral or parenteral medications, including carbonic anhydrase inhibitors (eg, acetazolamide), parenteral mannitol, or oral glycerol. If underlying causes are identified, treatment should be modified to treat the underlying cause (eg, adding topical steroids and cycloplegics in inflammatory causes). Eyelid closure and gentle punctal occlusion may reduce systemic side effects. Please see **Table 46.1** for an overview of commonly used medications for treatment of glaucomas.

If adequate IOP control is not obtained with medications, patients must be seen by an ophthalmologist for more aggressive and possibly invasive management. Anterior chamber paracentesis can be done to acutely lower IOP and improve penetration of topical medication, although the IOP

TABLE 46.1 Commonly Used Medications for Elevated IOP in the ED

Medication Class	Examples	Mechanism	Administration	Side Effects
Prostaglandin analogs	Latanoprost	Increase uveoscleral outflow	Topical	Darkening of iris or periorbital skin, periorbital fat atrophy, eyelash growth, reactivation of herpetic keratitis, elevated IOP if overdosed, macular edema
Beta-blockers	Timolol, betaxolol (more β-1 selective)	Aqueous suppression	Topical	Bradycardia, AV nodal blockade, bronchospasm, CNS depression, fatigue, masking hypoglycemia or thryotoxicosis
Alpha-2 agonists	Brimonidine, apraclonidine	Aqueous suppression, increase outflow	Topical	CNS depression, especially in children (lethargy, apnea, hypotension, bradycardia) Allergic reaction, dry mouth, conjunctival blanching
Rho kinase inhibitors	Netarsudil	Multifactorial 1. Aqueous suppression 2. Increased trabecular meshwork outflow 3. Decreased episcleral vascular pressure	Topical	Ocular injection, corneal verticillata, conjunctival hemorrhages, reticular bullous corneal epithelial edema
Miotics	Pilocarpine, echothiophate iodide	Increased trabecular meshwork outflow	Topical	Extensive (ie, headache, retinal detachment, inflammation, angle closure exacerbation, etc)
Carbonic anhydrase inhibitors	Topical: Dorzolamide, brinzolamide Oral: Acetazolamide (IV available), methazolamide	Aqueous suppression	Topical or Oral or IV	Corneal edema, metabolic acidosis, hypokalemia, malaise, nausea, paresthesia, sickle cell crisis, metallic taste, sulfa allergy or Steven-Johnson syndrome, angle closure, bone marrow suppression
Osmotic agents	Oral: Glycerol IV: Mannitol	Osmotic effect	IV or Oral	Respiratory/cardiac/renal failure from volume shifts, sickle cell crisis, nausea/bad taste, caution with glycerol in diabetic patients

lowering effects usually last for a few hours at most. Surgical intervention like filtering surgery or glaucoma drainage implant surgery may be required in refractory cases.

Traumatic glaucoma is treated similarly to other forms of open angle glaucoma in that IOP control is the mainstay of treatment. If a hyphema is present, topical steroids and cycloplegia should be added to reduce inflammation and prevent synechiae formation.

PREGNANCY AND PEDIATRICS

A few issues must be considered in pediatric populations and pregnant populations presenting with elevated IOP. Notably, only brimonidine, an alpha agonist, is a class B medication. Other glaucoma medications are categorized as Class C, generally because there are limited data studying the medications in pregnancy.[11]

The pediatric population itself brings its own unique challenges. Notably, the exam may be more difficult and limited, although new advances in technology like the iCare tonometer make obtaining IOP easier. However, given the malleability of pediatric eyes, IOP may be lower than anticipated because the eye may stretch in response to the elevated IOPs. Initial management with IOP medications including acetazolamide can be considered. Alpha agonists (eg, brimonidine) should be avoided in young patients because of a risk of central nervous system depression and apnea. Treatment in this population, ultimately, often requires surgical intervention with goniotomy, trabeculotomy, or more invasive glaucoma surgeries.

Finally, in patients presenting with nontraumatic hyphemas, one should consider sickle cell disease. Carbonic anhydrase inhibitors, especially systemic ones, are typically avoided or used with caution because they can induce acidosis, which can exacerbate sickling. Mannitol should also be used with caution as the dehydrating effect can induce a sickle crisis. These patients should be monitored closely by an ophthalmologist because they may require early surgical intervention.

TIPS AND PEARLS

- Although the differential diagnosis is broad, the initial management of glaucoma, regardless of the cause, is to decrease IOP, initially with topical or oral/intravenous medications.
- If IOP control is not obtained with medications, urgent evaluation by ophthalmology is required to prevent irreversible vision loss.
- Prostaglandin analogs have limited use in the acute setting because they may take time to reach peak effect and overdosing can paradoxically increase IOP.
- Beware of potential systemic effects of medications, especially when using beta-blockers, oral or IV carbonic anhydrase inhibitors, and mannitol.
- Avoid acetazolamide in patients with sickle cell disease. If necessary, in this population, methazolamide is preferred because it induces less systemic acidosis.
- Early detection, close follow-up and good adherence to medication are key factors to prevent blindness from glaucoma.

EVIDENCE

What is the risk of blindness?

Patients presenting to the emergency department are often concerned about the prognosis of their disease and may ask if they will go blind from glaucoma. Answering this question is difficult given the progressive and irreversible nature of glaucoma, but an evidence-based answer may provide some guidance. Notably, one major reason patients go blind from glaucoma is lack of diagnosis or late diagnosis, so patients presenting to the emergency department with a new diagnosis can be reassured that having the diagnosis decreases their risk of blindness. Even so, rates of blindness in at least one eye range from 26% to 38% over 10 to 20 years.[12,13] As such, it is important to reiterate with patients the importance of close, lifelong treatment and follow-up with their ophthalmologist to prevent blindness.

What is the benefit of IOP reduction?

Patients who are asymptomatic from their elevated IOP may question the need for lifelong treatment. Notably, two major reasons for permanent blindness from glaucoma is lack of adherence to medication and undetected disease.[12] Additionally, numerous studies, including the Collaborative Initial Glaucoma Treatment Study (CIGTS), the Ocular Hypertension Treatment Study (OHTS), the Advanced Glaucoma Intervention Study (AGIS), the Early Manifest Glaucoma Trial (EMGT), and the European Glaucoma Prevention Study (EGPS), have found that reducing IOPs with medications, lasers, and/or surgery lowers the risk of irreversible progression from glaucoma.

References

1. Hu CX, Zangalli C, Hsieh M, et al. What do patients with glaucoma see? Visual symptoms reported by patients with glaucoma. *Am J Med Sci.* 2014;348(5):403-409.
2. Dhawan M, Hans T, Sandhu PS, et al. Evaluation of vision-related quality of life in patients with glaucoma: a hospital-based study. *J Curr Glaucoma Pract*. 2019;13(1):9-15.
3. Chen Y, Lai Y, Wang J, et al. The association between glaucoma and risk of depression: a nationwide population-based cohort study. *BMC Ophthalmol*. 2018;18(1):146.
4. Coleman AL, Miglior S. Risk factors for glaucoma onset and progression. *Surv Ophthalmol.* 2008;53(6):S3-S10.
5. Grzybowski A, Och M, Kanclerz P, et al. Primary open angle glaucoma and vascular risk factors: a review of population based studies from 1990 to 2019. *J Clin Med.* 2020;9(3):761.
6. Quigley HA, Broman AT. The number of people with glaucoma worldwide in 2010 and 2020. *Br J Ophthalmol.* 2006;90(3):262-267.
7. Tham Y, Li X, Wong TY, et al. Global prevalence of glaucoma and projections of glaucoma burden through 2040: a systematic review and meta-analysis. *Ophthalmology*. 2014;121(11):2081-2090.
8. Sommer A, Tielsch JM, Katz J, et al. Racial differences in the cause-specific prevalence of blindness in east Baltimore. *NEJM*. 1991;325(20):1412-1417.
9. Girkin CA, McGwin G Jr, Long C, et al. Glaucoma after ocular contusion: a cohort study of the United States eye injury registry. *J Glaucoma.* 2005;14:470-473.
10. Kaushik S, Sukhija J, Pandav SS, et al. Blunt ocular trauma in one eye: a photo documentation. *Ann Ophthalmol (Skokie)*. 2006;38(3):249-252.
11. Sethi HS, Naik M, Gupta VS. Management of glaucoma in pregnancy: risks or choices, a dilemma? *Int J Ophthalmol*. 2016;9(11):1684-1690.
12. Susanna R Jr, De Moraes CG, Cioffi GA, Ritch R. Why do people (still) go blind from glaucoma? *Transl Vis Sci Technol*. 2015;4(2):1.
13. Hattenhauer MG, Johnson DH, Ing HH, et al. The probability of blindness from open-angle glaucoma. *Ophthalmology*. 1998;105:2099-2104.

CHAPTER 47

Angle Closure Glaucoma

Sandra Fernando Sieminski
Sanjay Mohan

THE CLINICAL CHALLENGE

Angle closure is a process that results from appositional closure of the iridocorneal angle, or drainage angle of the eye, leading to aqueous humor outflow obstruction and consequent increase in intraocular pressure (IOP). This increase in IOP can lead to progressive optic nerve damage and peripheral vision loss, which is a disease state known as glaucoma. Primary angle-closure (PAC) occurs when obstruction is a result of anatomic predisposition of the eye to have crowding of the angle, usually owing to a small eye or a large cataract. Secondary angle-closure is attributable to a coexisting ocular disease process (eg, inflammation, tumor, or hemorrhage), which causes physical occlusion of the angle owing to debris or scar tissue formation in the angle. In the United States, although more than 80% of glaucoma cases are open-angle in etiology, angle closure glaucoma accounts for a disproportionate number of patients with severe vision loss and thus accounts for more emergency department (ED) visits.[1]

The prevalence of angle closure glaucoma varies considerably among ethnic and racial groups. Inuit and Asian populations account for the highest rates, whereas lower rates are reported in African and European populations.[2] Other risk factors include female gender, farsightedness (hyperopia), having a shallow anterior chamber, use of medications that can induce angle narrowing (eg, pupil dilators, including alpha agonists and anticholinergic agents), advanced age (most common between ages of 55 and 65), cataracts, and family history.[2]

The challenge of this disease primarily posits in prevention and diagnosis. Much like open-angle glaucoma, closed-angle glaucoma is typically an asymptomatic disease process in which patients are unaware of this illness until advanced visual loss occurs. Whereas acute angle closure glaucoma presents with a change in vision or with severe acute symptoms, chronic angle closure glaucoma tends to be discovered incidentally.

Clinical presentation and symptoms result from the rapidity and degree of IOP elevation. Acute angle glaucoma is suggested by severe ocular or periocular pain, decreased vision, halos around lights, headache, nausea, and vomiting. In contrast, chronic angle glaucoma patients are asymptomatic because the rise in IOP is gradual and less severe.

PATHOPHYSIOLOGY

The distinguishing feature of angle closure glaucoma is that the iridocorneal angle, the junction between the iris and the cornea, which functions as the site of aqueous humor outflow, is obstructed. The most common cause of primary angle closure is referred to as "pupillary block." In order to understand the pathophysiology involved with pupillary block, it is important to understand the flow of aqueous in a nondiseased state (**Figure 47.1**). Aqueous humor is secreted from the ciliary body, a circumferential structure located behind the iris in the posterior chamber of the eye, and flows through the pupil to the anterior chamber of the eye. Eventually, the aqueous humor exits the

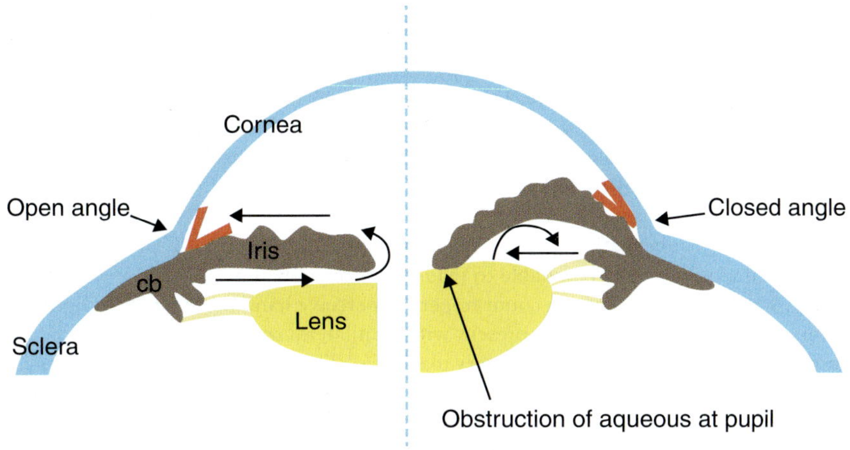

Figure 47.1: Left side of diagram indicates normal aqueous humor flow in nondiseased state. Right side of diagram indicates mechanism of pupillary block, causing obstruction at the iridocorneal angle. (Courtesy of Dr. Sandra Fernando Sieminski.)

anterior chamber through the iridocorneal angle, which is composed of multiple layers of tissue. The most superficial layer is called the trabecular meshwork, a sievelike tissue with the deepest layer, called the canal of Schlemm. Through the canal of Schlemm, the aqueous humor ultimately drains into the venous system.

In pupillary block, the flow of aqueous humor from posterior to anterior chamber is blocked at the pupil, typically because there is contact between the lens and the iris. As the lens opacifies and grows with age (ie, cataract), the propensity of pupillary block to occur increases. As the aqueous accumulates behind the iris, the pressure in the posterior chamber increases, causing the iris to bow anteriorly, creating an outlet obstruction and perpetuating the cycle of angle closure.

Outside of pupillary block, the etiology of angle closure glaucoma can be subdivided into three other groups: physiologic crowding of the angle, lens induced, and plateau iris syndrome.[3] Crowded angle tends to occur in patients with thicker iris tissue. In these cases, there is less space for aqueous humor to drain through the trabecular meshwork. With pupillary dilation, the iris is pulled peripherally and further crowds the iridocorneal angle. Lens-induced angle closure can occur either when a large, mature cataract pushes the iris forward and closes the angle or when the lens is subluxed anteriorly. In both cases, there may still be an element of pupillary block owing to the lens-iris contact, but the primary mechanism of angle closure is anterior displacement of the iris by the lens. In lens subluxation, the zonules, ligaments that suspend the lens in its anatomic position behind the iris, are loosened and cause the lens to displace anteriorly. Predisposing conditions for lens subluxation include trauma, Marfan syndrome, Ehlers-Danlos syndrome, and homocystinuria. Plateau iris syndrome is defined by an anterior insertion of the peripheral iris base onto the ciliary body. This positioning of the iris can cause narrowing of the iridocorneal angle that is not caused by pupillary block and can present as acute or chronic angle closure.[3]

Medication-induced angle closure glaucoma can be accounted for by a variety of mechanisms (pupillary block via miosis, angle crowding with mydriasis, and iridocorneal angle disruption secondary to ciliochoroidal effusion). Alpha-adrenergic agonists are mydriatic agents that are routinely administered by ophthalmologists and optometrists for pupillary dilation and funduscopic examination and are also found in a variety of over-the-counter cold and allergy medicines such as decongestants. Mydriasis induces thickening at the base of the iris that can potentially generate iridotrabecular contact and angle closure acutely. Anticholinergic agents such as atropine, tropicamide, and cyclopentolate target different muscles; however, all result in pupillary dilation and iridocorneal angle closure. Other medications that may precipitate angle closure glaucoma include beta$_2$ agonists, sulfonamide containing medications such as topiramate and trimethoprim-sulfamethoxazole, anticoagulants such as heparin and warfarin, and certain serotonergic agents.[4]

APPROACH/THE FOCUSED EXAM

In approaching a patient with suspected angle closure, it is important to elicit a thorough history. This includes history of eye surgery, medications, recent medical procedures, recent facial trauma, contact lens use, eye drop use, and prior occurrences of eye pain and/or redness. Patients may endorse symptoms such as halos around lights, blurry vision, headache over the brow, and nausea. Their symptom onset can be linked to starting a new medication or entering a dimly lit room, which causes pupillary dilation.[4]

As with any ocular pathology, visual acuity should be assessed. Given the degree of pain and discomfort, the patient may be unable to read letters on a Snellen chart, and if so, it should be determined whether the patient can count fingers or perceive hand movements or light. On gross inspection, the patient will classically present with a unilateral red eye, a fixed mid-dilated pupil, and some degree of corneal clouding secondary to edema.[4] There can also be focal redness surrounding the limbus (the junction between the cornea and the sclera), pigment granules or white flecks on the anterior surface of the cataract, iris atrophy or transillumination caused by iris ischemia from high IOP if this is not the patient's first episode of angle closure, and a shallow anterior chamber (the space between the cornea and the iris). Many of these features are seen in **Figure 47.2** of a patient presenting in angle closure after receiving laser iridotomy.

A light source should be used to assess for corneal clouding and pupillary reactivity. Instillation of a topical anesthetic is recommended before measurement of IOP (tonometry). Normal IOP generally ranges from 10 to 20 mmHg. In angle closure glaucoma, pressures can be well over 50 mm Hg.[4] Of note, if significant relief is achieved with the topical anesthetic alone, it may point to corneal pathology (eg, corneal abrasion, foreign body). Targeted evaluation should be performed thereafter (ie, slit-lamp examination and corneal staining).

The gold standard for measuring IOP is Goldmann applanation tonometry, although this method requires a special biomicroscope, called a slit lamp, with an attached tonometer, and it is technically challenging to obtain accurate measurements. Typically, IOP is measured in the emergency setting by a handheld device called a TonoPen (Reichert Technologies®, Buffalo, NY). This requires installation of a topical anesthetic and requires minimal training to obtain an accurate measurement. Newer handheld tonometry devices such as the iCare rebound tonometer (iCare, Tiolat Oy, Helsinki, Finland) offer the advantages of a disposable tip and no need for topical anesthetic to obtain a measurement. Historically, digital assessment of the globe has been suggested as a means to diagnose elevated IOP, particularly when the eye resists digital indentation and "feels hard."[5,6] This technique, however, is inaccurate and not recommended as standard practice.

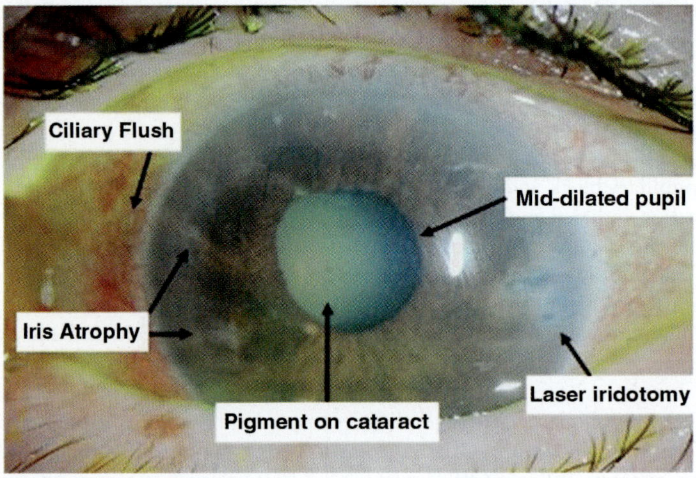

Figure 47.2: A patient presenting with angle closure glaucoma after receiving laser iridotomy. (Courtesy of Dr. Chuck Terranova.)

If there is access to a slit lamp, one can assess for anterior chamber depth using the Van Herick grading system. To perform this, the slit beam is offset approximately 60° from center on to the peripheral cornea. The thickness of the bright slit beam projected perpendicularly on the cornea and a second beam reflection appears on the iris. The thickness of the corneal beam is then compared with the depth of the peripheral anterior chamber (or the space between the two beams). The only method in which to directly view the angle is termed gonioscopy, in which a mirrored lens is placed on the eye. This is typically performed by an ophthalmologist at the slit lamp.

DIFFERENTIAL DIAGNOSIS

The differential diagnosis of angle closure glaucoma should include any cause of a painful red eye and/or headache. Often, the first step in the evaluation of ocular pathology is to determine whether symptoms are uni- or bilateral. Conjunctivitis, whether allergic, viral, or bacterial, can be unilateral and may progress to both eyes and is often associated with itchy or gritty sensations associated with tearing or discharge. Other infectious pathologies to consider include keratitis and uveitis (especially in the context of underlying autoimmune systemic diseases). Ocular trauma, including corneal abrasions, ulcers, or foreign bodies, should be evaluated for as well. Slit-lamp examination is often needed to assess for cell and flare and corneal disease processes that are not apparent with gross inspection.

It is imperative to consider nonocular pathologies as well. Because patients with angle closure glaucoma may appear systemically ill, complaining of headaches, nausea, and vomiting, a broad differential should be maintained. Primary headache disorders, including migraines, tension-type headaches, and cluster headaches, can be severely debilitating. In fact, cluster headaches, in particular, may present with monocular pain and autonomic features such as conjunctival injection, profuse tearing, or eyelid edema that can be mistaken for primary ocular pathology. Lastly, it is important to consider life-threatening disease processes such as meningitis and other etiologies of elevated intracranial pressures (eg, tumors, intracranial hemorrhage).

MANAGEMENT

For the patient in angle closure, the main management goals are to lower the IOP and relieve the pupillary block, if this is the suspected mechanism. Initially, topical antihypertensive drops can be started to lower IOP, but oftentimes systemic medications such as acetazolamide are necessary to significantly decrease the pressure and associated pain.[4]

A helpful guideline for initiating drops in acute angle closure glaucoma is to start with the "ABC's": alpha-adrenergic agonists (such as brimonidine 0.2%), beta-blockers (such as timolol 0.5%), and carbonic anhydrase inhibitors (such as dorzolamide 2%). These drops are administered in rapid succession in three rounds separated by 15 minutes.[7] A typical initial dose of acetazolamide is 500 mg orally or intravenously. The IOP and visual acuity should be reevaluated 1 hour after initial drops and acetazolamide have been administered.

Pilocarpine is controversial in the setting of angle closure. While it offers the advantage of miosis, which pulls the peripheral iris away from the angle, it can also increase vascular permeability, causing iris congestion and further narrowing of the angle.[8]

If these agents are unsuccessful at lowering the IOP, hyperosmotic agents such as mannitol can be considered. Mannitol should be administered at 1 to 2 g/kg over 45 minutes (a 500 mL bag of mannitol 20% contains 100 g of mannitol).[7] However, mannitol should be used with caution, because it can involve more severe systemic side effects such as cerebral edema and congestive heart failure. All systemic medications should be used with careful consideration of the patient's medical history.

Lowering intraocular pressure can alleviate pain and also help clear the corneal edema in order to perform more definitive therapy. The mainstays of treatment for angle closure are laser peripheral iridotomy (LPI) and lens extraction. In LPI, a laser such as an Nd-YAG or argon is applied to the peripheral iris to create a small full thickness opening.[8] This opening allows the sequestered aqueous fluid in the posterior chamber to flow anteriorly, bypassing the pupil and allowing the iris to decompress posteriorly. This procedure is typically performed by an ophthalmologist with a

YAG (yttrium aluminum garnet) or argon laser. These lasers are sometimes available in the ED or can be transported to the ED in emergency situations. If they are not readily available, an ophthalmologist should be consulted immediately to begin arrangements for the prodedure.

Lens extraction, or cataract surgery, can definitively alleviate the angle closure mechanism, whether it is caused by pupillary block or phacomorphic angle closure. This surgical procedure is done in the operating room and can be scheduled urgently in the case of sight threatening increased IOP and/or failure to relieve the angle closure with LPI.

In the emergency setting, it is important to know when to refer urgently to ophthalmology for an intervention such as an LPI. Generally speaking, any patient with suspected angle closure and high IOP should have an ophthalmology consultation. If IOP can successfully be lowered in the ED, this consultation could theoretically be delayed until the following day, but, ideally, the ophthalmologist should be notified on the same day. Urgent evaluation and definitive treatment such as an LPI is to avoid irreversible ischemic damage to intraocular structures that can be caused by high IOP.

TIPS AND PEARLS

- **Knowing the patient's refractive error is key in assessing their risk of angle closure.** Most patients with acute angle closure glaucoma are hyperopic, or farsighted. Angle closure is rare in patients who are myopic, or nearsighted, or who are emmetropic, or do not wear glasses. A simple way to assess this is to look at print or an object through the patient's glasses. If the object is magnified, the patient is hyperopic. Keep in mind that all over-the-counter reading glasses will magnify images, and this discussion pertains mainly to patients' prescription glasses.
- **It is unlikely for a patient who has had cataract surgery to have angle closure.** This is because the intraocular lens implant is far thinner than the crystalline (natural) lens. After cataract surgery and intraocular lens implantation, the convex surface of the cataract is eliminated, and aqueous can flow freely through the pupil and out of the drainage angle anteriorly. One can assess for pseudophakia (when a patient has had cataract surgery and has an artificial lens) by shining a penlight across a patient's pupil moving from laterally to medially. In pseudophakic patients, there is a shiny, reflective appearance to the pupil, whereas a phakic patient (natural lens/cataract) will exhibit a dark, jet black appearance to the pupil if there is no cataract formation and a yellow or milky appearance to the pupil if there is a cataract present. **Figures 47.3** and **47.4** demonstrate this difference in the same patient, who is pseudophakic in her right eye (Figure 47.3) and phakic in the left (Figure 47.4).

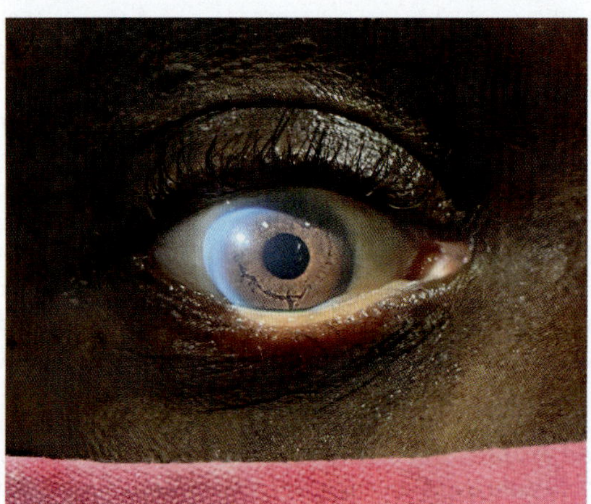

Figure 47.3: Pseudophakic eye: reflective appearance to pupil. (Courtesy of Dr. Sandra Fernando Sieminski.)

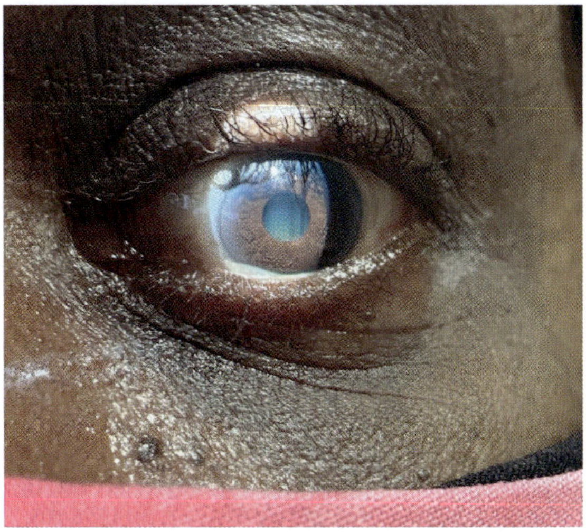

Figure 47.4: Phakic eye: milky appearance to pupil. (Courtesy of Dr. Sandra Fernando Sieminski.)

- **Looking at the contralateral eye can provide useful information.** Typically, patients who present with acute angle closure have a predisposition for angle closure in the contralateral eye. This is because there is usually a very high level of symmetry between eye measurements such as axial length, lens thickness, and anterior chamber depth.[9] Therefore, if a patient presents with suspected acute angle closure but corneal edema precludes an adequate view of the anterior chamber, one can assess the likelihood of angle closure if the contralateral eye has a large cataract or a shallow anterior chamber.
- **Remember the ABC's of IOP lowering:** Alpha-adrenergic agonists, beta-blockers, and carbonic anhydrase inhibitors.

EVIDENCE

Why is there such a large ethnic variation in the prevalence of angle closure glaucoma?

Asians have the highest prevalance of primary angle closure glaucoma (PACG) with the exception of the Inuit people. It is unclear why Asians have this predeliction, given the lack of high-quality epidemiologic data. There are theories that Asian populations are more prone to having a plateau iris, an anteriorly positioned ciliary body, or a shallow anterior chamber, all of which places them at higher risk for angle closure glaucoma; however, this has not been borne out in the literature.[10]

Do dilating drops precipitate angle closure?

The evidence is mixed. In the Baltimore Eye Survey, which surveyed 4870 multiracial urban patients who were dilated for a screening ophthalmologic examination, none developed acute angle closure glaucoma. However, 38 of those patients who were referred for definitive ophthalmologic examination were found to have occludable angles, or angles that appeared very narrow.[11] In patients who had narrow angles and visually significant cataract, Zhao et al. found the risk of precipitating angle closure was very low. In this study, 78 patients at risk were dilated and observed for 6 hours post dilation. There were some patients who had an increase in IOP post dilation but none developed acute angle closure glaucoma. They hypothesized that the dilating agents (0.5% tropicamide and 0.5% phenylephrine) caused relaxation of the ciliary muscle, leading to posterior displacement of the lens-iris diaphragm and a deepening of the angle.[12] In contrast, Chua et al. found that 1 in 5 acute angle closure glaucoma cases found in an active surveillance study in Scotland were precipitated by dilating drops for retinal examination.[13] However, the overall rate of angle closure in Scotland is 2.2 out of 100 000 people. This remains an area of controversy without definitive answers. But the overall low incidence of angle closure induced from dilating drops in the literature should reassure practitioners that dilating a patient is unlikely to harm them, unless there is a high suspicion of angle closure.

References

1. Weinreb RN, Aung T, Medeiros FA. The pathophysiology and treatment of glaucoma: a review. *JAMA*. 2014;311(18):1901-1911.
2. Prum BE, Herndon LW, Moroi SE, et al. Primary angle closure preferred practice pattern® guidelines. *Ophthalmology*. 2016;123(1):P1-P40.
3. Yang MC, Lin KY. Drug-induced acute angle-closure glaucoma: a review. *J Curr Glaucoma Pract*. 2019;13(3):104-109.
4. Flores-Sánchez BC, Tatham AJ. Acute angle closure glaucoma. *Br J Hosp Med (Lond)*. 2019;80(12):C174-C179.
5. Rojanapongpun P, Suwanpimolkul O. Acute intraocular pressure rise. In: Shaarawy T, Sherwood M, Hitchings R, Crowston J, eds. *Glaucoma*. 2nd ed. Elsevier; 2015:598-608.
6. Baum J, Chaturvedi N, Netland PA, Dreyer EB. Assessment of intraocular pressure by palpation. *Am J Ophthalmol*. 1995;119(5):650-651.
7. Ehlers JP, Shah CP. *The Wills Eye Manual: Office and Emergency Room Diagnosis and Treatment of Eye Disease*. Lippincott Williams & Wilkins; 2008.
8. Chan PP, Pang JC, Tham CC. Acute primary angle closure-treatment strategies, evidences and economical considerations. *Eye*. 2019;33:110-119.
9. Li Y, Bao FJ. Interocular symmetry analysis of bilateral eyes. *J Med Eng Technol*. 2014;38(4):179-187.
10. Zhang X, Liu Y, Wang W, et al. Potential risk factors for acute primary angle closure. *Surv Ophthalmol*. 2017;62(5):635-647.
11. Patel KH, Javitt JC, Tielsch JM, et al. Incidence of acute angle closure glaucoma after pharmacological mydriasis. *Am J Ophthalmolol*. 1995;120(6):709-717.
12. Zhao M, Sun Q, Oatts J. Changes in intraocular pressure and angle structure after dilation in primary angle-closure suspects with visually significant cataract. *Ophthalmology*. 2021;128(1):39-47.
13. Chua PY, Day AC, Lai KL, et al. The incidence of acute angle closure in Scotland: a prospective surveillance study. *Br J Ophthalmol*. 2018;102(4):539-543.

CHAPTER 48

Pupils

Paul Y. Ko
Melissa W. Ko

THE CLINICAL CHALLENGE

A comprehensive understanding of a quick yet thorough pupillary exam is essential, because recognition of abnormal pupillary findings may be the first sign of an underlying or impending serious neurologic condition. Reliable automated measurement of pupils, or pupillometry, is now commonly utilized in intensive care settings because abnormal changes in pupil reactivity may be an early indicator of elevations in intracranial pressure (ICP).[1]

Some clinicians often reflexively write the acronym "PERRLA" as shorthand for the pupils being equally round and reactive to light and accommodation without too much thought about the localization of the accommodation. When you observe pupils that do not react to light, but do react to near response, that is termed "light-near dissociation." Conditions with light-near dissociation that more commonly present in the emergent setting will be discussed in the "Differential Diagnoses" section.

PATHOPHYSIOLOGY

The functions of the pupil include titrating the quantity of light reaching the retina, increasing the depth of field, and minimizing spherical aberrations. Whereas the dilator muscle of the iris contracts to enlarge the pupil, the sphincter muscle contracts to constrict the pupil. The normal pupillary light reflex is a parasympathetically mediated response that results in bilateral pupillary constriction when light is shined into the eyes. The afferent arc of the pupillary light reflex begins when light enters the eyes, causing retinal photoreceptors to hyperpolarize, leading to pathways that activate retinal ganglion cells (RGC). The activated RGC axons travel through the optic nerve, chiasm, and optic tract to reach the pretectal nuclei located in the midbrain. Through interneurons, the pretectal nuclei connect to the Edinger-Westphal nuclei, where efferent parasympathetic fibers leave the midbrain within CN III and enter the subarachnoid space. The pupillary fibers generally run along the external surface within the third nerve, making them susceptible to compression or infiltration. Hence, as noted later in this chapter, compression of the third nerve by a posterior communicating artery aneurysm (PCoA) oftentimes manifests with pupillary involvement, clinically presenting as an ipsilateral mydriatic pupil along with ptosis and motility defects.

The near pupillary response, where a pupil will constrict when a patient views a near target, includes the triad of pupillary constriction, accommodation (lens shape change), and convergence of the eyes. The supranuclear control of the near response is unknown but is thought to be cortical in origin with downstream connections to the superior colliculus (accommodation/miosis), mesencephalic reticular formation (accommodation/vergence), and raphe interpositus (visual fixation).[3] The Edinger-Westphal nuclei mediate the last step of pupillary miosis in the near response.

Anisocoria

The causes of anisocoria are broad, and it is important to consider the various potential etiologies and correlate them with the patient's clinical presentation. Physiologic anisocoria, also known as simple anisocoria, can be seen in up to 19% of the population at any given time,[2] although the difference is usually less than 0.4 mm between the two pupils. This is the most common cause of anisocoria. The patient has normal pupillary functions on testing with little to no difference in net change of the pupil size between light and dark settings (**Figure 48.1**). Viewing an old photograph or a driver's license to see if the anisocoria was present previously can be helpful and reassuring.[3]

A structural defect in the iris can cause abnormal pupillary shape and anisocoria. There are various congenital conditions that can lead to this, particularly in the pediatric population. Additionally, acquired ocular defects causing anisocoria include trauma, inflammatory changes (eg, iritis), iris sphincter atrophy, an intraocular tumor, or angle-closure glaucoma.[3] This is often suggested by the clinical presentation (ie, vision loss, ocular pain, or redness associated with acute glaucoma).

APPROACH/THE FOCUSED EXAM

Every pupil exam begins with inspection. An estimate of pupillary size in both eyes can be done quickly with direct visualization. Pupillary size is often difficult to gauge, so use of a pocket eye chart is helpful to document (in mm) the size of the pupil in bright and dimly lit settings. Specific care should be taken to identify the shape of the pupils and, potentially, any difference in size. Any potential pupillary shape that is not round should warrant further investigation with a slit-lamp evaluation.[3]

The examination of the pupil's reactivity to light should be evaluated. In a dim setting, direct the patient to look off into the distance to avoid the miosis that occurs with near viewing. Using a bright flashlight, observe the direct response of the pupil to the light and repeat with the fellow eye. Observe the consensual response of each eye. The briskness of the pupils' reactivity to light should be noted (3+ normal brisk reaction, 2+ slightly sluggish, 1+ sluggish). Reactivity to light testing is followed by the swinging flashlight test. The swinging flashlight test is performed by rapidly alternating the light source (1-second intervals) between each eye to assess for a relative afferent pupillary defect (RAPD). The RAPD is detected by an asymmetric pupil response to direct light. In a patient with a RAPD, when the light is swung to the abnormal eye, both pupils dilate owing to less afferent input reaching the midbrain.[3] When the light is swung back to the normal eye, both eyes will constrict. This should direct the examiner to consider a unilateral optic nerve or retinal process in the eye that dilates with direct light (**Figure 48.2**). Less frequently, one can see an RAPD with chiasmal, optic tract, or midbrain lesions. Oftentimes, the RAPD is graded with a numerical system whereby 1+RAPD OD means there is initial constriction, but early redilation of the affected pupil;

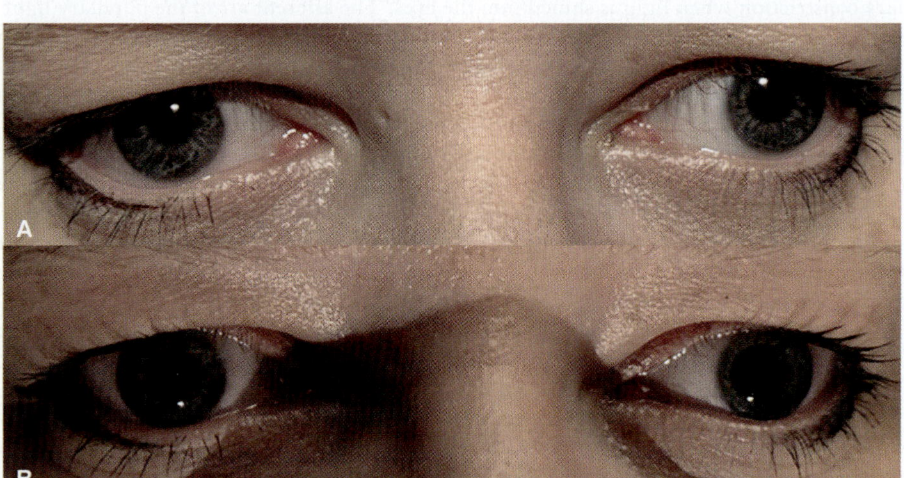

Figure 48.1: Physiologic anisocoria. The net difference in pupillary size is relatively the same in (A) bright light and (B) the dark.

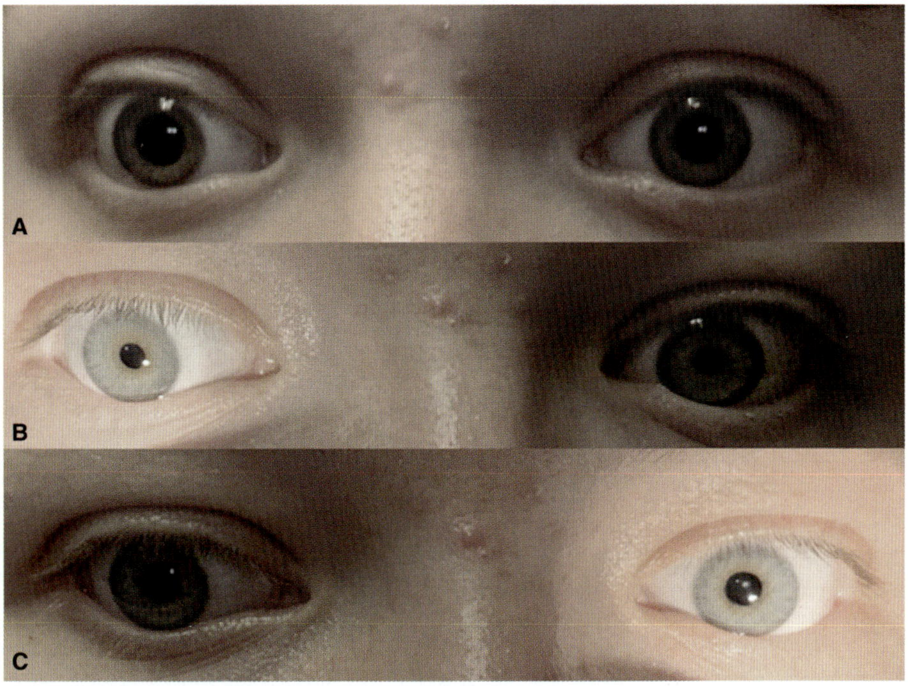

Figure 48.2: Afferent pupillary defect (left eye). A, Pupil sizes are equal at rest in ambient lighting. B, Bright light directed at the good right eye leads to brisk bilateral response of pupillary constriction. C, Bright light directed at the affected left eye with optic neuropathy results in a relative weaker pupillary constriction and both eyes dilated.

2+ RAPD translates to no initial pupil movement, then dilation; 3+ indicates immediate redilation; and 4+ means the pupil is amaurotic (blind).[3] A general approach to the patient with anisocoria is outlined in **Figure 48.3**. Of note, the testing strategies using pharmacologic ophthalmic drops noted in the approach are primarily for reference. The clinical assumption is that the ED or urgent care physician observing these pupillary abnormalities will involve an ophthalmologist or neuro-ophthalmologist in timely consultation for guidance in diagnosis, management, and treatment of the pupillary abnormalities. Therefore, the management strategies listed in what follows will focus primarily on settings when neuroimaging is considered critical and time sensitive such that delay in recognition may cause permanent neurologic deficits.

DIFFERENTIAL DIAGNOSIS AND ASSOCIATED MANAGEMENT

The approach to anisocoria begins with identifying whether the small pupil is abnormal or the larger pupil is abnormal and is helpful in identifying the differential etiologies.

When the Abnormal Pupil Is Small

The small pupil is deemed abnormal when it does not dilate as well as the larger one in dim light. The etiology of an abnormal small pupil anisocoria can include ocular (eg, iridocyclitis or prior ocular surgery), pharmacologic (eg, owing to a constricting drop such as pilocarpine), or neurologic (ie, dysfunction from the ipsilateral sympathetic system as in Horner syndrome).[4,5]

Horner Syndrome

Horner syndrome results from a lesion along the sympathetic pathway, which begins in the brain at the level of the hypothalamus and extends through the brainstem and upper spinal cord before making a U-turn at the lung apex and routing onto the internal carotid artery toward the orbit. It has the classic clinical presentation triad of ptosis, miosis, and anhidrosis. The examiner may also note dilation lag, which is the observation that in a dim setting the involved sympathetically denervated pupil takes longer to reach a dilated resting state in the dark compared with the normal

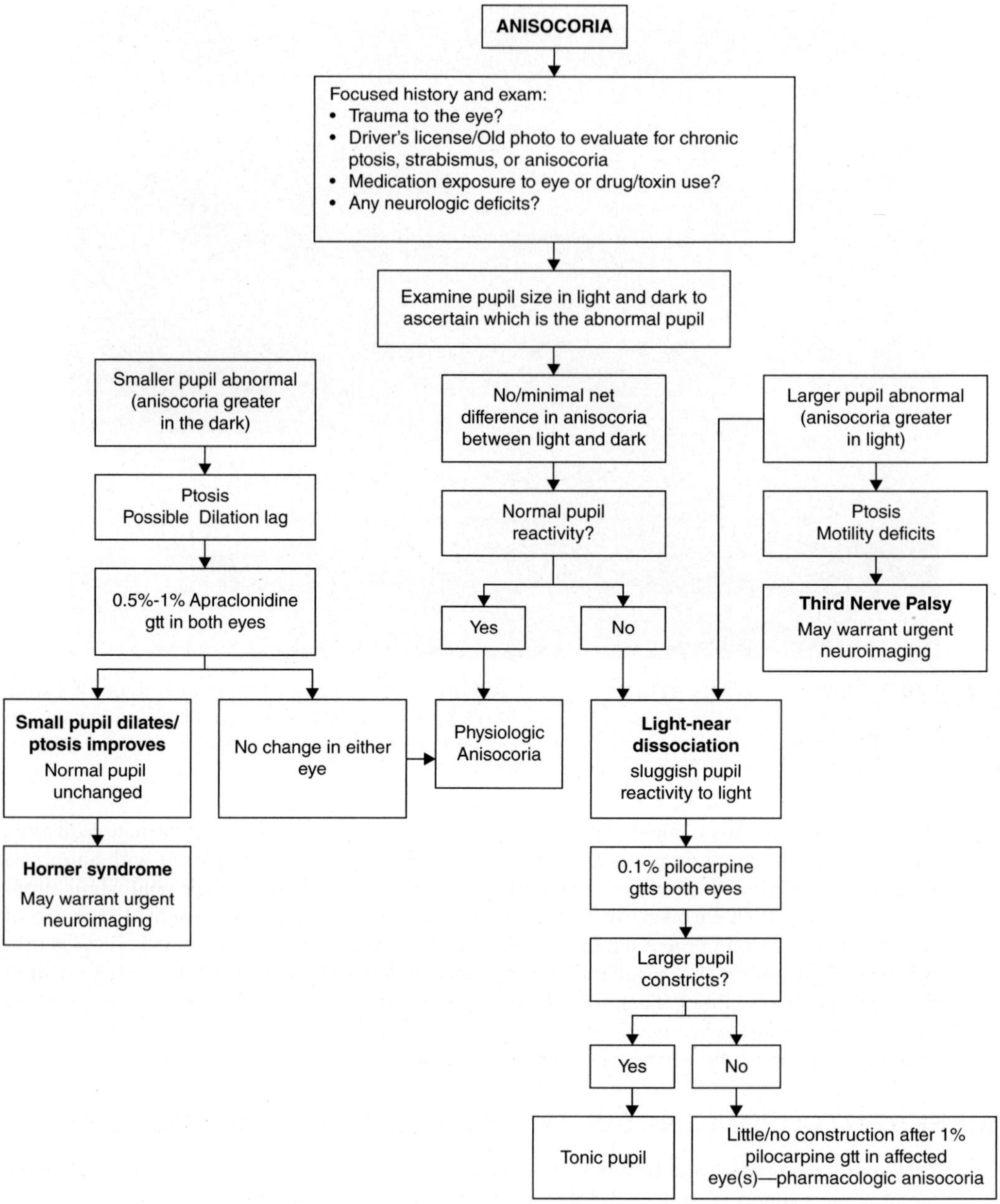

Figure 48.3: A general approach to the patient with anisocoria.

pupil, which quickly dilates when the lights are turned off. The ptosis noted in Horner syndrome is typically mild and does not obstruct the visual axis of the patient. Visual acuity is not affected in Horner syndrome. The cause of a Horner can be unknown (up to 40% of presentations), a first order central lesion, a second-order preganglionic etiology, or a third-order postganglionic etiology.

A common cause of a primary/first-order central lesion would be a stroke, tumor, or demyelinating lesion of the central system. The most common cause is a lateral medullary infarction that may be seen in Wallenberg syndrome (**Figure 48.4**). Patients often present with severe ataxia and vertigo. There may also be associated abnormal eye movement and the classic sensory loss (pain/temperature loss in the ipsilateral face and contralateral trunk). A thorough neurologic exam will usually identify other central presentations in this etiology. If there is injury to the spinal cord that

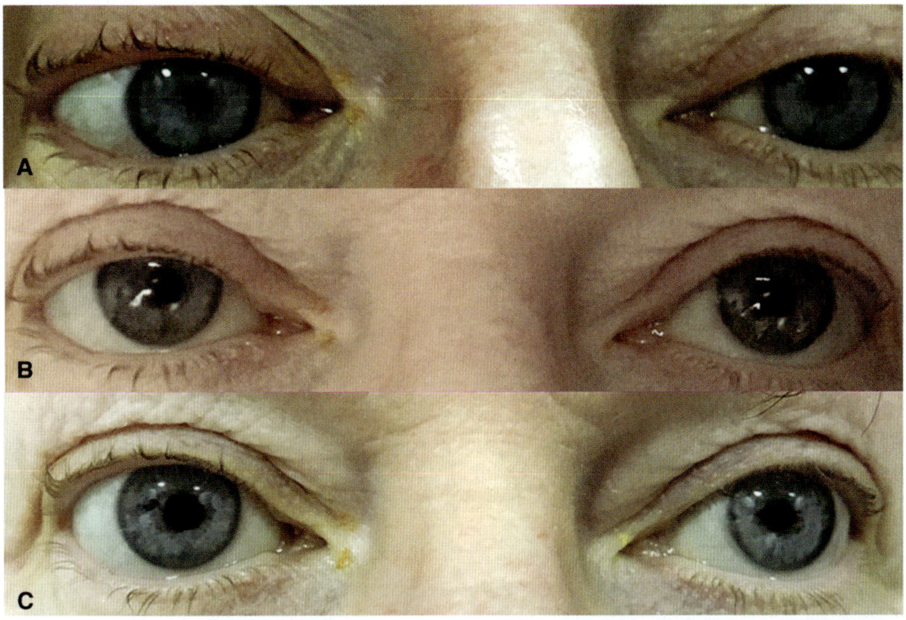

Figure 48.4: Right Horner syndrome caused by Wallenberg stroke. Patient presented with diplopia, dysarthria, ataxia, and numbness. A, In bright light, note the right miotic pupil (examiner lifting ptotic right lid). B, In dim light, the anisocoria is more apparent. C, Following topical administration of 0.5% apraclonidine to both eyes, the alpha-adrenergic receptor agonist leads to pupillary dilation of the affected right eye and resolution of ptosis owing to sympathetic stimulation of hypersensitive alpha-1 receptors on the pupillary dilator muscle. The normal left pupil does not react to the apraclonidine.

impacts the descending sympathetic pathway (C9-T2), this can also lead to an acquired Horner syndrome ipsilateral to the spinal cord process. Trauma, syringomyelia, infarction, myelitis and tumors with accompanying clinical features of a sensory level, urinary or bowel issues, quadriparesis/paraparesis, and Babinski signs may be present.

Second-order Horner (preganglionic etiology) can be seen with trauma or surgery of the spinal cord, lung apex, or thoracic outlet region. A second-order Horner can also be seen with pharmacologic etiology in an obstetric patient who recently received a lumbar epidural anesthesia, and this is usually temporary and self resolves within a few hours.[3]

A third-order (postganglionic etiology) Horner should cause one to consider lesions of the internal carotid artery such as carotid artery dissection, thrombosis, or cavernous sinus aneurysm. This is considered a neurologic/neuro-ophthalmic emergency because there can be complications from stroke. Internal carotid artery dissection should be ruled out in a patient with a Horner and ipsilateral headache. Often, there is a recent history of neck trauma, although these dissections can occur spontaneously.

Of note, a Horner can also be seen in a patient with cluster headache, often presenting with a headache, unilateral eye pain, and lachrymation. When present, these symptoms typically do not last more than a few hours. In infants and children, congenital cases of Horner syndrome may be associated with iris heterochromia (iris color is lighter) on the involved side. A Horner in a child should cause one to think about a congenital, birth trauma; congenital infection; neuroblastoma, and vascular etiologies.

When the Abnormal Pupil Is Large

Third Nerve Palsy

The third nerve palsy (TNP) is considered a potential neurologic/neuro-ophthalmic emergency because it may indicate the presence of a PCoA compressing against the oculomotor nerve or uncal herniation. When describing a TNP, it can be either complete or partial and pupil involving or sparing. A complete TNP has ipsilateral ptosis with motility deficits including ipsilateral inability to elevate, adduct, or depress the involved eye. When lifting the ptotic lid, the examiner will often see a mydriatic pupil with a "down and out" eye (**Figure 48.5**) owing to unopposed and intact abduction and hypodeviation. Partial TNP refers to incomplete palsies of eye motility. As suggested by the description, a pupil involving TNP describes a pupil that is mydriatic and less reactive to light, whereas pupil sparing is a normal-sized and reactive pupil. Although aneurysmal compression typically causes a painful and complete TNP, because there can be pupil sparing or partial TNPs owing to an aneurysm, one must have a high degree of clinical suspicion. Although more than a third of patients with a PCoA develop a TNP, 90% of such patients present with TNP and subarachnoid hemorrhage *before* aneurysmal rupture.[6] Ordering an urgent CT angiogram of the head *and* directing the reading neuroradiologist to specifically evaluate for a PCoA or aneurysm caused by TNP is critical because small ones can be missed.

Uncal Herniation

When a patient has a TNP and altered mental status, this should raise concern for uncal herniation. The uncus, located at the anterior and medial portion of the temporal lobe, can compress the third nerve in settings of rising ICP. The first sign of uncal herniation is ipsilateral pupillary dilation. As the condition progresses, the patient's level of consciousness will further decrease, and an initial

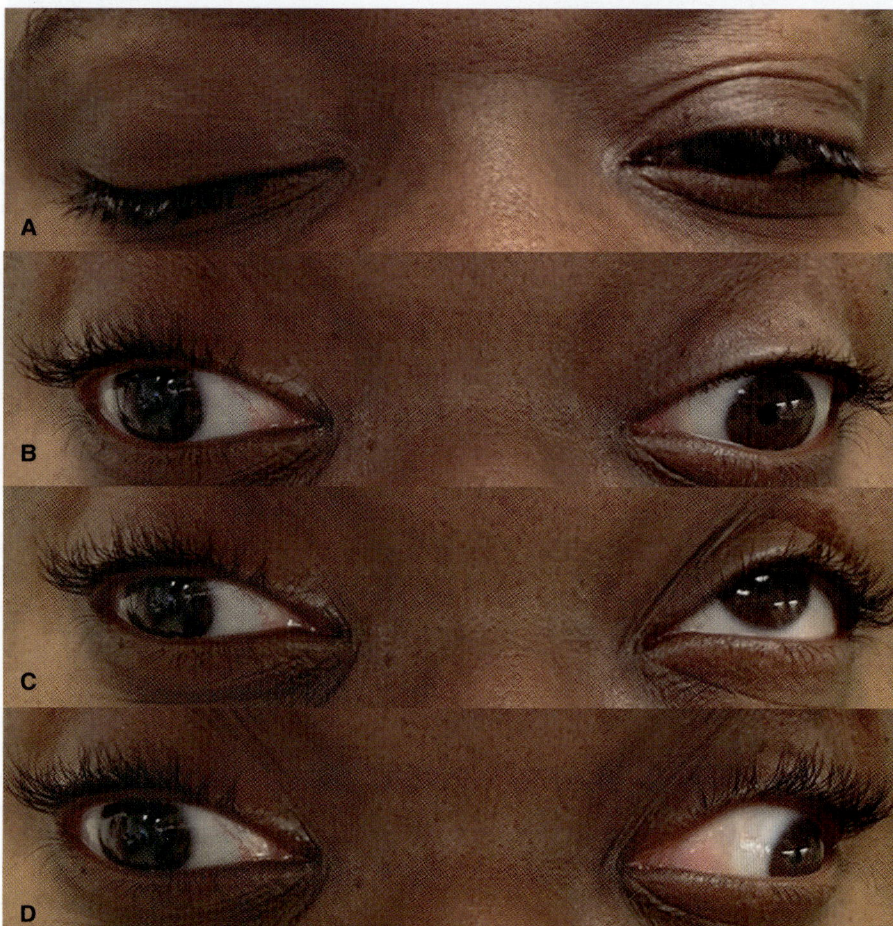

Figure 48.5: Pupil-involving third nerve palsy owing to a posterior communicating artery aneurysm (A). The ptotic right eyelid is being elevated, demonstrating the "down and out" exotropic and hypotropic right eye with a dilated right pupil (B-D).

partial TNP becomes complete along with ipsilateral hemiplegia and a Babinski response. One should monitor the contralateral pupil because it may become increasingly involved, first as mid-position with less reactivity to light, then miotic, and, finally, dilated. Oval-shaped pupils can also be seen as brain herniation progresses.

Tonic Pupils

A tonic pupil (Adie pupil) is one that does not readily constrict to light but does accommodate to near response. It is caused by parasympathetic denervation at the level of ciliary ganglion and is one of the key items on the differential diagnosis for light-near dissociation. Most cases of a tonic pupil are idiopathic in etiology and more commonly affect women with a mean age in the 30s. Other causes include inflammation or infection, ischemia, trauma (both surgical and nonsurgical), toxicity (eg, quinine), local anesthesia (eg, inferior dental block), or paraneoplastic syndromes. A tonic pupil can be distinguished from other etiologies via pharmacologic testing with dilute pilocarpine drops in both eyes. If the involved pupil is a tonic pupil, there will be iris sphincter denervation hypersensitivity to the cholinergic properties of dilute pilocarpine, but the unaffected eye will have little or no response at dilute concentrations. An Argyll Robertson pupil (seen in neurosyphilis) may be confused with a tonic pupil.[5] With an Argyll Robertson pupil, the affected pupil(s) is small, whereas the classic tonic pupil is large. Although both conditions demonstrate light-near dissociation, the Argyll Robertson pupil will constrict to accommodation and quickly redilate when removed from the near response. In contrast, a tonic pupil stays constricted and only dilates slowly when exposed to the dark. A tonic pupil is generally benign and no treatment is needed.

Pharmacologically Dilated Pupil

When a healthy, fully oriented and neurologically intact patient presents with a dilated pupil (greater than 7-8 mm) that does not react to light *or* near testing, consider exposure of the eye (accidental or intentional) to a pharmacologic agent. Careful history taking for possible exposure to sympathomimetic or anticholinergic medications/agents may reveal the source. Common agents include ipratropium, atropine, or scopolamine patches. Topical administration of 1% pilocarpine will fail to constrict pharmacologically dilated pupils (30 minutes after instillation in eyes) but will constrict normal pupils, mydriatic pupils caused by TNP, and tonic pupils. Of note, patients with a traumatic injury to the iris or acute narrow-angle glaucoma will not constrict with pilocarpine. Additionally, if the pharmacologic medication is starting to wear off, the involved pupil will constrict with pilocarpine. Unlike a tonic pupil, which has light-near dissociation with reaction to near intact, the pharmacologically dilated pupil will not constrict with near targets. One can readily distinguish the pharmacologically dilated pupil from a TNP because there should be exam findings of ptosis and motility deficits with a TNP.

TIPS AND PEARLS

- Be sure you are standing symmetrically in front of the patient and aligned with the patient's visual axis. If the light source is too close to either the right or the left eye, it may lead you to a false RAPD.
- Do not confuse hippus, a benign, rhythmic variation of dilation and contraction of the pupils, with an RAPD. The pupil size is never fully at rest but can have normal small transient fluctuations in pupil size that can become more apparent when an examiner uses a flashlight.
- The authors prefer to perform the swinging flashlight across the bridge of the nose rather than swing under the chin of the patient because subtle early release of a pupil or a subtle RAPD may be missed in the time you are swinging under the chin.
- Even if the patient has only one working pupil, you can still check for an RAPD by observing the consensual response of the "good" contralateral eye. For example, if a patient has a fixed and dilated pupil with poor vision on the right, swing the light to the right "bad" eye while observing the good left pupil. If the left pupil dilates as a consensual response to the direct light on the right eye, this reveals a right RAPD detected on reverse testing.
- Although Horner syndrome and TNP are both associated with ptosis, the ptosis of a Horner is mild, whereas the ptosis of a TNP is severe and covers the patient's visual axis.

EVIDENCE

Do patients with third nerve palsies require neuroimaging, even when the patient has known vascular risk factors for stroke?

A prospective article by Tamhankar et al.[7] looked at this very question. It was a multicenter observational case series of 109 patients presenting with isolated third, fourth, or sixth cranial nerve palsies and found that the presence of one or more vascular risk factors (ie, diabetes, hypertension, hyperlipidemia, smoking, stroke, or coronary artery disease [CAD] history) was significantly associated with a microvascular cause of the palsies. Up to 10% of these patients (with no other medical conditions associated) were found to have a cause including midbrain infarct, neoplasm, inflammation, pituitary apoplexy, or giant cell arteritis. Therefore, the authors of this study recommended that in these patients those with vascular risk factors, neuroimaging (ie, magnetic resonance angiography [MRA] brain or CT head angiogram), and laboratory workup should be considered.

Do patients with Horner syndrome require neuroimaging studies?

A retrospective study by Sadaka et al.[8] evaluated 200 adult patients with Horner syndrome presenting in an outpatient setting. In this cohort, MRI imaging showed causative lesions in about 12% and idiopathic in 69%. Approximately 9% of the patients imaged had a serious pathology such as carotid dissection or brain or neck mass. Of those patients with serious pathology, only approximately a third had acute symptoms and/or pain. This study suggested that although most patients presenting with Horner syndrome are idiopathic and have no serious underlying etiology, the importance of ruling out serious pathology, even in the absence of acute symptoms, may be warranted, particularly in those presenting with acute onset of symptoms and/or pain.

References

1. Jahns FP, Miroz JP, Messerer M, et al. Quantitative pupillometry for the monitoring of intracranial hypertension in patients with severe traumatic brain injury. *Crit Care*. 2019;23(1):155. doi:10.1186/s13054-019-2436-3. PMID: 31046817; PMCID: PMC6498599.
2. Lam BL, Thompson HS, Corbett JJ. The prevalence of simple anisocoria. *Am J Ophthalmol*. 1987;104(1):69.
3. Liu GT, Galetta SL. The neuro-ophthamologic examination (including coma). *Ophthalmol Clin North Am*. 2001;14:23-39.
4. Chambers DJ, Bhatia K. Horner's syndrome following obstetric neuraxial blockade—a systematic review of the literature. *Int J Obstet Anesth*. 2018;35:75-87. doi:10.1016/j.ijoa.2018.03.005. Epub 2018 Mar 17. PMID: 29657082.
5. Thompson HS, Kardon RH. The Argyll Robertson pupil. *J Neuro-Ophthalmol*. 2006;26(2):134-138. doi:10.1097/01.wno.0000222971.09745.91
6. Kupersmith MJ. *Neuro-vascular Neuro-ophthalmology*. Springer-Verlag; 1993:1-554.
7. Tamhankar MA, Biousse V, Ying GS, et al. Isolated third, fourth, and sixth cranial nerve palsies from presumed microvascular versus other causes: a prospective study. *Ophthalmology*. 2013;120(11):2264-2269. doi:10.1016/j.ophtha.2013.04.009. Epub 2013 Jun 6. PMID: 23747163; PMCID: PMC3795864.
8. Sadaka, A, Schockman, SL, Golnik KC. Evaluation of Horner syndrome in the MRI era. *J Neuro-Ophthalmol*. 2017;37(3):268-272. doi:10.1097/WNO.0000000000000503

CHAPTER 49

Diplopia

Zoe Williams
Jonathan Strong

THE CLINICAL CHALLENGE

Diplopia—colloquially referred to as "double vision"—is a challenging chief complaint in the emergency and urgent care setting. It is also an infrequent chief complaint in the emergency and urgent care setting, representing 0.1% of all ED visits.[1] Diplopia may occur from a wide spectrum of pathologies including many benign causes (e.g. decompensated phoria, convergence or divergence insufficiency, and microvascular disease) as well as vision- or lifethreatening causes (e.g. stroke, cerebral aneurysm, brain tumor, intracranial hemorrhage, thyroid eye disease, giant cell arteritis, myasthenia gravis, meningitis, cavernous sinus thrombosis, or increased intracranial pressure). Structural lesions causing diplopia may localize to the cortical, subcortex, brainstem, subarachnoid, cavernous sinus or orbital level. A comprehensive review of all causes of diplopia is beyond the scope of this chapter, but several important causes to consider in the emergency and urgent care settings are listed in **Table 49-1**.

The clinician should first determine whether the diplopia is monocular or binocular. Monocular diplopia is confirmed when covering the unaffected eye does not resolve the diplopia. This strongly suggests a single eye problem such as dry eye, refractive error, corneal pathology, cataract, or retinal disease. These patients warrant a thorough eye exam, but monocular diplopia is generally not an emergency.

In contrast, binocular diplopia resolves with occlusion of either eye indicating misalignment of the visual axes. This chapter describes the evaluation of binocular diplopia (henceforth referred to as diplopia) with an emphasis on identifying emergent disease entities that clinicians must consider.

PATHOPHYSIOLOGY

A brief review of the neuroanatomy of eye movement is helpful to recognize patterns of extraocular muscle weakness, identify cranial nerve (CN) palsies, and localize structural lesions. The eye moves in three axes: horizontal (adduction and abduction), vertical (supraduction and infraduction), and torsional (intorsion and extorsion).

CN III (oculomotor nerve) originates from the dorsal midbrain and innervates four of the six extraocular muscles: the medial rectus, inferior rectus, inferior oblique muscles (inferior division), and superior rectus (superior division). Motor fibers of the superior division also innervate the levator muscle of the eyelid. In addition, CN III contains parasympathetic fibers on the periphery that control pupil constriction, making them susceptible to compressive lesions. Patients with a complete CN III palsy present with ptosis and the inability to supraduct, infraduct, or adduct the eye. As a result, the affected eye will display exotropia and hypotropia (the "down and out" position) (**Figure 49.1**). An incomplete CN III palsy will present with varying degrees of weakness in each of the extraocular muscles and/or levator palpebrae. It is important to note that complete and incomplete refer only to the motor function of CN III. The parasympathetic fibers act independently, and thus patients with complete or incomplete CN III palsy may or may not have pupil involvement.

CN IV (trochlear nerve) possesses the longest intracranial length, making it particularly susceptible to injury. It originates from the dorsal midbrain and ultimately innervates a single extraocular muscle, the superior oblique. A patient with CN IV palsy may display hypertropia and excyclotorsion in the affected eye; however, these deficits are often not readily apparent on gross examination owing to the compensatory effect of other extraocular muscles (**Figure 49.2**). To diagnose an isolated unilateral CN IV palsy, the examiner should assess whether the hypertropia in the affected eye worsens with gaze toward the contralateral side and with head tilt toward the ipsilateral side (the Parks-Bielschowsky method). One should note, however, that the sensitivity

TABLE 49.1 Selected Causes of Diplopia

Demyelinating disease Guillain-Barré syndrome (Miller Fisher variant) Multiple sclerosis	**Neuromuscular junction disease** Botulism Myasthenia gravis
Hematologic Intracranial hemorrhage Cavernous sinus thrombosis	**Toxic, metabolic** Wernicke-Korsakoff syndrome Tick paralysis Neurotoxic envenomation (eg, coral snake)
Infectious Meningitis Orbital cellulitis Intracranial abscess Invasive fungal infection (eg, mucormyosis)	**Traumatic** Decompensated phoria Extraocular muscle entrapment/orbit fracture Direct extraocular muscle injury Orbital compartment syndrome/retrobulbar hematoma CN injury (direct or secondary to mass effect or elevated ICP) Carotid-cavernous fistula
Inflammatory, infiltrative, vasculitic Tolosa-Hunt syndrome Orbital myositis Giant cell arteritis Granulomatosis with polyangiitis Sarcoidosis	**Vascular** Ischemic stroke Microvascular ischemia Intracranial aneurysm Cervical artery dissection
Neoplastic Primary intracranial tumor (including pituitary apoplexy) Metastatic disease (including perineural spread and carcinomatous meningitis) Tumors of the cavernous sinus or orbital apex	**Other** Recurrent painful ophthalmoplegic neuropathy (ophthalmoplegic migraine) Thyroid eye disease Elevated ICP (including idiopathic intracranial hypertension) Spontaneous intracranial hypotension Adult divergence insufficiency Heavy eye syndrome Convergence insufficiency

ICP, intracranial pressure.

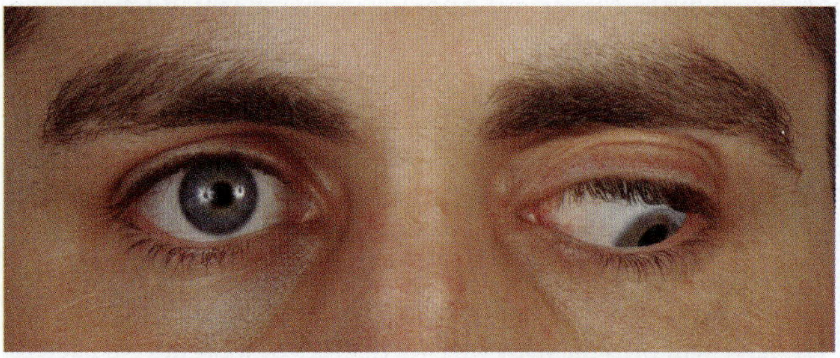

Figure 49.1: Left oculomotor (CN III) nerve palsy. (From Agur AM, Dalley AF. *Moore's Essential Clinical Anatomy*. 6th ed. Wolters Kluwer; 2020. UnFigure 8.11.)

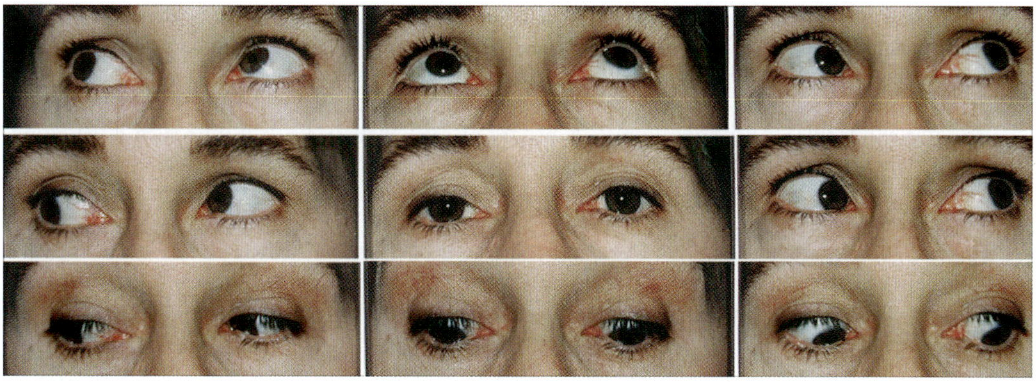

Figure 49.2: Trochlear nerve palsy of the left eye. (Images courtesy of Jason Peragallo, MD. In: Sherman SC, Ross C, Nordquist E, Wang E, Cico S, eds. *Atlas of Clinical Emergency Medicine*. 1st ed. Wolters Kluwer; 2016. Figure 2.19.)

and specificity of this combination of findings is limited.[2–4] If the hypertropia does not follow this characteristic pattern, one should consider alternative causes.

CN VI (abducens nerve) originates from the pons and ultimately innervates the lateral rectus muscle. A patient with an isolated unilateral CN VI palsy will display esotropia most apparent on ipsilateral gaze and/or inability to abduct the affected eye fully (**Figure 49.3**). Elevated intracranial pressure caused by structural lesions or idiopathic intracranial hypertension may cause traction on CN VI as it travels along the clivus, resulting in unilateral or bilateral CN VI palsy.

Diplopia in the setting of head trauma may be caused by decompensated phoria, convergence insufficiency, CN palsies (CN III, IV, VI paresis) attributable to stretch injury, hemorrhage of a preexisting brain lesion with resultant compressive injury, intracranial hemorrhage, direct extraocular muscle damage, extraocular muscle entrapment attributable to orbital fracture, orbital compartment syndrome secondary to retrobulbar hematoma, or a direct carotid-cavernous fistula. Usually direct carotid-cavernous fistulas will present with other ocular signs such as arterialization of the conjunctival vessels, chemosis, proptosis, and elevated intraocular pressure in addition to diplopia; however, diplopia is occasionally the only finding. Thus, patients should be asked if they have an audible bruit suggestive of a carotid-cavernous fistula.

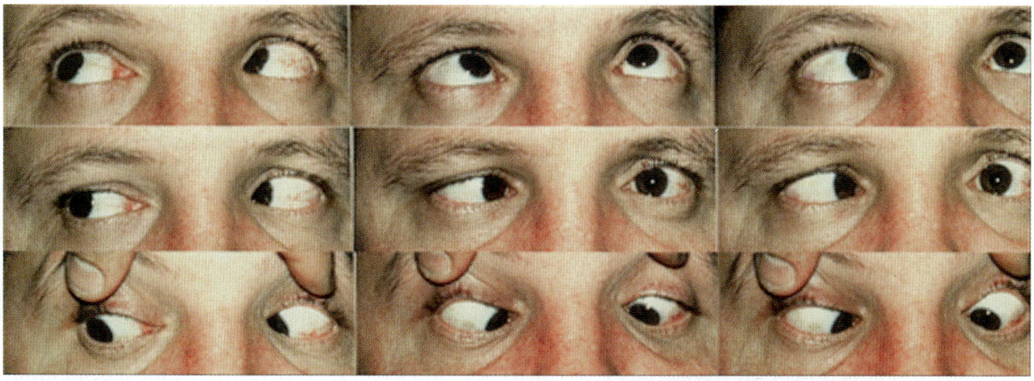

Figure 49.3: Left CNVI (abducens nerve) palsy. (Images courtesy of Jason Peragallo, MD. In: Sherman SC, Ross C, Nordquist E, Wang E, Cico S, eds. *Atlas of Clinical Emergency Medicine*. 1st ed. Wolters Kluwer; 2016. Figure 2.1.)

Patients with a history of malignancy, including skin cancer, particularly those with progressive facial numbness, paresthesias, or weakness, should be suspected to have diplopia attributable to perineural spread. Patients suffering from chronic alcoholism may develop Wernicke encephalopathy characterized by altered mental status, gait ataxia, and oculomotor dysfunction (ie, nystagmus and/or extraocular muscle weakness). A history of cardiovascular risk factors such as smoking, hypertension, hyperlipidemia, or diabetes is supportive of microvascular ischemia or vertebrobasilar insufficiency, although it is important not to assume cardiovascular risk factors exclude other serious neurologic disease.[5]

Giant cell arteritis may cause diplopia in patients over age 50. Associated systemic symptoms of giant cell arteritis (GCA) include jaw claudication, scalp tenderness, headaches, neck pain, ear pain, sudden hearing loss, myalgias, unexplained weight loss, fevers, or malaise. Rarely, patients with GCA may present with diplopia and without systemic symptoms.[5,6]

APPROACH/THE FOCUSED EXAM

History

The first step in evaluating a patient with binocular diplopia is to determine whether the patient has isolated diplopia or diplopia with additional neurologic deficits suggestive of a posterior circulation stroke. Patients presenting with acute onset diplopia in combination with altered mental status, bulbar weakness, vertigo, ataxia, or "crossed" brain stem signs (ipsilateral CN deficits with contralateral limb weakness or sensory loss) should be considered to have a brainstem stroke until proven otherwise.

The evaluation of patients with diplopia in the absence of acute onset brainstem symptoms begins with a focused history. The clinician should first determine the orientation of the diplopia (horizontal, vertical, or oblique) and whether the diplopia worsens in a particular direction of gaze. CN palsies and restrictive processes (such as thyroid eye disease or muscle entrapment by orbital fractures) cause incomitant diplopia, that is, diplopia that worsens in a particular direction of gaze corresponding with the affected extraocular muscle(s). By contrast, neuromuscular disorders such as myasthenia gravis may cause comitant (the same in all gaze directions) or incomitant diplopia.

The onset and timing of diplopia can also aid in diagnosis. Intermittent diplopia that worsens with fatigue and later in the day (diurnal fluctuation) is suggestive of myasthenia gravis. Slowly progressive diplopia may suggest a compressive cause (eg, inflammatory, infectious, neoplastic, or vascular lesions), whereas intermittent diplopia may be caused by a decompensating phoria, myasthenia gravis, or vertebrobasilar insufficiency.

Pain associated with diplopia can be seen in a wide variety of conditions. Pain localizing to the eye, periorbital area, or retrobulbar region—particularly pain that worsens with eye movement—suggests pathology of the cavernous sinus, orbit and/or extraocular muscles such as Tolosa-Hunt syndrome, thyroid eye disease, orbital pseudotumor, trochleitis, infection, or malignancy. Microvascular ischemia and optic neuritis can also cause pain in a similar distribution. Headache can be seen in giant cell arteritis, cavernous sinus thrombosis, pituitary apoplexy, intracranial aneurysm, cervical artery dissection, meningitis, malignancy, intracranial hemorrhage, and a variety of other conditions. Severe or thunderclap headache should prompt consideration of aneurysmal subarachnoid hemorrhage, which may be associated with aneurysmal compression of cranial nerves, most commonly CN III. However, it is important not to exclude serious neurologic conditions such as aneurysm if the patient has painless diplopia, because pain is an unreliable finding in many conditions.[7]

External Eye Exam

External examination for ptosis, aberrant regeneration, lid retraction, lid lag, lateral flare, enophthalmos, or proptosis can assist with localization of the pathology causing diplopia. Ipsilateral ptosis with decreased levator function in the setting of limited supraduction, infraduction, and/or adduction of the ipsilateral eye is consistent with a CN III paresis. Aberrant regeneration (eyelid elevation during adduction or infraduction of the eye, or pupillary constriction during adduction, supraduction or infraduction of the eye) is consistent with CN III paresis that is compressive or traumatic in etiology. Eyelid retraction (elevation of the upper lid margin above the superior limbus) or lid lag on downgaze (upper eyelid does not follow eye movement in downgaze) can be a sign of thyroid eye disease. Bilateral upper eyelid retraction can also be seen in dorsal midbrain syndrome. Proptosis may be a sign of thyroid eye disease or can be caused by cavernous sinus or orbital processes. Enophthalmos can be seen with orbital floor fractures or infiltrative/neoplastic disease involving the orbit.

Pupil Exam

Pupillary assessment should be performed to evaluate for anisocoria, an afferent pupillary defect or an efferent pupillary defect. Evaluation for anisocoria is performed in both bright and dim light. If the right and left pupil size are more unequal in bright light, this suggests a problem with pupillary constriction (parasympathetic dysfunction) in the eye with the larger pupil. If there is decreased pupillary constriction to light directed in the eye and a decreased consensual response to light directed into the contralateral eye, this is consistent with an efferent pupillary defect. An efferent pupillary defect in the setting of vertical or oblique diplopia with ipsilateral ocular motility limitation of adduction, supraduction or infraduction signifies a pupil involving CN III paresis, which requires urgent evaluation for a cerebral aneurysm. If, by contrast, the anisocoria is greatest in the dark, this suggests sympathetic dysfunction of the smaller pupil consistent with a Horner syndrome. A Horner syndrome in conjunction with a contralateral CN IV paresis localizes to the ipsilateral dorsal midbrain, whereas a Horner syndrome and an ipsilateral CN VI paresis localizes to the ipsilateral cavernous sinus.

After assessing for anisocoria, assessment for an afferent pupillary defect should be performed. If an afferent pupillary defect is found ipsilateral to a CN palsy or palsies causing diplopia, this signifies an orbital apex process as the cause.

Ocular Motility

Ocular motility is assessed by evaluating ocular versions (movement of both eyes) and ductions (movement of each eye separately). Versions should be assessed by asking the patient to follow the examiner's finger in right gaze, left gaze, up gaze, down gaze, up and right, up and left, down and right, and down and left. In addition, the patient should be asked to follow the examiner's finger in toward their nose to assess convergence. The ductions of each eye should be tested with monocular occlusion of the contralateral eye. In cases of suspected restrictive myopathy from thyroid eye disease or orbital fracture with entrapment, an ophthalmologist may perform forced ductions.

Saccadic testing is performed by asking the patient to look quickly from primary gaze to the examiner's finger presented to the right, left, up, and down. Slow hypometric saccades are suggestive of CN paresis. Slow saccades can also be seen with cerebellar pathology such as spinocerebellar ataxia or neurodegenerative disease such as Parkinson disease or progressive supranuclear palsy.[7] In addition, inaccuracy of saccades with over- or undershooting with corrective eye movement to target (saccadic dysmetria) should be noted because this may signify cerebellar dysfunction. Lastly, pursuit is assessed with the patient following the examiner's finger at a slow speed from primary gaze to the cardinal gazes. It should be noted whether the patient has the ability to maintain the same speed of eye movements as the examiner's finger movement (normal gain) or whether corrective "catch-up" saccades are needed. Abnormal gain can be a sign of cerebellar dysfunction or lesions of the frontal, temporal, or parietal lobes. It should be noted whether the patient has any nystagmus, because this can be of localizing value.

If there is limited motility, oculocephalic maneuver can be performed to determine whether the pathology is occurring at a prenuclear versus nuclear/infranuclear level. The oculocephalic maneuver is performed by having the patient look at the examiner's nose while the examiner moves the patient's head slowly to the right, left, upward, and downward while assessing for movement of the eyes in the opposite direction (ie, eyes move leftward on right head turn, rightward on left head turn, downward with upward movement of the head, and upward with downward movement of the head). If the limitation of ocular motility resolves with oculocephalic maneuver, this indicates a prenuclear level pathology that is overcome with stimulation of the vestibular system. If the limitation of ocular motility does not resolve with oculocephalic maneuver, the pathology localizes to either the nuclear or the infranuclear level.

Ocular Alignment

Ocular alignment should be measured in primary gaze, right gaze, left gaze, up gaze, down gaze, and at near using alternate cover testing with prism. If there is a vertical misalignment, alternate cover testing with prism should also be performed in right and left head tilt to determine whether the ocular misalignment follows the pattern of a CN IV palsy. A hyperdeviation worsening in contralateral gaze and ipsilateral head tilt is consistent with a CN IV palsy but may also be caused by a skew deviation. Laying the patient flat and having him or her fixate at a target on the ceiling with repeat alternate cover testing with prism can differentiate a CN IV paresis (ocular misalignment does not improve) from a skew deviation (ocular misalignment improves).

Anterior Segment Exam

Engorged, tortuous, "arterialized" episcleral vessels extending are highly suggestive of a carotid-cavernous fistula. There may be additional signs of chemosis and conjunctival injection as well as elevated intraocular pressure. The presence of ocular inflammation may suggest orbital pseudotumor or an alternate inflammatory, infectious (including herpes zoster), or neoplastic cause.

Cranial Nerve Testing

All patients with diplopia should undergo careful CN examination. It is essential to test, at a minimum, CN V, VII, and VIII to assist with localization of the level of pathology. Multiple cranial nerves may be affected bilaterally by a brainstem lesion or a subarachnoid level process such as infectious, inflammatory, or carcinomatous meningitis. Unilateral involvement of multiple cranial nerves suggests a cerebellopontine angle (CN VI, VII, VIII), brainstem, cavernous sinus (CN III, IV, V_1 and V_2, VI), or orbital (CN III, IV, V_1, VI) process. If CN III, IV, V_1, and VI paresis are associated with ipsilateral proptosis, a cavernous sinus or orbital process should be suspected. The presence of an ipsilateral decrease in visual acuity and CN III, IV, and VI pareses suggests an orbital apex process.

Posterior Segment Exam

All patients over age 50 presenting with new onset diplopia should have a dilated funduscopic exam to ensure there are no signs of ocular ischemia to suggest giant cell arteritis. Signs of ocular ischemia include cotton wool spots, retinal arteriolar occlusion, or ischemic optic neuropathy. Optic disc exam is also useful in the assessment of suspected orbital apex syndrome because there may be associated optic disc edema versus optic disc pallor with long-standing compression. All patients presenting with CN IV paresis or CN VI paresis should have a funduscopic exam to rule out papilledema.

Laboratory Testing

When considering GCA as the etiology of diplopia, laboratory testing with sedimentation rate, C-reactive protein, and complete blood count with platelets is appropriate. If there is any suspicion for giant cell arteritis, the patient should be empirically treated with high-dose corticosteroids pending temporal artery biopsy, and ophthalmology should be consulted to assess for any signs of ocular ischemia.

DIFFERENTIAL DIAGNOSIS

The differential diagnosis for diplopia is vast. Structural lesions at the cortical, subcortical, brainstem, cerebellum, subarachnoid, cavernous sinus, or orbital level may produce diplopia. Clinicians should narrow the differential diagnosis by localizing pathology according to the patient's history and exam findings. **Table 49.2** summarizes the localization of diplopia based on symptoms and signs as well as the suggested neuroimaging and further workup for each localization.

MANAGEMENT

Patients with an isolated ocular motor nerve palsy (ie, a single CN III, IV, or VI palsy) without other neurologic deficits often require urgent neuroimaging to assess for serious neurologic disease. Patients with isolated ocular motor nerve palsy determined to be caused by microvascular ischemia

TABLE 49.2 Localization of Pathology Causing Diplopia

Localization	Signs	Etiologies	Workup
Prenuclear/nuclear	Altered mental status, hemiparesis, upper or lower extremity sensory loss, facial weakness/sensory loss, imbalance, or ataxia	Neoplastic, ischemic, demyelinating, inflammatory, infectious	MRI brain without and with gadolinium.
Brainstem/subarachnoid space	Multiple cranial nerves with bilateral involvement	Neoplastic, ischemic, demyelinating, or inflammatory/infectious lesions OR infectious, inflammatory, or carcinomatous meningitis	MRI brain without and with gadolinium. Lumbar puncture with cell count and differential, total protein, glucose, Gram stain, aerobic culture, cytology, and flow cytometry.
Brainstem/cavernous sinus/orbit	Multiple cranial nerves with unilateral involvement: CN III, IV, V_1 and V_2, VI (brainstem or cavernous sinus) CN III, IV, V_1, VI (orbit)	Neoplastic, ischemic, demyelinating, inflammatory, infectious, vascular	MRI brain and orbits without and with gadolinium.
Cavernous sinus/orbit	CN III, IV, V_1, and VI pareses with ipsilateral proptosis	Neoplastic, inflammatory, infectious, vascular	MRI brain and orbits without and with gadolinium and with fat suppression. MRA head if carotid-cavernous fistula is suspected.
Orbital apex	CN III, IV, V_1, and VI pareses and decrease in visual acuity	Neoplastic, inflammatory, infectious	MRI orbit without and with gadolinium and with fat suppression or CT orbit with contrast

CT, computed tomography; MRI, magnetic resonance imaging; MRA, magnetic resonance angiography

can be managed expectantly with close outpatient follow-up with an ophthalmologist. Others with underlying structural lesions often require hospital admission for further evaluation and treatment.

Patients with pathology that localizes to the cortical, subcortical, brainstem, cerebellum, subarachnoid, cavernous sinus, or orbital level most often require neuroimaging and specialist consultation. An urgent magnetic resonance imaging (MRI) of brain without and with gadolinium is indicated if there is a concern for a prenuclear or brainstem level process. Patients with multiple bilateral CN palsies should undergo MRI brain without and with gadolinium to assess for CN or leptomeningeal enhancement followed by lumbar puncture for infectious, inflammatory, or carcinomatous meningitis. Multiple unilateral CN pareses suggests a brainstem, cavernous sinus (CN III, IV, V_1 and V_2, VI) or orbital (CN III, IV, V_1, VI) process and, therefore, MRI brain and orbits without and with gadolinium is indicated. If there is associated ipsilateral proptosis, a cavernous sinus or orbital process should be suspected. If a potential carotid-cavernous fistula is suspected, angiography is indicated. An ipsilateral decrease in visual acuity and CN III, IV, and VI pareses suggests an orbital apex process, which is usually secondary to a neoplastic, inflammatory, or infectious process but may also be caused by thyroid eye disease with restrictive myopathy. MRI or computed tomography (CT) orbits is indicated for evaluation of orbital apex processes. It is helpful to include contrast for possible neoplastic processes. If thyroid eye disease with apical compression of the optic nerve is suspected, contrast is not needed.

TIPS AND PEARLS

- Microvascular ischemia is among the most prevalent causes of isolated CN III, IV, and VI palsy in adults over the age of 50. Most patients recover spontaneously over weeks to months.[8] Several studies have demonstrated that clinical exam findings and the presence of cardiovascular risk factors cannot reliably differentiate patients with microvascular ischemia from those with serious neurologic disease.[5,7,9]
- All patients presenting with partial CN III paresis or pupil-involving complete CN III paresis need urgent neuroimaging to rule out aneurysm, mostly commonly posterior communicating artery followed by the internal carotid artery and basilar artery.[10]
- Clinicians should consider elevated intracranial pressure in all patients presenting with unilateral or bilateral CN VI palsy. A funduscopic exam assessing for papilledema should be performed in these patients.
- All patients above the age of 50 presenting with diplopia require evaluation for GCA.
- Children presenting with a new CN palsy should undergo MRI of the brain with gadolinium enhancement to rule out a compressive lesion.
- Internuclear ophthalmoplegia (INO) is an ocular motility disorder of horizontal conjugate gaze. When a patient with INO attempts to look away from the affected side, there is impaired ipsilateral eye adduction and nystagmus of the contralateral eye on abduction. This may occur with conjugate gaze toward one or both sides. Convergence is usually preserved. INO occurs owing to a lesion in the medial longitudinal fasciculus of the brainstem, most commonly from multiple sclerosis or ischemic stroke.

EVIDENCE

What is the prevalence of serious neurologic illness in patients presenting with diplopia?

Patients presenting to the ED frequently have serious neurologic disease such as stroke (16.1%), multiple sclerosis (6.5%), brain tumor (4.2%), cerebral aneurysm (2.7%), or myasthenia gravis (2.3%).[1] Another study reported a low prevalence of serious neurologic illness (3.5%) among patients presenting to a specialty eye hospital with dedicated emergency services.[11]

What is the role of noncontrast head CT (NHCT) in patients presenting with isolated diplopia?

Only one study has evaluated the utility of NHCT among patients with isolated diplopia (diplopia without other signs or symptoms).[1] The diagnostic yield of NHCT among these patients was 0%. Most of these patients (89.9%) were thought to have primary diplopia or diplopia caused by microvascular ischemia if cardiovascular risk factors were present. The remaining patients (10.1%) were diagnosed with multiple sclerosis, ischemic stroke, myasthenia gravis, brain tumor, and carotid-cavernous fistula. It is important to note that this study excluded trauma patients for which NHCT plays an important role. NHCT may also be considered if there is concern for acute intracranial hemorrhage or if the patient has a contraindication to MRI.

What is the best approach to neuroimaging in patients presenting with isolated CN IV or VI palsy?

Experts are divided in regard to early versus deferred neuroimaging for patients presenting with isolated CN IV or CN VI palsy. Previous studies have supported the historical practice of deferring neuroimaging in selected patients lacking high-risk features (**Table 49.3**).[12,13] However, this practice has been called into question by two studies demonstrating that a significant proportion of patients with isolated CN IV or CN VI palsy (14%-16.5%) have structural lesions evident on MRI that may dictate a change in early management.[5 9] Therefore, the decision to defer early neuroimaging in a patient without high-risk features should be made on an individual basis according to

TABLE 49.3 High-Risk Features That Warrant Early Neuroimaging in Patients with Isolated CN III, IV, and VI Palsies

Age <50 yr
CN III palsy with pupil dysfunction, partial motor dysfunction, or aberrant regeneration[a]
History of cancer
History of head trauma
Absence of cardiovascular risk factors
Other neurologic signs or symptoms
Lack of resolution within 3 mo

[a] Aberrant regeneration is characterized by (1) eyelid elevation occurring with eye adduction or infraduction or (2) pupil constriction occurring with eye adduction, supraduction, or infraduction.

Adapted from Murchison AP, Gilbert ME, Savino PJ. Neuroimaging and acute ocular motor mononeuropathies: a prospective study. *Arch Ophthalmol.* 2011;129;301-305.

pretest probability of serious neurologic disease, patient and clinician preferences, and the ability to obtain close outpatient follow-up. The preferred imaging modality is MRI of the brain and orbits with gadolinium enhancement.

References

1. Nazerian P, Vanni S, Tarocchi C, et al. Causes of diplopia in the emergency department: diagnostic accuracy of clinical assessment and of head computed tomography. *Eur J Emerg Med.* 2014;21:118-124.
2. Demer JL, Kung J, Clark RA. Functional imaging of human extraocular muscles in head tilt dependent hypertropia. *Invest Ophthalmol Vis Sci.* 2011;52:3023-3031.
3. Manchandia AM, Demer JL. Sensitivity of the three-step test in diagnosis of superior oblique palsy. *J AAPOS.* 2014;18:567-571.
4. Kono R, Okanobu H, Ohtsuki H, Demer JL. Absence of relationship between oblique muscle size and bielschowsky head tilt phenomenon in clinically diagnosed superior oblique palsy. *Invest Ophthalmol Vis Sci.* 2009;50:175-179.
5. Tamhankar MA, Biousse V, Ying GS, et al. Isolated third, fourth, and sixth cranial nerve palsies from presumed microvascular versus other causes: a prospective study. *Ophthalmology.* 2013;120:2264-2269.
6. Ross AG, Jivraj I, Rodriguez G, et al. Retrospective, multicenter comparison of the clinical presentation of patients presenting with diplopia from giant cell arteritis vs other causes. *J Neuroophthalmol.* 2019;39:8-13.
7. Fang C, Leavitt JA, Hodge DO, Holmes JM, Mohney BG, Chen JJ. Incidence and etiologies of acquired third nerve palsy using a population-based method. *JAMA Ophthalmol.* 2017;135:23-28.
8. Park UC, Kim SJ, Hwang JM, Yu YS. Clinical features and natural history of acquired third, fourth, and sixth cranial nerve palsy. *Eye (Lond).* 2008;22:691-696.
9. Chou KL, Galetta SL, Liu GT, et al. Acute ocular motor mononeuropathies: prospective study of the roles of neuroimaging and clinical assessment. *J Neurol Sci.* 2004;219:35-39.
10. Chen H, Wang X, Yao S, et al. The aetiologies of unilateral oculomotor nerve palsy: a clinical analysis on 121 patients. *Somatosens Mot Res.* 2019;36:102-108.
11. Comer RM, Dawson E, Plant G, Acheson JF, Lee JP. Causes and outcomes for patients presenting with diplopia to an eye casualty department. *Eye (Lond).* 2007;21:413-418.
12. Murchison AP, Gilbert ME, Savino PJ. Neuroimaging and acute ocular motor mononeuropathies: a prospective study. *Arch Ophthalmol.* 2011;129:301-305.
13. Patel SV, Mutyala S, Leske DA, Hodge DO, Holmes JM. Incidence, associations, and evaluation of sixth nerve palsy using a population-based method. *Ophthalmology.* 2004;111:369-375.

CHAPTER 50

Optic Neuropathies: Ischemic, Inflammatory, Infectious, or Compressive

Mitchell B. Strominger
Victoria M. Hammond

THE CLINICAL CHALLENGE

Optic neuropathy is the general term that describes vision loss secondary to a disease process involving the prelateral geniculate optic nerves. Patients present with the primary complaint of acute or chronic vision loss in one or both eyes depending on the primary diagnosis. The visual defect occurs either centrally or peripherally secondary to a visual field abnormality. Occasionally, patients might also notice a decrease in color vision and have nonocular symptoms such as pain on eye movement or headaches. Clinically, it is challenging because the differential for causes of optic neuropathy is broad, taking into account age, systemic complaints, and other medical disorders.

PATHOPHYSIOLOGY

Optic neuropathies can be ischemic, inflammatory, infectious, or compressive.

Ischemic Optic Neuropathy

Ischemic optic neuropathy can be separated into its two most common forms: arteritic anterior ischemic optic neuropathy (AAION) and nonarteritic anterior ischemic optic neuropathy (NAAION).

Nonarteritic Anterior Ischemic Optic Neuropathy

NAAION is by far the most common form of an acute ischemic optic neuropathy that presents for acute evaluation in the emergency and urgent care settings. It is typically seen in patients older than 50, most of whom have underlying vascular risk factors, including hypertension and diabetes. The onset of vision loss is sudden and classically altitudinal, meaning the patient's visual field loss respects the horizontal meridian. The inferior field is more commonly affected than the superior field.

Patients often notice vision loss when wakening in the morning, which may be related to the normal diurnal fluctuation in blood pressure and potentially exacerbated in those who take antihypertensives at bedtime. Other risk factors include the use of amiodarone, phosphodiesterase (PDE) inhibitors, and sleep apnea.[1-3] NAAION can also be seen perioperatively, most notably after coronary artery bypass grafting and prolonged spinal-fusion surgery, with the patient being in the prone position.

Arteritic Anterior Ischemic Optic Neuropathy

AAION is less frequent than NAAION but more visually devastating if not recognized and treated emergently. Most cases occur secondary to giant cell arteritis (GCA) and should not be missed. GCA is an inflammatory vasculitis most commonly occurring in the arteries of the head, scalp, and arms. The mean age of patients with AAION is 70 years and rarely presents in patients under 50. Thus, for patients with acute vision loss, it is imperative to take a comprehensive history for other signs of GCA, including temporal headache, scalp tenderness, jaw claudication, anorexia, weight loss, fever, and associated polymyalgia rheumatica. Workup for GCA includes inflammatory markers (erythrocyte sedimentation rate [ESR] and C-reactive protein [CRP]) and referral for temporal artery biopsy.

Infectious Optic Neuropathy

Infections can directly involve the optic nerve, leading to an optic neuropathy. Vision loss occurs as a result of optic nerve head swelling and often hemorrhage. Primary infection of the optic nerve may lead to exudation into the macula in a star pattern. Retinal vasculitis can also occur, causing exudation, flame hemorrhages, and ischemic cotton wool spots. This combined disorder of the optic nerve and retinal vasculature is called neuroretinitis.[4] Inflammation as well can occur in the vitreous (vitritis), and, depending on the organism (eg, tuberculosis), choroidal lesions can be seen. Common causes of infectious optic neuropathy include Bartonella and toxoplasmosis, but syphilis, Lyme, tuberculosis, cytomegalovirus, and herpes simplex virus must also be considered. Each of these has characteristic involvement of the optic nerve, retina, and vitreous, which is beyond the scope of this chapter. However, primary optic nerve involvement can occur without retina involvement in Bartonella and syphilis. In addition, optic nerve swelling from meningitis may cause an optic perineuritis.

Inflammatory Optic Neuropathy

Optic neuritis broadly describes any inflammatory condition involving the optic nerve, although it most commonly refers to inflammation caused by a demyelinating disease. Neuromyelitis optica spectrum disorder (NMOSD) is a form of optic neuritis associated with transverse myelitis and other brain stem lesions. Symptoms include unexplained hiccups, nausea or vomiting, and diencephalic syndrome. Unfortunately, the visual prognosis is poorer in NMOSD and tends to recur, leading to severe visual impairment. Myelin oligodendrocyte glycoprotein antibody disease (MOGAD) is another more recently described demyelinating central nervous system disorder that appears to be different than MS. Its presentation, however, is similar to NMOSD, with optic neuritis, transverse myelitis, or both. Magnetic resonance imaging (MRI) findings are similar, especially involving the brainstem, but can have dramatic improvement or resolution over time. Compared to NMOSD, MOGAD patients tend to be younger, lack female predominance, can present with acute disseminated encephalomyelitis (ADEM), and have a better outcome.

Other causes that overlap in the ischemic or infiltrative category include autoimmune processes such as systemic lupus erythematous, associations with inflammatory bowel disease, sarcoidosis, and Wegener.[5]

Compressive Optic Neuropathy

Compressive lesions of the optic nerve can occur anywhere from behind the globe to the chiasm and optic tract. The degree and location of compression correlates with the symptoms. The most common causes include optic nerve sheath and intracranial meningioma, anterior communicating artery aneurysm, and pituitary adenoma. Other infiltrative tumors should also be considered, such as optic nerve glioma in neurofibromatosis type 1 and metastatic carcinoma. Classically, patients describe a more chronic progressive peripheral vision loss. In the cases of central fiber compression, or with an acutely expanding lesion such as compressive thyroid orbitopathy, an expanding intracranial aneurysm, or pituitary apoplexy, patients may have a more acute vision loss.

APPROACH/THE FOCUSED EXAM

Nonarteritic Anterior Ischemic Optic Neuropathy

Unless bilateral, the examination of a patient with NAAION reveals a relative afferent pupillary defect. Funduscopic exam demonstrates an edematous optic nerve with areas of hemorrhage (**Figure 50.1**). On direct ophthalmoscopy, the optic nerve head may appear small and crowded with no cup. Owing to acute disc edema, this trait may be appreciated only in the uninvolved eye and is known as a "disc at risk." The diagnosis is essentially a clinical diagnosis after other inflammatory and infectious etiologies have been ruled out. These cases can be bilateral and more severe and occur in the retrobulbar portion of the optic nerve. Therefore, these cases present a clinical challenge because exam and/or photography of the optic nerve head may appear normal. Depending on the location within the nerve, MRI with gadolinium may or may not show enhancement.

Arteritic Anterior Ischemic Optic Neuropathy

Vision loss is typically severe and central, with acuities worse than 20/200 in most patients. On funduscopic examination, the disc has "pallid" swelling (**Figure 50.2**), which is whiter and more ischemic, appearing in distinction to the hemorrhagic findings in NAAION. Other areas of retinal vascular ischemia can be seen as cotton wool spots.

Infectious Optic Neuropathy

Vision loss in infectious optic neuropathy is similar to the other optic neuropathies. It is typically relatively acute with central acuity affected. On examination, the visual acuity is decreased but can range from mild to severe. There is an afferent pupillary defect with decreased color vision. The optic nerve is swollen most often with associated hemorrhages or exudates. As described previously, concurrent retinal vasculitis leads to macular exudation in a star configuration, retinal flame hemorrhages, and cotton wool spots.

Inflammatory Optic Neuropathy

Optic neuritis presents with primarily central vision loss of variable degree along with a decrease in color vision. Patients may describe pain on eye movement that precedes the vision loss. Ocular examination demonstrates an afferent pupillary defect. The degree of optic nerve swelling depends

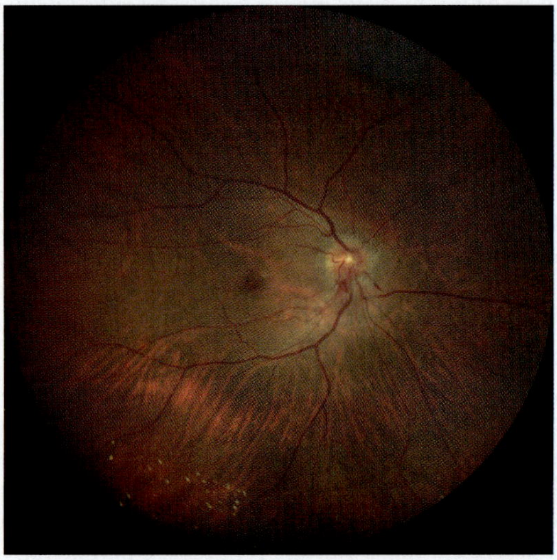

Figure 50.1: Fundus photograph of right eye demonstrating segmental hemorrhagic disc swelling in patient with NAAION (nonarteritic anterior ischemic optic neuropathy) from hypertension.

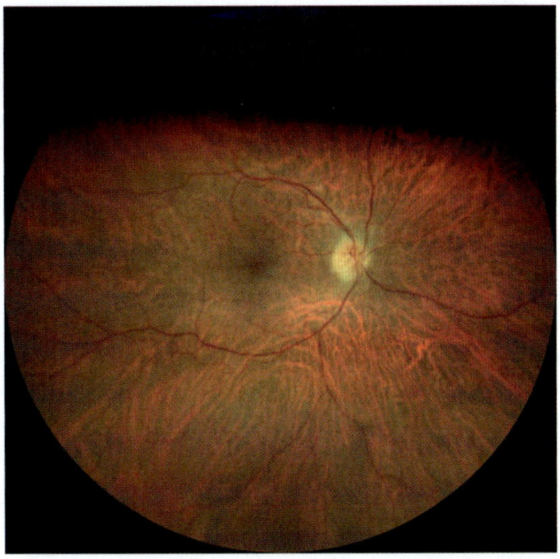

Figure 50.2: Fundus photograph of right eye demonstrating pallid disc swelling in AAION (arteritic ischemic optic neuropathy) from giant cell arteritis.

on the primary location of inflammation. When the nerves appear edematous, this is sometimes called papillitis. If the inflammation is posterior to the globe, it is termed retrobulbar. In this instance, there might be slight nerve swelling, but it is out of proportion to the amount of vision loss. Optic neuritis can be either isolated or part of a demyelinating disorder such as multiple sclerosis (MS), warranting a complete history for other neurologic symptoms.

Compressive Optic Neuropathy

Unless affecting both eyes, examination reveals an afferent pupillary defect. On fundoscopy, the nerves will typically exhibit some aspect of pallor owing to the slowly progressive course. In cases with acutely expanding lesions, the nerve will be swollen. Additionally, these lesions can also affect nearby structures, and, therefore, a thorough examination of the efferent oculomotor system is critical and may help localize the site of the lesion. Proptosis and a restrictive orbitopathy suggest an orbital process. Abnormalities of cranial nerves III and IV suggest a process involving the wall of the cavernous sinus, whereas the addition of a CNVI nerve palsy suggests cavernous sinus involvement. Trigeminal neuralgia can be seen in lesions extending intracranially via the foramen ovale. Systemic diagnoses such as a history of hyperthyroidism, polycystic kidney disease, hypothalamic pituitary axis abnormalities, and a family history of intracranial aneurysm can help with determining the cause.

MANAGEMENT

Nonarteritic Anterior Ischemic Optic Neuropathy

Unfortunately, there is no specific treatment for NAAION except the modification of underlying risk factors such as hypertension and diabetes. Over time, the swelling resolves, but areas of optic atrophy develop. Studies suggest that 40% of patients have some improvement in visual function, but the degree is variable.[6] The risk of other eye involvement over 5 years is approximately 20%, and rarely does it recur in the same eye.[7] Theoretically, treatment for sleep apnea and the administration of low-dose aspirin may decrease the risk, but evidence is limited.

Arteritic Anterior Ischemic Optic Neuropathy

Given the high risk of permanent vision loss and progression to the other eye (95% if untreated), recommendations include intravenous methylprednisolone (1 g/d for the first 3 to 5 days), followed by a slow taper of oral prednisone (1 mg/kg/d) over months while monitoring clinical symptoms,

ESR, and CRP.[8] Tocilizumab has recently been approved for use in GCA to allow for a more rapid steroid taper, reducing long-term side effects.[9] Patients need referral for temporal artery biopsy to occur within 1 week without compromising the sensitivity. Unfortunately, given the severity of ischemia and typically delayed presentation, visual recovery is poor despite aggressive treatment.

Infectious Optic Neuropathy

Treatment is aimed at the underlying cause, including treatment for meningitis if that is the primary infectious process taking place.

Inflammatory Optic Neuropathy

The evaluation includes laboratory testing to help exclude other autoimmune disorders (eg, ESR, CRP, antinuclear antibody [ANA], angiotensin converting enzyme [ACE], antineutrophil cytoplasmic antibody [ANCA]) and chest X-ray (CXR) to exclude sarcoidosis. MRI of the brain with gadolinium is the best test to determine the presence of a demyelinating disease. NMSOD and MOGAD patients may have characteristic findings on the brainstem. When considering NMSOD, an associated positive aquaporin-4 antibody test (AQP4-IgG) is diagnostic. MOG-IgG testing is now available and is becoming more routine along with AQP4-IgG.

In multiple sclerosis, the extent of periventricular white mater lesions consistent with demyelination can estimate the risk of developing multiple sclerosis and guides use of immunomodulation therapy. According to the ONTT (optic neuritis treatment trial), patients without lesions had a 25% 5-year risk of developing MS versus 72% with at least one lesion.[10] More recently, demyelinating optic neuritis is being subclassified and has both prognostic and therapeutic implications.

Treatment of acute vision loss in optic neuritis is high-dose intravenous methylprednisolone (1 g/d) for three days, followed by oral prednisone taper. This is according to the ONTT guidelines.[11] In the long term, recovery can occur without treatment. However, in the ONTT intravenous steroids sped recovery by 2 weeks. Patients treated with oral prednisone alone demonstrated a higher recurrence rate, and it is therefore not recommended. Other therapies may be initiated after the ED in steroid nonresponsive patients with NMSOD, including plasmapheresis, intravenous immunoglobulin, azathioprine, mycophenolate, or rituximab. Disease-modifying therapies used to treat multiple sclerosis are numerous and require consultation.

Compressive Optic Neuropathy

The main diagnostic test is neuroimaging, preferably an MRI of the orbits with gadolinium and including the suprasellar and chiasmal regions. Treatment depends on the type of lesion and can include coiling or clipping for aneurysm, tumor excision, radiation therapy, or chemotherapy.

PEDIATRIC ISSUES

Although children are not at risk for NAAION or AAION, they may have an underlying systemic disorder such as SLE predisposing them to an ischemic event. Children are susceptible to infections, especially Bartonella or Lyme. Compression of the optic nerve can occur from tumors more commonly seen in the pediatric population such as craniopharyngioma or glioma.

Demyelinating optic neuritis is rare in children when compared to adults, and presenting symptoms are variable among the two populations. The mean age at presentation for prepubertal children ranges from 9 to 11 years.[12] Pediatric optic neuritis has an increased rate of bilateral involvement (up to 72% in children under 10 years of age), poorer initial visual acuity, and more anterior optic nerve involvement (papillitis). Thus, optic nerve edema may be more evident on fundus examination when compared to adults. Studies have found that pain with eye movements is less common in children. Recovery of vision tends to be better in children. Diagnostic testing is similar to that in adults. However, an argument can be made to image the entire neuro-axis, looking for spinal demyelinating lesions at the same time as brain MRI, because this often requires sedation. Younger children are more likely to have a systemic illness or presentation after viral infection, post vaccine, or associated with ADEM. Older children and adolescents are more likely to have associated MS, NMO, or anti-MOG.[13] Thus, diagnosing NMO-SD can lead to more aggressive treatment with long-term immunosuppression to prevent recurrences and morbidity. We now know that many patients diagnosed with ADEM were probably anti-MOG positive. Because there are limited data regarding treatment of demyelinating pediatric optic neuritis, guidelines from adult studies are used, which include intravenous corticosteroids.[14]

In the differential diagnosis of a young adolescent that presents with painless, sequential, bilateral central vision loss is the miochondrial disorder Lebers Optic Neuropathy. In prepubescent patients with slowly progressive vision loss, autosomal dominant optic atrophy is a consideration.

TIPS AND PEARLS

- In patients over 50 years old, a full review of symptoms for GCA is critical, with appropriate laboratory testing and referral for biopsy when indicated.
- The typical presentation for demyelinating optic neuropathy is sudden central decrease in vision, decrease in color vision, an afferent pupillary defect, and pain on eye movement.
- Optic disc pallor suggests either a prior episode or an enlarging compressive lesion.
- Initial treatment of optic neuritis (except NAAION) is 1 g intravenous methylprednisolone daily for 3 days.

EVIDENCE

What is the effect on intravenous methylprednisolone on the treatment of optic neuritis?

The most robust study on the treatment and prognosis of demyelinating optic neuropathy was the ONTT. This multicenter trial involved 15 centers and randomized patients into receiving oral prednisone (1 mg/kg/d for 14 days), intravenous methylprednisolone (250 mg every 6 hours for 3 days), followed by oral prednisone 1 mg/kg/d for 11 days, or oral placebo. The mean age of patients was 32 years, and at 6 months all groups showed good visual recovery. However, patients in the intravenous methylprednisolone group recovered quicker, and those in the oral prednisone group were twice as likely to develop recurrent optic neuritis. Also, the 5-year risk for definite MS was 52% in those patients with one or more asymptomatic white matter lesions on MRI comparted with a 5-year risk of only 16% in patients with normal MRI. Thus, following the ONTT the treatment recommendations were to use intravenous corticosteroids. More recent studies have looked at using bioequivalent oral prednisone at 1250 mg day for 3 days (50 mg tablets at 25 tablets per day for 3 days) and have shown equal efficacy.[15]

What is the recommended dose of corticosteroids in the treatment of AAION from giant cell arteritis?

The dose of corticosteroids in patients with optic neuropathy and vision loss from giant cell arteritis has also been studied. Comparison has been looked at between oral prednisone typically 1 mg/kg/d versus intravenous methylprednisolone 1000 mg per day for 3 days, followed by oral prednisone taper similar to the ONTT. These studies support the use of pulse intravenous methylprednisolone, and the current recommendation is at a dose of 15 mg/kg/d. Changing to an oral prednisone taper is dependent on patient response, and in some instances intravenous is continued for upward of 5 days.[8]

References

1. Danesh-Meyer HV, Levin LA. Erectile dysfunction drugs and risk of anterior ischaemic optic neuropathy: casual or causal association? *Br J Ophthalmol*. 2007;91(11):1551-1555.
2. Liu B, Zhu L, Zhong J, Zeng G, Deng T. The association between phosphodiesterase type 5 inhibitor use and risk of non-arteritic anterior ischemic optic neuropathy: a systematic review and meta-analysis. *Sex Med*. 2018;6(3):185-192.
3. Mojon DS, Hedges TR 3rd, Ehrenberg B, et al. Association between sleep apnea syndrome and nonarteritic anterior ischemic optic neuropathy. *Arch Ophthalmol*. 2002;120(5):601-605.
4. Purvin V, Sundaram S, Kawasaki A. Neuroretinitis: review of the literature and new observations. *J Neuro-Ophthalmol*. 2011;31:58-68.

5. Henderson AD, Tian J, Carey AR. Neuro-ophthalmic manifestations of sarcoidosis. *J Neuroophthalmol*. 2020. doi:10.1097/WNO.0000000000001108. Published online ahead of print, Oct 26, 2020.
6. Hayreh SS, Zimmerman MB. Nonarteritic anterior ischemic optic neuropathy: natural history of visual outcome. *Ophthalmology*. 2008;115(2):298-305.e292.
7. Newman NJ, Scherer R, Langenberg P, et al. The fellow eye in NAION: report from the ischemic optic neuropathy decompression trial follow-up study. *Am J Ophthalmol*. 2002;134(3):317-328.
8. Chan CC, Paine M, O'Day J. Steroid management in giant cell arteritis. *Br J Ophthalmol*. 2001;85(9):1061-1064.
9. Villiger PM, Adler S, Kuchen S, et al. Tocilizumab for induction and maintenance of remission in giant cell arteritis: a phase 2, randomized, double-blind, placebo-controlled trial. *Lancet*. 2016;387(10031):1921-1927.
10. Newman NJ. The optic neuritis treatment trial (Commentary). *Ophthalmology*. 2020;127(4):S172-S173.
11. Trobe JD, Sieving PC, Guire EK, Fendrick AM. The impact of the optic neuritis treatment trial on the practices of ophthalmologists and neurologists. *Ophthalmology*. 1999;106(11):2047-2053.
12. Boomer JA, Siatkowski RM. Optic Neuropathy in adults and children. *Semin Ophthalmol*. 2003;18(4):174-180.
13. Chang MY, Pineles SL. Pediatric optic neuritis. *Semin Pediatr Neurol*. 2017;24(2):122-128.
14. Bonhomme GR, Mitchell EB. Treatment of pediatric optic neuritis. *Curr Treat Options Neurol*. 2012;14(1):93-102.
15. Morrow SA, Fraser JA, Day C, et al. Effect of treating acute optic neuritis with bioequivalent oral vs intravenous corticosteroids. *JAMA Neurol*. 2018;75(6):690-696.

CHAPTER 51

Papilledema

Abbe Craven
Brian Milman

THE CLINICAL CHALLENGE

Papilledema describes optic disc edema secondary to elevated intracranial pressure (ICP). Recognition of papilledema is important because if untreated or undertreated, papilledema can result in irreversible vision loss. Additionally, undiagnosed elevated ICP can lead to significant morbidity and mortality. The presence of papilledema should prompt an investigation of the etiology of increased ICP (eg, neoplasm, hydrocephalus, or idiopathic intracranial hypertension [IIH]).

PATHOPHYSIOLOGY

The Monro-Kellie doctrine describes the relationship between blood, brain, and cerebrospinal fluid (CSF) within the cranium. Because the total volume within the cranium is fixed, an increase in the volume of blood, cerebral tissue, or CSF must be compensated for by a decrease in the others, or elevated ICP will occur. Therefore, increase in intracranial volume, decrease in intracranial space, increase in CSF production, decrease in CSF absorption, or CSF obstruction can all increase ICP. The differential diagnosis of papilledema is focused on pathophysiology that results in one or more of these five phenomena.

APPROACH/THE FOCUSED EXAM

Signs and symptoms of elevated ICP are listed in **Table 51.1**. The most common symptom of increased ICP is headache, often described as holocranial, worse in the morning, and worse with Valsalva or bending over. Visual dysfunction may be present but can be subtle initially. One of the most common visual symptoms associated with papilledema is transient visual obscurations (TVOs). These are often described as a darkness, graying out of vision, or flickering of vision lasting for just a few seconds. TVOs may be provoked by the same changes in body position that worsen headache or pulse-synchronous tinnitus. Other forms of transient vision loss should be carefully differentiated from TVOs and are addressed in other chapters.

VISUALIZATION OF THE OPTIC NERVE

Direct Ophthalmoscopy

Visualization of the optic disc is critical in the assessment of the patient with suspected papilledema and is the gold standard for evaluating for optic disc edema and papilledema. Fundoscopy may show optic disc hyperemia, retinal hemorrhages, distention of the retinal veins, loss of pulsations of the retinal veins, and optic disc elevation. Fundoscopy can be challenging to interpret because optic disc edema may be difficult to differentiate from other optic disc abnormalities such as pseudopapilledema, crowded optic disc morphology, and optic disc drusen. The direct ophthalmoscope

TABLE 51.1 Signs and Symptoms Associated With Papilledema
Headaches
Pulse-synchronous tinnitus
Nausea
Vomiting
Horizontal binocular diplopia
Visual dysfunction
Transient visual obscurations
Enlargement of physiologic blind spot
Visual field deficits
Vision loss up to and including blindness

is commonly found in emergency departments (EDs), although limited training, uncertainty in interpreting results, and other time demands may lead to reluctance in performing the exam. The PanOptic ophthalmoscope is another instrument sometimes found in EDs. The direct ophthalmoscope has a 5° field of view, whereas the PanOptic ophthalmoscope has a 25° field of view. In a study of 36 emergency medicine residents, participants were significantly more likely to identify pathology using a PanOptic ophthalmoscope compared with a direct ophthalmoscope.[1] If the optic disc cannot be visualized by direct ophthalmoscopy and visualization of the optic disc is necessary, pupillary dilation may be considered. Pupillary dilation can be accomplished with short-acting mydriatic eye drops. Atropine should not be considered for diagnostic purposes because the effect on vision and pupillary dilation can last days to weeks. In patients with narrow angle anatomy, diagnostic pupillary dilation may precipitate an attack of angle closure glaucoma.

Nonmydriatic Fundus Camera

Nonmydriatic fundus camera photography is a tool that can increase the ability to visualize the optic disc and fundus without the need for pupillary dilation (**Figure 51.1**). Although some EDs have retinal cameras, most do not, although this may change with decreased cost and increased portability. Bruce et al demonstrated successful use of nonmydriatic ocular fundus photography by a nurse practitioner in the ED with high patient satisfaction with the technique. The median time

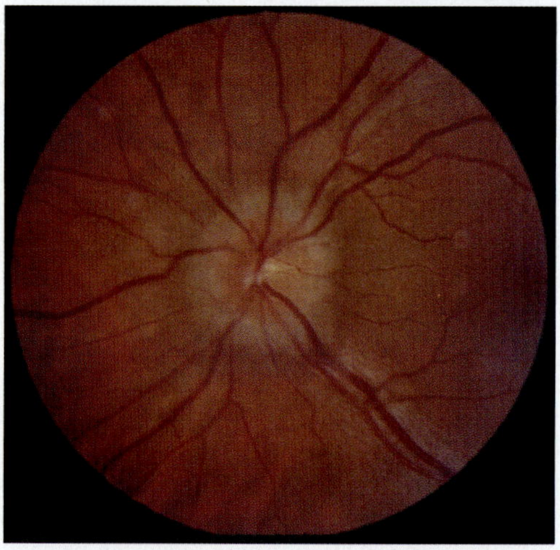

Figure 51.1: Photo of disc edema in the left eye. (This image was originally published in the Retina Image Bank. Lambert MH, Photographer. Papilledema. Retina Image Bank. 2015; 23145. © the American Society of Retina Specialists.)

of image acquisition was 1.9 minutes.[2] Interpretation of images can be performed on-site by an experienced clinician or remotely by a tele-consultant.

Point-of-Care Ultrasound

Although most of the published studies enrolled few patients, ultrasound measurement of optic nerve sheath diameter (ONSD) and optic disc height (ODH) is potentially useful in screening for papilledema and increased ICP.[3] To measure the ONSD, a high-frequency linear transducer is placed in a transverse orientation over the eye. The ONSD appears as a hypoechoic area posterior to the globe. The width should be measured 3 mm back from the globe. Measurement of ONSD can be seen in **Figure 51.2**.

Neuroimaging

When optic disc edema has been identified, or workup for papilledema/elevated ICP is required, neuroimaging is critical. Computed tomography (CT) is often the initial study because of its accessibility. However, magnetic resonance imaging (MRI) of the brain is the most sensitive study for intracranial pathology causing elevated ICP. Magnetic resonance venography (MRV) can also be performed simultaneously to evaluate for venous thrombosis. MRI may also demonstrate findings that can independently raise concern for increased ICP and papilledema (**Table 51.2**). These soft signs are not always present, and, therefore, their absence does not reliably exclude the presence of papilledema, and these findings may be present in individuals who do not ultimately have papilledema or increased ICP. Direct visualization of the optic disc is the only reliable way to exclude optic disc edema.

Lumbar Puncture/CSF Analysis

In cases of papilledema where no abnormal structural finding is detected on neuroimaging, lumbar puncture should be considered as the next diagnostic step. Opening pressure (OP) should be measured, because even in cases where elevated ICP is not initially suspected (eg, meningitis), failure to

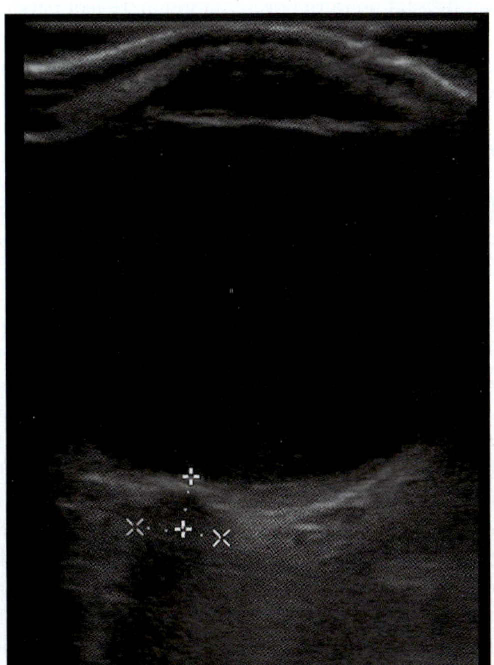

Figure 51.2: Measurement of optic nerve sheath diameter on point-of-care ultrasound. The calipers labeled "+" measure 3 mm back from the globe. The calipers labeled "X" measure the diameter of the optic nerve sheath. (Courtesy of Nima Sarani, MD, University of Kansas Medical Center.)

TABLE 51.2 MRI Findings Seen with Increased ICP
Enlargement or tortuosity of optic nerve sheath
Flattening of the posterior sclera
Empty sella
Narrowing or stenosis of dural venous sinuses

ICP, intracranial pressure; MRI, magnetic resonance imaging.

identify this and the resultant papilledema may result in vision loss. The most accurate measurements are obtained when the procedure is performed with the patient in the lateral decubitus position.

DIFFERENTIAL DIAGNOSIS

Papilledema Secondary to Increased Intracranial Volume

Intracranial mass lesions can increase ICP, leading to papilledema. In slowly developing or small mass lesions, compensatory mechanisms can often prevent an increase in ICP high enough to cause papilledema. However, quickly progressive or large masses are likely to increase ICP. Mass lesions, especially infratentorial masses, may also obstruct ventricular outflow, leading to papilledema. The reported incidence of papilledema in a series of patients with known intracranial masses ranged from 28% to 80%.[4]

Cerebral hemorrhage also often causes elevated ICP. Subarachnoid hemorrhage (SAH), subdural hematoma, epidural hematoma, and intraparenchymal hemorrhage are all associated with papilledema. In the acute trauma setting, the absence of papilledema does not reliably exclude elevated ICP.

Papilledema Secondary to Obstruction of Cerebral Venous Drainage

Occlusion of a cerebral venous sinus with a thrombus is known as cerebral venous sinus thrombosis (CVST). Papilledema is present on initial presentation in 54% of patients with CVST.[5] CVST may result from infection, trauma, surgery, hypercoagulability, malignancy, and drugs. It is important that these patients are evaluated for papilledema because severe cases may result in vision loss from prolonged elevated ICP during recovery.

Papilledema Secondary to Infection

Cerebral edema and impaired CSF absorption may occur in the setting of meningitis (bacterial, aseptic, or Lyme). Although ICP is often elevated, especially in the setting of bacterial or cryptococcal meningitis, papilledema is rare. In one series of patients with meningitis, the incidence of papilledema was 2.5%.[4]

Papilledema in Idiopathic Intracranial Hypertension

IIH presents a challenge because it is a diagnosis of exclusion but must remain high on the differential diagnosis in the setting of papilledema. Additionally, papilledema may be one of the only positive exam findings in patients with IIH. Cranial nerve VI palsy is occasionally encountered in IIH.

Diagnostic criteria for IIH are classically defined by the modified Dandy criteria (**Table 51.3**). It is important to differentiate IIH from all other secondary causes of intracranial hypertension, including intracranial mass, CVST, infection, drug-induced (particularly tetracycline class antibiotics such as minocycline and vitamin A derivatives, including isotretinoin and all trans retinoic acid [ATRA] chemotherapy). Hormonal contraceptive use (particularly estrogen containing) had previously been thought to be a risk factor for increased ICP, but outside of prothrombotic risk resulting in CVST it does not appear to have a direct association.[6] IIH most commonly affects obese adolescents and adult women but may be seen in nonobese individuals, pediatric age groups, and rarely older adults. Papilledema in IIH is typically bilateral, but asymmetric and unilateral papilledema can occur. Timely diagnosis of IIH is imperative because of the risk of irreversible vision loss. When papilledema is present and secondary to IIH, up to 40% of patients may develop permanent vision loss.[7]

TABLE 51.3 Modified Dandy Criteria for IIH Diagnosis

Presence of signs and symptoms of increased intracranial pressure (such as headache, vision change, and papilledema)
Absence of localizing findings on neurologic exam except those that are known to occur secondary to increased intracranial pressure (may have CN VI palsy)
Normal neuroimaging except for those findings that can be seen incidentally as a result of increased ICP (empty sella, dilated optic nerve sheath, venous sinus stenosis)
Evidence of increased cerebrospinal fluid pressure measured during properly positioned lumbar puncture (>25 cmH_2O in adults)
Normal CSF profile
Awake and alert
No other cause of increased intracranial pressure identified

CSF, cerebrospinal fluid; IIH, idiopathic intracranial hypertension.

MANAGEMENT

The most important management consideration in papilledema is protection of the patient's vision. Ultimately, management of papilledema is directed at the underlying cause. For cases of intracranial mass lesion, infection, and CVST, definitive treatment is undertaken via directed surgical or medical management. Although treating the underlying cause will improve the papilledema eventually, if the patient is already losing or has lost vision due to severe papilledema, they may require additional specific treatment (diuretics, lumbar puncture [LP], optic nerve sheath fenestration [ONSF], neurosurgical shunting) to protect their vision while the underlying condition is managed. These techniques are the same as treatment for primary intracranial hypertension or IIH.

IIH Management

There are several medical and surgical interventions available for treatment of IIH. Weight loss is particularly therapeutic for this condition, especially in obese individuals. Although weight loss can be highly effective, if the patient's vision is at risk, medical or surgical intervention is necessary to protect the vision while working toward this goal. There is no standardized therapy or set of guidelines for initial IIH management. Decisions are based on patient presentation, risk of vision loss, individual patient and physician preferences, and, in the case of surgical interventions, local availability and expertise.

The cornerstone of medical therapy is the use of carbonic anhydrase inhibitors, particularly acetazolamide. Acetazolamide has a wide dosing range for IIH, from 250 mg to 4 g daily. Most initial dosing recommendations will fall toward the middle of this range. Dosing is individualized and should be managed in consultation with neurology or ophthalmology.

Side effects are very common on acetazolamide, and it is important to discuss with patients the expectation of side effects prior to commencing therapy. Paresthesias in the hands, feet, and around the mouth are extremely common. Other side effects include urinary frequency, nephrolithiasis, GI upset, and altered taste of carbonated beverages. Mild, asymptomatic metabolic acidosis is common. Blood dyscrasia is very rare but has been reported. Hypokalemia (occasionally severe) can occur, and patients should be counseled that they should be monitored for this and aware of the symptoms of hypokalemia.

Topiramate has carbonic anhydrase inhibitor activity and can be used as adjunct therapy or primary therapy in some cases and provide additional benefit with weight loss efforts. Migraine control is an additional secondary benefit of topiramate in those with a comorbid migraine disorder, which is common in IIH. Topiramate is associated with fetal malformation and is contraindicated in pregnancy or in patients who may become pregnant. Topiramate may also result in a form of acute angle closure glaucoma, which can be bilateral and present in those with no other glaucoma or angle closure risk factors. Additional diuretic therapy such as furosemide is sometimes employed as an adjunct but rarely as primary therapy.

There are three primary surgical interventions for IIH. CSF diversion (VP or LP shunt) and ONSF are the two most common and effective treatments with overlapping protective roles in reducing ICP and papilledema. Venous sinus stenting is a more recent intervention that has shown benefit for some patients; however, investigations are ongoing to establish the role of venous sinus stenting in the treatment of IIH.[8] Surgery is not typically a first-line treatment of IIH except in the cases of fulminant or late IIH presentation, where the patient's vision is already severely compromised or at imminent risk of decompensation over a short time.

Prior to the advent of modern medical and surgical management of IIH, serial lumbar puncture was a cornerstone of IIH management. This provides only short-term and inconsistent ICP reduction. Most patients with IIH will have a single LP in the course of their illness to establish their diagnosis, but subsequent LP can be considered in individual cases, for example, to help evaluate for infection or shunt dysfunction, and rarely as a therapeutic temporizing measure.

TIPS AND PEARLS

- ED physicians are more successful in visualizing the optic disc when using a PanOptic ophthalmoscope or nonmydriatic retinal photography compared with a direct ophthalmoscope.
- Papilledema can result in insidious vision loss. All patients with papilledema should be counseled on this risk and the need to follow up with an ophthalmologist shortly after discharge.
- Ultrasound may be helpful as a diagnostic tool.
- Neuroimaging, particularly MRI and MRV, are important in ruling out underlying structural etiologies of increased ICP.
- In patients where elevated ICP is suspected and a structural abnormality is not identified, lumbar puncture with OP and CSF analysis is the next step in evaluation.
- IIH is a diagnosis of exclusion.
- IIH can be managed medically with weight loss, acetazolamide, topiramate, or a combination of these methods. A discussion of medication side effects with patients is imperative.

EVIDENCE

Are POCUS and MRI reliable for detecting significant papilledema?

In one study that was done in the neurointensive care unit in patients undergoing invasive ICP monitoring, the sensitivity and specificity of point-of-care ultrasound (POCUS) measured ONSD for detecting ICP greater than 20 mm Hg using an ONSD cutoff of 4.8 mm was 96% and 94%, respectively. When the ONSD cutoff was increased to 5.2 mm, the sensitivity and specificity for detecting elevated ICP was 67% and 98%, respectively.[9] This study reported a higher sensitivity and specificity than others and is of unclear application to the ED setting because it enrolled patients undergoing invasive ICP monitoring rather than undifferentiated patients presenting to the ED. An area of controversy is what diameter of the optic nerve sheath to use for a threshold for determining elevated ICP. Proposed values from different prospective studies have ranged from 4.8 to 6.0 mm, all reporting different sensitivities and specificities. Although 5.0 mm is a threshold that many clinicians use, false positives and false negatives will occur when using ONSD to identify elevated ICP.

Another study compared POCUS-measured ODH obtained by an emergency physician to the dilated fundoscopic exam performed by a neuro-ophthalmologist attending physician. A cutoff value of 0.6 mm ODH was 82% sensitive and 76% specific for clinically apparent papilledema and a cutoff value of 1.0 mm was 73% sensitive and 100% specific.[10] However, a recent study looking at novice emergency physicians demonstrated a sensitivity of 46.9% (95% CI 32.5%-61.7%) and specificity of 87.0% (95% CI 82.8-90.5) when compared with ophthalmologist-performed fundoscopy.[11]

In studies comparing MRI to ultrasound, there is a high correlation between both methods for measuring ONSD.[12] The advantage of MRI is the ability to identify other orbital and cerebral pathology as well as the ability to look for other signs of increased ICP. MRI is an important tool in the evaluation of the patient with suspected increased ICP, but papilledema can be present with negative MRI. In cases of shunted hydrocephalus, CSF outflow obstruction, or parenchymal edema, signs of increased ICP on MRI may be absent.

References

1. Petrushkin H, Barsam A, Mavrakakis M, Parfitt A, Jaye P. Optic disc assessment in the emergency department: a comparative study between the panoptic and direct ophthalmoscopes. *Emerg Med J*. 2011;29(12):1007-1008.
2. Bruce BB, Lamirel C, Biousse V, et al. Feasibility of nonmydriatic ocular fundus photography in the emergency department: phase I of the FOTO-ED study. *Acad Emerg Med*. 2011;18(9):928-933.
3. Robba C, Santori G, Czosnyka M, et al. Optic nerve sheath diameter measured sonographically as non-invasive estimator of intracranial pressure: a systematic review and meta-analysis. *Intensive Care Med*. 2018;44:1284-1294.
4. Rigi M, Almarzouqi SJ, Morgan ML, Lee AG. Papilledema: epidemiology, etiology, and clinical management. *Eye Brain*. 2015;7:47-57.
5. Liu KC, Bhatti MT, Chen JJ, et al. Presentation and progression of papilledema in cerebral venous sinus thrombosis. *Am J Ophthalmol*. 2020;213:1-8.
6. Kilgore KP, Lee MS, Leavitt JA, Frank RD, McClelland CM, Chen JJ. A population-based, case-control evaluation of the association between hormonal contraceptives and idiopathic intracranial hypertension. *Am J Ophthalmol*. 2019;197:74-79.
7. Chen JJ, Thurtell MJ, Longmuir RA, et al. Causes and prognosis of visual acuity loss at the time of initial presentation in idiopathic intracranial hypertension. *Invest Ophthalmol Visual Sci*. 2015;56(6):3850-3859.
8. Nicholson P, Brinjikji W, Radovanovic I, et al. Venous sinus stenting for idiopathic intracranial hypertension: a systematic review and meta-analysis. *J Neurointerv Surg*. 2019;11(4):380-385.
9. Rajajee V, Vanaman M, Fletcher JJ, Jacobs TL. Optic nerve ultrasound for the detection of raised intracranial pressure. *Neurocrit Care*. 2011;15(3):506-515.
10. Teismann N, Lenaghan P, Nolan R, Stein J, Green A. Point-of-care ocular ultrasound to detect optic disc swelling. *Acad Emerg Med*. 2013;20(9):920-925.
11. Wilson CL, Leaman SM, O'Brien C, et al. Novice emergency physician ultrasonography of optic nerve sheath diameter compared to ophthalmologist fundoscopic evaluation for papilledema. *J Am Coll Emerg Physicians Open*. 2021;2(1):e12355.
12. Shirodkar CG, Munta K, Rao SM, Mahesh MU. Correlation of measurement of optic nerve sheath diameter using ultrasound with magnetic resonance imaging. *Indian J Crit Care Med*. 2015;19(8):466-470.

Index

Note: Page numbers followed by *f* denote figures and *t* denote tables.

D

E

F

G

J

K

L

M

N

O

P

R

S

T

U

V